Drug Therapy in Dermatology

BASIC AND CLINICAL DERMATOLOGY

Series Editors

ALAN R. SHALITA, M.D.

Distinguished Teaching Professor and Chairman
Department of Dermatology
State University of New York
Health Science Center at Brooklyn
Brooklyn, New York

DAVID A. NORRIS, M.D.

Director of Research
Professor of Dermatology
The University of Colorado
Health Sciences Center
Denver, Colorado

1. Cutaneous Investigation in Health and Disease: Noninvasive Methods and Instrumentation, *edited by Jean-Luc Lévêque*
2. Irritant Contact Dermatitis, *edited by Edward M. Jackson and Ronald Goldner*
3. Fundamentals of Dermatology: A Study Guide, *Franklin S. Glickman and Alan R. Shalita*
4. Aging Skin: Properties and Functional Changes, *edited by Jean-Luc Lévêque and Pierre G. Agache*
5. Retinoids: Progress in Research and Clinical Applications, *edited by Maria A. Livrea and Lester Packer*
6. Clinical Photomedicine, *edited by Henry W. Lim and Nicholas A. Soter*
7. Cutaneous Antifungal Agents: Selected Compounds in Clinical Practice and Development, *edited by John W. Rippon and Robert A. Fromtling*
8. Oxidative Stress in Dermatology, *edited by Jürgen Fuchs and Lester Packer*
9. Connective Tissue Diseases of the Skin, *edited by Charles M. Lapière and Thomas Krieg*
10. Epidermal Growth Factors and Cytokines, *edited by Thomas A. Luger and Thomas Schwarz*
11. Skin Changes and Diseases in Pregnancy, *edited by Marwali Harahap and Robert C. Wallach*
12. Fungal Disease: Biology, Immunology, and Diagnosis, *edited by Paul H. Jacobs and Lexie Nall*

Library of Congress Cataloging-in-Publication Data

Drug therapy in dermatology / edited by Larry E. Millikan.
p. ; cm.—(Basic and clinical dermatology ; 18)
Includes index.
ISBN 0-8247-0306-5 (alk. paper)
1. Dermatopharmacology. 2. Skin—Diseases—Chemotherapy. I. Millikan, Larry E., 1936-II. Series.
[DNLM: 1. Skin Diseases—drug therapy. 2. Dermatologic Agents—therapeutic use. WR 650 D794 2000]
RL801.D78 2000
616.5′061—dc21

00-038332

ISBN: 0-8247-0306-5

This book is printed on acid-free paper.

Headquarters
Marcel Dekker, Inc.
270 Madison Avenue, New York, NY 10016
tel: 212-696-9000; fax: 212-685-4540

Eastern Hemisphere Distribution
Marcel Dekker AG
Hutgasse 4, Postfach 812, CH-4001 Basel, Switzerland
tel: 41-61-261-8482; fax: 41-61-261-8896

World Wide Web
http://www.dekker.com

The publisher offers discounts on this book when ordered in bulk quantities. For more information, write to Special Sales/Professional Marketing at the headquarters address above.

Current printing (last digit):
10 9 8 7 6 5 4 3 2 1

PRINTED IN THE UNITED STATES OF AMERICA

Drug Therapy in Dermatology

edited by

Larry E. Millikan

Tulane University Medical Center
New Orleans, Louisiana

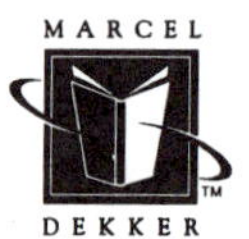

Marcel Dekker, Inc. New York • Basel

13. Immunomodulatory and Cytotoxic Agents in Dermatology, *edited by Charles J. McDonald*
14. Cutaneous Infection and Therapy, *edited by Raza Aly, Karl R. Beutner, and Howard I. Maibach*
15. Tissue Augmentation in Clinical Practice: Procedures and Techniques, *edited by Arnold William Klein*
16. Psoriasis: Third Edition, Revised and Expanded, *edited by Henry H. Roenigk, Jr., and Howard I. Maibach*
17. Surgical Techniques for Cutaneous Scar Revision, *edited by Marwali Harahap*
18. Drug Therapy in Dermatology, *edited by Larry E. Millikan*
19. Scarless Wound Healing, *edited by Hari G. Garg and Michael T. Longaker*

ADDITIONAL VOLUMES IN PREPARATION

Cosmetic Surgery: An Interdisciplinary Approach, *edited by Rhoda S. Narins*

Series Introduction

The latest addition to the Basic and Clinical Dermatology series, *Drug Therapy in Dermatology,* edited by Larry E. Millikan, is unique in that it not only represents a comprehensive review of an important and practical subject, but also adds an important international perspective to dermatological therapy. Many well-known and respected authorities in the field have contributed chapters to this volume, which should make it the standard reference book in the field. As such, I trust it will become a valuable addition to every dermatologist's library.

Alan R. Shalita
SUNY Health Science Center
Brooklyn, New York

Preface

One of the most useful resources for me as a resident at the University of Michigan was the wonderful book by Lerner and Lerner on dermatological therapy. This text provided a scientific yet practical clinical overview of therapy at a time when much of dermatology was based on anecdotal therapeutics. This book is long since out of print, but Aaron Lerner's stature as a scientist certified its value in my mind. Books on therapy in our specialty are infrequently published and, I feel, much needed. *Drug Therapy in Dermatology* covers dermatological therapy as espoused by an international group of experts. Readers from all around the world will find useful information with which to enhance their therapeutic skills.

It has been my intent to provide a source of therapeutic guidance using a two-pronged approach. First, groups and categories of drugs are summarized by international experts who provide sound guidance in appropriate therapeutic choices, optimal follow-up in therapy, and expectations for drug effects. Second, this book contains chapters that are dedicated to common and major dermatological diseases and that review therapy for such conditions as acne and psoriasis. This approach provides at least two points of view from different experts in the field. These chapters explore complex dermatological diseases, considering multiple therapeutic approaches and providing expert guidance for the selection, initiation, and follow-up of drug therapies.

Inasmuch as this book has an international authorship, the reader should keep in mind that dosages, along with appropriate indications, may vary from country to country. These authors discuss when a given therapy should be used, but again there may be regional variations. A second caveat is that when using any drug, the changes brought about by drug interactions are of key importance.

This book makes no attempt to be comprehensive, and indeed the pace at which our understanding of many of the issues discussed here is expanding makes it nearly impossible to be simultaneously comprehensive and current. Knowledge can be supplemented by using such tools as the *Physician's Desk Reference* (in the United States) and the Internet, which contain up-to-date sources for additional information. When referring to an Internet source for the current status of any given drug, it is important to determine the time of the last revision as well as whether the information conflicts with other available data.

I hope that this volume will become a most useful addition to the dermatologist's library.

Larry E. Millikan

Contents

Contributors

Mohamed Amer, M.D. Department of Dermatology, Zagazig University, Zagazig, Egypt

Angela N. Anigbogu, Ph.D. Department of Dermatology, University of California at San Francisco, San Francisco, California

Joel E. Bernstein, M.D. Winston Laboratories, Inc., Vernon Hills, Illinois

John Berth-Jones, M.D. Department of Dermatology, Walsgrave Hospital, University of Warwick, Coventry, United Kingdom

Grazia Campanile University of Florence, Florence, Italy

Jose Contreras-Ruiz, M.D. Department of Pediatric Dermatology, National Institute of Pediatrics, Mexico City, Mexico

J Carl Craft, M.D. Anti-Infective Venture, Abbott Laboratories, Abbott Park, Illinois

W. J. Cunliffe, M.D. Department of Dermatology, Leeds General Infirmary, Leeds, United Kingdom

Rodney P. R. Dawber Department of Dermatology, Churchill Hospital, Oxford, United Kingdom

Anne M. Farrell Department of Dermatology, Churchill Hospital, Oxford, United Kingdom

Ilaria Ghersetich University of Florence, Florence, Italy

Maria Goula University of Athens, A. Syngros Hospital, Athens, Greece

Malcolm W. Greaves, M.D., Ph.D. Department of Clinical Dermatology, St. Johns Institute of Dermatology, St. Thomas' Hospital, London, United Kingdom

Pearl E. Grimes Vitiligo and Pigmentation Institute of Southern California, and University of California at Los Angeles, Los Angeles, California

Giuseppe Hautmann University of Florence, Florence, Italy

Ranella J. Hirsch, M.D. Department of Dermatology, State University of New York Health Science Center at Brooklyn, Brooklyn, New York

David P. Jacobus, M.D. Jacobus Pharmaceutical Company, Inc., Princeton, New Jersey

Andreas D. Katsambas, M.D. Department of Dermatology and Venereology, University of Athens, A. Syngros Hospital, Athens, Greece

Francisco A. Kerdel, Ph.D. Department of Dermatology, University of Miami School of Medicine, Miami, Florida

John Y. M. Koo, M.D. Department of Dermatology, University of California at San Francisco Medical Center, San Francisco, California

Torello Lotti, M.D. Department of Dermatology, University of Florence, Florence, Italy

Howard I. Maibach, M.D. Department of Dermatology, University of California at San Francisco, San Francisco, California

Jack Maloney University of California at San Francisco Medical Center, San Francisco, California

Larry E. Millikan, M.D. Tulane University Medical Center, New Orleans, Louisiana

Warwick L. Morison Department of Dermatology, Johns Hopkins University, Baltimore, Maryland

Constantin E. Orfanos, M.D. Department of Dermatology, University Medical Center Benjamin Franklin, The Free University of Berlin, Berlin, Germany

Lawrence Charles Parish, M.D. Department of Dermatology and Cutaneous Biology, Jefferson Medical College of Thomas Jefferson University, Philadelphia, Pennsylvania

Kyrill Pramatarov, M.D. Department of Dermatology, Medical University, Sofia, Bulgaria

Glenn Russo, M.D. Department of Dermatology, Tulane University School of Medicine, New Orleans, Louisiana

Alan R. Shalita, M.D. Department of Dermatology, State University of New York Health Science Center at Brooklyn, Brooklyn, New York

Joseph P. Shrum, M.D. Derpartment of Dermatology, Tulane Medical Center, New Orleans, Louisiana

Richard D. Sontheimer, M.D. Department of Dermatology, University of Iowa College of Medicine, and University of Iowa Health Care, Iowa City, Iowa

Snejina Vassileva, M.D. Department of Dermatology, Medical University, Sofia, Bulgaria

Christos C. Zouboulis, M.D. Department of Dermatology, University Medical Center Benjamin Franklin, The Free University of Berlin, Berlin, Germany

1

Topical Corticosteroid Therapy

Angela N. Anigbogu and Howard I. Maibach
University of California at San Francisco
San Francisco, California

Corticosteroids are used orally and parenterally, intralesionally and topically. Topical corticoids represent a major chemotherapeutic class in dermatology and have been used for decades to treat skin diseases. The risks associated with topical corticoids parallel the benefits of their therapeutic power. Their efficacy/toxicity is related to their potency and percutaneous penetration. This chapter reviews topical corticoids and their place in dermatology.

I. HISTORICAL PERSPECTIVES

Soon after their introduction 4 decades ago, it became apparent that these compounds had a wide-ranging application to human diseases, particularly in conditions involving inflammation. These drugs, whether administered orally or topically, are effective in many inflammatory conditions. Topical application is, however, preferred, with a view to minimizing their systemic side effects. The references cited here are not meant to cover the entire literature on topical corticoids and their use.

Cortisone, the first glucocorticoid to be introduced in the early 1950s in the acetate form, had no topical activity [1], even though it has been shown to be absorbed to the same degree as hydrocortisone after topical application [2]. Furthermore, cortisone is converted to hydrocortisone at least in vitro [3]. Hydrocortisone, which became available 1 to 2 years later, was shown to be efficacious in eczematous dermatoses [4]. The success associated with hydrocortisone led to the design and development of other, more potent analogues. The fluoro deriva-

TABLE 1 Structural Modifications Improving the Efficacy of Topical Corticoids

Reduction of keto group at position 11
Insertion of double bond at positions 1 and 2
Fluorination at position 6 and/or 9
Hydroxylation/methylation at position 16
Esterification at positions 16, 17, or 21
Removal of the 17 α- or 21-hydroxyl group
Addition of 16 α-hydroxy substituent

tives of hydrocortisone and prednisolone were also active topically but had strong mineralocorticoid activity. The first major advance in topical glucocorticoid therapy came with the introduction of triamcinolone acetonide in the late 1950s, followed shortly after by flucinonolone acetonide. Betamethasone-17-valerate was introduced in the late 1960s and was found to be more active than triamcinolone acetonide and flucinonolone acetonide. The early 1970s saw the introduction of the 21-acetate derivative of fluocinolone acetonide, which had more biological activity than the others. Since the late 1970s, many more potent, topically active glucocorticoids have been introduced, including desoximetasone, clobetasol propionate, and betamethasone-17-dipropionate. A list of topical glucocorticoids available on the U.S. market is shown in Table 1.

In the early years following their introduction, topical corticosteroids were widely misused, often prescribed for the wrong conditions or in the wrong potencies. Reports of local and serious systemic side effects were rampant both in the lay media and scientific publications leading to the emergence of the so-called "corticophobia" in patients and practitioners. Nowadays, however, there are stricter guidelines for the safe and effective use of steroids.

II. PHARMACOLOGY

A. Chemistry and Structure Activity Relationships

Corticosteroids, like other steroid hormones, have a basic skeletal structure (Fig. 1a). Anti-inflammatory corticoids with a 2-carbon chain attached to the 17 position are called C21 steroids. Modifications have led to compounds of varying potencies and side effects. Cortisone, the first corticosteroid to be introduced (Fig. 1b), is devoid of topical activity. Reduction of the carbonyl group on position 11 yields hydrocortisone (Fig. 1c). A double bond inserted between positions 1 and 2 of hydrocortisone (Fig. 1d) yields prednisolone, which is even more potent. Addition of fluoro groups at positions 6 and/or 9 increases the potency of both

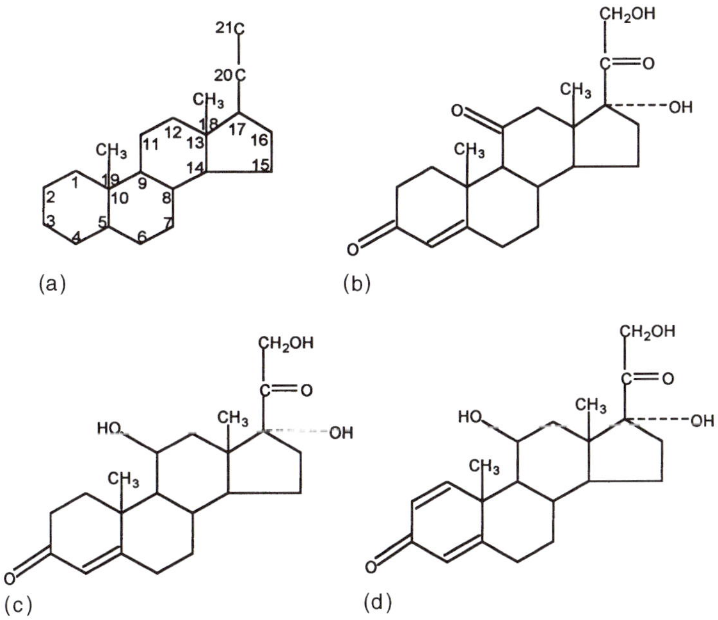

FIGURE 1 The basic steroid skeleton and modifications yielding mildly acting topical steroids: (a) basic steroid skeleton, (b) cortisone, (c) hydrocortisone, and (d) prednisolone.

steroids. This modification, however, produces strong mineralocorticoid activity. Further substitution by an α-hydroxyl, α-methyl, or β-methyl group at position 16 effectively eliminates this problem.

An ideal topical corticoid should permeate the stratum corneum and reach an adequate concentration in the epidermis without crossing the dermis to reach the systemic circulation. This may be achieved by increasing the lipophilicity of the topically active steroids, which results in an alteration of the partition coefficient. One such way of increasing lipophilicity is by esterification (e.g., at the 21-hydroxyl group, yielding compounds such as prednisolone 21-stearoylglycolate; with butyric acid at the 17 position of hydrocortisone, yielding hydrocortisone butyrate; with valeric acid at the 17 position of betamethasone, yielding the valerate; or by removing the 17-α- or 21-hydroxyl group to yield desoxysteroids such as fluorometholone and desoxymethasone). Addition of a 16-α-hydroxy substituent produces an acetonide such as triamcinolone acetonide and fluocinolone acetonide. Chlorination of 21-desoxybetamethasone 17-propionate at the 21 position yields clobetasol 17-propionate, a most potent topical corticoid. A summary of the typical modifications producing topical steroids of greater potencies ap-

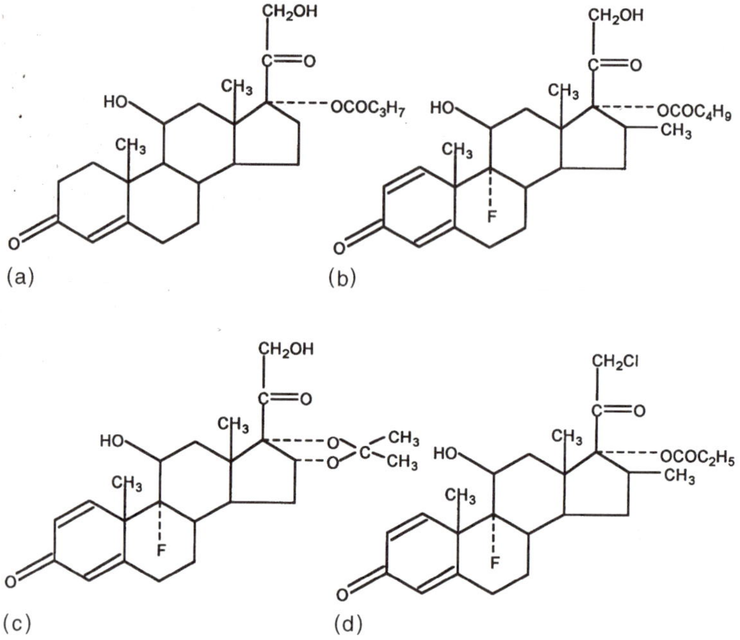

FIGURE 2 Further modifications yielding more potent topical steroids: (a) hydrocortisone 17-butyrate, (b) betamethasone 17-butyrate, (c) triamcinolone acetonide, and (d) clobetasol 17-propionate.

pears in Table 1 and the structures of some of the potents arising from these chemical modifications are shown in Figure 2.

B. Mechanism of Action

Corticosteroids, being lipophilic in nature, permeate the skin by passive diffusion, the rate of which is directly related to the extracellular concentration. The extracellular concentration is determined by many factors, including the concentration applied, percutaneous penetration, metabolic inactivation, and removal into the systemic circulation. Even though the precise sequence of cellular and subcellular events leading to the observed effects of topical corticoids remains unclear, these compounds are known to act in four ways: anti-inflammatory, immunosuppressive, antimitotic, and vasoconstrictive.

C. Actions at the Molecular Level

Following penetration of the cell membrane, topical corticoids bind with specific cytoplasmic receptors. These receptors have been demonstrated in all target tissues including the skin [5,6]. After modification, the corticoid-receptor complex enters the nucleus, where it interacts with DNA to alter the production of mRNA induced locally by RNA-polymerase. This mRNA moves into the cytoplasm, where it attaches to ribosomes and acts as a template for protein synthesis.

1. *Anti-Inflammatory and Immunosuppressive Effects*

Since inflammation is the endpoint of the immune response, the anti-inflammatory and immunosuppressive effects of corticosteroids may overlap. Corticosteroids effectively suppress inflammation caused by infectious, mechanical, radiant, immunological, or chemical agents. They inhibit many aspects of the inflammatory response, a major focus being the reduction of neutrophil and monocyte recruitment into the involved areas [7]. Corticosteroids also affect leukocytes and macrophages by reducing adherence, migration, and phagocytosis [8,9]. They may also inhibit the later manifestations of inflammation: capillary proliferation, fibroblast proliferation, collagen deposition, and cicatrization [10]. There is also evidence that glucocorticoids induce the synthesis of a protein that inhibits phospholipase A_2 and thus diminishes the release of arachidonic acid from phospholipids. This, in turn, decreases the formation of prostaglandins, leukotrienes, and related compounds that play a key role in the inflammation process [11,12]. The reduction in arachidonic acid release had previously been demonstrated in psoriatic skin [13].

2. *Antimitotic Effects*

Glucocorticoids may produce some of their therapeutic benefit by affecting cell differentiation. Glucocorticoids have been found to be antimitotic to several tissues and cells. It is believed that the effect of glucocorticoids in psoriasis is in part due to their antimitotic activities. Many have been shown to inhibit fibroblast replication [14], hydrocortisone has been shown specifically to delay the onset of DNA synthesis in mouse fore-stomach mucosa [15]. This has been demonstrated both in vivo and in vitro and in both normal and diseased skin. Hydrocortisone and triamcinolone have been shown to decrease mitosis in human skin in vitro [16,17], and a decrease in the rate of mitosis has been demonstrated with corticosteroids in psoriasis therapy [18,19].

3. *Vasoconstrictive Effects*

Shortly after their introduction, glucocorticoids were noted to cause vasoconstriction in certain vascular beds. This vasoconstrictive property of glucocorticoids may contribute to their anti-inflammatory effects. The mechanisms by which they cause vasoconstriction remains *sub judice*, but is thought to be related to their inhibition of natural vasodilators, histamine, bradykinins, and prostaglandins [20,21]. Some have suggested that corticosteroids potentiate norepinephrine [22]; others suggest that glucocorticoids actually cause the release of norepinephrine

[23]. Corticosteroids are thought also to have a direct effect on vascular endothelial cells.

The use of the standard laser Doppler velocimetry (LDV) was not able to demonstrate the vasoconstrictive effect of topical corticoids even in the presence of skin blanching visible to the eye [24,25]. The CIRD group were, however, able to correlate the clinical effect of topical steroids with LDV measurements by using a double laser [26]. LDV data obtained from patients with plaque-type psoriasis treated with clobetasol propionate showed that the technique was useful in following normalization of blood flow during treatment [27]. Recently, laser Doppler perfusion imaging was used successfully to evaluate the vasoconstrictive effects of topical corticosteroids as a means of assessing potency [28].

4. Effects on Mast Cells and Immediate Reactivity

The effect of topical application of corticoids on human mast cells has been examined [29]. Two potent corticoids, clobetasol-17-propionate and fluocinonide, produced greater than 85% decrease in histamine content over a 6-week course of treatment. Examination of biopsies taken after the treatment by electron microscopy revealed marked mast-cell depletion. Histamine levels did not decline until after 3 weeks of treatment. This thus suggests that corticoids are not immediately harmful to mast cells. The first signs of cells containing sparse amounts of mast-cell granules became apparent 14 days post-treatment. By 3 months, histamine levels returned to normal. This work suggested a possible treatment for one human mast-cell disease, urticaria pigmentosa, and a possible additional mechanism of action of corticoids.

D. Bioassay

Of importance in the discussion of the efficacy of any pharmacological agent is the method, validity, and exactness of its mensuration.

The main screening method is the vasoconstrictor assay of McKenzie and Stoughton [30] and other modifications of the assay [31,32]. The method based on the empirical, but unexplained, relationship between the ability of a corticoid to cause vasoconstriction and its therapeutic efficacy utilizes serial dilutions of an alcoholic solution of a test corticoid and a standard reference corticoid applied to the forearm; the weakest dilution producing vasoconstriction is considered the endpoint. There are statistical methods for treating the data [33]. Even though the relevance of the vasoconstricting actions of topical corticoids to their therapeutic efficacy is not obvious, they have been ranked for potency based on the degree of skin blanching they produce. It is likely that their increased effects are tied to their potency.

A more recent development is an intradermal vasoconstrictor assay that distinguishes vasoconstrictor potency from the complicating aspects of percutaneous penetration [34]. An additional assay method involves the application of corticoids to damaged skin [35]. A review of various modifications of the vasoconstrictor assay methods and results arising from the tests has been done [36].

The ability of corticoids to inhibit cell division provides the basis of an in vitro fibroblast inhibition assay [14,37,38] and an epidermal mitotic assay in vivo in humans [17,39,40]. These assay methods may prove particularly valuable in identifying corticosteroids useful in the therapy of psoriasis and other dermatoses associated with increased cell proliferation. These compounds cannot readily be identified by the vasoconstrictor assay since their mechanism of action is different.

Attempts have been made to develop screening methods utilizing a more realistic model of diseased skin. This involves the induction of inflammation by tape stripping, mustard oil and nitric acid, croton oil, tetrahydrofurfuryl alcohol, ultraviolet light, kerosene, histamine, cantharidin, and carrageen [34,41–48]. Each of these models has its own drawbacks. The natural disease process of allergic contact dermatitis offers the most attractive model for testing corticosteroids [49].

The demonstration of actual relative clinical efficacy is done by applying the product to small areas of psoriatic plaques; the clinical clearing allows the determination of clinical activity and dosage-response relationships [50]. A detailed description of the plaque assay for the determination of topical drug activity has been made [51]. Assessment of efficacy is made by visual scoring for erythema and infiltration, laser Doppler velocimetry, ultrasound measurements and/or histopathological examination from punch biopsies.

As an alternative, a double-blind paired comparison or parallel clinical observations of the test corticoid compared to either a placebo vehicle or reference compound is done as a test of efficacy. The interpretation of such studies requires knowledge of the natural history of the dermatoses being treated. In the first few days of treatment, there are marked differences in activity but with time (1–2 weeks), both sides tend to equalize. The inclusion of dermatoses not readily responsive to corticoids may lead to the bias of a "no difference" result. Indeed, most errors in this bioassay lead to such a false "no difference" result.

The Food and Drug Administration has recently released a guidance document for topical corticosteroid bioequivalence testing requiring a dose-vasoconstriction response estimation using the Minolta chromameter. The procedure was evaluated and compared to visual data using two formulations containing 0.12% betamethasone 17-valerate [52]. The results showed that while visual data showed the expected rank order of AUC values for most dose durations, the chromameter did not show similar results. The instrument determined the ED_{50} values for both preparations to be 2 h, but it was concluded that, at short dose durations, the instrument may not be sensitive enough to distinguish between weak blanching responses and normal skin for the purposes of bioequivalence assessment.

E. Percutaneous Penetration

Following topical application, glucocorticoids penetrate the stratum corneum and are absorbed into the epidermis. The efficacy and toxicity are directly related to corticoid penetration. Corticoids may act on the epidermis (as in their antimitotic effect in psoriasis), the dermis, or both. In each case, it is therefore unlikely that molecules residing only in the stratum corneum contribute to their therapeutic effects.

The rate of absorption is influenced by the status of the skin, chemical structure of the corticoid, and such other factors as formulation and formulation vehicle. All topical corticoids applied to diseased skin will be absorbed to some degree into the systemic circulation. When administration is chronic or when large areas of skin are involved, the absorption may be sufficient to cause systemic effects including adrenocortical suppression.

Several methods have been employed to quantify the percutaneous penetration of topical corticoids. A standard method is the vasoconstrictor assay, which measures the effect of a corticoid on blood vessels and allows the determination of the extent of its penetration from different vehicles or a comparison of the extent of penetration of different corticoids [30]. Other methods measure in vivo the rate of disappearance of radiolabeled corticoid from the surface of the skin with surface counting or its penetration into the dermis with isolation from urine or feces.

Regardless of the method employed, data obtained show that topical corticoids are minimally absorbed from healthy skin. On the forearm, approximately 1% of the applied dose of hydrocortisone penetrates [53,54]. Other corticoids for which data exist are not necessarily absorbed to a greater degree than hydrocortisone [55], suggesting they may owe their increased efficacy to their potency rather than enhanced penetration. To put this in perspective, only 1% of corticoids applied to healthy skin is therapeutically active with approximately 99% being wasted either by being rubbed off, washed off, or exfoliating with the stratum corneum.

F. Metabolism

The hydrolysis of betamethasone 17- and 21-valerates by hepatic and cutaneous esterases have been studied [56,57]. The 17-ester was found to be resistant to both esterases, while the 21-ester was rapidly hydrolyzed to the free steroid alcohol. The resistance of the 17-ester to enzymic hydrolysis may lead to a more pronounced reservoir effect. This may explain why 17-steroid esters are more potent than 21-esters. Following topical application, the 17-ester corticoids, by being resistant to cutaneous esterases, form better reservoirs and act longer. Hydrocortisone 17-butyrate has been reported to be converted to the 21-butyrate [58,59] and subsequently to hydrocortisone by esterase activity. In penetration studies, no biotransformation of desonide in the skin was observed [60]. In vitro, desonide is, however, rapidly metabolized in the liver to yield five metabolites, two of which show affinity to glucocorticoid receptors.

III. CLINICAL FORMULATIONS

A. Potency of Corticoids

Topical corticoids form a vast range of compounds and formulations with varying effects. Table 2 groups topical corticoids according to their relative potency. The relative potencies are based on the vasoconstrictor assay under open-testing methods [61]. The formulations in each group are only roughly equipotent. It is to be emphasized that the relative potency be considered carefully in choosing the formulations for an individual patient. While the least potent corticoids, such as hydrocortisone, may be sufficient in certain conditions, and for long-term maintenance therapy, it may be ineffective in certain diseases such as psoriasis and in certain sites such as palms and soles where the skin is thickened. Furthermore, the greater the potency, the greater the therapeutic efficacy and likelihood of more adverse effects. It is important when reading relative vasoconstriction data to verify whether the experiment refers to the use of occlusion, to a simple solvent vehicle like alcohol, rather than the final formulation, or to open testing, with or without a guard to protect wipe-off for variable times. The relative rankings can be varied significantly by manipulating these factors.

B. Superpotent Formulations

Superpotent formulations include clobetasol propionate, optimized betamethasone diproprionate, and difluorosone. In this most active class, clobetasol ointment appears more potent than the optimized formulation of betamethasone diproprionate ointment.

Attempting to develop application schedules that would maintain efficacy and decrease local and systemic toxicity led many investigators to explore intermittent dosing. In a multicenter study, 334 psoriasis patients were managed with three application schedules. The first utilized a conventional twice-daily application. The second employed twice-daily applications only on days 1 to 4, 8 to 9, and 12 and 14; whereas the third schedule had thrice-daily dosing on the same days. The first schedule induced 94% clearing and the second and third (intermit-

TABLE 2 List of Topical Corticoids Available in the United States Ranked According to Their Potencies

Drug	Potency
Lowest potency	
Hydrocortisone	0.25–2.5%
Methylprednisolone acetate (Medrol)	0.25%
Dexamethasone[a] (Hexadrol)	0.04%
Dexamethasone[a] (Decaderm)	0.1%
Methylprednisolone acetate (Medrol)	1.0%
Prednisolone (meti-Derm)	0.5%
Betamethasone[a] (Celestone)	0.2%
Low potency	
Fluocinolone acetonide[a] (Fluonid, Synalar)	0.01%
Betamethasone valerate[a] (Valisone)	0.01%
Flurometholone[a] (Oxylone)	0.025%
Aclometasone dipropionate (Aclovate)	0.05%
Triamcinolone acetonide[a] (Aristocort, Kenalog, Triacet)	0.025%
Clocortolone pivalate[a] (Cloderm)	0.1%
Flumethasone pivalate[a] (Locorten)	0.03%
Intermediate potency	
Hydrocortisone valerate (Westcort)	0.2%
Mometasone furoate (Elocon)	0.1%
Hydrocortisone butyrate (Locoid)	0.1%
Betamethasone benzoate[a] (Benison, Flurobate, Uticort)	0.025%
Flurandrenolide[a] (Cordran)	0.025%
Betamethasone valerate[a] (Valisone)	0.1%
Desonide (Tridesilon, Desowen)	0.05%
Halcinonide[a] (Halog)	0.025%
Desoximetasone[a] (Topicort L.P.)	0.05%
Flurandrenolide[a] (Cordran)	0.05%
Triamcinolone acetonide[a]	0.1%
Fluocinolone acetonide[a]	0.025%
High potency	
Betamethasone dipropionate[a] (Diprosone)	0.05%
Amcinonide[a] (Cyclocort)	0.1%
Desoximetasone[a] (Topicort)	0.25%
Triamcinolone acetonide[a]	0.5%
Fluocinolone acetonide[a] (Synalar-HP)	0.2%
Diflorasone diacetate[a] (Florone, Maxiflor)	0.05%
Halcinonide[a] (Halog)	0.1%
Fluocinonide[a] (Lidex, Topsyn)	0.05%
Highest potency	
Betamethasone dipropionate[a] in optimized vehicle (Diprolene)	0.05%
Diflorasone diacetate[a] in optimized vehicle (Psorcon)	0.05%
Clobetasol propionate[a] (Temovate)	0.05%

[a] Fluorinated steroids.

tent applications) 75% and 59%, respectively [62]. Even more extended, intermittent dosing—once weekly—has proven effective.

A larger study found that 75% of psoriasis patients remained in remission with clobetasol applied twice weekly.

These corticoids are grouped together and since they are unique in being a class of compounds that are not only superpotent but must be used with caution [63], they have the potential for significant topical and systemic side effects far in excess of other currently utilized formulations.

Because of the increased risk of systemic and local toxicity from the superpotents, considerable clinical investigation is underway to define application schedules that maximize efficacy and minimize adverse effects. This research depends on clinical observations; that is, ascertaining the least frequent application that will maintain a disease (usually psoriasis) under control [63]. Too few studies have been completed to generalize prudently; nevertheless, we suspect that each superpotent corticoid and specific vehicle may not be the same as the other. Furthermore, none of the studies utilized fundamental studies of dermatopharmacokinetics to separate drug delivery from biological result. We hope that meticulous experimental design will lead to dermatopharmacokinetics and biological (efficacy) intermittent studies that maximize efficacy and minimize toxicity, so that intermittent dosing will permit greater use of the superpotents.

Ascertaining the optimal intermittent schedule has yet to be achieved; this golden grail might be attained more efficiently by combining knowledge of the basic dermatopharmacokinetics with the classical approaches of clinical studies. Until the appropriate kinetic data become available with these potent agents, we cannot be certain how much less systemic exposure occurs with the intermittent exposures than with daily or twice-daily dosing.

C. Vehicles

The potency of topical corticoids can be further enhanced by enhancing percutaneous absorption. One way of optimizing absorption is by altering the formulation vehicle. It was thought that penetration of the skin by a therapeutic agent was not influenced by the vehicle in which it was applied [64]. It is now clear, however, that some vehicles enhance the penetration and biological activity of therapeutic agents [61]. The release of glucocorticoids from gels, creams, films, and ointments have been measured in a number of in vitro experiments [65–68]. It is important for vehicles to be free of the three S's, namely, sting, stench, and stain.

The major classes of vehicles are powders, creams, ointments, aerosols, and lotions. Important considerations in choosing vehicles are (1) solubility of the therapeutic agent in the vehicle; (2) rate of release of the agent from the vehicle; (3) ability of the vehicle to hydrate the stratum corneum, thus enhancing penetration; (4) stability of the therapeutic agent in the vehicle; and (5) interactions, chemical and physical, of the vehicle, stratum corneum, and therapeutic agent.

There are some general rules for the use of topical glucocorticoids in relation to the vehicle.

1. The ointment bases tend to give better activity than cream or lotion vehicles [61]. This has been clearly demonstrated in physiological studies of vasoconstriction.
2. Vehicles that are designed specifically for the corticoid with regard to rate of release from the vehicle and degree of solubility of the corticoid in the vehicle are more likely to be successful in clinical application.
3. Lotion vehicles are more cosmetically acceptable to patients than are ointments. Cream vehicles are widely accepted by patients, but may be less effective than ointments containing the same corticoid.
4. Hairy areas are best treated with lotions, mousses, or aerosol vehicles; this is particularly true of the scalp.
5. Compounded formulations of triamcinolone acetonide, hydrocortisone acetate, or fluocinonide [68] with an adhesive base are useful in mucous-membrane applications.
6. Other than patient acceptability, there are no stringent rules against the use of any particular vehicle on the cutaneous surface of any particular area. Contrary to the myth, there is no harm in applying powders to dry areas or ointments to wet areas. Ointment vehicles, however, do tend to hydrate the stratum corneum and are more soothing to dry skin than are powders, lotions, and many creams. In the future, the main consideration will be which vehicles deliver the greatest biological activity of the steroid.
7. Novel vehicles, including gels, may not retain their optimal drug delivery qualities if they are diluted, even with the same base.
8. The properties of the vehicle, compatibility with the type of lesion, and patient acceptance may be important determinants of therapeutic efficacy, along with drug delivery and vasoconstrictor potency. For example, when creams are indicated, one cream may be more efficacious than another, based on the vehicle properties. There are lubricating creams as well as less oily creams, the latter sometimes being more effective in intertriginous lesions.

IV. ADVERSE EFFECTS

A. Systemic Adverse Effects

Table 3 lists adverse effects associated with topical corticoid therapy. All absorbable topical corticoids possess the ability to produce adrenal suppression (69,70).

Table 3 Adverse Effects Associated with Topical Corticoid Therapy

Local
Atrophy
Corticoid atrophy
Striae
Ulcerations
Ectasia
Purpura
Stellate pseudoscars
Nonhealing wounds
Infections
Granuloma gluteal infantum
Tinea incognito
Scabies incognito
Ophthalmic
Ocular hypertension
Glaucoma
Cataracts
Pharmacological
Corticoid addiction
Corticoid rebound
Tachyphylaxis
Dermatological
Corticoid acne
Cortical rosacea
Allergic contact dermatitis
Perioral dermatitis
Hypopigmentation
Masking underlying cutaneous diseases
Generalized
Weight gain
Cushing's syndrome
Electrolyte inbalance
Hypertension
Diabetes
Pseudoprimary aldosteronism
Growth retardation

Adapted from Ref. 107.

The degree of suppression is related to potency. Comparative quantitative studies employed the FDA diseased-skin protocol. As little as 14 g per week of clobetasol has induced suppression. Optimized betamethasone diproprionate is somewhat less suppressive, requiring over 49 g per week to significantly reduce plasma cortisol. Incomplete data with difluorosone suggest that it may be even less suppressive. Fortunately, plasma cortisol usually returns to normal within 3 days when the superpotents are discontinued—at least in short-time application studies (62).

Certain factors increase the penetration and therefore the tendency to suppression; application to large surface areas, occlusion, inflamed skin, and higher concentrations. In general, patients that do have adrenal suppression demonstrate a laboratory test abnormality rather than a clinical state such as Addison's disease. There are, however, cases of severely impaired stress response to topical corticoids [71]. Fewer of the predisposing factors listed above are required to produce suppression in children [72–74]. Of major concern in children is growth retardation associated with excessive and prolonged use of topical corticoids [75,76].

Iatrogenic Cushing's syndrome is seen in patients after prolonged use of potent corticoids [77–81].

B. Local Adverse Effects

1. *Skin Atrophy*

This is the most commonly encountered side effect associated with potent topical corticoids and they can produce severe cosmetic disability in addition to clinical problems. Corticoids cause thinning of both epidermis and dermis [82] and sometimes subcutaneous tissue. Clinical presentations may include depressed, shiny, often wrinkled skin and telangiectasia [83–85]. The skin is extremely fragile, with tears and bruises occurring easily (corticoid purpura). Atrophic striae was recognized early in patients being treated for inguinal intertrigo [86]. Excessive application of a corticoid for pruritus ani may result in a tender and troublesome perianal atrophoderma [87,88]. Severe subcutaneous atrophy has been reported in the diaper area of an infant treated with a potent corticoid for 14 months. Atrophy of a distal digit resulting in a ''pencil-sharpened'' appearance has been reported following vigorous occlusive corticoid therapy [89]. The use of corticoids on ulcerated lesions can delay wound healing and may exacerbate the condition [90].

Although it has generally been assumed that the atrophogenicity of various corticoids is directly related to their potency, recent evidence suggests that there could be a dissociation between anti-inflammatory and atrophogenic effects for some corticoids. The final determination of the atrophogenicity of each corticoid awaits studies utilizing specific assays designed to measure epidermal and dermal atrophy.

2. Steroid Face, Rosacea, and Perioral Dermatitis

Prolonged application of potent steroids on the face may result in erythema and telangiectasia, the so-called "steroid face," partly as a result of corticoid-induced capillary dilatation and partly due to atrophy of dermal connective tissue leading to the loss of vascular support tissue. In the particularly susceptible patient, this could result after only a few applications of a potent or moderately potent formulation. Potent corticoids are known to exacerbate preexisting rosacea [91]. Prolonged application of potent steroids can also induce a rosacealike condition presenting with erythema, papules, pustules, and telangiectasia on the cheeks, nose, and forehead [92,93].

A similar condition, perioral dermatitis, is more commonly seen in adult women [94], even though it has also been observed in children [95]. The features include erythema, papules, pustules, and scaling in the perioral region. All three conditions described show marked improvement with the withdrawal of topical steroids and a long course of oral tetracyclines.

3. Corticoid Acne

Topical corticoids can worsen preexisting acne vulgaris [96], and can also induce an acneform eruption [97–99]. The most commonly affected sites are the face, chest, and upper arms. The clinical features include predominantly monomorphic eruption of red papules and pustules around the hair follicles. Steroid acne is seen more frequently with the most potent formulations, but can sometimes occur with less potent corticoids used with occlusion. When it is associated with occlusion therapy, it is important to distinguish it from bacterial folliculitis. Gram's stain of the pus in bacterial folliculitis reveals gram-positive cocci (*Staphylococcus aureus*), and gram-positive pleomorphic rods (*Propionibacterium acnes*) appear in steroid acne. The acnegenic effects of corticoids have been attributed to degeneration of the follicular epithelium leading to the extrusion of the follicular contents [97].

4. Allergic Contact Dermatitis

It seems paradoxical that corticoids, used in treating allergic disorders, can themselves produce contact dermatitis. True contact allergy to steroids is not rare. Most such clinical examples are probably not diagnosed, since the clinician rarely thinks of the possibility. In a study of contact dermatitis, which involved patients patch-tested in the Finsen Institute (Copenhagen), 21 patients were contact sensitive to hydrocortisone, and several were sensitive to triamcinolone and betamethasone [100]. A more recent study reported the incidence of contact dermatitis in 2.4% of 2742 patients patch-tested with desonide [101]. Other studies have shown the incidence of allergy to several corticosteroids in many patients, suggesting the possibility of cross-reactions between corticoids, especially those with common chemical structures [102,103]. It has been suggested that many cases of hypersensitivity to corticosteroids occur in patients with stasis dermatitis, even though it is also seen in other types of dermatitis [104]. Some of these patients may have been sensitive to impurities in the corticoid, which is of clinical significance, since the impurities are present in commercially available material. When a physician sees a patient who is not responding to a topical corticoid, or who first responds and then relapses, patch-testing for delayed hypersensitivity should be considered. Since the topical corticoids themselves are not irritating, high concentrations can be used for testing. Although this may change as more experience is obtained, the patch-test recommendation is 25% hydrocortisone in petrolatum. Remember that vehicle systems may contain topical sensitizers, such as preservatives, and bases, such as lanolin. Sensitivity to these materials is generally overlooked and must be watched for carefully [105].

Data on contact sensitization to the fluorinated corticoids are not sufficiently conclusive to make a firm recommendation on suitable patch-test concentrations. Approximately 1% in petrolatum may prove suitable. Transient vasodilation rather than vasoconstriction occurs occasionally with patch-testing using fluorinated corticoids.

5. Hypertrichosis

Local hypertrichosis due to topical corticoid application though usually subclinical is not uncommon [106]. It is seen mainly in females applying potent corticoids on the face. Such subjects may be predisposed to hirsutism [107]. Hypertrichosis has also been reported in children [108]. The mechanism by which corticoids promote the coarser growth of vellus hair is not known.

6. Hypopigmentation

Although more common with intralesional injections of corticoids, hypopigmentation, nevertheless, occurs following topical corticoid therapy. African Americans are more at risk. It is thought that corticoids interfere with melanin synthesis. However, the condition is reversible and repigmentation occurs rapidly following cessation of steroid therapy [109].

7. Ophthalmological Side Effects

Topical corticoids used in the treatment of irritant dermatitis involving the eyelids may cause conjunctival sac contamination during therapy. In most cases, complications resulting from this contamination are not serious, but it is important to be aware of potentially serious problems, including blindness. Cases of glaucoma, ocular hypertension, and cataracts induced by application of corticoids to the periorbital region have been reported [110–115]. A recent study concluded that ocular hypertensive response to topical dexamethasone occurred more frequently, more severely, and more rapidly in children than in adults [116].

8. Masking and Aggravation of Cutaneous Infections

Corticoids suppress the normal inflammatory response associated with ineffective processes and perhaps exacerbate these conditions. In dermatophyte infections, this has been termed ''tinea incognito'' [117,118]. Similar difficulties have been noted in scabies infestations, with reported conversions from ordinary scabies to crusted type [119]. *Candida albicans* infections may be exacerbated by topical corticoids [120]. The prolongation of herpetic infections and molluscum contagiosum treated with topical corticoids have been reported [121,122]. Topical glucocorticoids were recently demonstrated to inhibit transcription of all genes encoding antibacterial peptides in frog skin, resulting in an increase in viable bacteria [123]. The authors suggest that since human skin was recently found to produce two different antibacterial peptides, LL-37 and β-defensin, topical corticosteroids applied to human skin may also inhibit the transcription of the genes coding for these peptides, thus resulting in undesirable cutaneous infections.

9. Provocation of Erythema Craquelé

Following the discontinuation of a long-term course of potent topical corticoids, an erythematous pattern of superficial fissuring of the epidermis, resembling erythema craquelé, has been seen in susceptible individuals. Although most of these cases are reported to follow occlusive therapy, one subject developed the reaction following 6 weeks of application without occlusion. No correlation has been established between the development of erythema craquelé and skin thinning as measured with the Harpenden caliper technique. It is hypothesized that the topical corticoids induce a functional abnormality that predisposes the skin to desiccation and the development of the erythema craquelé. A similar reaction was reported previously, although in the earlier report a correlation appeared to exist between the degree of atrophogenicity and the inflammatory reaction.

V. CURRENT APPROVED INDICATIONS

Table 4 lists the diseases that are responsive and those less responsive to topical steroids. Also included are those that are generally not responsive to topical steroids and require intralesional therapy with injections of insoluble corticoids. The very responsive diseases generally require low- to medium-potency corticoids. For less responsive diseases, higher potency corticoids, higher concentrations, and occlusion may be necessary.

VI. THERAPEUTIC PROTOCOLS

A. Dosage and Concentration

Physicians rarely prescribe oral or parenteral preparations without due consideration to dosage; yet most physicians prescribe topical corticoids with little or no

TABLE 4 Indications for Topical Corticoids

Very responsive
Atopic dermatitis
Seborrheic dermatitis
Lichen simplex chronicus
Pruritis ani
Later phase of allergic contact dermatitis
Later phase of irritant dermatitis
Nummular eczematous dermatitis
Stasis dermatitis
Psoriasis, especially of the face and genitalia
Less responsive
Discoid lupus erythematosus
Psoriasis of the palms and soles
Necrobiosis lipoidica diabeticorum
Sarcoidosis
Lichen striatus
Pemphigus
Familial benign pemphigus
Vitiligo
Granuloma annulare
Least responsive (intralesional injection required)
Keloids
Hypertrophic scars
Hypertrophic lichen planus
Alopecia areata
Acne cysts
Prurigo nodularis
Chondrodermatitis nodularis helicus

thought as to the number of milligrams of material per surface area of skin. There is a dose-response relationship, with increasing efficacy closely following increased dosage. Severalfold differences in dosage can override differences in potency among halogenated analogues. Therefore, it is important to estimate the quantity required by the patient in any given condition.

Increasing the concentration of any given corticoid will often produce increased efficacy. Fortunately, most manufacturers provide a standard or regular concentration yielding the desired therapeutic result for most patients. For instance, triamcinolone acetonide is available in 0.025%, 0.1%, and 0.5% formulations. The bulk of patients with corticoid-responsive dermatoses need only the 0.025% formulations; by increasing this to 0.1%, all but a few percentage of probable responders will respond. For the patient with more resistant lesions, however, the 0.5% formulations may provide the difference between therapeutic success and failure. For certain uncommon instances, such as psoriasis of the palms and soles, even higher concentrations, 1% triamcinolone acetonide, may be compounded.

The standard trade concentrations suffice for most patients. In the more resistant diseases, higher concentrations should be considered. For instance, approximately 1% of a 0.25% hydrocortisone solution is absorbed from the forearm. Increasing the amount applied per unit area of skin tenfold increases the amount absorbed four times. Other methods of increasing effectiveness will be described in the section on ''Occlusion''; some have previously been discussed in the section on ''Vehicles.'' Increased efficacy, however, must be balanced against increased risk of adverse effect (see Sec. IV).

Regional differences in response are based mainly on the differences in penetration of skin in various areas. Thus, areas with increased permeability, such as the scrotum, eyelids, ears, scalp, and face respond far better to topical corticoids than such areas as the dorsa of the hands, extensor surfaces of knees and elbows, and the palms and soles [124].

B. Occlusion

Occlusion with an impermeable film, such as plastic wrap, constitutes a most effective method of enhancing penetration, yielding approximately a tenfold increase [125]. Specifically, with occlusion, penetration of hydrocortisone on the forearm increases from 1% of applied dose to 10%. This tenfold increase constitutes an important clinical advantage; even with the more potent analogues, occlusion in the resistant case will often produce a successful result. There are, however, obvious problems associated with occlusion therapy—the plastics are sometimes uncomfortable, warm, and troublesome to apply. Side effects encountered with occlusion include miliaria, bacterial, and candidal infection. The incidence of side effects correlates directly with the duration of occlusion and, for this reason, the plastic should generally be worn for no more than 12 h a day.

Occlusion has the added advantage of keeping the drug on the skin by preventing rubbing off onto clothing. Occlusion is also particularly useful in pruritic skin diseases because it limits access to the skin and, therefore, scratching, which may worsen the condition.

We have some data delineating the effect of duration of occlusion on percutaneous penetration. Limited studies show that there is a direct correlation; the longer the occlusion, the greater the effect. Since there is a measurable enhancement of penetration after several hours of occlusion, it is now recommended that patients utilize occlusion for relatively shorter periods. For instance, many patients apply the wrap after work and remove it when they retire, approximately 6 h, thus avoiding the discomfort of sleeping in plastic.

Initial methods of occlusion were homemade. Now, for convenience, plastic gloves, booties, arm and leg wraps, and whole-body plastic exercise suits have been adapted for this purpose. Premedicated corticoid tape (flurandrenolide) is also available and is convenient for providing occlusion to small areas.

Recent studies in dermatopharmacokinetics of hydrocortisone force a clinical reevaluation of the mechanism of action of occlusion [126]. The original study [125] demonstrated a tenfold enhancement in penetration by utilizing a 96-h period of occlusion. The current occlusion study utilizes a more realistic, 24-h therapeutic time period, and does not reveal penetration enhancement. Yet occlusion increases biological activity in the standard 16-h blanching assay; and, clinically, some disease entities fail to respond without it. Understanding this phenomenon may provide important new pharmacological insights.

C. Frequency of Application

Previously, a patient applied topical corticoids 3 to 4 times daily. Studies on the percutaneous absorption of hydrocortisone failed to reveal a significant increase in absorption applied on a repetitive basis compared to a single dose [127]. Clinical trials of various corticoids suggest that less frequent applications are equally effective [128,129]. In view of the relatively slow process of corticosteroid absorption, a phenomenon referred to as the ''reservoir effect'' [130], there may be no advantage to frequent application. A similar pharmacodynamic slow-release curve has been noted with many organic compounds [131].

A multiple-dose hydrocortisone study conducted in humans [131], in which radiolabeled hydrocortisone was applied on days 1 and 8 and unlabeled material on days 2 through 7 and 9 through 14, with the sites of application being washed daily 1 h prior to the next application, showed no significant increase in penetration, in contrast to the earlier study in the rhesus monkey [127].

Acute tolerance (tachyphylaxis) to vasoconstriction and antimitotic effects and suppression of epidermal DNA synthesis by topical corticoids have been demonstrated [133,134]. This suggests that the resistance clinically observed after prolonged use might be prevented by less intensive therapy, such as daily application with short resting periods between treatment courses [90,135].

Another study examining corticoid tachyphylaxis used fluocinolone acetonide under occlusion to the forearm and induced wheal and flare to histamine with the prick technique [136]. By the eighth day, the wheal was nonexistent, adding now a third tachyphylaxis phenomenon.

Clement and coworkers also examined tachyphylaxis by utilizing the DNA synthesis, hairless mouse epidermis model to determine a treatment schedule for continuous epidermal suppression [137]. With all the twice-daily treatment regimens, tachyphylaxis occurred but not with the 72-h application of certain corticoids. In this study, vehicles appeared to play a role in determining the speed of tachyphylaxis. Clearly, this model deserves additional work to aid in unraveling the clinical relevance of tachyphylaxis.

D. Anatomical Variation

There are regional variations in percutaneous absorption of compounds [138]. These variations are determined by factors including hair follicle density, thickness of the stratum corneum, and vasculature of the region. There is a distinct difference in the penetration of hydrocortisone in different anatomical sites. This suggests that for areas of higher penetrability such as the face, scalp, scrotum, axilla, and the groin, smaller doses are required and occlusion is not needed [139].

In flexural areas of the skin in which hydration may occur, absorption may be increased. Absorption through diseased skin with an increased blood supply may also increase. Little quantitative information is, however, available on how much penetration is increased in diseased skin. In initial studies, it was noted that skin with only minimally involved atopic dermatitis allowed for a severalfold increase in penetration; psoriatic plaques had no significant increase, whereas exfoliative psoriatic skin had little barrier to penetration. This important subject needs additional investigation, which should be of practical value in dermatopharmacology.

E. Intralesional Therapy

In certain disease conditions where the limited penetration of corticoids pose a problem, intralesional injection of relatively insoluble corticoids, such as triamcinolone acetonide, triamcinolone diacetate, and betamethasone acetatephosphate can be used. When they are injected into the lesion, measurable amounts remain in place and are gradually released for 3 to 4 weeks. This figure is estimated from the duration of the transient adrenal suppression and by examination of biopsies to ascertain the duration of the local antimitotic response [121]. This form of therapy is particularly beneficial in certain lesions generally unresponsive to topical corticoids, such as alopecia areata. Intralesional corticoid injections have been reported to be effective in the early treatment of infantile capillary hemangiomas of the eyelids. As with all corticosteroid use in the periocular region, due caution must be exercised.

In intralesional therapy, dosage is critical and requires strict attention to decrease the incidence of local atrophy, a term that is a partial misnomer. The involved sites are depressed and often atrophic because of inhibition of collagen synthesis, but fortunately, unlike most atrophic states, the condition is often self-limited and reversible in time. The dosage of the triamcinolone salts is generally limited to 1 mg per treatment site (that is 0.1 mL of a 10 mg/mL suspension). Many physicians prefer to increase the dilution to increase the volume of solution injected into each site.

REFERENCES

1. Goldman L, Thompson RG, Trice ER. Cortisone acetate in skin disease: Local effect in skin from topical applications and local injections. AMA Arch Dermat Syph 1952; 19:101–102.
2. Feldmann RJ, Maibach HI. Percutaneous penetration of steroids in man. J Invest Dermatol 1968; 52:89–94.
3. Hsia SL, Hao YL. Transformation of cortisone to cortisol in human skin. Steroid 1967; 10:489–500.
4. Sulzberger MB, Witten VH. The effect of topically applied compound F in selected dermatoses. J Invest Dermatol 1957; 19:101–102.
5. Ballard PL, Baxter JD, Higgins SJ, Rousseau GC, Tomkins GM. General presence of glucocorticoid receptors in mammalian tissues. Endocrinology 1974; 94:998–1002.
6. Epstein EH, Bonifas JM. Glucocorticoid receptors of the human epidermis. J Invest Dermatol 1982; 78:144–146.
7. Parrillo JE, Fauci AS. Mechanisms of glucocorticoid action on immune processes. Ann Rev Pharmacol Toxicol 1979; 19:179–201.
8. Vernon-Roberts B. The effects of steroid hormones on macrophage activity. Int Rev Cytol 1969; 25:131–159.
9. Thompson J, van Furth R. The effect of glucocorticosteroids on the kinetics of mononuclear phagocytes. J Exp Med 1970; 131:429–442.
10. Haynes RC, Muraud F. Adrenocorticotropic hormone; adrenocortical steroids and their synthetic analogs; inhibitors of adrenocortical steroid biosynthesis. In: Gilman AG, Goodman LS, Rall TW, Murad F, eds. The Pharmacological Basics of Therapeutics. New York: Macmillan, 1985:1459–1489.
11. Blackwell GJ, Carnuccio R, DiRosa M, Flower RJ, Parente L, Persico P. Macrocortin: a polypeptide causing the anti-phospholipase effect of glucocorticoids. Nature 1980; 287:147–149.
12. Hirata F, Schiffmann E, Venkatasubamanian K, Salomon D, Axelrod J. A phospholipase A_2 inhibitory protein in rabbit neutrophils induced by glucocorticoids. Proc Natl Acad Sci USA 1980; 77:2533–2536.
13. Hammarström S, Hamberg M, Duell EA, Stawiski MA, Anderson TF, Voorhees JJ. Glucocorticoids in inflammatory proliferative skin disease reduces arachidonic and hydroxy eicosatetranoic acids. Science 1977; 197:994–996.
14. Berliner DL, Ruhmann AG. Comparison of the growth of fibroblasts under the influence of 11 β-hydroxy and 11-keto corticosteroids. Endocrinology 1966; 78: 373–382.
15. Frankfort OS. Effect of hydrocortisone, adrenaline and actinomycin D on transition of cells to the DNA synthesis phase. Exp Cell Res 1968; 52:222–232.
16. Reaven EP, Cox AJ. Behavior of adult human skin in organ culture. J Invest Dermatol 1968; 50:118–128.
17. Fisher LB, Maibach HI. The effect of corticosteroids on human epidermal mitotic activity. Arch Dermatol 1971; 103:39–44.
18. Baxter DL, Stoughton RB. Mitotic index of psoriatic lesions treated with anthralin, glucocorticosteroid and occlusion only. J Invest Dermatol 1970; 54:410–412.

19. Fry L, McMinn RMH. The action of chemotherapeutic agents on psoriatic epidermis. Br J Dermatol 1968; 80:373–383.
20. Altura BM. Role of glucocorticoids in local regulation of blood flow. Am J Physiol 1966; 211:1393–1397.
21. Juhlin L, Michaelsson G. Cutaneous vascular reactions to prostaglandins in healthy subjects and in patients with urticaria and atopic dermatitis. Acta Dermatol Venereol 1969; 49:251–261.
22. Ginsburg J, Duff RS. Influence of intra-arterial hydrocortisone on adrenergic responses in the hand. Br Med J 1958; 2:424–428.
23. Solomon LM, Wentzel HE, Greenberg MS. Studies in the mechanism of steroid vasoconstriction. J Invest Dermatol 1965; 44:129–131.
24. Amantea M, Tur E, Maibach H, Guy R. Preliminary skin blood flow measurements appear unsuccessful for assessing topical corticosteroid effect. Arch Dermatol Res 1983; 275:419–420.
25. Smith EW, Maibach HI. A preliminary comparison of laser Doppler velocimeter and visual ranking of corticosteroid-induced skin blanching. In: Berardesca E, Elsner P, Maibach HI, eds. Bioengineering of the Skin: Cutaneous Blood Flow and Erythema. Boca Raton: CRC Press, 1995:217–223.
26. Bisgaard H, Kristensen J, Sondergaard J. New technique for ranking vascular corticosteroid effects in humans using laser Doppler velocimetry. J Invest Dermatol 1986; 86:275–278.
27. Berardesca E, Vignoli GP, Farinelli N, Vignini M, Distante F, Rabbiosi G. Noninvasive evaluation of topical calcipotriol versus clobetasol in the treatment of psoriasis. Acta Dermatol Venereol (Stockh) 1994; 74:302–304.
28. Sommer A, Veraart J, Neumann M, Kessels A. Evaluation of the vasoconstrictive effects of topical steroids by Laser-Doppler-Perfusion-Imaging. Acta Dermatol Venereol (Stockh) 1998; 78:15–18.
29. Lavker R, Scheckter N. Cutaneous mast cell depletion results from topical corticosteroid usage. J Immunol 1985; 135:2368–2373.
30. McKenzie SW, Stoughton RB. Method for comparing percutaneous absorption of steroids. Arch Dermatol 1962; 86:608–610.
31. Christe GA, Moore-Robinson M. Vehicle assessment-methodology and results. Br J Dermatol 1970; 82 (suppl 6):93–98.
32. Barry BW, Woodford R. Comparative bioavailability of proprietary topical corticosteroid preparations; Vasoconstrictor assays on thirty creams and gels. Br J Dermatol 1974; 91:323–338.
33. Place V, Giner-Velazquez J, Burdick K. Precise evaluation of topically applied corticosteroid potency. Arch Dermatol 1970; 101:531–537.
34. Sutton P, Feldmann R, Maibach HI. Vasoconstrictor potency of corticoids: Intradermal injection. J Invest Dermatol 1971; 57:371–376.
35. Wells GC. The effect of hydrocortisone on standardized skin surface trauma. Br J Dermatol 1957; 69:11–18.
36. Smith EW, Meyer E, Haigh JM, Maibach HI. The human skin blanching assay as an indicator of topical corticosteroid bioavailability and potency. In: Bronaugh R, Maibach HI, eds. Percutaneous Absorption; Mechanisms—Methodology—Drug Delivery. New York: Marcel Dekker, 1989:443–460.

37. Ponec M, DeHaas C, Bachra BN, Poland MK. Effects of glucocorticosteroids on primary human skin fibroblasts. Inhibition of the proliferation of cultured primary human skin and mouse L 929 fibroblasts. Arch Dermatol Res 1977; 259:117–123.
38. Saarni H, Jalkanen M, Kopsu-Hauu VK. Effects of five anti-inflammatory steroids on DNA synthesis by normal skin fibroblasts in vitro. Arch Dermatol Res 1980; 258:217–219.
39. Du Vivier A, Bible R, Miicuriye R, Stoughton RB. An animal model for the screening drugs for antipsoriatic properties using hydroxy apatite to rapidly isolate DNA from the epidermis. Br J Dermatol 1976; 94:1–6.
40. Du Vivier A, Marshall RC, Brookes LG. An animal model for evaluating the local and systemic effects of topically applied corticosteroids on epidermal DNA synthesis. Br J Dermatol 1978; 93:305–308.
41. Scott A, Kalz F. The effect of the topical application of corticotrophin, hydrocortisone and fluocortisone on the process of cutaneous inflammation. J Invest Dermatol 1956; 26:361–378.
42. Witkowski JA, Kligman AM. A screening test for anti-inflammatory activity using human skin. J Invest Dermatol 1959; 32:481–483.
43. Schlagel CA, Northan JI. Comparative anti-inflammatory efficacy of topically applied steroids on human skin. Proc Soc Exp Biol Med 1959; 101:626–632.
44. Altmeyer P. Modification of experimental UV erythema by external steroids—a reflex photometric study. Arch Dermatol Res 1977; 258:203–209.
45. Zaynoun S, Kurban A. Evaluation of the efficacy of topical corticosteroids. Br J Dermatol 1974; 90:85–90.
46. Reddy BSN, Singh G. A new model for human bioassay of topical corticosteroids. Br J Dermatol 1976; 94:191–193.
47. Boris A, Hurley JF. Assessment of topical anti-inflammatory activity in rats with cantharidin-induced inflammation. J Invest Dermatol 1977; 68:161–164.
48. Sugio K, Tsurufuji S. Mechanism of anti-inflammatory action of glucocorticoids reevaluation of vascular constriction hypothesis. Br J Pharmacol 1981; 73:605–608.
49. Kaidbey KH, Kligman AM. Assay of topical corticosteroids. Arch Dermatol 1976; 112:808–810.
50. Dumas KJ, Schultz JR. The psoriasis bioassay for topical corticosteroid activity. Acta Derm-Venereol 1972; 52:43–48.
51. Lauerma AI, Maibach HI. Psoriasis small plaque assay for assessment of topical drug activity. In: Roenigk HM, Maibach HI, eds. Psoriasis, 3rd ed. New York: Dekker, 1998:727–730.
52. Demana PH, Smith EW, Walker RB, Haigh JM, Kanfer I. Evaluation of the proposed FDA pilot dose-response methodology for topical corticocteroid bioequivalence testing. Pharm Res 1997; 14:303–308.
53. Malkinson FD, Ferguson EH. Percutaneous absorption of hydrocortisone-1-C^{14} in two human subjects. J Invest Dermatol 1955; 25:281–283.
54. Feldmann RJ, Maibach HI. Percutaneous penetration of hydrocortisone in man. II. Effect of certain bases and pretreatments. Arch Dermatol 1966; 94:649–651.
55. Feldmann RJ, Maibach HI. Percutaneous penetration of steroids in man. J Invest Dermatol 1968; 52:89–94.

56. Cheung YW, Po ALW, Irwin WJ. Cutaneous biotransformation as a parameter in the modulation of the activity of topical corticosteroids. Int J Pharmacol 1985; 26: 175–179.
57. Kubota K, Ademola J, Maibach HI. Metabolism of topical drugs within the skin, in particular glucocorticoids. In: Korting HC, Maibach HI, eds. Topical glucocorticoids with increased benefit/risk ratio. Basel: Karger, 1993:61–66.
58. Misaki T, Yamada M, Hiroi R, Komori M, Washitake M, Ozawa Y, Kayama I, Yoshizawa H. Enzymic hydrolysis of hydrocortisone diesters in skin. Yakuzaigaku 1982; 42:92–98.
59. Kitano Y. Hydrolysis of hydrocortisone 17-butyrate 21-propionate by cultured human keratinocytes. Acta Dermatol Venereol (Stockh) 1986; 66:98–102.
60. Andersson P, Brattsand R, Edsbäker S, Käsllström L, Ryrfeldt A. In vitro biotransformation of glucocorticoids in the liver and skin homogenate fraction from man, rat and hairless mouse. J Steroid Biochem 1982; 16:787–795.
61. Stoughton RB. Bioassay systems for topically applied glucocorticoids. Arch Dermatol 1972; 106:825–827.
62. Cornell R, Stoughton R. Review of super-potent corticosteroids. Semin Dermatol 1987; 6:72–76.
63. Prawer SE, Katz HI. Guidelines for using superpotent topical steroids. Am Fam Phys 1990; 41:1531–1538.
64. Rothman S. Physiology and Biochemistry of the Skin. Chicago: University of Chicago Press, 1954.
65. Ostrenga J, Haleblian J, Poulsen B, Fernel B, Mueler N, Shastri S. Vehicle design for a new topical steroid, fluocinonide. J Invest Dermatol 1971; 56:392–399.
66. Malone T, Haleblian JK, Poulsen BJ, Burdick KH. Development and evaluation of ointment and cream and cream vehicles for a new topical steroid, flucurolone acetonide. Br J Dermatol 1974; 90:187–195.
67. Borodkin S, Tucker FE. Drug release from hydroxylpropyl cellulose-polyvinyl acetate films. J Pharm Sci 1974; 63:1359–1364.
68. Lozada F, Silverman SL. Topically applied fluocinonide in the adhesive base in the treatment of oral vesiculo-erosive diseases. Arch Dermatol 1980; 116:898–901.
69. Scoggins RB, Kliman B. Relative potency of percutaneously absorbed corticosteroids in the suppression of pituitary-adrenal function. J Invest Dermatol 1965; 45: 347–355.
70. Carr RD, Tarnowski WM. Percutaneous absorption of corticosteroids: adrenocortical suppression with total body inunction. Acta Dermatol Venereol 1968; 48:417–428.
71. Pascher F. Systemic reactions to topically applied drugs. Int J Dermatol 1978; 17: 768–775.
72. Feiwel M, James VHT, Barnett ES. Effect of potent topical steroids on plasma cortisol levels of infants and children with eczema. Lancet 1969; 2:485–487.
73. Munro DD. The effect of percutaneously absorbed steroids on hypothalamic-pituitary-adrenal function after intensive use in patients. Br J Dermatol 1976; 94(suppl 12):67–76.
74. Weston WL, Sams WM, Morris HG. Morning plasma cortisol levels in infants

treated with topical fluorinated glucocorticosteroids. Paediatrics 1980; 65:103–106.
75. Vermeer BJ, Heremans GFP. A case of growth retardation and Cushing's syndrome due to excessive application of betamethasone-17-valerate ointment. Dermatologica 1974; 149:299–304.
76. Bode HH. Dwarfism following long-term topical corticosteroid therapy. J Am Med Assoc 1980; 244:813–814.
77. Keipert JA, Kelly R. Temporary Cushing's syndrome from percutaneous absorption of betamethasone 17-valerate. Med J Aust 1971; 1:542–544.
78. May P, Stein ES, Ryter RJ, Hirsh FS, Michel B, Levy RP. Cushing's syndrome from percutaneous absorption of triamcinolone cream. Arch Intern Med 1976; 136: 612–613.
79. Himathongkam T, Dasanabhairochona P, Pitchayayothin N, Sriphrapradanc A. Florid Cushing's syndrome and hirsutism induced by desoximethasone. J Am Med Assoc 1978; 239:430–431.
80. Nilsson JE, Gip LS. Systemic effects of local treatment with high doses of potent corticosteroids in psoriatics. Acta Dermatol Venereol 1979; 59:246–248.
81. Stoughton RCD, August PS. Cushing's syndrome and pituitary-adrenal suppression due to clobetasol propionate. Br J Med 1975; 2:419–421.
82. Kirby JD, Munro DD. Steroid-induced atrophy in an animal and human model. Br J Dermatol 1976; 94:111–119.
83. Stenmovic DU. Corticosteroid-involved atrophy of the skin with telangiectasia: a clinical and experimental study. Br J Dermatol 1972; 87:548–556.
84. Fisher DA. Adverse effects of topical corticosteroid use. West J Med 1995; 162: 123–126.
85. Koivukangas V, Karvonen J, Risteli J, Oikarinen A. Topical mometasone furoate and betamethasone-17-valerate decrease collagen synthesis to a similar extent in human skin in vivo. Br J Dermatol 1995; 132:66–68.
86. Epstein EH, Epstein WL, Epstein JH. Atrophic striae in patients with inguinal intertrigo. Arch Dermatol 1963; 87:450–457.
87. Goldman L, Kitzmiuer K. Perianal atrophoderma from topical corticosteroids. Arch Dermatol 1973; 107:611–612.
88. Johns AM, Bower BD. Wasting of napkin area after repeated use of fluorinated steroid ointment. Br Med J 1970; 1:347–348.
89. Tavenbaum MH. Topical steroid atrophy: ''a disappearing digit.'' J Am Med Assoc 1972; 220:125.
90. Miller JA, Munro DD. Topical corticosteroids: clinical pharmacology and therapeutic use. Drugs 1980; 19:119–134.
91. Sneddon IB. Adverse effect of topical fluorinated corticosteroids in rosacea. Br Med J 1969; 1:671–673.
92. Leyden JJ, Thew M, Kligman AM. Steroid rosacea. Arch Dermatol 1974; 110: 619–622.
93. Litt JZ. Steroid-induced rosacea. Am Fam Phys 1993; 48:67–71.
94. Sneddon IB. Perioral dermatitis. Br J Dermatol 1972; 87:430–434.
95. Weber G. Perioral dermatitis, an important side effect of corticosteroids. Dermatologica 1976; 152 (suppl 1):161–172.

96. Fulton JE, Kligman AM. Aggravation of acne vulgaris by topical application corticosteroids under occlusion. Cutis 1968; 4:1106–1109.
97. Kaidbey KH, Kligman AM. The pathogenesis of topical steroid acne. J Invest Dermatol 1974; 62:31–36.
98. Plewig G, Kligman AM. Induction of acne by topical steroids. Arch Dermatol Forsch 1973; 247:29–52.
99. Hurwitz RN. Steroid acne. J Am Acad Dermatol 1989; 21:1179–1181.
100. Alani MD, Alani SP. Allergic contact dermatitis to corticosteroids. Ann Allergy 1972; 30:181–185.
101. Vestergaard L, Andersen KE. Contact allergy to local steroids. Contact allergy to corticosteroids among consecutively tested patients with eczema. Ugeskrift 1997; 159:5662–5666.
102. Ohi T. Contact dermatitis due to topical steroids with a conceivable cross reactions between topical steroid preparations. J Dermatol 1996; 23:200–208.
103. McKenna DB, Murphy GM. Contact allergy to topical corticosteroids and systemic allergy to prednisolone. Contact Dermatitis 1998; 38:121–122.
104. Wilkinson SM. Hypersensitivity to corticosteroids. Clin Exp Dermatol 1994; 19: 1–11.
105. Fisher AA, Pascher F, Kanof N. Allergic contact dermatitis due to ingredients of vehicles. Arch Dermatol 1971; 104:286–290.
106. Bertolino AP, Freedberg IM. Disorders of epidermal appendages and related disorders: Hair. In: Fitzpatrick TB, Eisen AZ, Wolff K, Freedberg IM, Austen KF, eds. Dermatology in General Medicine. New York: McGraw-Hill, 1987:671–695.
107. Bondi EE, Kligman AM. Adverse effects of topical corticosteroids. Prog Dermatol 1980; 14(abstr 4).
108. Takeda K, Arase S, Takahashi S. Side effects of topical corticosteroids and their prevention. Drugs 1988; 36(suppl 5):15–23.
109. Lavker RM, Schechter NM, Lazarus GS. Effects of topical corticosteroids on human dermis. Br J Dermatol 1986; 115(suppl 3):101–107.
110. Bigger JF, Palmberg PF, Becker B. Increased cellular sensitivity to glucocorticoids in primary open-angle glaucoma. Invest Ophthalmol 1972; 11:832–837.
111. Howell JB. Eye diseases induced by topically applied steroids. Arch Dermatol 1976; 112:1529–1530.
112. Nielsen NV, Sorensen PN. Glaucoma induced by application of corticosteroids to the periorbital region. Arch Dermatol 1978; 114:953–954.
113. Vie R. Glaucoma and amaurosis associated with long-term application of topical corticosteroids to the eyelids. Acta Derm Venereol 1980; 60:541–542.
114. Wilson FM. Adverse external ocular effects of topical ophthalmic medications. Surv Ophthalmol 1979; 24:57–58.
115. Renfro L, Snow JS. Ocular effects and systemic steroids. Dermatol Clin 1992; 10(suppl 3):505–512.
116. Kwok AK, Lam DS, Ng JS, Fan DS, Chew SJ, Tso MO. Ocular-hypertensive response to topical steroids in children. Ophthalmology 1997; 104:2112–2116.
117. Ive FA, Marks R. Tinea incognito. Br Med J 1968; 3:149–152.
118. Solomon BA, Glass AT, Rabbin PE. Tinea incognito and over-the-counter potent topical steroids. Cutis 1996; 58(suppl 4):295–296.

119. Wishart J. Norwegian scabies: a Christ Church epidemic. Aust J Dermatol 1972; 13:127–131.
120. Maibach HI. Topical corticoid therapy: a round table discussion. Part II. Cutis 1979; 24:633–638.
121. Hellier FF. Profuse mollusca contagiosa of face induced by corticosteroids. Br J Dermatol 1971; 85:398.
122. Hill CJ, Rosenberg A. Adverse effects from topical steroids. Cutis 1978; 21:624–628.
123. Simmaco M, Boman A, Mangoni ML, Mignogna G, Miele R, Barra D, Boman HG. Effect of glucocorticoids on the synthesis of antimicrobial peptides in amphibian skin. FEBS Newslet 1997; 416:273–275.
124. Mckenzie AW, Stoughton RB. Method for comparing percutaneous absorption of steroids. Arch Dermatol 1962; 89:741–746.
125. Feldmann RJ, Maibach HI. Penetration of ^{14}C-hydrocortisone through normal human skin: the effect of stripping and occlusion. Arch Dermatol 1965; 91:661–666.
126. Bucks DAW, Maibach HI, Guy R. Occlusion does not uniformly enhance penetration in vivo. In: Bronaugh RL, Maibach HI, eds. Percutaneous Absorption; Mechanisms—Methodology—Drug Delivery. New York: Marcel Dekker, 1989:77–94.
127. Wester RC, Noonan PK, Maibach HI. Frequency of application of percutaneous absorption of hydrocortisone. Arch Dermatol 1977; 113–622.
128. Fredrickson T, Lassus A, Bleeker J. Treatment of psoriasis and atopic dermatitis with halcinonide cream applied once, two–three times daily. Br J Dermatol 1980; 102:575–577.
129. Sudilovsky A, Muir JG, Bocobo FC. A comparison of single and multiple applications of halcinonide cream. Int J Dermatol 1981; 20:609–613.
130. Vickers CFH. Existence of reservoir in the stratum corneum. Arch Dermatol 1963; 88:20–23.
131. Feldmann RJ, Maibach HI. Percutaneous penetration of steroids in man. J Invest Dermatol 1968; 52:89–94.
132. Bucks D, Maibach H, Guy R. Percutaneous absorption of steroids: Effect of repeated applications. J Pharm Sci 1985; 74:1337–1339.
133. Du Vivier A, Stoughton RB. Acute tolerance to effects of topical glucocorticoids. Br J Dermatol 1976; 94(suppl 12):25–32.
134. Du Vivier A, Phillips H, Hehir M. Applications of glucocorticosteroids: The effects of twice-daily vs once-every-other-day applications on mouse epidermal cell DNA synthesis. Arch Dermatol 1982; 118:305–308.
135. Barry BW, Woodford R. Vasoconstrictor activities and bioavailabilities of seven proprietary corticosteroid creams assessed using a non-occluded multiple dosage regimen: clinical considerations. Br J Dermatol 1977; 97:555–560.
136. Singh G, Singh P. Tachyphylaxis to topical steroid measured by histamine-induced wheal response. Int J Dermatol 1986; 25:324–326.
137. Clement N, Phillips H, Du Vivier A. Is steroid tachyphylaxis preventable? Clin Exp Dermatol 1985; 10:22–29.
138. Cronin E, Stoughton RB. Percutaneous absorption: regional variations and the effect of hydration and epidermal stripping. Br J Dermatol 1962; 74:265–272.

139. Feldmann RJ, Maibach HI. Regional variation in percutaneous penetration of ^{14}C cortisol in man. J Invest Dermatol 1967; 48:181–183.

SUGGESTED READINGS

Review Articles

Robertson DB, Maibach HI. Topical Corticosteroids; Efficacy-toxicity ratios favorable as a chemotherapeutic class. Hosp Form 1981; 16:1130–1139.

Robertson DB, Maibach HI. Topical glucocorticoids. In: Anti-Inflammatory Steroid Action Basic and Clinical Aspects. New York: Academic Press, 1989:494–524.

Yohn JJ, Weston WL. Topical glucocorticosteroids. Curr Probl Dermatol 1990; 2:31–63.

Books

Maibach HI, Surber C. Topical Corticosteroids. New York: Karger, 1992.

Korting HC, Maibach HI. Topical Glucocorticosteroids with Increased Benefit/Risk Ratio. New York: Karger, 1993.

2

Topical Antibiotics

W. J. Cunliffe
Leeds General Infirmary
Leeds, United Kingdom

I. INTRODUCTION

The major skin diseases treated topically with antibiotics are acne, rosacea, and infections caused by *Staphylococcus aureus* (*S. aureus*). This chapter will focus particularly on the topical therapies prescribed in such diseases. The first section will discuss topical antibiotics prescribed for acne. It is relevant to summarize briefly the etiology of acne so that the use of such topical therapies is put into context of the overall disease and its therapeutic options. Acne is a disorder of the pilosebaceous duct and four major etiological factors need to be considered. Androgens control the seborrhea, a characteristic feature of acne [1]. In most patients, this represents an end-organ hyperresponse of the pilosebaceous gland to circulating androgens [2]. Androgens, along with other factors such as sebaceous lipid composition, local cytokines, and retinoids, influence the development of comedones, which represent ductal accumulation of ductal keratinocytes [3,4]. Acne is not an infectious disease, but colonization of the ducts with the commensal organism *Propionibacterium acnes* (*P. acnes*) probably play a central feature in the development of the inflammatory papules, pustules, and nodules [5,6]. The inflammation initially represents a type IV (lymphocytic) response to cytokines produced by the ductal keratinocytes and ductal microorganisms [7,8]. It is likely that topical antibiotics prescribed in acne act predominantly through their effect on the growth and function of *P. acnes* [9,10]. However, an effect on inflammation and comedogenesis may be important [11,12].

II. GENERAL PRINCIPLES OF THERAPY

Prescribing topical antibiotics alone is not the optimum way of treating acne patients. Treatment procedures involve patient discussion, assessment of the severity, and appropriate therapy based on the history, severity, lesion type, and the psychological effects of the disease [13].

The cause of the disease should be discussed as should the likely success of therapy. Patient leaflets are usually helpful. The patient should be told that, in mild cases, acne will last for 4 to 6 years, but in severe cases the natural history could be in excess of 20 years. However, the patient should be informed that if the acne has not responded well to reasonable courses of oral antibiotics and appropriate topical therapy, then oral isotretinoin can be prescribed—and this therapy is a guaranteed success [14]. Because of its cost and teratogenicity, many patients will initially receive the standard therapy (i.e., a variety of alternative oral and topical therapies). With such therapies, either alone or in combination, there is little improvement after 1 month of therapy; there should be 30% improvement at 2 months, 50% improvement at 6 months, and 80% improvement at 8 months.

A. Acne grading

Grading is very helpful in the assessment of acne in the clinic. A grading scale similar to that shown in Figures 1 to 6 is recommended. Good light and palpation, as well as inspection, are required [15]. The acne can be graded on a 0–10 scale on the face, back, and chest. Relatively little practice is required to become reasonably proficient, and it does not necessarily matter if the physician's grading scale varies somewhat from published ones, as long as the observer is consistent. Lesion counts are essential for clinical trials but not for use in the day-to-day clinic [15].

B. Choice of Acne Therapy

Patients with mild acne (Figs. 1 and 2) usually receive topical therapy; patients with moderate acne usually receive oral and topical therapies; patients with severe acne should immediately receive oral isotretinoin. The severity assessment should include not just the extent of the inflammatory and comedonal lesions but also the presence of scarring, the psychological effects of the disease, and the lack of success with previous treatment [13].

The most widely used topical therapies in acne are benzoyl peroxide, antibiotics, and azaleic acid and retinoids, either alone or in combination. Patients with predominantly inflamed lesions should receive topical benzoyl peroxide, antibiotics, or azaleic acid.

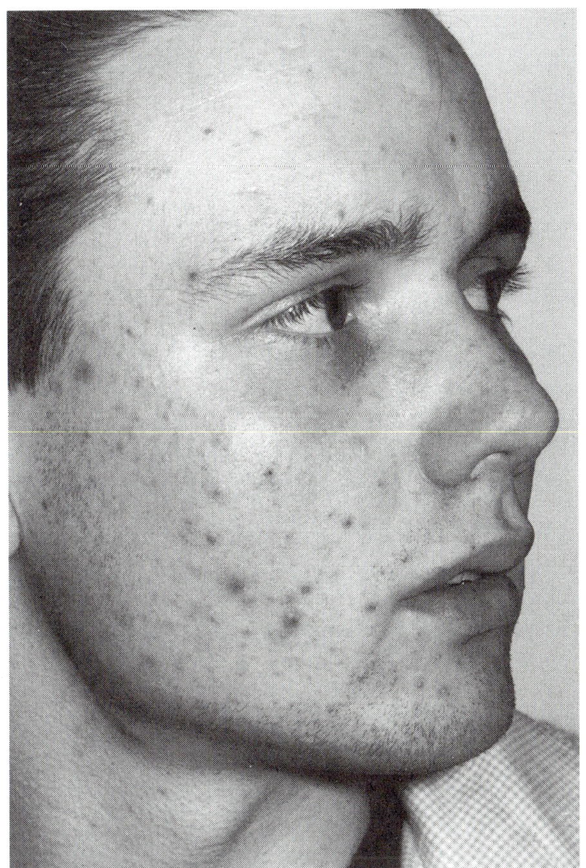

FIGURE 1 Patient with mild acne.

C. Topical Antibiotics for Acne

Topical antibiotics prescribed in acne are usually tetracycline, erythromycin, and clindamycin [16–21]. There is less evidence to support the benefit of topical chloramphenicol and fucidic acid in acne. Fucidin and neomycin are, in worldwide terms, only available in a few countries [22,23]. Topical antibiotics are prescribed in concentrations of 1 to 4% in a cream, gel, or lotion base. Table 1 summarizes some of the formulations and presentations of commonly used products. Combination antibiotics include erythromycin with zinc [24,25] or with benzoyl peroxide [26,27]. Topical tetracycline is probably the least effective topi-

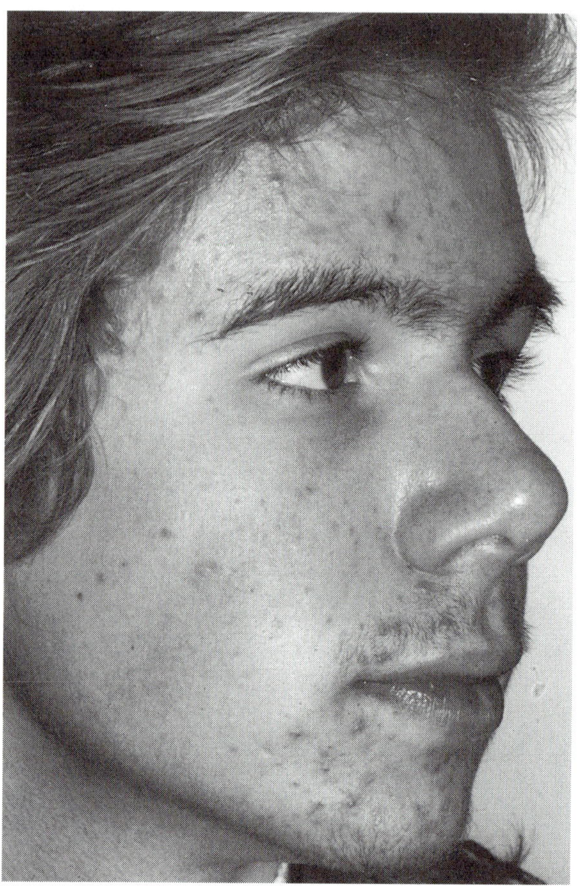

Figure 2 Patient with mild acne.

cal antibiotic and combination of antibiotics with zinc or benzoyl peroxide are marginally better than single therapies [24,26]. Newer topical antibiotics for acne include Nadifloxacillin [28,29].

1. Mechanisms of Action

Most drugs are bactericidal. This can be demonstrated by measuring the reduction in surface and/or follicle *P. acnes* [9,10,25]. It is quite likely that an effect on follicular *P. acnes* may be more relevant than simply an effect on surface *P. acnes*. Unfortunately, there are relatively little data to show the effect on follicular

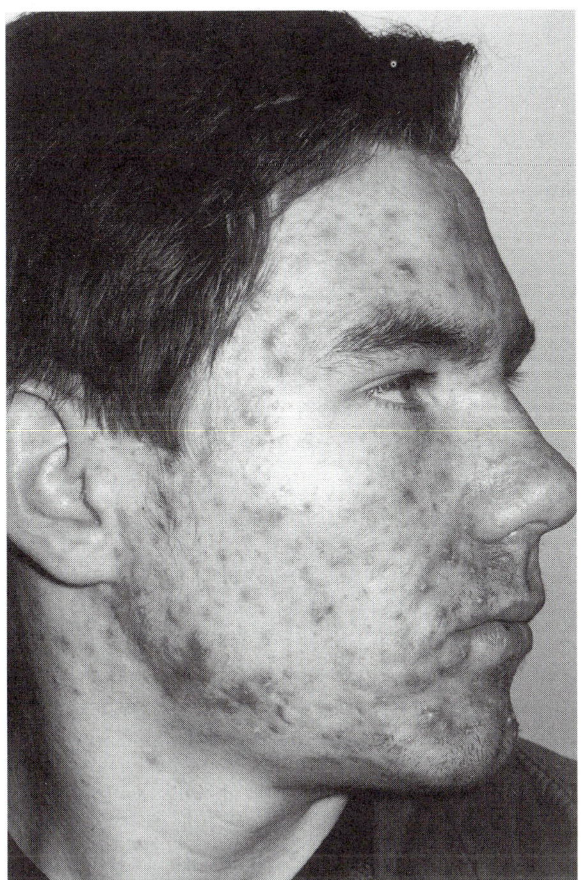

FIGURE 3 Patient with moderate acne.

organisms. *P. acnes* function can be measured by showing a decrease in surface lipid free fatty acids. Sebaceous triglycerides are hydrolyzed to free fatty acids by bacterial lipases; antibiotic therapy in less than optimum doses may have no effect on the numbers of *P. acnes* but may show a decrease in surface lipid free fatty acids [25].

Topical antibiotics do not directly affect sebum production [30], but they may possibly influence comedogenesis. However, an erythromycin–zinc complex (Zineryt®) has been shown to reduce the output of sebum from certain follicles [31]. This may be due to an indirect effect on comedogenesis. The didac-

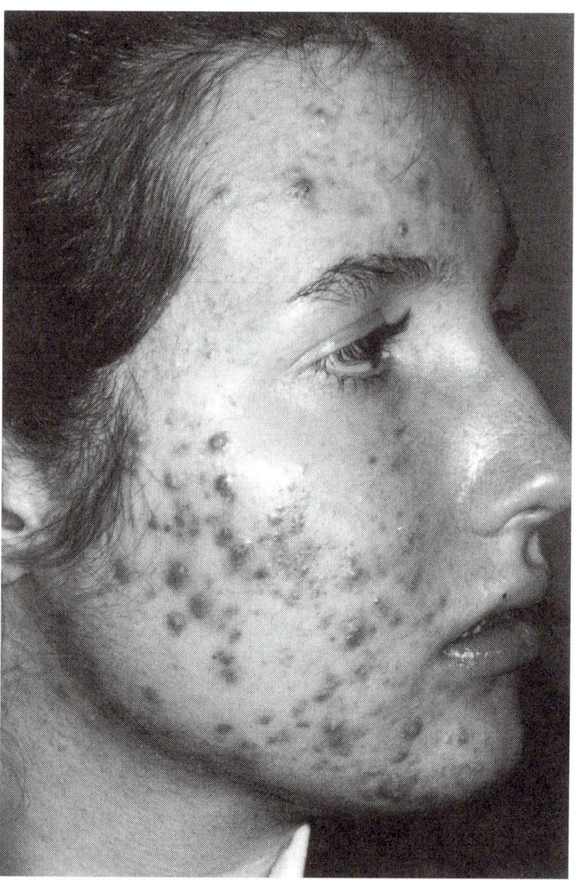

FIGURE 4 Patient with moderate acne.

tic teaching on acne therapy frequently suggests that if comedones are the most clinically significant feature, then retinoids are the preferred topical therapy. Conversely, it is generally believed that antimicrobial therapies should be used if inflamed lesions predominate. However, virtually all clinical trials of topical antibiotics in acne show that topical antibiotics significantly reduce comedones [17,18,21,28]. Whether this is a direct effect on ductal keratinocytes or an indirect effect on *P. acnes* is not known. In vitro studies with minocycline (orally) do show a reduction in keratinocyte proliferation. There are no similar data with topical antibiotics.

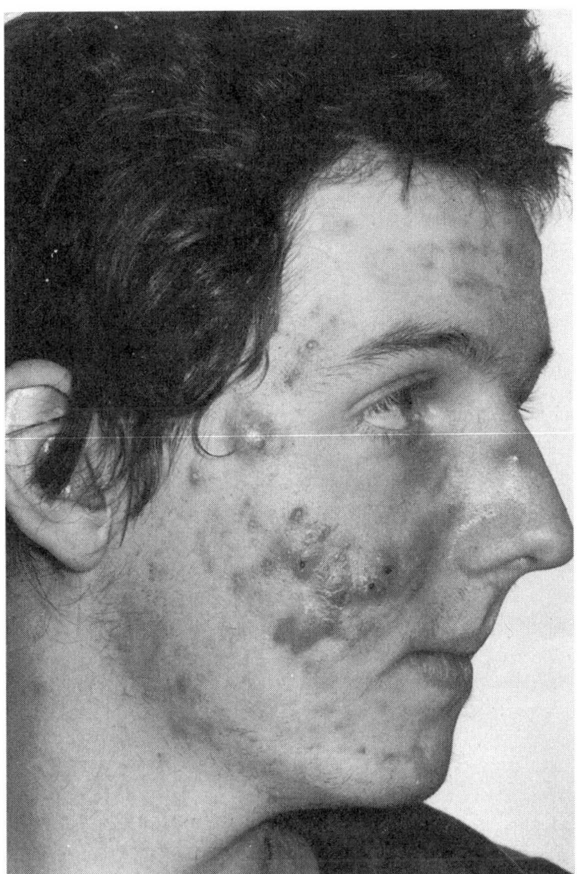

FIGURE 5 Patient with severe acne.

In general, many antibiotics have effects on downregulating inflammation. For example, it is known that antibiotics will reduce chemotaxis, reduce the proliferation of stimulated mononuclear cells, reduce reaction oxygen species, and affect IL-α production by ductal keratinocytes [12,32,33]. Most studies on the anti-inflammatory effects relate to oral antibiotics. There are very few data on the anti-inflammatory role of topical antibiotics. Topical potassium iodide is a way of inducing follicular inflammation and this inflammation can be reduced with topical erythromycin [11].

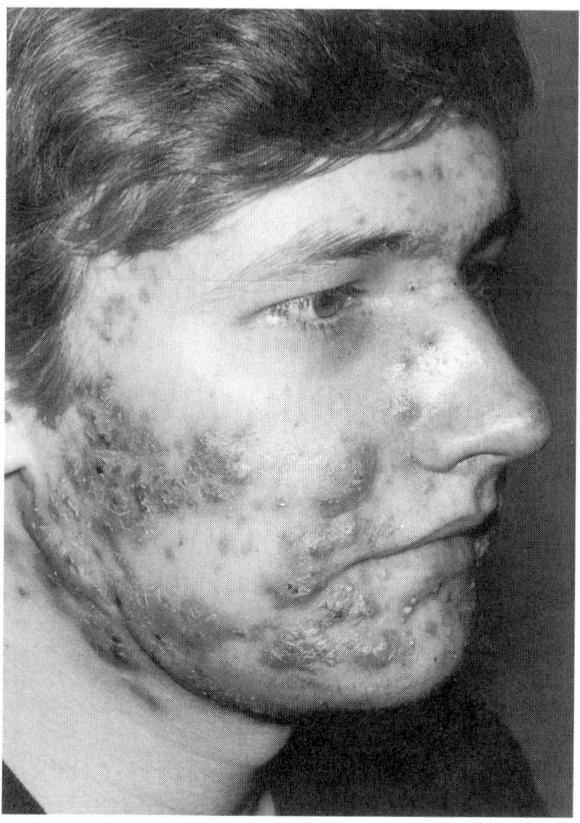

Figure 6 Patient with severe acne.

Table 1 Summary of Some Topical Therapies Used to Treat Acne in the United Kingdom

Anticomedonal	Combination Therapy	Anti-inflammatory
Adapalene	Benzoyl Peroxide + Erythromycin (Benzamycin Gel™)	Adapalene
All-trans retinoid acid	Isotretinoin + Erythromycin (Isotrexin®)	Azelaic acid
Azelaic acid	Zinc Acetate + Erythromycin (Zineryt®)	Benzoyl Peroxide
Isotretinoin		Clindamycin
		Erythromycin
		Tetracycline

III. ABSORPTION, METABOLISM, AND EXCRETION

When discussing the mode of action of drugs it is important to know about their absorption, localization, metabolism, and excretion. Unfortunately, there is precious little information for topical antibiotics in acne. Clearly, they must be absorbed and localized to their site of action in the skin, otherwise they simply would not work. There are only limited data as to where precisely in the skin the drug is absorbed. Topical tetracycline has been shown to be localized in the follicle [34], but its presence at that site does not necessarily imply a biological activity. Such inference can be made by measuring the number and function of follicular organisms. In in vitro studies on excised human skin, a topically applied erythromycin–zinc complex is concentrated in the stratum corneum [35]. To have a direct inflammatory role, perifollicular localization is necessary, but data are lacking.

Excretion of the drug could be into the follicle, by the transepidermal route or by systemic absorption. What limited studies have been performed clearly show that there is likely to be very little systemic absorption after the application of topical antibiotics. After the application of topical tetracycline, a plasma concentration of 1.7 mg/mL was found: this compares to 200 mg/mL after taking 500 mg of oral tetracycline twice daily [36]. Absorption after application of 2% erythromycin to the face, back, and chest of patients with moderate-to-severe acne for 1 month revealed virtually no systemic absorption whatsoever (E.A. Eady, personal observation).

The percutaneous absorption of clindamycin has been reported to occur following topical application of clindamycin hydrochloride [37], with clindamycin being detected in the urine; however, evidence suggests that absorption does not occur to a significant extent when clindamycin phosphate is used. Serum levels of clindamycin were below measurable limits following topical application of clindamycin hydrochloride and the appearance of clindamycin in the urine may reflect a kidney concentrating action.

The matter of systemic uptake of clindamycin following its topical application has been directly addressed in two major studies. In the first of these, Algra et al. [38] investigated the safety of a 1% hydroalcoholic solution of clindamycin hydrochloride in 18 patients. Blood samples taken 1 to 9 h after topical application of this solution were assayed for traces of clindamycin in order to determine the extent, if any, of systemic absorption.

It was reported that no measurable levels of clindamycin were present in any serum sample tested, and none of the patients complained of gastrointestinal side effects.

In the second study relating to possible systemic absorption of topically applied clindamycin, Siegle et al. [39] examined 32 patients (aged 15 to 29 years) who had been involved in a randomized double-blind study of this agent in comparison with its vehicle over an 8-week period. Assays were performed on stool and urine samples for organisms of the *Bacteroides fragilis* group, for *C. difficile* and its toxin, as well as for levels of clindamycin. Positive *C. difficile* cultures were determined in 7 out of 32 patients at various times during the study. In only two patients were the cultures positive at the end of the study, one of whom was receiving vehicle. Clindamycin was not detected in urine or stool of any patient in the trial.

There is also negligible absorption of topical nadifloxacillin associated with its use in patients with acne [29].

In support of the zero or insignificant absorption of topical antibiotics is the relative lack of clinical complication, such as might exist if significant systemic absorption had occurred. For example, gastrointestinal problems such as nausea, colic, or diarrhea are hardly ever recorded. There are very few cases of pseudomembranous colitis associated with the topical application of clindamycin [41], and there are no reports of vaginal candidiasis secondary to topical application of antibiotics.

This lack of systemic absorption would support the safe use of topical antibiotics for acne in pregnancy but virtually all companies state in their documentation that there are no human data to confirm for certain the safety of such products in pregnancy. The ABPI guidelines indicate there is no evidence of hazard from erythromycin in human pregnancy; it has been in wide use for many years without apparent ill consequences [42]. Data on the excretion of topical antibiotics into breast milk are also lacking, and thus use while breast feeding is not advised.

IV. DRUG INTERACTIONS

As with other pharmacokinetic data, little is known about drug interactions with other topical therapies. Benzoyl peroxide is a very reactive substance, so perhaps it is best avoided as a codrug unless specifically formulated for such use, as in Benzamycin® (benzoyl peroxide and erythromycin). Likewise, there are no data on the possible interaction of topical acne therapies and other oral therapies. However, in order to minimize the risk of *P. acnes* resistance, it may be prudent not to coprescribe different types of oral and topical antibiotics.

V. CLINICAL USE OF TOPICAL ANTIBIOTICS IN ACNE

Didactic teaching suggests that patients with mixed lesions (i.e., inflammatory and comedonal) should be prescribed anticomedonal therapy at night and anti-inflammatory therapy in the morning. Topical therapy should be prescribed alone in mild acne (Figs. 1 and 2), in conjunction with appropriate oral acne therapy in moderate disease (Figs. 3–5), and as a maintenance therapy after oral therapy has been discontinued. Thus, in many acne patients, topical therapy is necessary for many years. It is also necessary to stress to the patient that, when appropriate, topical therapy must be applied to acne on the trunk as well as on the face. Also, topical therapy should not just be applied to the spots but to the whole site prone to acne, because the apparently normal skin of acne patients in an acne-prone area is likely to have many microcomedones [43].

A. Which Antibiotic and Why?

A detailed analysis of 144 clinical trials of topical antimicrobial therapy in 1990 rejected over 50% because of poor trial design [44]. Adequate conclusions could not be drawn from the remaining data because of the different protocols, but benzoyl peroxide is a successful treatment and is probably similar in activity to topical erythromycin and clindamycin, with topicycline possibly being less effective. The benefit of topical erythromycin may be improved by combining it with either zinc [24,25] or benzoyl peroxide [26,27]. Comparative studies of topical antibiotics with oral antibiotics were often biased, less oral antibiotic was used than is currently recommended. In general, topical therapy appears less effective than adequate oral treatment. Topical chloramphenicol and pucidic acid preparations are also available in the United Kingdom [22,23]. Chloramphenicol proved less effective than benzoyl peroxide in a single study. Since 1991 there has not been a systemic review of the topical antibiotic acne literature and a few new formulations have emerged. Nadifloxacillin is widely used as a topical agent for acne in Japan; studies show its superiority to placebo and equivalence with 2% erythromycin cream [28,29]. It has not been introduced into European countries or the United States. Comparative studies published since 1991 suggest that topical Benzamycin® is more effective than Zineryt®, but this is based only on one publication [45]. One new product is the combination of clindamycin and benzoyl peroxide which appears to be more effective than either product alone [46]. The likely reason for this increased benefit of topical antibiotics combined with benzoyl peroxide is a reduction in *P. acnes* resistance [47]. The significance of *P. acnes* resistance is discussed in detail in Section VI. It is unlikely that combinations of antibiotics with topical retinoids reduce the risk of resistance. Such combinations include isotretinoin with erythromycin (Isotrexin®) and isotretinoin with clindamycin (Velac[a]). Both products, in particular the isotretinoin/clindamycin preparation, show some greater benefit than monotherapy [48,49].

VI. P. ACNES RESISTANCE

There is an alarming increase in resistance to *P. acnes* [50–53], and the relationship between *P. acnes* resistance and clinical failure is not straightforward [51]. It is important to note that if a strain of *P. acnes* is reported as being resistant, it does not necessarily imply that the patient is resistant to therapy. For there to be clinical resistance, the concentration of that antibiotic at the relevant skin site must be less than the minimum inhibitory concentration (MIC) of that same *P. acnes* strain grown from that same patient. The absence of a simple relationship between clinical response and *P. acnes* resistance is in part explained by variation in comedonal levels of antibiotic after topical application [54]. There is, however, evidence to show some correlation between *P. acnes* resistance and clinical failure [51]. Furthermore, many antiacne drugs have additional nonantimicrobial anti-inflammatory mechanisms of action [12,31,32]. Thus the relationship between clinical response to topical antibiotics and clinical failure is complex. Whether oral or topical antibiotics or both are equally involved in inducing *P. acnes* resistance is not known.

In 1997, 61% of patients referred to special acne clinics had resistant *P. acnes* [53]. Resistance is most frequently seen to erythromycin and clindamycin, and less so to tetracycline and doxycycline (Fig. 7). Multiple resistance is seen in 22% of patients. Resistance to minocycline is rare (<5%). There is also a significantly greater number of resistant *P. acnes* on the skin of close contacts of acne patients compared with controls [55]. Given the fact that the resistance is due to point mutations in the target site, 23s ribosomal rRNA (for erythromycin and clindamycin) [56], it is likely that *P. acnes* resistance is going to last for many, many years. For tetracycline, the target site is 16s ribosomal rRNA [57]. It is likely that, of all topical antimicrobial therapies, topical benzoyl peroxide and a combination of erythromycin and benzoyl peroxide are associated with the least resistance; in vitro and in vivo, both therapies can significantly reduce *P. acnes* resistance [47]. Benzoyl peroxide also significantly reduces *P. acnes* resis-

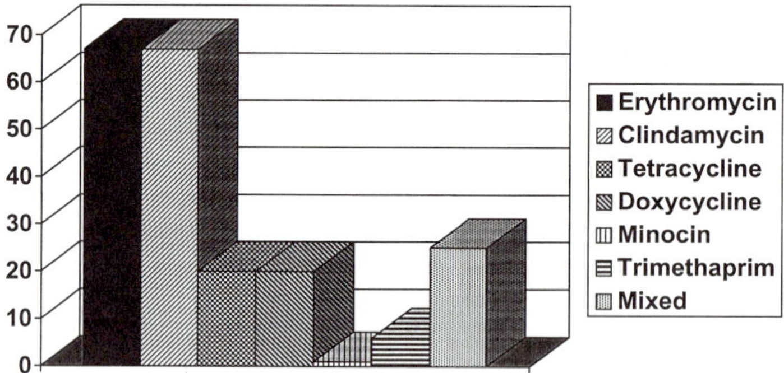

FIGURE 7 *P. acnes*-resistant profile.

tance [47]. Physicians should avoid prescribing dissimilar oral and topical antibiotics as this may encourage resistance.

VII. SIDE EFFECTS OF TOPICAL ANTIBIOTICS

Many topical preparations produce a primary irritant dermatitis (Fig. 8) [58,59] and the patient must be warned not to stop treatment prematurely as a result of this. Indeed, with some preparations such as benzoyl peroxide and certain retinoids, the total absence of such skin irritation should lead the physician to suspect that the topical therapy is not being used correctly. If a primary irritant reaction occurs, the product should not be used for a few days and the dermatitis should be treated with moisturizers or a weak steroid ointment. Thereafter, the acne preparation can be restarted at a somewhat reduced frequency of application. Some topical therapies have a comparatively less irritating profile than others. For example, azaleic acid is relatively non irritant [60]; and certain antibiotic/benzoyl peroxide combinations (such as erythromycin and benzoyl peroxide) are less irritating than benzoyl peroxide alone [26,27], presumably because of the anti-inflammatory action of the antibiotic. An allergic contact dermatitis is extremely rare. Combined benzoyl peroxide preparations bleach clothes and hair and the patient must be informed of these inconvenient side effects. Topical tetracycline may give a light yellow color to the skin and can fluoresce under disco lights—a temporary, but interesting, phenomenon for a 15-year-old!

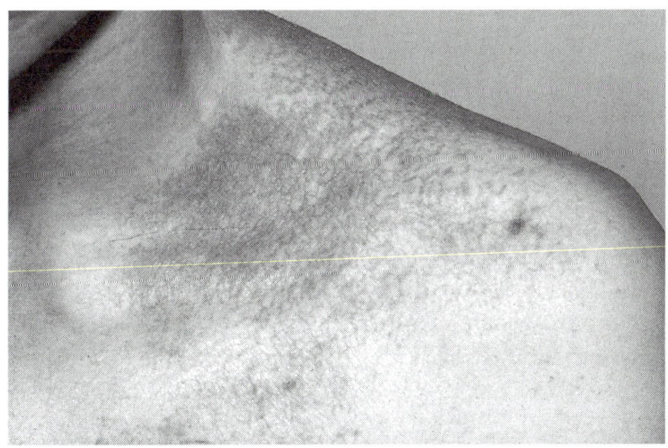

FIGURE 8 Typical primary irritant dermatitis.

VIII. TOPICAL METRONIDAZOLE AND ROSACEA

Topical antibiotics do not help the telangiectatic component of rosacea; they only influence the inflammatory aspects of the disease. Topical metronidazole is the major topical antibiotic used for patients with rosacea. Topical antibiotics such as those used in acne are much less frequently prescribed, although there is evidence of some beneficial effect for erythromycin and tetracycline [61]. As for acne, the pharmacokinetic data on the use of such drugs in rosacea are very limited. It is likely that the benefit of such drugs in rosacea relates much more to an anti-inflammatory, rather than antibacterial, action.

The most widely used topical antibiotic therapy in rosacea is metronidazole [62–68]. Its benefit alone or in combination with oral tetracyclines is overwhelming. The drug should be applied twice daily to all affected sites, including perilesional skin. Duration of therapy with topical metronidazole varies but may be needed for 2 to 4 years, most often months. Comparative studies are limited, but in less than severe disease topical metronidazole may be equally beneficial with oral tetracyclines [64]. However, a follow-up study to assess the relapse rate after treatment of rosacea with either oral tetracycline or 1% metronidazole cream once daily for 4 months of treatment with 1% metronidazole cream showed significantly fewer relapses compared with 250 mg oxytetracycline taken orally twice daily for 2 months [65]. No significant difference was found between 2 months of treatment with 1% metronidazole cream once daily and oxytetracycline therapy [64].

A. Absorption, Metabolism, and Excretion

As with other topical antibiotics, there are limited data on cutaneous absorption, metabolism, and excretion. Systemic absorption is minimal [67,69,70]. The systemic concentration of metronidazole following topical administration of 1 g of 0.75% gel to 10 patients with rosacea ranged from 25 ng/mL (limit of detection) to 66 ng/mL, with a mean C_{max} of 40.6 ng/mL. The corresponding mean C_{max} following the oral administration of a solution containing 30 mg of metronidazole was 850 ng/mL (equivalent to 212 ng/mL if dose corrected). The mean T_{max} for the topical formulation was 6.0 h compared to 0.87 h for the oral solution.

Oral metronidazole is degraded into at least five metabolites with potential biological activity, among which the major urinary product, the 2-hydroxymethyl derivative, is approximately one-third to ten times more active as an antibacterial agent than metronidazole. Percutaneous absorption of metronidazole and its metabolites was investigated in serum of patients suffering from rosacea, who were treated with 1% metronidazole cream and placebo cream once or twice daily for 1 and 2 months, the average amount of cream being 0.5 to 1.0 g, corresponding to 5 to 10 mg metronidazole a day. Metronidazole and its major metabolite, OH-metronidazole, were analyzed in 24-h urine specimens. In 14% of the serum samples, only traces of metronidazole or substances interfering with the analysis were found. Results ranged from 20 to 45 ng/mL serum, corresponding to a sensitivity limit of the method used of about 50 ng/mL serum. Traces of metronidazole were even found in one patient treated with the placebo cream, corresponding well to the analysis of pooled donor serum in which a chromatographic pattern like that of metronidazole occasionally is found. The hydroxy metabolite of metronidazole was found in the 24-h urine specimen from only one patient; however, detection of untransformed metronidazole was impossible in the urine investigated. Serum samples and 24-h urine specimens were analyzed according to a high-performance liquid chromatography (HPLC) method first described by Hackett and Dusci [70].

B. Mechanisms of Action

The effect of antimicrobial agents on leukocyte chemotaxis has been studied in in vitro systems, and a marked suppression of chemotaxis for tetracyclines, erythromycin, and clindamycin was demonstrated. It has even been postulated that the capacity of these agents to inhibit leukocyte migration may account, in part, for their efficacy in inflammatory skin diseases like acne vulgaris and rosacea.

During the last decade, studies have shown that metronidazole impedes leukocyte chemotaxis and selectively suppresses some aspect of cell-mediated immunity. The favorable effect of metronidazole in the treatment of Crohn's disease and in skin ulcers should, therefore, probably be interpreted as an influence on the host defense mechanism and not as a drug effect on anaerobic bacteria.

The antibiotics generally prescribed for the treatment of rosacea (tetracyclines, erythromycin, and metronidazole) possess an inhibitory influence on the immunological defense mechanism. Therefore, it is not improbable that the major effect of topically applied metronidazole is the same.

C. Side Effects of Metronidazole

As with other topical antibiotics, side effects consist of a primary irritant dermatitis. In placebo-controlled studies, irritant reactions were observed in about 10%, equally distributed between 1% metronidazole cream and the cream base [63]. The same rates of reactions were found in patients included in the clinical trials. No allergic reactions were observed, which corresponds well to a low frequency of allergic reactions to imidazole derivatives. About 5% of the patients included in the studies of 1% metronidazole cream complained about skin irritation, dryness, and stinging. These complaints did not interfere with the beneficial effect on rosacea lesions. As with all topical facial products, contact with the eyes should be avoided.

A disulfiramlike reaction has been reported in a small number of patients taking oral metronidazole and alcohol concomitantly but not following topical therapy. The safety of topical metronidazole in pregnancy and lactation has not been adequately established, and topical metronidazole should not be used in these circumstances.

IX. MUPIROCIN (BACTROBAN®)

Bactroban® is available as a sterile ointment containing the antibiotic mupirocin (2% w/w) in a water-soluble polyethylene glycol base.

A. Mechanisms of Action

Mupirocin possesses a high level of bactericidal activity against staphylococci (including multiply resistant strains), streptococci, and certain Gram-negative species [72]. It has a novel chemical structure and mode of action, unrelated to those of other available antibiotics, which involves competitive inhibition of bacterial iso-leucyl transfer-RNA synthetase [73]. Mupirocin is not available for systemic administration and bacterial cross-resistance to other available antibiotics would not be expected to arise.

B. Absorption, Metabolism, and Excretion

Skin penetration studies indicate that Bactroban® exhibits good penetration through diseased skin, but penetration through healthy skin is relatively low [74]. Any mupirocin absorbed into the systemic circulation through damaged skin is rapidly metabolized to an inactive derivative, monic acid [75].

C. Clinical Studies

Bactroban® ointment is indicated for the topical treatment of bacterial skin infections such as impetigo, folliculitis, and furunculosis. Its successful use in the treatment of a range of bacterial skin infections has been well documented [71–83]. White et al. [75] reported overall clinical success rates of 97% (Bactroban) and 93% (Fucidin) in their study, which included a total of 390 assessable patients. Bactroban was found to be significantly more effective in the treatment of acute primary skin infections and in the treatment of a subgroup of patients with impetigo. Similar clinical success rates have been reported by Langdon and Mahaptra [76], whereas Morley and Munot [77] reported an overall clinical response rate of 86% for both Bactroban and Fucidin. More detailed analysis of their results also revealed no significant difference between the two products in cases of primary or secondary skin infections.

The clinical efficacy of Bactroban and neomycin has also been compared by several investigators. For example, Kennedy et al. [78] evaluated their relative efficacy in the treatment of impetigo and found Bactroban to be at least as effective as 1% neomycin. A later study by Wilkinson and Carey [79] compared Bactroban with topical Neosporin and showed Bactroban to be the more effective agent in terms of both clinical and bacteriological efficacy.

The comparative clinical efficacy of Bactroban and oral antibiotics in the treatment of skin infections has been evaluated in several studies [80–82]. Villiger et al. [80] describe a comparison between Bactroban and oral flucloxacillin or erythromycin in a group of 200 patients presenting with skin infections. In this study, Bactroban was found to be as effective as oral flucloxacillin and more effective than oral erythromycin. In a similar multicenter study, Maddin [81] found Bactroban to be at least as effective as oral erythromycin and superior to oral cloxacillin and topical Neosporin.

Bar David and Dagan [82] compared topical mupirocin (t.i.d.) with erythromycin 50 mg/kg daily in the treatment of impetigo in children. At the end of the study, 10/43(23%) evaluable patients in the erythromycin group and only 1/46 (2%) in the mupirocin group were considered treatment failures ($p < 0.05$). Four patients in the erythromycin group had to be withdrawn due to gastrointestinal side effects. The authors noted a marked difference in favor of mupirocin in the clinical course of the disease and concluded that mupirocin is an appropriate choice, particularly in areas where erythromycin resistance is high.

In addition to comparative studies, the efficacy of Bactroban has also been demonstrated in open studies. For example, Bork et al. [83] describe a multicenter study involving a total of 1391 general practice patients with superficial skin infections, in which a clinical success rate of 96% was recorded; 73% of patients were cured and 22.5% showed marked clinical improvement following a course of Bactroban.

D. Side Effects

Bactroban™ appears to be almost devoid of side effects [25]. An irritant dermatitis is exceptionally uncommon and an allergic contact dermatitis is very rare.

XI. FUSIDIC ACID

Topical fusidic acid (Fucidin) is available alone as a cream, gel, or intertulle, or combined with steroids. The combined steroid–antibiotic is mainly prescribed in eczema; the antibiotic alone is prescribed alone in *S. aureus* infections and acne.

A. Mechanisms of Action

Fusidic acid is an antimicrobial agent that acts as an inhibitor of protein synthesis in the microorganism [84,85]. It interferes with the translocation step by stabilizing the ribosome-guanosine diphosphate-elongation factor G complex. This prevents binding of aminoacyl tRNA to the ribosome and thereafter stops transfer of additional amino acids to the growing polypeptide [86].

The activity of fusidic acid in infections is dependent upon the drug reaching concentrations in the tissues above the MIC for the particular organism. Concentrations of fusidic acid between 0.03 and 0.12 $mg.L^{-1}$ inhibit virtually all strains of *Staphylococcus*. In vitro studies in which the concentration of fusidic acid was increased did not appear to change the rate of killing of the organisms but did decrease the rate of development of resistance in *S. aureus* [86].

B. Absorption, Metabolism, and Excretion

There are very little data on cutaneous absorption, metabolism, and excretion after topical therapy, but it is likely that there is very little absorption [87]. After oral administration of fusidic acid, it undergoes extensive metabolism in the liver and is primarily excreted in the bile as metabolites with weak or no bioactivity. Three metabolites predominate: glucuronic acid conjugate; dicarboxylic acid metabolite; and hydroxy metabolite [88].

C. Clinical Studies

Fusidic acid, when used alone against infections, is available as a cream or an ointment containing 2% fusidic acid. Fucidin ointment contains 2% fusidate sodium. Excipients in the cream include potassium sorbate, butylated hydroxyanisole, polysorbate 60, and white soft paraffin; excipients in the ointment include lanolin and white soft paraffin; and excipients in the gel include parabens, polysorbate 80, and triethanolamine. Fucidin intertulle is also available, which is a medicated dressing consisting of sterile gauze squares impregnated with Fucidin ointment. The topical treatment is recommended for skin infections caused by *S. aureus*, *Streptococcus pyogenes*, and *Corynebacterium minitissimum*. Impetigo is its most common indication.

The efficacy of topical fusidic acid has been established over many years. Some of the early clinical studies were uncontrolled [89,90]. This is not surprising since they were conducted many years ago, but there are several good comparative studies worthy of comment. For example, in impetigo, fusidic acid ointment was shown to be significantly more effective than its vehicle [91]. Another comparative study in the same indication showed that fusidic acid was superior to a neomycin/bacitracin combination [92]. The comparative clinical and bacteriological efficacy of fusidic acid and mupirocin has been investigated in several clinical studies [93–99]. In one study, mupirocin appeared more effective than fusidic acid with respect to bacteriological clearance [96]. However, this finding was not confirmed in other comparative studies [94–96]. Overall it thus appears that the two preparations are likely to be equally effective in routine clinical use.

Topical fusidic acid has also been compared with oral antibiotics in the treatment of superficial infections [100,101]. It was found to be at least as effective and, in one study, it was found to be superior to oral antibiotics [101]. Systemic therapy is necessary when there is evidence of systemic spread of infection or in debilitated or immunocompromised patients, but in the typical patient with a localized, superficial infection, topical fusidic acid is appropriate. Fusidic acid is available in combination with betamethasone valerate, hydrocortisone acetate or butyrate, or triamcinolone benetonide for use in eczema and dermatitis associated with, or likely to be associated with, *S. aureus* infection [102,103].

The combination of fusidic acid and hydrocortisone has been compared with hydrocortisone alone in atopic eczema [102]. Combined therapy was significantly more effective in eradicating bacterial pathogens (almost exclusively *S. aureus*) and the clinical response appeared better in patients given the combination. Overall, fusidic acid/hydrocortisone treatment was significantly superior to the hydrocortisone alone on combined clinical and bacteriological assessments. Fusidic acid and hydrocortisone have been shown to produce a faster clinical improvement than combined hydrocortisone and miconazole in clinically infected eczema, and the fusidic acid combination had advantages in terms of bacteriological efficacy and patient acceptability [103].

Fusidic acid/betamethasone combination has been evaluated in the treatment of infected eczema [104–107]. Again, the combination was considered superior to the corticosteroid alone [104]. Fusidic acid/betamethasone and neomycin/betamethasone have been shown to be equally effective [106,107]. Comparative efficacy with a gentamicin/betamethasone combination was also established [108]. A 4-week study comparing fusidic acid/betamethasone and a clioquinol/betamethasone combination in patients with clinically infected hand eczema demonstrated equal clinical effectiveness but a significantly better bacteriological outcome was seen with fusidic acid/betamethasone [108]. Patient acceptability for the fusidic acid cream was superior to that of the clioquinol cream [108] because of the lack of staining with fusidic acid.

D. Side Effects

Shanson, after reviewing the published literature on the use of topical fusidic acid in treating skin infections, concluded that short courses were unlikely to be epidemiologically harmful [109]. During more than 35 years of extended usage of fusidic acid, the level of microbiological resistance has remained low [109–111].

There is no cross-resistance between fusidic acid and other antibiotics used clinically [111,112]. This is probably due to the fact that fusidic acid belongs to a group of its own, the fusidanes, which have a very different structure from all other classes of antibiotics, such as the beta-lactams, aminoglycosides, and macrolides, thus reducing the likelihood of having the same mechanism of resistance. In 1999, the increasing prevalence of fusidic resistance to *S. aureus* in patients with atopic eczema has been reported [113]. The incidence of allergic reactions to fusidic acid is low [114] and cross-allergy has not been seen.

REFERENCES

1. Pochi PE, Straus JS. Sebum production, casual sebum levels, titratable acidity of sebum and urinary fractional 17-ketosteroid excretion in males with acne. J Invest Dermatol 1964; 43:383–388.
2. Walton S, Cunliffe WJ, Keczkes K. Clinical, ultrasound and hormonal markers of androgenicity in acne vulgaris. Br J Dermatol 1995; 133:249–253.
3. Plewig G, Fulton JE, Kligman AM. Cellular dynamics of comedo formation in acne vulgaris. Arch Dermatol Forsch 1971; 242:12–29.
4. Knaggs HE, Holland DB, Morris C. Quantification of cellular proliferation in acne using the monoclonal antibody of Ki-67. J Invest Dermatol 1994:89–92.
5. Webster GF. Inflammation in acne vulgaris. J Am Acad Dermatol 1995; 33:247–253.
6. Marples RR. The microflora of the face and acne lesions. J Invest Dermatol 1974; 62:326–331.
7. Strauss JS, Kligman AM. The pathologic dynamics of acne vulgaris. Br J Dermatol 1960; 50:779–790.
8. Norris JF, Cunliffe WJ. A histological and immunocytochemical study of early acne lesions. Br J Dermatol 1988; 118:651–659.
9. Gloor M, Kraft H, Franke M. Effectiveness of topically applied antibiotics on anaerobic bacteria in the pilosebaceous duct. Dermatologica 1984; 157:96–104.
10. Bernstein JE, Shalita AR. Effects of topical erythromycin on aerobic and anaerobic surface flora. Acta Dermatol Venereol (Stockh) 1980; 60:537–538.
11. Esterly NB, Koronsky JS, Furey NL, et al. Neutrophil chemotaxis in patients with acne receiving oral tetracycline. Arch Dermatol 1984; 120:1308–1313.
12. Eady EA, Ingham E, Walters CE. Modulation of comedonal levels of interleukin-1 in acne patients treated with tetracyclines. J Invest Dermatol 1993; 101:86–91.
13. Olsen TC. Therapy of acne. Med Clin North Am 1982; 66:851–871.
14. Leyden JJ. New understandings of the pathogenesis of acne. J Am Acad Dermatol 1995; 32:15–25.
15. Burke BM, Cunliffe WJ. The assessment of acne vulgaris—the Leeds technique. Br J Dermatol 1984; 111:83–92.
16. Stoughton RB. Topical antibiotics for acne vulgaris. Arch Dermatol 1979; 115: 486–489.
17. Feucht CL, Allen BS, Chalker DK. Topical erythromycin with zinc in acne. A double-blind controlled study. J Am Acad Dermatol 1980; 3:483–489.
18. Norris JF, Hughes BR, Basey AJ, Cunliffe WJ. A comparison of the effectiveness of topical tetracycline, benzoyl peroxide gel and oral oxytetracycline in the treatment of acne. Clin Exp Dermatol 1991; 16:31–33.
19. Cratton D, Raymond CP, Guertin-Larochelle S. Topical clindamycin versus systemic tetracycline in the treatment of acne. Results of a multiclinic trial. J Am Acad Dermatol 1982; 1:50–53.

20. Swinyer LJ, Baker MD, Swinyer TA. A comparative study of benzoyl peroxide and clindamycin phosphate for treating acne vulgaris. Br J Dermatol 1989; 119: 615–622.
21. Schatner L, Pestana A, Kittles C. A clinical trial comparing the safety and efficacy of a topical erythromycin-zinc formulation with a topical clindamycin formulation. J Am Acad Dermatol 1990; 22:252–260.
22. Cunliffe WJ, Burke B, Dodman B. Chloramphenicol and benzoyl peroxide in acne: a double-blind clinical study. Practitioner 1980; 224:952–954.
23. Parrah AJ, Gray PL. An open multicentre study to compare Fucidin lotion and oral minocycline in the treatment of mild-moderate acne of the face. Eur J Clin Res 1996; 8:97–107.
24. Habbema L, Koopmans B, Menke HE. A 4% erythromycin and zinc combination (Zineryt) versus 2% erythromycin (Eryderm) in acne vulgaris; a randomized, double-blind comparative study. Br J Dermatol 1989; 121:497–502.
25. Strauss JS, Stranieri AM. Acne treatment with topical erythromycin and zinc; effect on Propionibacterium acnes and free fatty acid composition. J Am Acad Dermatol 1984; 11:86–89.
26. Chalker DK, Shalita A, Smith JG, Swann RW. A double-blind study of the effectiveness of a 3% erythromycin and 5% benzoyl peroxide combination in the treatment of acne vulgaris. J Am Acad Dermatol 1983; 9:933–936.
27. Shalita AR, Chalker DK, Ellis CN, et al. A multicenter, double-blind controlled study of the combination of erythromycin/benzoyl peroxide, erythromycin alone and benzoyl peroxide alone in the treatment of acne vulgaris. Cutis 1992; 49:1–4.
28. Vogt K, Hahn H, Hermann J, et al. Antimicrobial evaluation of nadifloxacillin, (OP.7251) a new topical quinolone in acne vulgaris. Drug 1995; 49(2):266–268.
29. Gollnick HPM, Vogt K, Hermann J, et al. Topical quinolone OPC7521, a clinical microbiological study in acne. Eur J Dermatol 1994; 4:210–215.
30. Exner JH, Comite H, Dahod S, Pochi PE. Topical erythromycin/zinc effect on acne and sebum excretion. Curr Ther Res Clin Exp 1983; 34:762–767.
31. Piérard-Franchimont C, Goffin V, Visser JN, Jacoby H, Piérard GE. A double-blind controlled evaluation of the sebosuppressive activity of topical erythromycin-zinc complex. Eur J Clin Pharmacol 1995; 49:57–60.
32. Webster GF, Leyden JJ, McGinley KJ. Suppression of poly-morphonuclear leukocyte chemotactic factor production in Propionibacterium acnes by submorphonuclear leukocyte chemotactic factor production in Propionibacterium acnes by sub-minimal inhibitory concentrations of tetracycline, ampicillin, minocycline and erythromycin. Antimicrob Agents Chemother 1982; 21:770–777.
33. Akamatsu H, Asada M, Koumura J. Effect of doxycycline on the generation of reactive oxygen species: a possible mechanism of action of acne therapy with doxycycline. Acta Dermatol Venereol (Stockh) 1992; 72:178–179.
34. Van Hoogdalem EJ, Van Den Hoven WE, Van Den Berg TP, Hespe W. Dermal pharmacokinetics of topically applied zinc-erythromycin in rats and man; preliminary results. Pharm Weekbl Sci Ed 1990; 12:D5.
35. Penetration of tetracycline into the human skin. Unpublished data. Monmouth Pharmaceuticals, 1998.

36. Barza M, Goldstein JA, Kane A, et al. Systemic absorption of clindamycin hydrochloride after topical application. J Am Acad Dermatol 1982; 7:208–214.
37. Rietschel RL, Duncan SH. Clindamycin phosphate used in combination with tretinoin in the treatment of acne. Int J Dermatol 1983; 22:41–43.
38. Algra RJ, Rosen T, Waisman M. Topical clindamycin in acne vulgaris: safety and stability. Arch Dermatol 1977; 113:1390–1391.
39. Siegle RJ, Fekety R, Sarbone PD, Finch RN, Deery HG, Voorhees JJ. Effects of topical clindamycin on intestinal microflora in patients with acne. J Am Acad Dermatol 1986; 15:180–185.
40. Parry MF, Rha CK. Pseudomembranous colitis caused by topical clindamycin phosphate. Arch Dermatol 1986; 122:583–584.
41. Milstone EB, McDonald AJ, Scholhamer F. Pseudomembranous colitis after topical application of clindamycin. Arch Dermatol 1981; 117:154–155.
42. ABPI Compendium of Data Sheets. London: Data Pharmaceutical Publications, Ltd., 1998, p. 1413.
43. Holmes RL, Williams M, Cunliffe WJ. Pilo-sebaceous duct obstruction and acne. Br J Dermatol 1972; 87:327–332.
44. Eady EA, Cove JH, Joanes DN. Topical antibiotics for the treatment of acne: a critical evaluation of the literature on their clinical benefit and comparative efficacy. J Dermatol Treat 1990; 1:215–216.
45. Chu A, Huber FJ, Plott RT. The comparative efficacy of benzoyl peroxide, 5% erythromycin gel, 3% gel and erythromycin 4% zinc 1-2% solution in the treatment of acne vulgaris. Br J Dermatol 1997; 136:235–238.
46. Lookingbill DP, Chalker DK, Lindholm JS, Katz HI, Kempers SE, Huerter CJ, Swinehart JM, Schelling DJ, Klauda HC. Treatment of acne with a combination clindamycin/benzoyl peroxide gel compared with clindamycin gel, benzoyl peroxide gel and vehicle gel: combined results of two double-blind investigations. J Am Acad Dermatol 1997; 37:590–595.
47. Eady EA, Farmery MR, Ross JI. Effects of benzoyl peroxide and erythromycin alone and in combination against antibiotic-sensitive and -resistant skin bacteria from acne patients. Br J Dermatol 1994; 131:331–336.
48. Stables G, Boorman G, Eady EA, Cunliffe WJ. The effects of combined topical erythromycin and retinoid (Isotrex) alone and in combination in the treatment of acne. Dermatology 1999 (In press).
49. Richter JR, Bousema KT, De-Boulle KLV, et al. Efficacy of a fixed clindamycin phosphate 1.2%, tretinoin 0.025% gel formulation (Velac) in the topical control of acne vulgaris. J Dermatol Treat 1998; 9:81–90.
50. Eady EA, Jones CE, Tipper JI. Antibiotic resistant propionibacteria in acne; need for policies to modify antibiotic usage. Br Med J 1993; 306:555–556.
51. Eady EA, Cove JH, Holland KT, Cunliffe WJ. Erythromycin resistant propionibacteria in antibiotic treated acne patients: association with therapeutic failure. Br J Dermatol 1989; 121:51–57.
52. Eady EA, Jones CE, Gardner KJ. Tetracycline-resistant propionibacteria from acne patients are cross-resistant to doxycycline but sensitive to minocycline. Br J Dermatol 1993; 128:556–560.
53. Eady EA. Bacterial resistance in acne. J Invest Dermatol 1997; 108:379.

54. Gardner KJ, Cunliffe WJ, Eady EA, Cove JH. Variation in comedonal antibiotic concentrations following application of topical tetracycline for acne vulgaris. Br J Dermatol 194; 131:649–654.
55. Miller Y, Eady EA, Vyakrnams S. One or two close contacts of antibiotic-treated acne patients carry resistant propionibacteria on their skin surface. J Invest Dermatol 1997; 108:379.
56. Ross JI, Eady EA, Cove JH, et al. Clinical resistance to erythromycin and clindamycin in cutaneous Propionibacteria isolated from acne patients is associated with mutations in 235 rRNA. Antimicrob Agents Chemother 1997; 41:1162–1165.
57. Ross JI, Eady EA, Cove JH, Cunliffe WJ. 16S rRNA mutation associated with tretracycline resistance in a gram-positive bacterium. Antimicrob Agents Chemother 1998; 42(7):1702–1705.
58. Sykes NL, Webster GF. Acne: a review of optimum treatment. Drugs 1994; 48: 59–70.
59. Cunliffe WJ. The conventional treatment of acne. Semin Dermatol 1983; 2:138–144.
60. Graupe K, Cunliffe WJ, Gollnick HP. Efficacy and safety of topical azelaic acid. Cutis 1996; 57(suppl 1):20–35.
61. Wilkin JH, Dewitts J. Treatment of Rosacea topical clindamycin versus oral tetracycline. Int Dermatol 1993; 32:65–67.
62. Kurkcuoglu N, Atakan N. Metronidazole in the treatment of rosacea. Arch Dermatol 1984; 120:837.
63. Neilsen PG. Treatment of rosacea with 1% metronidazole cream. A double-blind study. Br J Dermatol 1983; 108:327.
64. Neilsen PG. A double-blind study of 1% metronidazole cream versus systemic oxytetracycline therapy for rosacea. Br J Dermatol 1983; 109:63.
65. Neilsen PG. The relapse rate for rosacea after treatment with either oral tetracycline or metronidazole cream. Br J Dermatol 1983; 109:122–123.
66. Monk B. Topical metronidazole. A new treatment for Rosacea. Prescriber 1992; 3:17–18.
67. Stambaugh JE, Feop LG, Manthei RW. The isolation and identification of the urinary oxidative metabolites of metronidazole in man. J Pharmacol Exp Ther 1968; 161:373–381.
68. Neilson PG, Metronidazole treatment in rosacea. Int J Dermatol 1988; 27:1–5.
69. Arnold E. Dermal absorption of metronidazole from 1% cream: internal report. Copenhagen, Denmark: Dumex Ltd, 1984.
70. Hackett LP, Dusci LJ. Determination of metronidazole and tinidazole in human plasma using high-performance liquid chromatography. J Chromatogr 1979; 175: 347–349.
71. Sutherland R, Boon RJ, Griffin K. Antibacterial activity of Mupirocin (pseudomonic acid) a new antibiotic for topical use. Antimicrob Agents Chemother 1985; 27:495–498.
72. Mellows G. The mode of action of Mupirocin: inhibition of bacterial isoleucyl transfer-ribonucleic acid synthetase. Fortschr Antimicrob Antineoplast Chemother 1987; 6:169–173.

73. Jackson D, Tasker TGG, Sutherland R. Clinical pharmacology of Bactroban: pharmacokinetics, tolerance and efficacy studies. Excerpta Medica Curr Clin Pract Ser 1985; 1:54–67.
74. Baines PJ, Jackson D, Mellows G. Mupirocin: its chemistry and metabolism. R Soc Med Int Congr Symp Ser 1984; 8:13–22.
75. White DG, Collins PO, Rowsell RB. Topical antibiotics in the treatment of superficial skin infections in general practice—a comparison of Mupirocin with sodium fusidate. J Infect 1989; 18:221–229.
76. Langdon CG, Mahaptra KS. Efficacy and acceptability of fusidic acid cream and Mupirocin ointment in skin sepsis. Curr Ther Res 1990; 48:174–180.
77. Morley PAR, Munot LD. A comparison of sodium fusidate ointment and Mupirocin ointment in superficial skin sepsis. Curr Med Res Opin 1988; 11:142–148.
78. Kennedy CTC, Watts JA, Speller DCE. Bactroban ointment in the treatment of impetigo: a controlled trial against neomycin. Excerpta Medica Curr Clin Pract Ser 1985; 16:125–129.
79. Wilkinson RD, Carey WD. Topical Mupirocin versus topical neosporin in the treatment of cutaneous infections. Int J Dermatol 1988; 278:514–515.
80. Villiger JW, et al. A comparison of the new topical antibiotic Mupirocin (''Bactroban'') with oral antibiotics in the treatment of skin infections in general practice. Curr Med Res Opin 1986; 10:339–345.
81. Maddin S. Efficacy and tolerance of a novel, new topical antibiotic vs conventional systemic and topical treatment of primary and secondary skin infections. Contemp Dermatol 1987; June/July:32–39.
82. Bar David Y, Dagan R. Double-blind study comparing erythromycin and Mupirocin for treatment of impetigo in children: implications of a high prevalence of erythromycin-resistant stephylococcus aureus strains. Antimicrob Agents Chemother 1992; 36:287–290.
83. Bork K, et al. Efficacy and safety of 2% Mupirocin ointment in the treatment of primary and secondary skin infections: an open multicentre trial. Br J Clin Pract 1989; 43:284–288.
84. Tanaka N, Kinoshita T, Masukawa H. Mechanism of inhibition of protein synthesis by fusidic acid and related steroidal antibiotics. J Biochem 1969; 65:459–464.
85. Bodley JW, Zieve FJ, Lin L. Studies on translocation IV. The hydrolysis of a single round of guanosine triphosphate in the presence of fusidic acid. J Biol Chem 1970; 245:5662–5669.
86. Barber M, Waterworth PM. Antibacterial activity in vitro of fucidin. Lancet 1962; 1:931–932.
87. Vickers CFH. Percutaneous absorption of sodium fusidate and fusidic acid. Br J Dermatol 1969; 81:902–908.
88. MacGowan AP, Greig MA, Andrews JM, Reeves DS, Wise R. Pharmacokinetics and tolerance of a new film-coated tablet of sodium fusidate administered as a single oral dose to healthy volunteers. J Antimicrob Chemother 1989; 23:409–415.
89. Sobye P. Cutaneous *Staphylococcus aureus* infections treated with Fucidin ointment. Ugeskr Laeger 1966; 128:204–207.
90. Fleming JM, Mansfield AO. The place of a topical ointment in the treatment of common skin infections. Br J Clin Pract 1967; 21:529–531.

91. Yasuda T. Double-blind study as the method of evaluation of the effect of antibiotic ointments. An experience with a new antibiotic, sodium fusidate. Nifuka-No-Rinsho (Clin Dermatol) 1972; 13:343–357.
92. Cassels-Brown G. A comparative study of Fucidin ointment and Cicatrin cream in the treatment of impetigo. Br J Clin Pract 1981; 35:153–155.
93. Morley PAR, Munot LD. A comparison of sodium fusidate ointment and mupirocin ointment in superficial skin sepsis. Curr Med Res Opin 1988; 11:142–147.
94. Sutton JB. Efficacy and acceptability of fusidic acid cream and mupirocin ointment in facial impetigo. Curr Ther Res 1992; 51:673–678.
95. Langdon CG, Mahapatra KS. Efficacy and acceptability of fusidic acid cream and mupirocin ointment in acute skin sepsis. Curr Ther Res 1990; 48:174–180.
96. White DG, Collings PO, Rowsell B. Topical antibiotics in the treatment of superficial skin infections in general practice—a comparison of mupirocin with sodium fusidate. J Infect 1989; 18:221–229.
97. Ancill RJ. Double-blind comparison of mupirocin and fusidic acid in skin infections of the demented elderly. Can J Dermatol 1989; 1:19–22.
98. Lewis-Jones S, Hart CA, Vickers CFH. Bactroban ointment versus fusidic acid in acute primary skin infections in children. In: Dobson RL, Leyden JJ, Noble WC, Price JD, eds. Bactroban (mupirocin) Excerpta Medica 1985; 103–108.
99. Gilbert M. Topical 2% mupirocin versus 2% fusidic ointment in the treatment of primary and secondary skin infections. J Am Acad Dermatol 1989; 20:1083–1087.
100. Macotela-Ruiz E, Duran Bermudez H, Kuri Con FJ, et al. Evaluation of the efficacy and toxicity of local fusidic acid compared with oral dicloxacillin in skin infections. Med Cut I LA 1988; 16:171–173.
101. Pakrooh H. A comparison of sodium fusidate ointment (Fucidin) alone versus oral antibiotic therapy in soft-tissue infections. Curr Med Res Opin 1977/78; 5:289–294.
102. Ramsay CA, Savoie LM, Gilbert M, et al. The treatment of atopic dermatitis with topical fusidic acid and hydrocortisone acetate. J Eur Acad Dermatol Venereol 1996; 7(suppl 1):S15–22.
103. Poyner TF, Dass BK. Comparative efficacy and tolerability of fusidic acid/hydrocortisone cream (Fucidin H cream) and miconazole/hydrocortisone cream (Daktacort cream) in infected eczema. J Eur Acad Dermatol Venereol 1996; 7(suppl 1): S23–30.
104. Hjorth N, Schmidt H, Thomsen K. Fusidic acid plus betamethasone in infected or potentially infected eczema. Pharamatherapeutica 1985; 4:126.
105. Strategos J. Fusidic acid-betamethasone combination in infected eczema: an open, randomised comparison with gentamicin-betamethasone combination. Pharmatherapeutica 1986; 4:601–606.
106. Wilkinson JD, Leigh DA, Menday AP. Comparative efficacy of betamethasone and either fusidic acid or neomycin in infected or potentially infected eczema. Curr Ther Res 1985; 38:177–182.
107. Javier PR, Ortiz M, Torralba M, et al. Fusidic acid/betamethasone in infected dermatoses—a double-blind comparison with neomycin/betamethasone. Br J Clin Pract 1986; 40:235–238.
108. Hill VA, Wong E, Corbett MF. Comparative efficacy of betamethasone/clioquinol

(Betnovate C) cream and betamethasone/fusidic acid (Fucibet) cream in the treatment of infected hand eczema. J Dermatol Treat 1998; 9:15–19.
109. Shanson DC. Clinical relevance of resistance to fusidic acid in Staphylococcus aureus. J Antimicrob Chemother 1990; 25(suppl B):15–21.
110. Speller DCE, Johnson AP, James D, et al. Resistance to methicillin and other antibiotics in isolates of staphylococus aureus from blood and cerebrospinal fluid. England and Wales 1989–1995. Lancet 1997; 350:323–325.
111. Faber M, Rosdahl VT. Susceptibility to fusidic acid among Danish staphylococcus aureus strains and fusidic acid consumption. J Antimicrob Chemother 1990; 25(suppl B):7–14.
112. Moorhouse E, Fenelon L, Hone R, et al. Staphylococcus aureus sensitivity to various antibiotics–a national survery in Ireland 1993. Ir J Med Sci 1996; 165:42–43.
113. Ravenscroft J, Layton A, Bamham M. A study of positive reasons for increased Staphylococcus aureus fusidic acid resistance in Hemogate. Br J Dermatol 1999; 141(Suppl 155):57.
114. Wakelin SH, Shaw S, Marren S, et al. Allergic contact dermatitis to newer topical anti-staphylococcal agents. Br J Dermatol 1996; 135(suppl 47):17.

3

Systemic Antimicrobial Therapy

J Carl Craft
Abbott Laboratories
Abbott Park, Illinois

Lawrence Charles Parish
Jefferson Medical College of Thomas Jefferson University
Philadelphia, Pennsylvania

I. INTRODUCTION

Bacterial infections of the skin are among the most common reasons for patients to seek medical care. Treatment is usually initiated on a morphological basis whereby the physician recognizes the lesions associated with impetigo. Using epidemiological knowledge of the most common bacterial pathogens causing impetigo, the physician then makes a diagnosis and initiates empiric therapy. For uncomplicated skin infections, this is almost always appropriate. There are times when a specific etiology is absolutely necessary for the successful outcome of therapy. To determine the specific etiology, it is important to determine whether this is a primary infection, a secondary infection superimposed upon an underlying dermatitis or dermatosis, or a cutaneous manifestation of a systemic bacterial infection. Cultures then should be obtained prior to initiating therapy in order to determine the susceptibility of the infecting organism, should the empiric agent prove not to be successful.

In selecting an appropriate antimicrobial therapy from the many possible choices, several factors must be considered. These include host factors, such as site of infection, immune status, renal function, hepatic function, history of allergic reactions, and any other medications that the patient is taking. Drug factors that impact upon therapeutic choice are absorption, rate of excretion, protein binding, dosing frequency, antimicrobial spectrum, and cost. Because local susceptibility patterns can differ significantly, an understanding of the local resistance patterns of common skin pathogens is necessary. This chapter will concentrate on the issues relating to the choice of the most appropriate antimicrobial therapy and how these choices can best be made based on pharmacodynamic principles.

II. PHARMACODYNAMICS

Pharmacodynamics of an antimicrobial agent are the interactions of the time course of the drug concentration to the antimicrobial effects at the site of infection with any side effects of the drug [1]. The first two components, antimicrobial effect and the pharmacokinetics of the drug, are responsible for the success of treatment and will be discussed in depth. Side effects of therapy will only be mentioned when they are likely to impact upon the choice of therapies.

The first component is the antimicrobial activity of the agent. All antimicrobial agents produce their effect upon bacteria by binding to specific target sites of the bacteria. These targets sites include, for example, the penicillin binding protein of the bacterial cell wall, bacterial DNA topoisomerases (DNA gyrase), and bacterial ribosomes.

Antimicrobial activity is determined in vitro by determining the concentration of the antimicrobial agent that is necessary to occupy a critical number of bacterial sites causing the death of the bacteria. The minimum inhibitor concentration (MIC) of an antimicrobial is determined by placing twofold serial dilutions of a test antimicrobial in a series of tubes or wells of bacterial growth medium with an inoculum of the bacteria from the patient's infection. The series of tubes is then incubated overnight; the tubes are then observed for cloudy media as an indication of growth. The MIC is the lowest concentration of drug at which the microorganism tested does not show visible growth. The minimum bactericidal concentration (MBC) is the amount of antimicrobial needed to kill the organism. This is determined by taking an aliquot from each of the MIC tubes that showed no growth of bacteria following overnight incubation. The aliquot is plated on an agar plate and examined after overnight incubation. The MBC is equal to the lowest concentration of the drug that kills at least 99.9% of the original inoculum following overnight incubating. For bactericidal drugs, the MBC should be equal to or no more than 1 to 2 dilutions greater than the MIC. These commonly reported values give the physician an idea of whether the organism is susceptible to the antimicrobial agent, whether the antimicrobial is bactericidal or bacteriostatic, and what concentrations must be exceeded at the site of infection if therapy is to result in eradication of the infection [2]. They do not, however, adequately describe the rate and extent of the antimicrobial effect, the inoculum effect, the effects of subinhibitory concentrations [3], the postantibiotic effect [4], and the postantibiotic leukocyte effect [5]. These tests are experimental and not obtained routinely by the microbiology laboratory. They are used mainly to determine the activity of new antimicrobial agents before they are used in humans to define their activity or as research tools to gain a better understanding of how some antimicrobial agents work.

Pharmacodynamic parameters can be expressed as bacterial killing as a function of antimicrobial concentration at the site of infection and time of exposure of the bacteria to the drug [6–9]. Another term used is area under the curve (AUC), which is a product of the antimicrobial concentration and time. It should follow that bacterial killing is a function of AUC. The AUC can also be related to the MIC or MBC of the organism, and AUC/MIC becomes another important parameter. The importance of serum concentration and time (AUC) is dependent on how well the drug binds to the bacterial site. Antimicrobials can be categorized by two types of killing that are related to binding. Concentration-dependent bactericidal activity is observed for drugs that bind irreversibly or cause irreversible damage to the bind sites and time-dependent bactericidal activity is observed for the drugs that bind reversibly to the bacterial binding site (Table 1).

A. Concentration-Dependent Bactericidal Drugs

Drugs that work through concentration-dependent bactericidal activity show increased bacterial killing as the dose is increased above the MIC (Fig. 1). These drugs bind very tightly or irreversibly to the site of their activity. As the concentrations of the antimicrobials are increased above the MIC, the bacterial killing becomes very rapid, increasing as the concentration increases. Because the exposure time is not important to the bactericidal effects of these agents, the time portion of the equations can be ignored. The clinical response of patients treated with concentration-dependent bactericidal antibiotics increases as the serum concentration of drug exceeds the MIC [10]. No additional benefit is seen once the peak serum concentration exceeds the MIC by a factor of 10 [10]. At 10 times the MIC, all binding sites are exposed and killing is complete. As a result, in humans, antimicrobial agents with concentration-dependent killing are generally effective when given once daily in patients with normal renal function.

The length of therapy is dependent upon the location of the infection and the ability of the drug to obtain adequate concentrations at the site of infection. For example, uncomplicated urinary tract infections will respond to a single dose of an antimicrobial agent while bone infections may require weeks to months of intensive therapy. For these regimens, the dosing strategy employs the highest possible dose without causing toxicity [6].

B. Time-Dependent Bactericidal Active Drugs

Drugs that work through time-dependent bactericidal activity start to kill bacteria once the concentration of the antimicrobial exceeds the MIC. Bactericidal activity may increase as the antimicrobial concentration is increased up to 2 to 4 times the MIC, but increasing the concentrations above this level does not further in-

TABLE 1 Antimicrobial Agents Categorized by Pharmacodynamic Pattern of Bactericidal Activity

Concentration-dependent bactericidal activity	Drugs
Aminocyclitols	amikacin, gentamycin, kanamycin, netilimicin, streptomycin, tobramycin
Fluoroquinolones	ciprofloxacin, enoxacin, gatifloxacin, gemifloxacin, grepafloxacin, levofloxacin, lomefloxacin, moxifloxacin, norfloxacin, ofloxacin, sparfloxacin, trovafloxacin
Nitroimidazoles	metronidazole, tinidazole
Time-dependent bactericidal activity	
Penicillins	amoxicillin, amoxicillin/clavulanate, ampicillin, ampicillin/sulbactam, azlocillin, bacampicillin, carbenicillin, cloxacillin, dicloxacillin, mezlocillin, nafcillin, oxacillin, penicillin, piperacillin, piperacillin/tazobactam, ticarcillin, ticarcillin/clavulanate
Cephalosporins	cefazolin, cefepime, cefetamet pivoxil, cefixime, cefmetazole, cefotaxime, cefotetan, cefoxitin, cefpodoxime proxetil, cefprozil, ceftazidime, ceftibuten, cefuroxime, cephalexin, cephalothin, loracarbef
Carbapenems	imipenem, meropenem
Macrolides	azithromycin, clarithromycin, erythromycin, dirithromycin
Lincosamides	clindamycin, lincomycin
Streptogrammins	quinupristan/dalfopristan
Glycopeptide	vancomycin, teicoplanin
Rifamycins	rifamycin, rifabutin
Sulfonamides and trimethoprim	sulfamethoxazole/trimethoprim
Oxazolidones	linezolid
Tetracyclines	tetracycline, doxycycline, minocycline

crease the antimicrobial activity (Fig. 2). Time-dependent bactericidal drugs bind reversibly to the activity site and must be present to maintain activity. Bacterial killing takes place only when the concentration is high enough to maintain complete binding of the agent to the active site or when the binding site is actively involved in the survival of the organism. As the concentrations of the antimicrobial fall below the MIC, the binding sites are no longer completely occupied. This allows the organism to recover, and the bacteria will start to grow again. For these drugs, concentration only plays a minor part, because time is the most

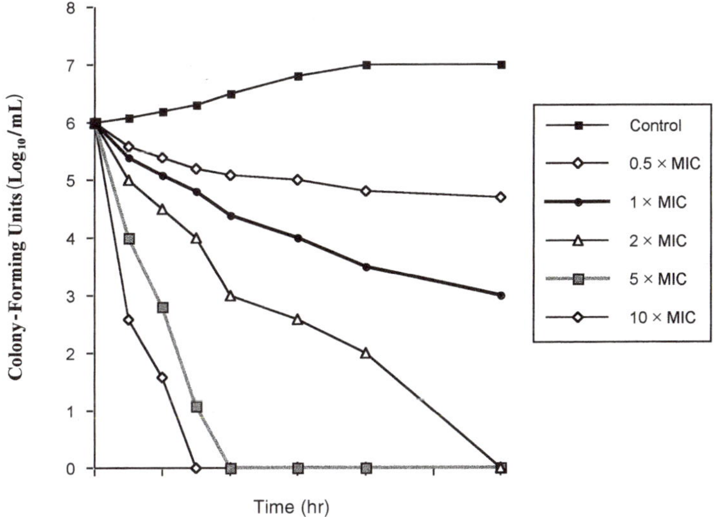

FIGURE 1 Time kill curves for *H. influenzae* exposed to ciprofloxacin at concentrations of 0, 0.5. 1, 2, 5, and 10 times the MIC (MIC = 0.01 μg/mL), showing increasing bactericidal activity as the concentration was increased.

important factor. The time above the MIC is the only part of the equation necessary to predict clinical success. The dosing strategy is to maximize the time that the serum concentration is above the MIC [6]. Time-dependent antimicrobials are generally effective if concentrations of the antimicrobials are above the MIC for more than 50% of the dosing interval due to the postantimicrobial effects [5,11] of some of these agents. The postantibiotic effect (PAE) is the time after the antimicrobial has been removed from the media until the bacteria starts to regrow. This recovery period varies, depending upon the organism and the antimicrobial agent, but it generally ranges from a few minutes to several hours. Antimicrobials with time-dependent bactericidal activity maintained above the MIC for the entire dosing period are both effective and less likely to be associated with the development of resistance [1].

C. Concentration at the Site of Infection

Antimicrobial concentrations are not equally distributed in the human body. For example, serum concentrations of antimicrobials will be greater than bone concentrations. Beta-lactams do not penetrate into the cell while macrolides are concentrated inside the cells. Skin and skin structure infections are localized to tissues that are generally well vascularized and the organisms are localized to the

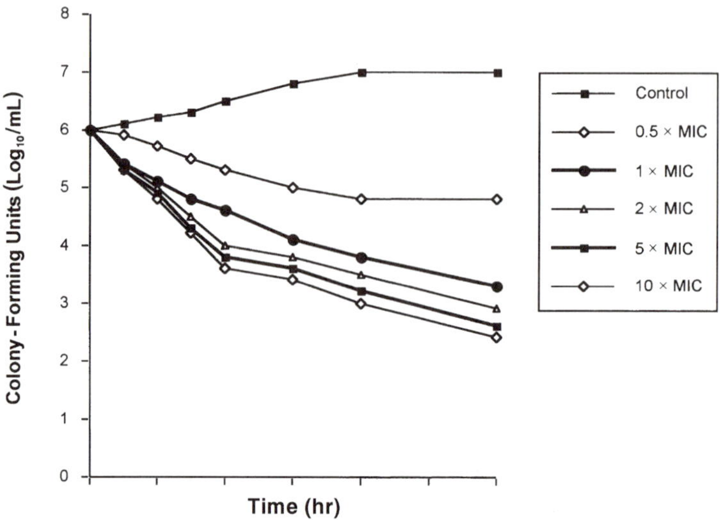

FIGURE 2 Time kill curves for *H. influenzae* exposed to amoxicillin at concentrations of 0, 0.5. 1, 2, 5, and 10 times the MIC (MIC = 0.1 μg/mL), showing increasing bactericidal activity as the concentration was increased to two times the MIC, but only small increases as the concentration was increased to five or ten times the MIC.

interstitial spaces between cells. The interstitial space is a dynamic site, but is in direct connection with the serum. Because of this situation, serum concentrations are generally predictive of the antimicrobial concentration at the site of skin infections. Patients with poor circulation, devitalized tissue, and bone infections will require larger doses than the serum concentrations would predict. Some infecting organisms can become intracellular, evading the antimicrobial activity of beta-lactams and other agents that do not penetrate into the cell. As an example, *Staphylococcus aureus* infection has both an extracellular and an intracellular component. The intracellular organisms are protected from antimicrobial agents that are either not present intracellularly or not effective intracellularly. In the patient with normal white-cell function, this is not important. However, this can be responsible for failure in immunocompromised patients with decreased white-cell function.

III. RESISTANCE

The increasing development of resistance in bacterial pathogens is the most ominous trend in medicine today [12–15]. Staphylococcal skin infections are frequently caused by strains that are resistant to all antimicrobial agents except vancomycin.

Within the past few years, however, *S. aureus* strains resistant to vancomycin have been isolated from patients, which leaves no therapeutic alternatives.

Mechanisms of resistance to antimicrobial agents include anything that gives the microorganism the ability to avoid the inhibitory or lethal effects of the antimicrobial agent. There are several ways in which a microorganism may demonstrate resistance. Constitutional resistance is the essential characteristic of a particular species of bacteria [12]. Examples are the lack of activity of metronidazole on aerobic bacteria because they have the molecular enzymes to handle free radicals such as oxygen, or the lack of activity of vancomycin on gram-negative bacteria because of the drug's inability to penetrate the gram-negative outer membrane.

Circumstantial resistance is the appearance of resistance in a clinical setting to an organism that is susceptible to the antimicrobial [12]. This occurs when an agent has activity against a pathogen (as demonstrated by susceptibility testing) but is not effective due to poor absorption from the gastrointestinal tract. This can also be seen in the patient whose infection is in tissues that cannot be reached by the antimicrobial agent due to pharmacokinetics. This occurred in children treated for *Haemophilus influenzae* septic arthritis with intravenous cefuroxime. These patients developed meningitis while on treatment against organisms susceptible to cefuroxime but with CSF concentrations inadequate to control the infection.

Acquired resistance occurs when a susceptible organism becomes tolerant to an antimicrobial agent or class of agents [12]. This requires a change in the bacterial genetic material. Table 2 lists mechanisms of resistance and the antimicrobial agents affected.

Pharmacodynamics can be used to predict whether antimicrobial use will result in the development of resistance [1]. Antimicrobial agents with concentration-dependent bactericidal activity kill bacteria very rapidly when the concentration exceeds the MIC by a factor of 10, but the killing becomes much slower near the MIC. This was seen with the fluoroquinolones for *S. aureus*, where the MIC_{90} ranged from 0.5 to 2.0 μg/mL and peak serum concentrations for the flouroquinolones ranged from 1.0 to 4.0 μg/mL. The peak serum-to-MIC ratio for many of these agents was frequently equal to or less than 1 and the development of quinolone-resistant *S. aureus* was seen soon after they became widely used [26]. The time-dependent bactericidal antimicrobial agents have similar problems [1]. Resistance can develop when the concentration of drug at the site of infection drops below the MIC for any length of time. These agents are generally active and do not induce resistance if the concentration is above the MIC for greater than 50% of the dosing time. Another problem that was predicted by pharmacodynamic modeling was for time-dependent agents with long half-lives. These agents with long half-lives and high tissue concentration may provide suboptimal concentrations in the upper respiratory tract for days to weeks following

Table 2 Mechanisms of Resistance to Antimicrobial Agents

Resistance mechanism	Examples	Ref.
Inactivation	Aminoglycoside-modifying enzymes	16
	Beta-lactamases	17
	Choramphenicol-inactivating enzymes	18
Binding site modification	Penicillin binding proteins	18
	DNA gyrase modification to decrease quinolone binding	18
	Methylation of ribosome modification of macrolide binding site	19
Efflux mechanism	Macrolide efflux	20–22
	Tetracycline efflux due to tetA	23
Membrane permeability	Beta-lactams OmpF	24
	Quinolone OmpF	14
Cytoplasmic membrane transport	Aminoglycosides transport mechanism due to decrease energy	25

even a single dose. This can have a selective effect on the growth and transmission of resistant strains [27].

Selection of resistant microorganisms can be kept to a minimum by using pharmacodynamics to choose antimicrobial agents. For concentration-dependent agents, agents that have peak concentrations greater than 5 to 10 times the MIC of the microorganism should be used. For time-dependent agents, an agent whose concentrations will exceed the MIC for greater than 50% of the time should be selected.

IV. SELECTING SYSTEMIC ANTIMICROBIALS FOR TREATING SKIN INFECTIONS

The variety of antimicrobials available to treat skin infections is large and growing. Choosing the best agent for the individual patient requires information about the most likely infecting organisms or a definite diagnosis based on culture and susceptibility. The pharmacokinetic data necessary to make a decision based on sound pharmacodynamic principles are present in sources such as the *Physicians' Desk Reference* (PDR). The PDR contains information on the following areas of interest to the treating physician: *clinical pharmacology*, including the peak serum concentration (C_{max}) and half-life for the dose of antibiotic selected; *microbiology*, including a list of susceptible organisms that have been successfully treated; *indications and usage*, which gives a list of all approved indications (if not listed, there are usually no data or the agent is not effective for that indication); and *contraindication, precautions and adverse reaction*, which should be checked for any problems that the patient may expect during treatment that are not part of the underlying illness.

Concentration-dependent bactericidal agents can be selected if the C_{max} is 5 to 10 times the MIC of the infecting organism. Time-dependent bactericidal agents will require more work. The C_{max} and half-life will indicate whether the agent will be present in the serum above the MIC for at least 50% of the dosing interval. If not, then another agent should be used or the dosing frequency increased to increase the time above the MIC. A brief description follows of the available antimicrobial agents; they are listed by class, in order of usefulness for treating skin infection and the type of pharmacodynamic activity to expect when using them.

Clinical selection of an antimicrobial agent becomes dependent upon the clinician's perception of the available agents, which is sometimes colored by the pharmaceutical company representive. While the pharmacodynamics might be appropriate, the physician may perceive that the agent has poor skin and skin structure penetration. The unwanted side effects could affect acceptance by dermatological patients, who are often less sick with an infection than their renal or pulmonary counterparts. The choice for the dermatologist is also determined by the type of administration. In the outpatient setting, oral administration would be preferred. Sometimes, topical application will suffice.

A. Beta-Lactams

No group of antibiotics has had such an enormous effort in discovery and development of new agents as the beta-lactams. The large number of resulting compounds has made it difficult to remember which ones are the most appropriate for the treatment of skin and skin structure infections. The categorization of beta-lactams by generation suggests that the newer generation formulations are superior to the older ones; this is not always true. This is evident in treating skin infection where the major pathogens are *S. aureus* and *Streptococcus pyogenes*, because many of the newer generation agents have lost good gram-positive activity in order to gain improved gram-negative activity.

The beta-lactam antibiotics (penicillins, penems, carbapenems, monobactams, cephalosporins, oxycephams, and oxa-beta-lactams) act by binding reversibly to the penicillin binding proteins (carboxypeptidases, endopeptidases, and transpeptidases). This inhibition of the cell wall synthesis is dependent on active replication of the bacteria. Resistance to the beta-lactams has been primarily through the production of beta-lactamase enzymes that hydrolyze the beta-lactam ring. This mechanism is important because it can be transferred from bacteria to bacteria on plasmids that can also amplify the activity by increasing the numbers of copies of that gene carried by the bacteria. Most of the research in beta-lactams has been in modifying the molecule to combat specific types of beta-lactamases.

More recently, there has been an increase in resistance to the beta-lactams by modification of the penicillin binding proteins [28,29]. This process is chromosomally mediated and is not rapidly disseminated from organism to organism but is the process by which *Staphylococcus* has become resistant to methicillin [29]. A similar resistance pattern has become a therapeutic problem in treating *Streptococcus pneumoniae*, which has become resistant to the standard penicillin and cephalosporin therapies [28]. Fortunately, *S. pyogenes* has not become resistant to penicillin to date, which makes penicillin the drug of choice for treating skin infection secondary to the group A beta-hemolytic streptococci. Other rare mechanisms of resistance include decreased permeability of the bacterial outer membrane to the beta-lactams seen occasionally but with limited clinical implications for patients outside of intensive care units [30].

Beta-lactam antibiotics have many properties in common. They are among the least toxic and best tolerated antibiotics used today. Their pharmacokinetics are generally similar, with short half-lives and primary renal clearance. The antimicrobial activity observed can best be described as time-dependent bacterial killing [6]. Therefore, it is important to keep the serum concentration above the MIC of the infecting organism for greater than 50% of the dosing period. With the short half-lives of these compounds, this can be done in two ways: (1) giving very large doses infrequently (once or twice daily); or (2) giving smaller doses more frequently (Fig. 3). There has been a trend in antimicrobial therapy to de-

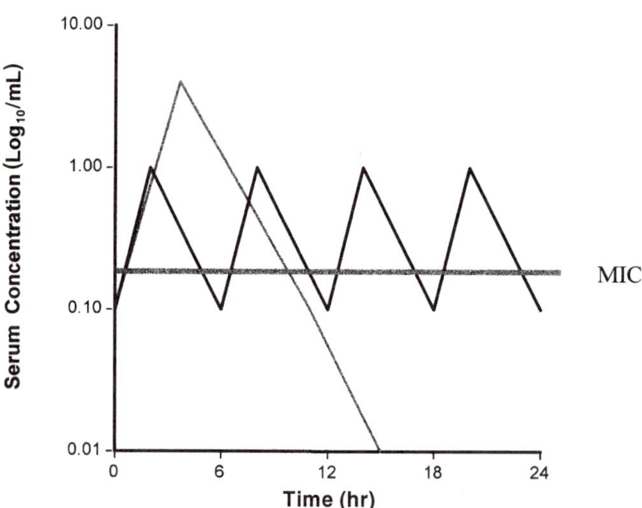

FIGURE 3 Time above the MIC is compared for a theoretical single large daily dose to four daily doses equal to the single daily dose. The time above the MIC is maximized by giving four daily doses compared to the single dose.

crease the frequency of dosing to obtain better patient compliance. This has occurred at the same time that resistance to beta-lactams has become critical. It is still possible today to treat intermediate penicillin-resistant *S. pneumoniae* with oral amoxicillin by increasing the total daily dose and giving the doses every 4 to 6 h (this will not work with the highly resistant strains). Table 3 separates the different beta-lactams by their utility in treating the most common skin infections caused by *S. aureus* (not methicillin-resistant *Staphylococcus aureus* [MRSA]) and group A beta-hemolytic streptococci.

I. Penicillins

Penicillin G and the acid stable penicillin V are natural penicillins that are still active against *S. pyogenes*, one of the major pathogens responsible for skin infections. Neither is active against *S. aureus*, the other major cause of skin infection.

The semisythetic aminopenicillins (ampicillin, amoxicillin, and bacampicillin) have the same activity as penicillin. The additional gram-negative activity was useful until the mid-1970s, when resistance became a major problem. Amoxicillin is still a good choice for the treatment of *S. pyogenes* skin infections because of the good oral absorption. Ampicillin is seldom used because of its lower absorption from the gastrointestinal tract, which results in increased diarrhea.

The isoxazolyl penicillins (cloxacillin, dicloxacillin, nafcillin, and oxacillin) are active against both *Staphylococcus* and *S. pyogenes* but are not active against MRSA. Nafcillin is only available as an intravenous formulation, while oxacillin has poor oral absorption; thus it is best used as intravenous therapy for Staphylococcus. Dicloxacillin is the best absorbed of the orally available antistaphylococcal penicillins and can be used to treat uncomplicated skin infections.

The carboxypenicillins (carbenicillin, ticarcillin) and the acylureidopenicillins (piperacillin, mezlocillin, azolocillin) have added additional gram-negative activity to the penicillins, in particular antipseudomomal activity, but they are only available as intravenous formulations with less activity against *S. aureus*. They are useful for treating skin infections caused by *Pseudomonas* when combined with an aminoglycoside. They are not useful for treating *Staphylococcal* infections.

The addition of a beta-lactamase inhibitor to the penicillins has greatly improved their spectrum of activity. The most useful of these agents is the orally available amoxicillin/clavulanate. This is the most useful of the penicillins for treating skin infections because of its activity against *S. pyogenes*, *S. aureus*, and many common gram-negative causes of skin infection. Ampicillin/sulbactam is only available as an intravenous formulation but is similar to amoxicillin/clavulanate in its activity. Ticarcillin/clavulanate and piperacillin/tazobactam are useful in treating very serious skin infections due to *S. aureus*, and many gram-negative organisms including *Pseudomonas aeruginosa*. Rapid development of resistance to *Pseudomonas* during treatment requires the addition of an aminoglycoside or

TABLE 3 Comparison of Oral Beta-Lactams for Activity Against Gram-Positive, Gram-Negative, *S. aureus* and Use in Treating Skin Infections

Class	Oral antimicrobial	Activity gram-positive	Activity gram-negative	Activity *S. aureus*	Comments
Penicillins					
	Amoxicillin	++++	++	–	Good for *S. pyogenes* proven infection
	Amoxicillin/clavulanate	++++	+++	+++	Good empirical choice for treatment of skin infection
	Ampicillin	++++	++	–	Not well absorbed but similar to amoxicillin
	Cloxacillin	++++	+	+++	Good activity but poor pharmacokinetics
	Dicloxacillin	++++	+	+++	Good empirical choice for treatment of skin infection
	Penicillin	++++	+	–	Not well absorbed but similar to amoxicillin
Cephalosporins					
first generation	Cefazolin	++++	++	+++	Best empirical choice for skin infections
	Cephalexin	++++	++	+++	Similar to cefazolin but shorter half-life
second generation	Cefuroxime axetil	+++	+++	++	Can be used but less active than first generation
	Cefprozil	+++	+++	++	Can be used but less active than first generation
	Loracarbef	+++	+++	++	Can be used but less active than first generation
third generation	Cefixime	++	+++	+	Avoid using this agent—decreased gram-positive activity
	Cefpodoxime proxetil	++	+++	+	Avoid using this agent—decreased gram-positive activity
	Cefetamet pivoxil	++	+++	+	Avoid using this agent—decreased gram-positive activity

quinolone to the regimen. They are also active against anaerobic bacteria commonly found in diabetic foot ulcers.

2. Cephalosporins

First-generation cephalosporins are very good drugs for the treatment of skin infections because of their activity against *S. pyogenes* and *S. aureus*. Each additional generation has produced agents that are much more active against gram-negative organisms but less active against skin pathogens [27]. Cefadroxil and cephalexin are good agents for treatment of skin infection. They are orally available and have very good activity against pathogens causing uncomplicated skin infections. Cefadroxil has the best pharmacokinetics, a longer half-life than most cephalosporins, and can be given twice a day for most skin infections while maintaining concentrations above the MIC for greater than 50% of the dosing period. Other orally available cephalosporins (second-generation cephalosporins cefuroxime, loracarbef, and cefprozil) can be used to treat skin infections but are less active against *S. pyogenes* and *S. aureus*, and are more expensive than cefadroxil. Third-generation oral agents (cefixime, cefpodoxime proxetil, cefetamet pivoxil, and ceftibuten) have decreased activity to *S. pyogenes* and *S. aureus*, and should not be used to treat uncomplicated skin infections.

Cephalothin and cefazolin are first-generation intravenously available agents that can be used for more serious *S. aureus* infection. The spectrum is limited and they have no activity against MRSA. Intravenous cefoxitin and cefotetan are the most active cephalosporins against anaerobic bacteria; while maintaining good *S. aureus* activity they can be used to treat serious skin infections when anaerobic organisms are considered to be involved. Ceftazidime is the most active cephalosporin against *P. aeruginosa* and can be used to treat skin infection caused by this pathogen. Rapid development of resistance to *Pseudomonas* during treatment requires the addition of an aminoglycoside or quinolone to the regimen.

3. Carbapenams

Imipenem and meropenem are the most potent and have the broadest spectrum of the beta-lactam antimicrobical agents. They are not active against most MRSA, but they are active against *P. aeruginosa*. Unfortunately, resistance can develop rapidly during therapy. These agents can be used to treat some serious skin infections, but therapy should be guided by susceptibility testing to warrant the usc of these very potent agents. There are no oral carbapenems available, but they are in development and may have utility in skin infections.

4. Monobactams

Monbactams differ from beta-lactams because of the monocyclic nucleus [31]. However, they work through the same mechanisms. Aztreonam is the only approved member of this group of agents, but it has little use in treating skin infection. Its activity is primarily gram-negative, with little or no activity against gram-positive bacteria. It has not been able to find its therapeutic niche, because most other agents have a broader spectrum of activity. The other agents used to treat serious gram-negative infections are much more potent.

B. Glycopeptides

Vancomycin is a tricyclic glycopeptide that is active only against gram-positive bacteria. Its bactericidal activity against multiplying gram-positive bacteria is principally through binding to the D-alanyl-D-alanine precursor units of the peptidoglycan of the bacterial cell membranes [32]. Vancomycin may also impair bacterial RNA synthesis in some bacteria.

Vancomycin is bactericidal against *S. aureus*, many coagulase-negative *Staphylococcus spp.*, aerobic *Streptococcus spp.* (beta-hemolytic, viridans, and pneumococci), *Corynebacterium spp.*, *Bacillus spp. Clostrium spp.*, *Peptococcus spp.*, and *Enterococcus spp.* Vancomycin has been the last resort for treating skin infections due to MRSA and other multiply resistant organisms, but this has changed recently, with the isolation of MRSA strains resistant to vancomycin.

Systemic administration of vancomycin is necessary to treat infections, oral vancomycin is not absorbed from the GI tract and is only used to treat psuedomembranous colitis. After intravenous injection of a 1-g dose of vancomycin, peak serum concentrations of approximately 40 μg/mL and serum trough concentrations of 10 μg/mL are seen [32]. The half-life in adults is generally about 6 h and twice-daily dosing is used except in patients with decreased renal function [32]. Dosing in patients with renal failure is best guided by measuring serum concentrations. The pharmacodynamics of vancomycin best fit with time-dependent killing, and the best results are seen when the serum concentration is maintained above the MIC of the infecting organism for greater than 50% of the dosing period.

Teicoplanin is very similar to vancomycin, but it is not available in the United States. Its advantages are said to be ease of administration and reduced toxicity based on limited clinical trials.

C. Fluoroquinolones

The quinolones are bactericidal against a wide spectrum of aerobic organisms, including *Enterobacteriaceae*, oxidative gram-negative bacilli, including *P. aeruginosa* and facultative gram-negative bacilli; *Neisseria spp.*; *Chlamydia spp.*; *Mycoplasma spp.*; *Legionella spp.*; some of the *Mycobacterium spp*; and *Staphylococcus spp.* (many MRSA are resistant to quinolones) [26]. Other than the newer quinolones, most have only modest activity against *Streptococcus spp.* and *Enterococcus spp.* Resistance to the quinolones results from mutation of a single amino acid substituent in a subunit of topoisomerase II; this is relatively rare, but it does happen when organisms are exposed to suboptimal therapy, particularly with *P. aeruginosa* and *Staphylococcus spp*. Resistance due to decreased membrane permeability of the outer membrane protein infrequently occurs [26].

Quinolones bind irreversibly to topoisomerase II of the bacterial DNA gyrase. This inhibits the activity of the bacterial DNA gyrase, causing rapid bacterial killing. This mechanism is essentially dose-dependent and maximal effect is achieved when the antibiotic concentration exceeds the MIC of the infecting organism by a factor of 4 to 5 times [6]. This has been a major problem for the quinolones in treating skin infections, because efficacy against *S. aureus* and *S. pyogenes* is limited by pharymacokinetics that prevent the drug from exceeding the MICs of these organisms by a factor of at least 4 to 5 times (Table 4). Because

Table 4 Comparison of the Fluoroquinolones by the Potential for Use in Treating Skin Infections

Quinolone	Treatment
Moxifloxacin, gatifloxacin, and gemifloxacin	Soon-to-be-approved quinolones with improved gram-positive activity, which may prove useful in treating skin infections.
Grepafloxacin	Not as potent as trovafloxacin but can be used to treat skin infections due to susceptible organisms. Concerns about phototoxicity and potential for cardiac arrhythmias may limit use.
Sparfloxacin	Phototoxicity and potential for cardiac arrhythmias limits use, although good activity against most *Staphylococcus* and *Streptococcus spp*.
Ciprofloxacin	Treatment of skin infections limited because of low blood levels of drug and decreased gram-positive activity, but preferred agent for *P. aeruginosa* and many gram-negative skin infections.
Ofloxacin and levofloxacin	Weak gram-positive activity. Levofloxacin is the pure s-entiomer of ofloxacin, which results in a twofold improvement in activity and reduced toxicity. These improvements are inadequate to consider it for general use for skin infections.
Lomefloxacin	Weak gram-positive activity and high potential for phototoxicity; not useful in treating skin infections.
Enoxacin	Weak gram-positive activity and high potential for drug–drug interactions; no longer useful for skin infections.
Norfloxacin	Limited to treatment of urinary tract and gastrointestinal infections due to poor pharmacokinetics and weak antibacterial activity.

of this, *Staphylococcus* become resistant to the quinolones very rapidly, thus limiting their usefulness. The newer quinolones (gatifloxacin, gemifloxacin, grepafloxacin, moxifloxacin, and sparfloxacin) have better in vitro activity compared to their pharmacokinetic concentration and can be used against susceptible strains with more favorable results; however, they do not have activity against quinolone-resistant strains that have already developed [33]. They should probably be reserved for the most serious skin infections because of their broad spectrum of activity against gram-positive, gram-negative, and anaerobic bacteria and the concerns about superinfection and emergence of resistant microorganisms [34].

D. Macrolides, Azilides, Streptogrammins, and Lincosamides

The prototype macrolide, has long been the antibiotic of choice in skin infection. The macrolides, azilides, streptogrammins, and lincosamides work by binding reversibly to the 50S subunit of the ribosome. This binding results in translocation of aminocyl tRNA and stops the synthesis of proteins [35]. They are time-dependent antimicrobial agents that have pharmacokinetics with high intracellular and high tissue concentrations [36]. They are highly active against intracellular organisms because of their high intracellular concentrations. These compounds share the disadvantage of inducing resistance in *S. aureus*. Other mechanisms of resistance are seen for *S. pyogenes*, which also develop relatively rapidly if these agents are overused to treat skin infections. Because of this, they should be used sparingly for the occasional patient who needs treatment for an uncomplicated skin infection and is allergic to beta-lactams. It is probably best to obtain cultures and susceptibilities before starting treatment. Macrolides have activity against *Propionibacterium acnes* and also act as anti-inflammatory agents [37]. This dual activity has established a place for these as primary agents in the treatment of acne.

Clarithromycin is the most potent of the macrolides against environmental mycobacterium such as *Mycobacterium avium, M. marinium*, and others that occasionally cause skin infection. Used either as a single agent or in combination with other drugs, clarithromycin has been effective in these rare infections. It is also active against *M. lepre*, which is still present in the third-world nations. Treatment regimens for leprosy using clarithromycin are under investigation by the World Health Organization and National Institutes of Health.

Studies correlating rosacea to *Helicobacter pylori* infections of the gastric mucosa have resulted in treatment studies with clarithromycin. The results are promising, but the best treatment regimen has not been defined.

Azithromycin has a very long half-life, but low serum drug concentrations. Its long half-life is both its advantage and disadvantage [35]. Treatment can be accomplished with once-daily dosing for 5 days, which results in drug concentration lasting in tissues for several weeks. Skin blister concentrations are less than other macrolides. Adverse reaction can last until all drug is excreted from the body.

Dirithromycin is once-a-day erythromycin. The spectrum of activity is very similar to erythromycin, but does not include the coverage of azithromycin and clarithromycin. Because of this, it has not found a niche in the macrolide market.

Clindamycin and lincomycin have activity against anaerobic organisms as well as gram-positive aerobic organisms. Although they are not appropriate for most skin infections because of resistance problems, they can be very useful in treating skin infections such as decubitis ulcers, where anaerobic bacteria as well as aerobic bacteria may be involved. Psuedomembranous colitis has been a side effect limiting use in dermatology.

The streptogrammins are frequently active against *S. aureus* that are resistant to other agents; they can be used in these serious infections if they have been shown to have activity. At present, only intravenous formulations, which are a mixture of quinupristin and dalfopristin, are available. The combination of these two agents acts synergistically and provides bactericidal activity against MRSA. There is only limited experience with this agent in the treatment of serious skin infection. Orally available streptogrammins are under investigation but are several years away from clinical use.

E. Aminocyclitol

The aminocyclitol antimicrobials work by binding irreversibly to the 30S ribosomal subunit. This binding results in inhibition of protein synthesis in the bacterial cell and death of susceptible organisms. This activity can be referred to as dose-dependent killing [6]. Activity against an infecting organism can be predicted if the peak concentration of the drug at the site of infection is 5 to 10 times the MIC of the organism [10].

The aminocyclitol antibiotics include spectinomycin and the aminoglycosides (amikacin, gentamicin, kanamycin, neomycin, netilimicin, streptomycin, and tobramycin). None are available in an appropriate oral formulation because they are not absorbed from the gastrointestinal tract. Spectinomycin is only indicated for the treatment of urethritis, proctitis, and cervicitis caused by *Neisseria gonorrhoeae* and will not be discussed. The aminoglycoides are useful in treating skin and skin structure infections caused by *Escherichia coli*, *Klebsiella pneumoniae*, *P. aeruginosa*, *Enterobacter* and *Serratia spp*., *Proteus mirabilus*, *Proteus spp*., and *S. aureus*. They can be given either intravenously or intramuscularly. These agents are recommended to be given as a total daily dose based on a mg/kg dose divide every 8 to 12 h, but recent studies based on pharmacodynamics have shown that the aminoglycosides can be given as a single daily dose equal to that of the total daily dose given as two or three doses [6]. The single daily dose produces higher serum concentrations with less toxicity than seen with two or three daily doses. Renal function should be monitored and dosing adjustment made based on the patient's creatinine clearance.

Resistance to aminoglycosides is generally due to either enzyme degradation (acetylation, adenylylation, or phosphorylation) or reduced permeability mechanisms [16,25]. In general, these agents are used for complicated skin and skin structure infection with gram-negative organisms or difficult infection with MRSA. These complicated infections are best treated with combinations of an aminoglycoside and a beta-lactam with a beta-lactamase inhibitor such as ticarcillin/clavulanate. This is particularly important when treating *P. aeruginosa* infections.

F. Sulfonamides and Trimethoprim

Sulfonamides completely inhibit the synthesis of dihydropteroate. Resistance is the result of an isoenzymic dihydropteroate synthetase mutation that produces an isoenzyme with a higher affinity for ρ-aminobenzoic acid than for sulfonamides. The 2,4-diaminopyrimidines act by inhibiting the conversion of dihydrofolate to tetrahydrofolate [32], which is necessary for the synthesis of two-carbon fragments necessary for the formation of amino acids, pyrimidines, and purines for nucleic acid synthesis in bacteria. The combination of a sulfonamide with a 2,4-diaminopyrimidine should result in synergy because of their activity in the synthesis of tetrahydrofolate in the bacteria [32]. Trimethoprim is the only one of interest in the treatment of bacterial infection. The sulfonamides and 2,4-diaminopyrimidines are not very useful when given as single agents because of the development of resistance. The fixed combination of trimethoprim/sulfamethoxazole is a useful drug and can be used occasionally to treat skin infection due to *S. aureus* and *M. marinum* [32]. The sulfonamides are useful in treating acne.

G. Tetracyclines

The tetracyclines (tetracycline, oxytetracycline, doxycycline and minocycline) are bacteristatic. They bind loosely to the 30S ribosomal subunit and inhibit the access of tRNA to mRNA and the synthesis of proteins. Resistance to all tetracyclines develops rapidly and limits their use. Resistance bacteria have been shown to chemically modify the tetracyclines and to alter their cell walls to prevent entry of these agents through the inner cytoplasmic membrane. All dermatologists are familiar with the uses of tetracyclines in acne. Whether their activity in this disease is due to antibacterial activity or secondary to anti-inflammatory effects has not been proven. They will probably continue to be used for this indication until better agents are developed. Another member, minocycline, is highly effective in treating leprosy. Regimens with minocycline in combination with several other agents are currently being developed by the World Health Organization. Minocycline is occasionally active against MRSA and skin infections caused by these strains can be treated after obtaining susceptibility results. To prevent rapid development of resistance to minocycline, a second agent is recommended.

H. Rifamycins

The rifamycins are a group of complex macrolides that are primarily used to treat *Mycobacterium*, but have activity against *Staphylococcus spp*., *H. influenzae*, most *Enterobacteriaceae*, many anaerobic bacteria, *Legionella spp*., and *Chlamydia spp*. Rifampin is primarily used to treat *M. tuberculosis* infections, but can be used to treat skin infection due to *S. aureus* [32]. Unfortunately, rifamycins develop resistance rapidly and should never be used as single therapy. Combination therapy with another active agent such as trimethoprime/sulfamethoxazole can be useful for difficult infections. Rifabutin is only used as prophylaxis for *M. avium* infections in AIDS patients, but it can be considered as combination therapy in patients with atypical mycobacterium infections of the skin. Susceptibility should be determined before adding rifabutin to therapy since all rifamycins are enzyme inducers that may decrease the serum concentrations of other agents. The rifamycins can best be described as time-dependent antibiotics and the serum concentration must exceed the MIC of the infecting organism for more than 50% of the dosing period to be effective [6]. Treatment of acne with these agents should be discouraged because of the possible development of resistance; this is particularly important because these agents are used in the treatment of tuberculosis.

I. Oxazolidones

The oxazolidones are a new class of antibiotics developed by Pharmacia and Upjohn. The mechanism of action of these new agents is protein synthesis inhibition. The binding site is probably at the initiation step of protein synthesis, which differs from other agents such as the aminoglycosides, macrolides, and tetracyclines. They have a broad spectrum of activity against gram-positive organisms including common pathogens like *S. aureus*, *S. epidermidis*, *S. pyogenes*, *Enterococcus faecium*, *E. faecalis*, and *S. pneumoniae*. They are active in vitro against strains of bacteria resistant to penicillin, methicillin, cephalosporins, and vancomycin. The oxazolidones have not shown cross-resistance with other classes of antibiotics. They are in clinical trials for the treatment of community-acquired pneumonia and skin and soft tissue infections. Both oral and intravenous formulations of these drugs will be available. This group has a potential for being very useful in treating skin infections.

J. Nitroimidazoles

Metronidazole and tinadazole are antimicrobials with activity limited to anaerobic bacteria (*Bacteroides spp., Fusobacterium spp., Clostridium spp., Peptococcus spp.*). These agents are generally bactericidal against anaerobic bacteria probably because of their ability to produce free radicals within the bacteria. Metronidazole kills the organism without binding to any particular site, and is more representative of dose-dependent killing [6]. Both agents are rapidly and completely absorbed from the gastrointestinal tract and can be given orally or intravenously in the same dose. They are distributed in body water, where high tissue concentrations are seen.

Nitroimidazoles have limited usefulness in treating skin and skin structure infections except in rare cases like decubitus ulcers and bone infections. There are many other choices that also have anaerobic and gram-positive activity. Because of this, metronidazole is seldom used by dermatologists. Nitroimidazoles have activity against *H. pylori* and may have a place in the treatment of rosacea.

K. Chloramphenicol

Chloramphenicol was considered a wonder drug when introducted over 40 years ago. Most clinical pathogens at that time were susceptible to it and it was widely used. This was followed by a period of fear because of the rare possibility of developing aplastic anemia. It is still occasionally useful, but most clinically important bacteria have developed resistance to it. Chloramphenicol is not highly active against most skin pathogens, and is seldom needed because of the large number of safer and more active drugs today.

L. Polymyxins

Polymyxins are primarily active against gram-negative organisms, particularly *P. aeruginosa*. They are cationic detergents that cause disorganization of the lipid anionic cell membranes of both bacteria and human cells. The resulting nephrotoxicity and neurotoxicity of these compounds have limited their uses to topical application, although they are available as intravenous preparations. They have no place in the current systemic treatment of skin infections today.

V. SUMMARY

Antimicrobial therapy is an integral aspect of dermatological treatment. While laboratory confirmation of the pathogenic bacteria is desirable, it is not always feasible. By understanding the important aspects of the pharmacodynamics, an appropriate agent may be selected on an empiric basis. Adequate dosing is important not only to be effective but also to counter the growing problem of resistance.

Numerous groups of antimicrobials have been recognized since the seminal work of Domagk in the 1930s. The groups of significance to dermatologists include the beta-lactams, macrolides, azilides, streptogrammins, lincosamides, aminocycolitols, sulfonamides, tetracyclines, rifamycins, oxazolidones, nitroimadazoles, chloramphenicol, and polymyxins.

While usual dermatological therapy centers around erythromycin, the tetracyclines, and some penicillins, some of the newer quinolones and cephalosporins have seen increasing use by dermatologists and the trend will continue, making resource of the newer antibiotics an essential part of practice.

VI. REFERENCES

1. Levison, ME. Pharmacodynamics of antimicrobial agents. Infect Dis Clin North Am 1995; 9(3):483–495.
2. Woods GL. In Vitro testing of antimicrobial agents. Infect Dis Clin North Am 1995; 9:463–481.
3. Lorian V. Some effects of subinhibitory concentrations of antibiotics on bacteria. Bull NY Med 1975; 51:1046–1047.
4. Bundtzen RW, Gerber AU, Cohn DL, et al. Postantibiotic suppression of bacterial growth. Rev Infect Dis 1987; 3:28–29.
5. McDonald PJ, Wetherall BL, Pruul H. Postantibiotic leukocyte enhancement: Increased susceptibility of bacteria pretreated with antibiotics to activity of leukocytes. Rev Infect Dis 1981; 3:38.
6. Craig, WA. Pharmacokinetic/pharacodynamic parameters: Rationale for antibacterial dosing of mice and men. Clin Infect Dis 1998; 26:1–12.
7. Craig W. Pharmacodynamics of antimicrobial agents as a basis for determining dosing regimens. Eur J Clin Microbiol Infect Dis 1993; 12(suppl 1):6–8.
8. Craig W, Vogelman B. Changing concepts and new applications of antibiotic pharmacokinetics. Am J Med 1984; 77:24–25.
9. Vogelman B, Craig WA. Kinetics of antimicrobial activity. J Pediatr 1986; 108: 835–840.
10. Moore RD, Lietman PS, Smith CR. Clinical response to aminoglycoside therapy: importance of the ration of peak concentration to minimal inhibitory concentration. J Infect Dis 1987; 155:93–99.
11. Craig WA, Gudmundsson S. Postantibiotic effect. In: Lorian V, ed. Antibiotics in Laboratory Medicine, 4th ed. Baltimore: Williams and Wilkins, 1996:296–329.
12. Fraimow HS, Abrutyn E. Pathogens resistant to antimicrobial agents. Infect Dis Clin North Am 1995; 9:497–530.
13. Cohen ML. Epidemiology of drug resistance: Implications for a postantibiotic era. Science 1992; 257:1050–1055.
14. Neu HC: The crisis in antibiotic resistance. Science 1992; 254:1064–1073.
15. Tomasz A: Multiple antibiotic-resistant pathogenic bacteria. A report on the Rockefeller University workshop. N Engl J Med 1994; 330:1247–1252.
16. Shaw KJ, Rather PN, Hare RS, et al. Molecular genetics of aminoglycoside resis-

tance genes and familial relationships of the aminoglycoside-modifying enzymes. Microbiol Rev 1993; 57:138–163.
17. Bush K. Characterization of beta lactamases. Antimicrob Agents Chemother 1989; 33:259–263.
18. Spratt BG: Resistance to antibiotics mediated by target alterations. Science 1994; 264:388–393.
19. Davies J. Inactivation of antibiotics and the dissemination of resistance genes. Science 1994; 264:375–382.
20. Shortridge VD, Flamm RK, Ramer N, Beyer J, et al. Novel mechanism of macrolide resistance in *Streptococcus pneumoniae*. Diagn Microbiol Infect Dis 1996; 26:73–78.
21. Clancy J, Petitpas J, Dib-Hajj F, Yuan W, et al. Molecular cloning and functional analysis of a novel macrolide-resistance determinant, mefA, from *Streptococcus pyogenes*. Mol Microbiol 1996; 22(5):867–879.
22. Tait-Kamradt A, Clancy J, Cronan M, et al. mefE Is necessary for the erythromycin-resistant M phenotype in *Streptococcus pneumoniae*. Antimicrob Agents Chemother 1996; 41:2251–2255.
23. McMurry LM, Petrucci RE Jr, Levy SB. Active efflux of tetracycline encoded by four genetically different tetracycline resistance determinants in *E. coli*. Proc Natl Acad Sci USA 1980; 77:3974–3977.
24. Nakaido H. Prevention of drug access to bacterial targets: Permeability barriers and active reflux. Science 1992; 264:1064–1073.
25. Miller MH, Edberg SC, Mandel LJ, et al. Gentamicin uptake in wild type and aminoglycoside resistant small colony mutants of *Staphylococcus aureus*. Antimicrob Agents Chemother 1980; 18:722–729.
26. Hendershot EF. Fluoroquinolones. Infect Dis Clin North Am 1995; 9:715–730
27. Leach AJ, Shelby-James TM, Mayo M, et al. A prospective study of the impact of community-based azithromycin treatment of trachoma on carriage and resistance of *Streptococcus pneumoniae*. Clin Infect Dis 1997; 24:356–362.
28. Hakenbeck R, Tarpay M, Tomasz A. Multiple changes of penicillin-binding proteins in penicillin-resistant clinical isolates of *Streptococcus pneumoniae*. Antimicrob Agents Chemother 1980; 17:364–368.
29. Hartman BM, Tomasz A. Low-affinity penicillin binding protein associated with beta-lactam resistance in *Staphylococcus aureus*. J Bacteriol 1984; 158:513–514.
30. Costeron JW, Cheng KG. The role of the bacterial cell envelope in antibiotic resistance. J Antimicrob Chemother 1975; 1:363–367.
31. Ennis DM, Cobbs CG. The newer cephalosporins: Aztreonam and Imipenem. Infect Dis Clin of North Am 1995; 9:687–713.
32. Lundstrom TS, Sobel JD. Vancomycin, Trimethoprim-sulfamethoxazole and Rifamycin. Infect Dis Clin North Am 1995; 9:747–767.
33. Haria M, Lamb HM. Trovafloxacin. Drug 1997; 54:435–447.
34. Med Lett 1998; 40(1022):30–31.
35. Zuckerman JM, Kaye KM. The newer macrolides: azithromycin and clarithromycin. Infect Dis Clin North Am 1995; 9:731–745.
36. Bergfeld WF, Odom RB. New perspectives on acne. Clinician 1994; 12:14–15.

4

Oral Antifungal Therapy

Joseph P. Shrum and Larry E. Millikan
Tulane University Medical Center
New Orleans, Louisiana

I. GRISEOFULVIN

Griseofulvin, which is derived from species of the *Penicillium* mold, was first investigated for use as an antifungal for plants. Subsequently, griseofulvin was demonstrated to cure some dermatophyte infections in animals; in 1959, it was shown to be effective in the oral treatment of superficial fungal infections in humans [1,2].

A. Pharmacology

Griseofulvin consists of three connected carbon rings, one of which is a benzene ring with an attached chloride atom. Griseofulvin disrupts fungal cell division by inhibiting fungal RNA, DNA, microtubular assembly, and cell wall synthesis. Development of terminal hyphae is thus severely impaired [3].

Griseofulvin is poorly absorbed on an empty stomach, as it is insoluble in the aqueous medium of the upper gastrointestinal tract. Ingestion of griseofulvin after eating, especially a fatty meal, results in more rapid and greater serum levels of the drug [4].

Once absorbed, griseofulvin is primarily bound to serum albumin, with tissue distribution being determined by the plasma-free concentration. Following absorption, griseofulvin diffuses from both extracellular fluid and sweat in the epidermal cell layers into the stratum corneum [5].

Metabolism of griseofulvin occurs in the liver. Griseofulvin is reduced through hepatic demethylation to inactive compounds, including its major metabolite, 6-methyl griseofulvin. Subsequently, all these inactive compounds are excreted primarily by the kidneys [6,7].

B. Indications and Uses

Griseofulvin is fungistatic against species of *Microsporum, Epidermophyton*, and *Trichophyton*, common causes of fungal infections of the skin, hair, and nails [2]. Once a dermatophyte infection of one or more of these structures has been established, different formulations of griseofulvin may be administered. Microsize (microcrystalline) and ultramicrosize (ultramicrocrystalline) griseofulvin is available, with the latter being absorbed through the gastrointestinal tract with an efficiency 1.5 times that of microsized griseofulvin [8].

Today griseofulvin is used most frequently for the treatment of tinea capitis. While this condition may occur in adults, especially those who are immunosuppressed, it occurs most frequently in children and is usually due to *Trichophyton tonsurans*. Tinea capitis may be characterized by erythema and scale, ''black dot'' alopecia, or by an inflammatory kerion [8].

Children should be treated for tinea capitis with 15 to 20 mg/kg/day of griseofulvin microsize or, roughly, half the dose for griseofulvin ultramicrosize. Griseofulvin microsize may be given in a liquid formation, with a concentration of 125 mg/5 mL for 6 to 8 weeks. Kerion formation may require the concomitant use of oral antibiotics and steroids [8,9].

Prior to the availability of the newer azole antifungals, griseofulvin was the treatment of choice for tinea unguium, most frequently due to *Trichophyton rubrum*. However, duration of therapy is long (up to 18 months for toenails); compliance is poor; and the recurrence rate is high. While generally less expensive, griseofulvin therapy for tinea unguium has generally been replaced by the newer oral antifungals.

Dermatophyte infections at other body locations generally respond well to 4 to 6 weeks of therapy with griseofulvin. In adults, the required daily dose is 500 mg microsize (250–330 mg ultramicrosize) for skin and 1000 mg microsize (500–600 mg ultramicrosize) for hair and nails. In children, the doses are 5 to 10 mg/kg/day for cutaneous infections and 15 to 20 mg/kg/day for hair and nail infections [8,9]. Majocchi's granuloma, however, may require several months of treatment. Total length of therapy may also be influenced by KOH studies, fungal cultures, and the clinical picture. Recently, improved topical antifungals have to a large degree replaced systemic griseofulvin as a treatment for cutaneous fungal infections (Table 1).

Finally, griseofulvin has been reported to be an effective therapy for lichen planus [10,11]. The mechanism of action is unknown, and erosive oral lichen planus is more responsive than the cutaneous form [8].

Table 1 Indications for Topical Antifungals

Lamisil cream	Tinea pedis, tinea cruris, tinea corporis due to	*Epidermophyton floccosum*, *Trichophyton mentagrophytes*, or *Trichophyton rubrum*
Mentax cream	Tinea pedis, tinea cruris, tinea corporis due to	*Epidermophyton floccosum*, *Trichophyton mentagrophytes*, *Trichophyton rubrum*, and *Trichophyton tonsurans*
Nizoral cream	Tinea pedis, tinea cruris, tinea corporis due to	*Epidermophyton floccosum*, *Trichophyton mentagrophytes*, or *Trichophyton rubrum*
	Tinea versicolor caused by	Malassezia furfur (*Pityrosporum orbiculare*)
	Cutaneous candidiasis caused by *Candida spp*.	
	Seborrheic dermatitis	
Oxistat cream	Tinea pedis, tinea cruris, tinea corporis due to	*Epidermophyton floccosum*, *Trichophyton mentagrophytes*, or *Trichophyton rubrum*
Spectazole cream	Tinea pedis, tinea cruris, tinea corporis due to Cutaneous candidiasis Tinea versicolor	*Epidermophyton floccosum*, *Trichophyton mentagrophytes*, *Trichophyton rubrum*, *Trichophyton tonsurans*, *Microsporum canis*, *Microsporum audouini*, or *Microsporum gypseum*
Exelderm cream	Tinea cruris and tinea corporis due to	*Trichophyton rubrum*, *Trichophyton mentagrophytes*, *Epidermophyton floccosum*, and *Microsporum canis*
Loprox cream and lotion	Tinea pedis, tinea cruris, and tinea corporis due to	*Trichophyton rubrum*, *Trichophyton mentagrophytes*, *Epidermophyton floccosum*, *Microsporum canis*
	Candidiasis due to	*Candida albicans*
		Tinea versicolor
Lotrisone	Tinea pedis, tinea cruris, and tinea corporis due to	*Trichophyton rubrum*, *Trichophyton mentagrophytes*, *Epidermophyton floccosum*, and *Microsporum canis*
Mycostatin cream	Cutaneous or mucocutaneous myotic infections caused by	*Candida albicans* and other *Candida spp*.
Naftin cream and gel	Tinea pedis, tinea cruris, and tinea corporis due to	*Trichophyton rubrum*, *Trichophyton mentagrophytes*, *Epidermophyton floccosum*

C. Adverse Reactions

Adverse reactions to griseofulvin are few, relative to the number of patients treated with it. Cutaneous reactions included exfoliative erythroderma, flare of preexisting lupus, fixed drug eruption, phototoxicity, and urticaria. Other reactions reported are anaphylaxis, diarrhea, dizziness, headache, hepatotoxicity, nausea, vomiting, leukopenia, and proteinuria [12–14]. However, griseofulvin is a very safe medication and it is noteworthy that there has never been a death clearly caused by griseofulvin administration.

Well-demonstrated drug interactions include the inhibitory effect that griseofulvin may have on warfarin-type anticoagulants, and impeded absorption of griseofulvin that may be caused by phenobarbital [15,16].

Less well decided is the effect of griseofulvin and oral contraceptives. At present, it is wise to inform a patient on steroid birth control that some studies have shown interference by griseofulvin and other studies have not; the patient should then act accordingly [17].

II. KETOCONAZOLE (NIZORAL)

Ketoconazole, introduced initially in 1977, and in the United States in 1981, was the first orally available imidazole antifungal [18,19]. Ketoconazole has a broad spectrum of uses, and is effective against candidiasis, pityrosporosis, dermatophytosis, blastomycosis, coccidioidomycosis, cryptococcosis, and histoplasmosis [8].

A. Pharmacology

Ketoconazole, as an imidazole, inhibits sterol metabolism, with a preferential effect on ergosterol formation in the cells of fungi. By inhibiting fungal cytochrome P-450 and C-14 alpha-demethylase, the fungal cell wall becomes permeable, resulting in subsequent destruction of the fungus. Ketoconazole is not as fungal-specific as fluconazole and itraconazole. As a result, ketoconazole may interfere with human steroid metabolism in both the corticosteroid and androgen synthetic pathways. At higher doses, significant inhibition of androgen synthesis can result in gynecomastia and impotence [8,19].

Depending on several factors, an oral dose of ketoconazole has a wide range of bioavailability, with between 37 to 97% reaching the blood. Ketoconazole is a weakly dibasic imidazole derivative with optimal solubility at pH lower than 3. Patients with achlorhydria should ingest the drug with an acidified liquid. Patients who take antacids, anticholinergics, antiparkinsonian agents, and H_2-receptor antagonists should ingest ketoconazole 2 h prior to taking these other medications [8,19].

Ketoconazole has a strong keratin adherence; delivery occurs there within 2 h through eccrine sweat. Delivery occurs much more slowly (3–4 weeks) through the epidermal basal layer. Inhibitory concentrations of ketoconazole remain for at least 10 days following termination of the drug. Ketoconazole is widely distributed throughout urine, saliva, sebum, eccrine sweat, cerebrum, cerebrospinal fluids (CSF), and joint fluid. However, as ketoconazole is 99% plasma protein bound, relatively low levels are achieved in the CSF [8,19–22].

Ketoconazole is metabolized primarily by the cytochrome P-450 system in the liver with metabolites being excreted in the feces. Hepatotoxicity is rare but of serious concern, especially with a long-term regimen of therapy [23].

B. Indications and Uses

Ketoconazole has a broader spectrum of activity than griseofulvin, and is active against dermatophytes, dimorphic fungi, actinomycetes, phycomycetes, and yeasts [8].

Ketoconazole is the treatment of choice for chronic mucocutaneous candidiasis, promoting regression of mucosal, skin, and nail lesions and remission of symptoms [24].

Oral thrush may be treated with excellent results with 200 mg per day oral ketoconazole for 10 days [25].

Patients with extensive skin candidosis can be treated with ketoconazole, although topical therapy is usually effective [26,27].

Patients with severe recalcitrant dermatophyte infections can be treated with ketoconazole because the majority of cutaneous dermatophytes unresponsive to griseofulvin are responsive to ketoconazole [8]. The drug has been used for various types of tinea infections (i.e., faciei, corporis, cruris, unguium) with success; however, safer, more reliable medications are usually prescribed [28].

Because of its mechanism of action, ketoconazole interferes with all membrane biosynthesis, and thus ketoconazole has been studied as an agent to treat cutaneous leishmaniasis. While no complete cure has been achieved with ketoconazole, it has been shown to be effective against some types of cutaneous leishmaniasis [29].

Tinea versicolor is effectively treated with ketoconazole as well as many different treatment regimens [8,22].

Ketoconazole effectively treats *Pityrosporum* folliculitis. It has been shown to be effective against invasive fungi, including chromomycosis, histoplasmosis, blastomycosis, paracoccidioidomycosis, aspergillosis, and coccidioidomycosis [30,31].

Ketoconazole has been used to treat seborrheic dermatitis [32,33].

As noted earlier, ketoconazole is not as fungus-specific as some other antifungal agents and therefore it may interfere in human steroid metabolism in both the corticosteroid and androgen synthetic pathways. The antiandrogenic effect of ketoconazole has been used therapeutically to treat a variety of conditions, including Cushing disease, hirsutism, precocious puberty, and prostatic cancer [34–38]. Clearly, the severity of the underlying condition and the availability of alternate therapies should be weighed against the hepatotoxicity associated with high-dose, long-term ketoconazole treatment.

Ketoconazole is generally given in a dose of 200 to 400 mg a day, for as short as 1 week to as long as several months [39]. Dosing usually begins at 200 mg a day, with increases in dose and length of treatment dependent upon the severity of disease, patient response, and potential for hepatotoxicity [8].

Dosing regimens for treating tinea versicolor are most varied. Single-dose, once-weekly regimens and daily treatment for days to several weeks have been studied [38,40]. One study shows no difference in cure rate between a single 400-mg dose and a 10-day 200-mg dose of ketoconazole. As the author suggests, patient compliance and cost of treatment should be factored into the decision on how to treat [22].

C. Adverse Reactions

As stated previously, the most serious potential side effect from ketoconazole therapy is hepatotoxicity. The presumed mechanism for the hepatic injury caused by ketoconazole is a metabolic idiosyncrasy. Estimated incidence of symptomatic hepatic injury have ranged from 1:2000 to 1:50000 [8]. Patients may present with anorexia, icterus, malaise, nausea, or vomiting. Hepatotoxicity appears after approximately 2 weeks of therapy and occurs more commonly in elderly patients. In addition, transient elevation of serum transaminases occurs in approximately one-fifth of asymptomatic patients. These elevations have been reported to return to normal with cessation of therapy, as well as despite continuing ketoconazole therapy. For treatment schedules of less than 2 weeks, risk of hepatotoxicity is small. For more long-term therapy, appropriate screening and surveillance blood work should be obtained [41].

Other reported adverse reactions include urticaria and angioedema, pruritus, leukopenia, hemolytic anemia, thrombocytopenia, impotence, bulging fontanelles, papilledema, headaches, dizziness, drowsiness, nervousness, tremors, memory loss, depression, suicidal ideation, and paranoid delusions [42–46].

D. Drug Interactions

Ketoconazole increases the level of effect of astemizole, cisapride, corticosteroids, coumadin, cyclosporine, oral sulphonylureas, phenytoin, and terfenadine. The level or effect of ketoconazole is increased by cimetidine, and decreased by antacids, H_2-receptor antagonists, isoniazid, omeprazole, rifabutin, and rifampin [6,31].

Much press has been given to the coadministration of ketoconazole and, specifically, cisapride, astemizole, and terfenadine. The serious cardiovascular side effects, including prolongation of the Q-T interval and torsades de pointes, contraindicates coadministration of ketoconazole with these drugs [47–50].

Finally, the phenomenon of sticky hands reported in patients with psoriasis who are taking retinoids has also been known to occur in patients receiving ketoconazole and doxorubicin for androgen-independent prostate cancer [51].

Ketoconazole is a moderately priced medication. One 200-mg tablet may cost anywhere from $1 to $2 [19].

III. FLUCONAZOLE (DIFLUCAN)

Fluconazole (Diflucan) is a hydrophilic oral and intravenous synthetic triazole with an empirical formula of $C_{13}H_{12}F_2N_6O$. Initially introduced in Europe, then later in the United States, fluconazole is effective against both superficial and systemic fungi (Table 2).

A. Pharmacology

Triazoles (fluconazole, itraconazole, saperconazole), which are fungistatic, act by the same mechanism as the imidazoles. The mode of action of the triazoles is to inhibit the synthesis of ergosterol, the major sterol constituent of dermatophyte cell walls, which is vital for cellular growth [18,52].

The fungal enzyme cytochrome P-450-dependent C-14 alpha-demethylase catalyzes ergosterol synthesis from lanosterol. Imidazoles selectively inhibit the C-14 alpha-demethylation of lanosterol. Due to the absence of ergosterol synthesis and the accumulation of lanosterol, there is attenuation of the dermatophyte cell wall. Weakening of the fungal cell membrane results in its increased permeability, and prevents fungal cell growth and replication [53].

Since triazoles have less affinity for the mammalian cytochrome P-450 system than imidazoles, fluconazole does not have the detrimental effects on mammalian steroid hormone production of other antifungals [54,55], but still possesses strong antidermatophyte activity.

After oral intake, fluconazole has good absorption; after either oral or intravenous administration, there is little protein binding and the half-life is long enough to permit once-a-day dosing that is affected by neither food nor gastric pH [23].

Peak plasma concentrations in fasting normal volunteers occur between 1 to 2 h with a terminal plasma elimination half-life of approximately 30 h after oral administration [20,55]

Following either single or multiple oral doses for up to 14 days, fluconazole penetrates widely into most body fluids and body tissue. Since the drug is hydrophilic, it is therefore found mainly in body fluids. In addition, fluconazole has a high concentration in sweat; inhibitory levels of the drug are demonstrated in the stratum corneum within 1 to 3 days of administration [21,56,57].

Fluconazole is cleared primarily by renal excretion. Approximately 80% of the administered dose will appear in the urine as unchanged drug. Approximately 11% of the administered dose is excreted in the urine as metabolites. Patients who have renal insufficiency will require an adjustment in dose [55].

Although hydrophilic, long-term administration of fluconazole results in high levels of the drug in the skin and nails. Since higher levels are reached in eccrine sweat and in the dermis–epidermis than in serum, the drug reaches the stratum corneum both by sweat and by direct diffusion from the dermis–epidermis. Prolonged keratin levels result several months after discontinuation of fluconazole [56,57].

B. Indications and Uses

Fluconazole may be used for a wide variety of fungal infections. When first developed, its successful use for onychomycosis was anticipated because of its propensity to develop high levels of concentration in the horny layer of the skin. For onychomycosis, one study has demonstrated a 97% clinical response rate at the end of treatment and an 87% response at long-term follow-up using 150 mg once a week for 3 to 12 months [58,59]. Another study, using 300 mg once weekly or 100 to 200 mg on alternate days, had equally excellent results after 6 months and 3.7 months of treatment for toenail and fingernail infections, respectively [60].

As fluconazole is effective against most *Candida spp*., it is used in the treatment of yeast infections and, in fact, is a stronger inhibitor of the proliferation of *C. albicans* than of some dermatophytes [61].

Vaginal candidiasis can be treated with a single 150-mg oral dose of fluconazole, which is preferred for its ease of administration. Fluconazole reaches a maximum concentration in vaginal secretions 8 h after administration orally, and this level is sustained at least 24 h. Mucocutaneous candidiasis is a frequent complication in patients infected with human immunodeficiency syndrome (HIV), and fluconazole has been shown to be an effective treatment for oral thrush as well as esophageal and urinary candidiasis [19,62].

Children as well as adults with HIV infection have been safely and effectively treated with fluconazole for oropharyngeal candidiasis [63]. Fluconazole is effective against *Cryptococcus neoformans* and has become the drug of choice for maintenance therapy of cryptococcal meningitis in acquired immunodeficiency syndrome (AIDS) patients [53].

Resistance to fluconazole has been developing and is most apparent in immunocompromised hosts. Some cases of fluconazole resistance by *C. albicans* in AIDS patients have been associated with reduced intracellular accumulation of the drug [64]. Resistance develops especially in those patients taking long-term, low-dose fluconazole. Other resistant organisms have included *C. krusei*, *C. glabrata*, and *C. neoformans* [19,65].

With regard to other fungal infections, fluconazole is an alternative to amphotericin B in otherwise healthy individuals with associated infections [19]. Fluconazole has been used to treat cutaneous blastomycosis, cutaneous sporotrichosis, osteoarticular and visceral sporotrichosis, and chromoblastomycosis [66–69]. Fluconazole has been shown to be effective in the treatment of deep tropical mycoses. Successful therapy with fluconazole has been achieved for zygomycosis due to *Conidiobolus coronatus*, for African histoplasmosis, as well as for eumycetoma due to *Acremonium spp.* and *Pseudallescheria boydii* and *C. (Torulopsis) glabrata* [70]. Fluconazole has been reported to cure a case of protothecosis occurring in an immunocompetent individual [71]. In addition, fluconazole has been used to treat pityriasis versicolor using a single oral dose of 400 mg [72].

Fluconazole has been shown to be very effective in reducing fungal infections when used prophylactically in patients after chemotherapy or after radiation therapy following bone marrow transplantation [73,74].

C. Adverse Reactions

With regard to adverse reactions, fluconazole's side effects have occurred in about 10% of treated patients. Gastrointestinal complaints such as nausea, vomiting, abdominal pain, and diarrhea were commonly listed as side effects as were headaches [23,64]. Skin rash has been reported, including exfoliative erythroderma. Some patients have had elevated liver enzymes which returned to normal following cessation of treatment. Fluconazole has been associated with rare cases of fatal hepatotoxicity [20].

Finally, there have been two cases of thrombocytopenia reported in otherwise healthy adults treated for onychomycosis. These cases resolved after cessation of treatment, but may have been an idiosyncratic reaction to the fluconazole [75].

Some drug interactions have been noted with fluconazole. Fluconazole can increase the level or effect of astemizole, amitriptyline, caffeine, cyclosporine, phenytoin, sulfonylureas, terfenadine, theophylline, warfarin, and zidovudine. The level or effect of fluconazole is decreased by carbamazepine, isoniazid, phenobarbital, phenytoin, rifabutin, and rifampin. The level or effect of fluconazole is increased by cimetidine and hydrochlorothiazide [19,20,76].

Fluconazole is an expensive medicine. The cost of oral fluconazole is approximately four times that of oral ketoconazole (400 mg may cost $2–$4). The cost of intravenous fluconazole is 25 times as much. As fluconazole has a high bioavailability, the oral dose should be given whenever there is no overriding reason for giving the intravenous form [16].

IV. TERBINAFINE

A. Pharmacology

Terbinafine presently represents the first and only oral antifungal in the unique allylamine group of antifungals. Naftifine preceded it, and others are under development; they are primarily topical in nature, but possess many of the potent antifungal characteristics that terbinafine has. The drug acts at a unique step in the biochemical pathway, that of inhibition of the squalene epoxidase step. It blocks the production of 2–3 oxidosqualine, causing a buildup of precursors with significant fungicidal effects. It is the only oral antifungal that is listed as a cidal drug. It possesses minimum inhibitory concentrations (MIC) of 0.004 μg/mL for dermatophytes and minimum fungicidal concentrations (MFC) of 0.004 μg/mL [77].

In contrast, itraconazole's MICs for the same organisms are 0.078; MFCs are 0.595. This high potency confirmed in in vitro studies is the major reason for the drug's cidal capability. Thus far, in its extensive, widespread use, the drug appears to be very safe. In regard to absorption, the drug is lipophilic, but does not seem to be significantly altered by administration with meals. After an oral dosage, plasma levels will reach 0.8 to 1.5 μg/μL in 2 h; 85% of this is cleared from the plasma in 3 days, but, because of its lipophilicity, remains in the tissues.

Concern with the imidazoles centers around the cytochrome P-450 metabolism so critical with most oral antifungals. Allylamines are minimally metabolized by pathways other than the P-450 mechanism, which greatly adds to the safety of the drug. It is a pregnancy category B drug [78].

Excretion is slow. The T ½ of 16 h, and terminal T ½ of 80 to 100 h reflects with plasma levels [79]. Of even greater significance, however, with most effective antifungals is the binding in keratinized tissue. Faergemann has shed a great deal of light on this situation, looking at tissue distribution after 28 days of treatment [80]. This is of particular significance on tissues that are hard keratins, such as hair and nails. Here the incorporation of the drug into the keratinized tissue maintains MIC levels for long periods of time, up to 4 to 5 months in the nail plate in onychomycosis. While plasma levels rapidly fall after completion of course of treatment, cidal levels remain in both the stratum corneum and nails for longer than 3 months.

B. Indications and Uses

The U.S. Physician's Desk Reference (PDR) lists current indications as only onychomycosis. The dosage is 250 mg daily for 12 weeks, with a possible additional 4 weeks of therapy for severe involvement of the toenails. While this is the sole indication for the tablets, topical forms are used for a much broader range, suggesting future efficacy for the oral preparation. The cream is indicated for various forms of cutaneous tinea, tinea corporis, cruris, pedis, and the 1% solution is indicated for tinea versicolor, tinea pedis, tinea cruris, and tinea corporis. There are many studies reported in the literature of extended indications for the tablets in all the above-mentioned infections and tinea capitis, but none have fulfilled the rigorous studies for indication in the United States. Perhaps the most promising area is the use of terbinafine for the treatment of tinea capitis, with several studies now reporting excellent results (see Sec. IV.C). At the time of completion of this chapter it was assumed that approval for the treatment of tinea capitis would be forthcoming.

C. Clinical Studies in Onychomycosis

Clinical studies have been limited primarily to the two agents *T. rubrum* and *T. mentagrophytes* because they represent over 99% of dermatophyte-associated nail infections. Basic studies show that on 250 mg daily, one can very effectively treat infections (based on blood levels exceeding in vitro MICs) due to *Epidermophytin floccosum*, *Microsporum gypseum*, *Microsporum nanum*, *Trichophytin verrucosum*, *C. albicans*, and *Scopulariopsis brevicaulis*. The latter organism is of particular significance because in our experience it has been one of the more frequent molds associated with nail disease. "Associated" is an appropriate term, because there is still controversy in regard to cause and effect and direct versus incidental association of *Scopulariopsis* with nail dystrophy. Toenail studies, including the lion study (lion = Lamisil, itraconazole, onychomycosis) (data provided by Novartis Laboratories) [81], has shown in a comparison of continuous terbinafine versus intermittent itraconazole at 72 weeks very similar parallel curves, but highly statistically significant ($p = 0.0001$) differences between the two. Treatment with terbinafine gives a mycological cure rate at 16 weeks of 80.8%; at 12 weeks, 75.7%; 4-week therapy with itraconazole gives a 49.1% mycological cure rate; and three doses of itraconazole gives a 38.3% cure rate. Mycological cure is seen sooner with continuous terbinafine therapy at 24 to 25 weeks, as opposed to 36-week mycological cure with intermittent itraconazole dosage. Additionally, by week 72, the 100% clearing of the infected toenail was significantly higher for both the 12- and 16-week terbinafine groups when compared with intermittent itraconazole at 3 or 4 weeks. The lion study also reported no statistically significant differences in the safety profile of the two regimens. These data strongly support the use of terbinafine for the treatment of onychomycoses, especially those due to scopulariopsis and most dermatophytes. When dealing with other molds (Hendersonula/Scylatalidium), there is no absolute indication of the superiority of one drug over the other; however, the somewhat broader spectrum of the triazoles suggest that there may be a greater level of benefit with the use of itraconazole in patients with onychomycosis due to nondermatophytes.

While the best MICs are seen in the dermatophytes, the report by Cambon et al. (Novartis Research Institute) has extended the studies on effectiveness of terbinafine against other fungal organisms that have rarely been studied to this date [82]. When sufficient information becomes available from the appropriate studies, ultimate indications for systemic terbinafine use in subcutaneous and systemic mycoses may be broadened. Promising results in vitro against *Aspergillosis* and *Gypseum* suggest future utility in this area. Some case reports presented by Cambone et al. show curing of *Aspergillus fumigatus* infections at 500 mg daily for 3 months. Another dosage regimen of 5 to 15 mg/kg for 90 to 270 days results in an approximate 50% improvement, with three out of seven cases showing complete cure of *A. fumigatus* in the lungs. The use of the drug at 500 mg daily for 10 months also has been reported to clear osteomyelitis due to *A. fumigatus*. While the numbers of the patients in these studies are small because of the rarity of the disease and lack of active protocol at the present time, it seems that there is a potential for success in treating various forms of Aspergillosis. Similarly, the phaeohyphomycosis in these infections due to *Exophiala bipolaris*, *Dematiaceous fungi*, *Curvularia*, or *Alternaria* have all shown benefit, with marked improvement and approximately one-third (very limited numbers) showing clinical cure. Sixty-eight percent clinical and mycological cure in a year has been described by this same group in the treatment of *Fonsecaea pedrosoi* and *Cladosporium* and *Chromomycosis*. Marked improvement has also been seen in mycetoma, sporotrichosis, and cures or marked improvement in *Paracoccidioides*, *Rhizopus*, *Zygomycetes*, and *Pseudallescheria boydii*. Most intriguing are reports of effectiveness in the treatment of leishmaniasis. This may well be a very important treatment option in the future.

A number of other studies are currently looking at the treatment of tinea capitis with terbinafine. This is a critical step, because in the south our clinical experience has been that there is increasing resistance of the organism to griseofulvin, and most children with tinea capitis require long therapy with low incidence of clearing. Enough studies now have been reported to suggest that in the near future tinea capitis will be treated in adults with 250 mg daily. Patients weighing 100 pounds will take one-half of a tablet (or 125 mg daily), and patients weighing 40 pounds or less will take one-quarter of the tablet crushed (62.5 mg), and mixed with orange juice.

D. Duration of Therapy

Treatment of fingernail onychomycosis generally requires 12 weeks of 250 mg daily, and involvement of the toenails requires at least one additional month, and sometimes two. Reports of studies on the treatment of tinea corporis and cruris are premature, but we have found success using the standard pulse path for the treatment of these infections, and repeating in 2 weeks if necessary. The indications for these other fungal infections are not finalized and approved by the FDA at this time.

Future indications include the recently marketed Lamisil solution and the reports in the literature of its effectiveness against tinea versicolor. The most recent information from Novartis is that the 1% Lamisil solution is approved for topical therapy of pityriasis versicolor or tinea versicolor and tinea pedis, cruris, and corporis. In the last forms, the most effective and highest cure rates are due to those infections from *Trichophytin rubrum*, mentagaphytes, or *Epidermophyton floccosum*.

Current data suggest that this is an effective drug in the treatment of fungal infections and a very significant addition to the formulary of antimycotic agents.

E. Adverse Reactions

Of major significance in antifungal therapy are drug interactions relating to the cytochrome P-450 situation. With terbinafine, there is a much lower side-effect rate and profile. However, virtually all antifungal drugs have some reactions and the side-effect profile for Lamisil suggests that about 10% of patients will have some form of associated drug reaction, with most causing minimum morbidity and no significant mortality. Elevated, but transient, liver function tests have been reported in 3.3% of patients. Cholestasis has occurred in many patients, often presenting with pruritus then icterus, but when this is picked up early, it usually does not create any problems; however, clearance of the icterus may be slow [83]. Patients first present with pruritus and they are warned that this symptom requires evaluation. Of more serious nature are some of the bullous (erythema multiforme and Stevens–Johnson) reactions. Erythrodermia, urticaria, psoriasis, and pityriasis rosea have all been reported, but exact association is not entirely clear. All of these can vary in their medical and cosmetic significance. A recent, excellent review by Gupta [84] includes lists of types of reactions—exanthems, macular papular, purpuric, pustular, asteatotic, pigmentary reactions. Very significant problems can occur when toxic epidermal necrolysis or Stevens–Johnson syndrome are manifestations of the drug reaction. Four cases of hepatitis have been reported in 1993 [85]. Virtually every antifungal seems to have a low incidence of headache and taste disorders, and terbinafine also has been noted to cause some visual problems, including changes in the perception of the color green. Of greater significance and potential morbidity is the hematological side-effect potential, which includes decreases in lymphocyte counts of a transient note; this has been initially reported in clinical trials. There have also been occasional reports of thrombocytopenia and leukopenia in patients without other significant problems [84]. The exact incidence is not yet clear but this can be a life-threatening complication. As with nearly all antifungals, complaints of headache and GI symptoms including diarrhea, dyspepsia, abdominal pain, nausea, and flatulence have been reported.

F. Drug Interactions

While the incidence of significant problems with terbinafine are much less than with the triazoles or imidazoles, certain precautions should be considered in therapy. While cimetidine has an effect on pH and the absorption of the imidazoles and triazoles, a different problem occurs with terbinafine. Coadministration of terbinafine and cimetidine results in a 33% decrease in the clearance of terbinafine. Therefore, since cimetidine causes a decrease in absorption of the imidazoles and triazoles, concurrent administration with allylamines results in increased blood levels because it interferes with the clearance of the drug [86].

As with many of these drugs, interaction with cyclosporine is another key issue. This is of particular note with both the imidazoles and the allylamines, inasmuch as immunosuppressed patients and transplant patients often have significant fungal infections—skin, hair, and nails. The use/addition of terbinafine in the patient on cyclosporine results in a 15% increase in cyclosporine clearance, thereby altering the drug kinetics and potentially creating problems for the maintenance of effective blood levels of cyclosporine.

Use of cyclosporine and the imidazoles results in increased levels of either drug because of competitive interference with clearance, and significant potential for nephrotoxicity from cyclosporine results. This relates back to the Cyp 450 3A competitive excretion (see below) [87]. Concurrent administration of rifampin and terbinafine results in a 100% increase in terbinafine clearance, which could potentially create therapeutic failures. Last, interaction with terfenadine is a significant problem with the use of imidazoles and triazoles, and is also another point of caution for use with terbinafine. Coadministration results in a 16% decrease in terbinafine clearance [79].

The potential for terbinafine interactions with anticoagulants is minimal, an important consideration in therapeutic choices in elderly patients. Also, according to the pharmaceutical manufacturer, there are no significant prospective studies of drug interactions with oral contraceptives, hormone replacement therapy, hypoglycemics, theophylline, phenytoins, thiazide diuretics, beta-blockers, and calcium channel blockers, so coadministration with these commonly used drugs in elderly patients seems to be safe, but has not been studied enough to provide definitive answers at the present time.

V. ITRACONAZOLE

A. Pharmacology

Itraconazole is a member of the triazole family, related to the imidazoles such as ketoconazole. The other available triazoles are terconazole (topical vaginal) and fluconazole (vide supra). All of these drugs act at a different step in the fungal synthetic pathways than the allylamines. The azoles act on the pathway blocking conversion of lanosterol to ergosterol. While the accumulation of squalene associated with allylamines is toxic, resulting in rapid death or fungicidal activity, the function of itraconazole is slower, causing membrane leakage that is fungistatic only. Nonetheless, itraconazole is very effective with dermatophyte sensitivity of 0.1 μg per mL inhibiting growth of more than 90% of dermatophyte strains in vitro [78]. Absorption is increased by the presence of food, and therefore should be taken with full meals. Administration of the drug over a 3-week period of time at 200 mg per day results in a steady-state plasma concentration of 0.7 μg per mL, more than enough to inhibit the growth of most fungi. As with many of the antifungals, the lipophilic and keratinophilic nature of these drugs is key in their effectiveness. Itraconazole has a high affinity for keratinizing tissue and can be seen in concentrations in the nail within a week, which results from the drug reaching the nail through the matrix and through the dermal blood vessels in the nail bed. This drug is particularly useful because high levels of it remain in the keratinized tissue of the nail plate for as long as 6 months after discontinuation, both on 3-month daily schedules as well as pulsed therapeutic schedules [87]. Absorption is rapid with both the capsule and the solution. The capsules are best absorbed with meals (and gastric acidity necessary) while the solution is better absorbed under fasting conditions. Plasma levels of 127 mg/mL are achieved from a 100-mg dose and 272 mg/mL after a 200-mg dose. Pulse therapy lowers drug exposure by two-thirds compared with continuous (3-month) therapy, greatly enhancing the safety profile [88]. Metabolism of itraconazole in the body is through the P-450 3A4 enzyme, which is a significant factor in this drug's potential for interactions with other drugs of clinical significance. The drug is metabolized and then excreted in the feces and the urine. A metabolite hydroxy-itraconazole is also an active antifungal (88). It, like terbinafine, is a pregnancy category B drug.

B. Indications and Uses

The major indication for itraconazole or Sporanox has been that of onychomycosis. This represents a significant step forward in effectiveness, with a very broad spectrum azole drug, effective against dermatophytes and many other organs such as *Scopulariopsis*, *Hendersonula*, and molds [89]. While the original indications centered around a 12-week course of therapy, the recent approval of pulse therapy has provided for equal efficacy with greater safety and lower cost. Dosage of two tablets twice a day for 7 days out of the month, repeated monthly, has a very high cure rate, somewhere between 75 and 90%, according to various studies. The course of therapy for onychomycosis of the fingernails is generally 3 months, and the course of therapy for onychomycosis of the toenails is 4 months or more. The persistence of active drug in the nail plate for 6+ months allows continued therapy and greatly enhances the cure rate. The patient should be made aware of this at the onset of therapy. It is most important to educate the patient with regard to the kinetics of toenail growth and the fact that full growth of toenails in a senior citizen may be as long as 7 to 12 months, so that one can see progression of normal nail plate growing out over that period of time. In contrast, superficial white onychomycosis of the fingernails or other more dystrophic fungal infections will respond in half the time.

The other primary approved indication in the United States for itraconazole systemically has to do with patients who are immunocompromised, and the treatment for deep fungal infections, including histoplasmosis and blastomycosis. It is important to remember, especially in the immunocompromised population, the need for gastric acidity for absorption. Many AIDS patients are achlorhydric and, as a result, absorb the drug poorly. Recently, elaborate protocols using diluted hydrochloric acid sipped through a straw have been supplanted by the use of cola drinks [91]. This provides a simple and easy means to assure adequate absorption. The literature is replete with the use of the drug for most different fungal infections, but most reports are of anecdotal nature. The well-known MIC effectiveness of itraconazole in dermatophytes has been extended to other therapeutic studies. It seems to be very effective in the treatment of tinea corporis and tinea cruris [92], but indications and adequate studies for such have not been done in the United States at the present time. A difficult condition, Majocchi's granuloma, also has been reported to respond to itraconazole and this may prove to be a more effective approach to treatment than the traditional use of griseofulvin [93]. A significant problem is tinea capitis due to *Trichophyton tonsurans*. The previously mentioned problems with resistance to griseofulvin has heightened interest in the use of both itraconazole and terbinafine. It would appear from early studies that pulse therapy may be very effective in those patients who are so difficult to clear [94].

C. Adverse Reactions

The development of itraconazole represented a significant step forward from the problems associated with ketoconazole (i.e., problems with liver metabolism, liver disease, and the significant problems with nail/androgen/steroid metabolism). This was a major problem in the use of ketoconazole in the treatment of the deep mycoses, because prolonged high blood levels of ketoconazole had a very significant effect on androgens and AM serum cortisol, resulting in undesirable feminizing side effects in the male patient. The problem is minimized with itraconazole, making it generally a much safer drug than its predecessor. Usual expected reactions of significance include the omnipresent ''rash.'' This includes urticaria, photoallergic reactions, and pustulosis—which has been described in both itraconazole as well as terbinafine. The incidence of cutaneous reactions is

Table 2 Fluconazole Dose Chart

Oropharyngeal candidiasis	Loading: Maintenance:	200 mg 100 mg daily	14 days
Esophageal candidiasis	Loading: Maintenance:	200 mg 100 mg daily	21 days
Systemic candidiasis	Loading: Maintenance:	400 mg 200 mg daily	28 days
Acute cryptococcal meningitis	Loading: Maintenance:	400 mg 200 mg daily	10–12 weeks after cerebrospinal fluid becomes negative
Chronic cryptococcal		200 mg daily	For life, in patient w/HIV infection
Vaginal yeast infection		150 mg	One dose
Prevention of candidiasis		400 mg	Start several days in before the anticipated onset of neutrophil count rises above 1000 cells/mm^3

Source: Ref. 19.

more common in the immunocompromised patient. The overall incidence of patients having cutaneous reactions is less than 9%. Gastrointestinal reactions of highest incidence are nausea (10%) and vomiting (5%). Diarrhea has been reported, with incidence reported at about 3.3% [95]. Hepatic side effects occur in the range of 5%, with abnormalities including increased serum transaminases. Idiosyncratic reactions have been reported, but are much less frequent than that seen with ketoconazole [96]. Most other reactions occur at an incidence of less than 5%, and include headache (a universal side effect of every antifungal), dizziness, peripheral edema, mild hypertension, vomiting, diarrhea, abdominal pain, and pruritus. As noted above, the endocrine problems are much less than with ketoconazole, but some adrenal insufficiency has been reported in patients with very high doses of itraconazole (600 mg per day). Gynecomastia occurs in the higher dose in only 1% of patients, much less than with ketoconazole [96]. Similarly, impotence and decreased libido have been reported with high doses—400 mg per day or more—as well as hypertriglyceridemia and hypokalemia.

D. Drug Interactions

The previously mentioned cytochrome P-450 3A metabolism is a key to the major area of concern with itraconazole therapy. Drug interactions with drug–drug competition for the cytochrome system can result in toxicity, and serious interactions were in the past related to a combination of itraconazole with terfenadine (Sel-

TABLE 3 Cytochrome P-450 Drug Interactions Affecting Antifungals, Especially Imidazoles and Triazoles

Administration of antifungal with	Potential result
Anti-H_1	Astemizole[a]
	Terfenadine[a]
Anti-H_2	Cimetidine[b]
Antacids	Ranitidine[b]
Anti-seizure	Carbamazepine[c]
	Phenobarbital
	Phenytoin
Cisapride	[a]
Cyclosporine	Blood level increased → toxicity
Tacrolimus	Blood level increased → toxicity
Oral contraceptives	? Failure of contraceptives
Lovastatin-HMG COA inhibitors	[d]
Simvastatin-HMG COA inhibitors	[d]
Ethanol	Disulfiram-like activity
Midazolam	[d]
Triazolam	Serious toxicity (sedation)

[a] Cardiac toxicity, potentially fatal (torsade de pointes).
[b] Increased gastric pH → impaired absorption → therapeutic failure.
[c] Increased clearance I → therapeutic failure.
[d] Competes for clearance—results in potential drug toxicity.
Note: Always check pharmaceutical updates as the list has expanded greatly over 2 years.

TABLE 4 Partial List of Drugs Metabolized by Cyp450 3A4—Checklist for Consideration of Antifungal Therapy

Astemizole	Oral hypoglycemics
Carbamazepine	Phenobarbital
Cisapride	Phenytoin
Cyclosporine	Quinidine
Didanosine	Rifampin
Dioxin	Tacrolimus
H_2 receptor blockers	Terfenadine
Isoniazid	Triazolan
Lovastatin	Vincristine
Midazolam	Warfarin
Oral contraceptives	

dane®) or astemizole (Hismanal®); Seldane has since been withdrawn from the market in the United States. The interaction resulted in toxic levels of these antihistamines, with resultant cardiotoxicity. The drug interactions of significance are shown in Tables 2 and 3. As one can see from these tables, the list of potential interactions is very significant and mandates care in selecting patients for itraconazole therapy. This is particularly key with patients who are immunosuppressed related to HIV or organ transplantation. Patients with HIV or organ transplantations are also on a number of other medications, and very great care must be taken with the addition of itraconazole for the treatment of the often extensive tinea or candidiasis seen in these patients. Katz and Gupta have recently published a very useful overview [98]. The pulse approach with Sporanox therapy has been a major step forward in safety and cost. For these patients with onychomycosis or extensive tinea, it allows the use of the drug for 1 week out of the month, maximizing the keratophilic and lipophilic nature of the drug [94]. The binding to keratinized tissue allows a tissue effect for the whole month, while exposure to drug interactions and drug reactions is limited to only 1 week out of the month.

Also, the appropriate antifungal for cost-effective treatment of tinea versicolor still remains to be found. Ketaconazole has had a worldwide usage for this problem and, more recently, the use of itraconazole in short or pulse therapy has proved promising. Tinea versicolor can be extremely extensive and symptomatic in patients in tropical or subtropical climates. Adequate therapy to control this distressing and pruritic disorder still has not received attention and/or acceptance. Hopefully, in the future there will be a better approach to the treatment of tinea versicolor with the use of the imidazoles or possibly the use of terbinafine. Itraconazole, or Sporanox, is rapidly proving to be an extremely effective medication; drug interaction is the only caveat in considering it for therapy.

REFERENCES

1. Brian P. Control of fungal diseases of plants with griseofulvin. Trans St John's Hosp Dermatol Soc 1960; 45: 4–6.
2. Blank H, Roth F Jr, Smith J Jr, et al. The treatment of dermatomycoses with orally administered griseofulvin. Arch Dermatol 1959; 79: 259–266.
3. Brian P, Curtis P, Hemming H, et al. A substance causing abnormal development of fungal hyphae produced by Penicillium janozewskii: I. Biological assay, production and isolation of curing factor. Trans Br Mycol Soc 1946; 29: 173–187.
4. Crounse R. Human pharmacology of griseofulvin: the effect of fat intake on gastrointestinal absorption. J Invest Dermatol 1961; 529–532.
5. Epstein W, Shah V, Riegelman S. Griseofulvin levels in stratum corneum: study after oral administration in man. Arch Dermatol 1972; 106: 344–348.
6. Lesher J Jr, Smith J Jr. Antifungal agents in dermatology. J Am Acad Dermatol 1987; 17: 383–394.

7. Davies R. Griseofulvin. In: Speller DCE, ed. Antifungal Chemotherapy. Chichester: Wiley, 1980: 149–182.
8. Wolverton S, Wilkin J. Systemic Drugs for Skin Diseases. Philadelphia: W. B. Saunders Company, 1991.
9. Foged E, Jepsen L. Hair loss following kerion celsi: a follow-up examination. Mykosen 1984; 27: 411–414.
10. Sehgal V, Abraham G, Gauri-Bazaz M. Griseofulvin therapy in lichen planus: a double-blind controlled study. Br J Dermatol 1972; 87: 383–385.
11. Massa M, Rogers R III. Griseofulvin therapy in lichen planus. Acta Derm Venereol (Stockh) 1981; 61: 547–550.
12. Paget G, Walpole A. Some cytological effects of griseofulvin. Nature 1958; 182: 1320.
13. Lyell A. A review of toxic epidermal necrolysis in Britain. Br J Dermatol 1967; 79: 662–671.
14. Gris-PEG product information. In: Physicians' Desk Reference, 51st ed. Montvale, NJ: Medical Economics, 1997: 477.
15. Cullen S, Catalano P. Griseofulvin-warfarin antagonism. JAMA 1967; 199: 582–583.
16. Riegelman S, Rowland M, Epstein W. Griseofulvin phenobarbital interaction in man. JAMA 1970; 213: 426–431.
17. Van Dijke C, Weber J. Interaction between oral contraceptives and griseofulvin. Br Med J 1984; 288: 1125–1126.
18. Kauffman CA, Carver PL. Use of azoles for systemic antifungal therapy. Adv Pharmacol 1997; 39: 143–189.
19. Lee Y, Goldman M, Vidt D. The role of azole antifungal agents for systemic antifungal therapy. Cleveland Clin J Med 1997; 65: 99–106.
20. Suarez S. New antifungal therapy for children. Advances in Dermatology, Vol. 12. St. Louis: Mosby-Year Book, Inc., 1997.
21. Piérard G, Arrese J, Piérard-Franchimont C. Treatment and prophylaxis of tinea infections. Drugs 1996; 52(2): 209–224.
22. Fernandez-Nava H, Laya-Cuadra B, Tianco E. Comparison of single dose 400 mg versus 10-day 200 mg daily dose ketoconazole in the treatment of tinea versicolor. Int J Dermatol 1997; 36: 64–66.
23. Degreef H, DeDoncker P. Current therapy of dermatophytosis. J Am Acad Dermatol 1994; 31: S25–S30.
24. Kirkpatrick C, Petersen E, Alling D. Treatment of chronic mucocutaneous candidiasis with ketoconazole: preliminary results of a controlled, double-blind clinical trial. Rev Infect Dis 1980; 2: 599.
25. Petersen E, Alling D, Kirkpatrick C. Treatment of chronic mucocutaneous candidiasis with ketoconazole: a controlled clinical trial. Ann Intern Med 1980; 93: 791–795.
26. Jung E, Haas P, Bräutigan M, Weidinger G. Systemic treatment of skin candidosis: a randomized comparison of terbinafine and ketoconazole. Mycoses 1994; 37: 361–365.
27. Symoens J, Moens M, Dom J, et al. An evaluation of two years of clinical experience with ketoconazole. Rev Infect Dis 1980; 2: 674–687.
28. Cox F, Stiller R, South D, et al. Oral ketoconazole for dermatophyte infections. J Am Acad Dermatol 1982; 6: 455–462.

29. Ozgoztasi O, Baydar I. A randomized clinical trial of topical paromomycin versus oral ketoconazole for treating cutaneous leishmaniasis in Turkey. Int J Dermatol 1997; 36: 61–63.
30. Ford G, Ive F, Midgley G. Pityrosporum folliculitis and ketoconazole. Br J Dermatol 1982; 107: 691–695.
31. Jones H. Ketoconazole. In: Fleischmajer R, ed. Progress in Diseases of the Skin, Vol. 2. New York: Grune & Stratton, 1984: 217–249.
32. Wishner A, Teplitz E, Goodman P. Pityrosporum, ketoconazole, and seborrheic dermatitis. J Am Acad Dermatol 1987; 12: 140–141.
33. Ford G, Farr P, Ive F, et al. The response of seborrheic dermatitis to oral ketoconazole. Br J Dermatol 1984; 111: 603–607.
34. Chaban M, Mahler C. Clinical applications of ketoconazole in prostatic cancer. Prog Clin Biol Res 1985; 319–326.
35. Holland F, Fishman L, Bailey J, Fazekas A. Ketoconazole in the management of precocious puberty not responsive to LHRH-analogue therapy. N Engl J Med 1985; 312: 1023–1028.
36. Sonion N, Boscaro M, Merola G, Mantero F. Prolonged treatment of Cushing's disease by ketoconazole. J Clin Endocrinol Metab 1983; 57: 732–736.
37. Isik A, Gökmen O, Zeyneloglu H, Senoz S, Zorlu C. Low dose ketoconazole is an effective and a relatively safe alternative in the treatment of hirsutism. Aust NZ J Obstet Gynaecol 1996; 36: 2: 487–489.
38. Mahler C, Verhelst J, Denis J. Ketoconazole and liarozole in the treatment of advanced prostatic cancer. Cancer Suppl 1993; 71(3): 1068–1073.
39. Segal R, Trattner A, Alteras I, Ingber A, David M, Sandbank M. Once-weekly treatment with oral ketoconazole for superficial fungal infections. J Am Acad Dermatol 1993; 1: 126–127.
40. Borrelli D, Jacobs P, Nall L. Tinea versicolor: epidemiologic, clinical and therapeutic aspects. J Am Acad Dermatol 1991; 25: 300–305.
41. Chien R, Yang L, Lin P, Liaw Y. Hepatic injury during ketoconazole therapy in patients with onychomycosis: a controlled cohort study. Hepatology 1997; 25(1): 103–107.
42. González-Delgado P, Florido-Lopez F, Saenz de San Pedro B, Cuevas-Agusti M, Marin-Pozo J. Hypersensitivity to ketoconazole. Ann Allergy 1994; 73: 326–328.
43. Martindale W. The Extra Pharmacopoeia, 29th ed. London: The Pharmaceutical Press, 1989: 419.
44. Fisch R, Lahad A. Adverse psychiatric reaction to ketoconazole. Am J Psychiatry 1989; 146: 939–940. [Letter]
45. Hanash K. Neurologic complications of ketoconazole therapy for advanced prostate cancer. Urology 1989; 33: 466–467.
46. Finkelstein E, Amichai B, Halevy S. Paranoid delusions caused by ketoconazole. Int J Dermatol 1996; 35(1): 75. [Letter]
47. Chan-Tompkins NH, et al. Cardiac arrhythmias associated with coadministration of azole compounds and cisapride. Clin Infect Dis 1997; 24(6): 1285.
48. Tsai W, Tsai L, Chen J. Combined use of astemizole and ketoconazole resulting in torsade de pointes. J Formos Med Assoc 1997; 96(2): 144–146.

49. Thompson D, Oster G. Use of terfenadine and contraindicated drugs. JAMA 1996; 275(17): 1339–1341.
50. Perfect J, Lindsay M, Drew R. Adverse drug reactions to systemic antifungals. Prevention and management. Drug Saf 1992; 7(5): 323–363.
51. Polsen J, Cohen P, Sella A. Acquired cutaneous adherence in patients with androgen-independent prostate cancer receiving ketoconazole and doxorubicin: medication-induced sticky skin. J Am Acad Dermatol 1995; 32: 571–575.
52. Como JA, Dismukes WE. Oral azole drugs as systemic antifungal therapy. N Engl J Med 1994; 330: 263–272.
53. Kauffman CA, Carver PL. Antifungals in the 1990s. Drugs 1997; 53(4): 539–549.
54. Shaw JTB, Tarbit MH, Troke PF. Cytochrome P-450 mediated sterol synthesis and metabolism; differences in sensitivity to fluconazole and other azoles. Barcelona: J. R. Prous Science Publishers, 1987.
55. Grant SM, Clissold SP. Fluconazole: a review of its pharmacodynamic and pharmakinetic properties, and therapeutic potential in superficial and systemic mycoses. Drugs 1990; 39: 877–916.
56. Faergemann J, Godleski J, Laufen H, Liss R. Intracutaneous transport of orally administered fluconazole to the stratum corneum. Acta Derm Venereol (Stockh) 1995; 75: 361–363.
57. Faergemann J, Laufen H. Levels of fluconazole in serum, stratum corneum, epidermis (without stratum corneum) and eccrine sweat. Clin Exp Dermatol 1993; 18: 102–106.
58. Faergemann J, Laufen H. Levels of fluconazole in normal and diseased nails during and after treatment of onychomycoses in toe-nails with fluconazole 150 mg once weekly. Acta Dermatol Venerol (Stockh) 1996; 76: 219–221.
59. Montero-Gei F, Robles-Soto M, Schlager H. Fluconazole in the treatment of severe onychomycosis. Int J Dermatol 1996; 35: 587–588.
60. Assaf R, Elewski B. Intermittent fluconazole dosing in patients with onychomycosis: results of a pilot study. J Am Acad Dermatol 1996; 35: 216–219.
61. Wildfeuer A, Seidl H. Comparison of the in vitro activity of fluconazole against *Candida albicans* and Dermatophytes. Drugs Res 1995; 45: 819–821.
62. Laguna F, Rodríguez-Tudela J, Martínez-Suárez J, Polo R, Valencia E, Diaz-Guerra T, Dronda F, Pulido F. Patterns of fluconazole susceptibility in isolates from human immunodeficiency virus-infected patients with oropharyngeal candidiasis due to *Candida albicans*. Clin Infect Dis 1997; 24: 124–130.
63. Marchisio P, Principi N. Treatment of oropharyngeal candidiasis in HIV-infected children with oral fluconazole. Am J Clin Microbiol Infect Dis 1994; 13: 338–340.
64. Venkateswarlu K, Denning D, Manning N, Kelly S. Resistance to fluconazole in *Candida albicans* from AIDS patients correlated with reduced intracellular accumulation of drug. FEMS Microbiol Lett 1995; 131: 337–341.
65. Goa K, Barradell. Fluconazole. Drugs 1995; 50: 658–690.
66. Chodorowska G, Lecewicz-Torún B. Long-term observation of a case of cutaneous blastomycosis in Poland treated with fluconazole. Mycoses 1996; 39: 283–287.
67. Yoshida M, Hiruma M, Tezuka T. A case of sporotrichosis treated successfully with oral fluconazole 200 mg once weekly. Mycoses 1994; 37: 281–283.

68. Kauffman C, Pappas P, McKinsey D, Greefield R, Perfect J, Cloud G, Thomas C, Dismukes W, and the national Institute of Allergy and Infectious Diseases Mycoses Study Group. Treatment of lymphocutaneous and visceral sporotrichosis with fluconazole. Clin Infect Dis 1996; 22: 46–50.
69. Yang S, Liu C, Cheng N, Lee W, Liu C, Kuo B. Successful treatment of subcutaneous mycoses with fluconazole: a report of two cases. Clin Med J 1995; 56: 432–435.
70. Gugnani H, Ezeanolue B, Khalil M, Amoah C, Ajuiu E, Oyewo E. Fluconazole in the therapy of tropical deep mycoses. Mycoses 1995; 38: 485–488.
71. Kim S, Suh K, Chae Y, Kim Y. Successful treatment with fluconazole of protothecosis developing at the site of an intralesional corticosteroid injection. Br J Dermatol 1996; 135: 803–806.
72. Faergemann J. Treatment of pityriasis versicolor with a single dose of fluconazole. Acta Dermatol Venereol (Stockh) 1992; 72: 74–75.
73. Goodman JL, Winston DJ, Greenfield RA, et al. A controlled trial of fluconazole to prevent fungal infections in patients undergoing bone marrow transplantation. N Engl J Med 1992; 326: 845–851.
74. Slavin MA, Osborne B, Adams R, et al. Efficacy and safety of fluconazole prophylaxis for fungal infections after marrow transplantation—a prospective, randomized, double-blind study. Clin Infect Dis 1995; 171: 1545–1552.
75. Kalivas J. Thrombocytopenia caused by fluconazole. J Am Acad Dermatol 1996; 35:284. [Letter]
76. Morrison R, Wan J, Dorko C. A fluconazole/amitriptyline drug interaction in three male adults. Clin Infect Dis 1997; 24: 270–271. [Letter]
77. Leyden J. Pharmacokinetics and pharmacology of terbinafine and itraconazole. J Am Acad Dermatol 1998; 38: S42–47.
78. Package insert—Novartis Corp.
79. Hazen K. Fungicidal versus fungistatic activity of terbinafine and itraconazole: an in vitro comparison. J Am Acad Dermatol 1998; 38: S37–41.
80. Faergemann J, et al. Acta Dermatol Venerol (Stockh) 1990; 71: 322–326.
81. Evans EL, Sigurgeirsson B, Billstein S, et al. A double blind randomized study comparing cutaneous terbinafine with intermittent itraconazole for the treatment of toenail onychomycosis. Lion Study Group 1998 (data provided by Novartis).
82. Cambon N, Perez A, Ryder N. The therapeutic potential for terbinafine in subcutaneous and systemic mycoses. Poster presentation, European Academy of Dermatology and Venereology. Nice, France, October 6–11, 1998.
83. Dwyer C, White M, Sinclair T. Cholestatic jaundice due to terbinafine. Br J Dermatol 1997; 136: 976–977.
84. Gupta AJ. Cutaneous adverse effects with terbinafine therapy. Br J Dermatol 1998; 138: 529–532.
85. Lowe G, Green C, Jennings P. Hepatitis associated with terbinafine treatment. Br Med J 1993; 306: 248
86. Katz H. Systemic antifungal agents used to treat onychomycosis. J Am Acad Dermatol 1998; 38: 548–551.
87. Gupta A, DeDoncker P, Scher R. Itraconazole for the treatment of onychomycosis. Int J Dermatol 1998; 37: 303–308.

88. Heykants J, Van Peer A, Van de Volde V, et al. The clinical pharmacokinetics of itraconazole: an overview. Mycoses 1989; 32: 567–587.
89. De Doncker P, Seher R, Baran R, et al. Itraconazole Therapy is effective for Pedal onychomycosis caused by some nondermatophyte molds and in mixed infection wit dermatophytes and molds: a multicenter study with 36 patients. J Am Acad Dermatol 1997; 36: 173–177.
90. Sporanox—Drug information, Physicians Desk Reference, 1999.
91. Lange D, Hardin-Pava J, Wu J, et al. The effect of cola beverages on the bioavailability of itraconazole in the presence of H2 blockers. J Clin Pharmacol 1997; 37: 535–540.
92. Katsambas A, Antonion C, Frangoli E, et al. Itraconazole in the treatment of tinea corporis and tinea cruris. Clin Exp Dermatol 1993; 18: 322–325.
93. Gupta A, De Doncker P. Intermittent itraconazole is effective in the treatment of Majocchis granuloma: a clinical and pharmacokinetic evaluation and implications for possible effectiveness in tinea capitis. Clin Exp Dermatol 1998; 23: 103–108.
94. Gupta A, Alexis M, Rabaabee N, et al. Itraconazole pulse therapy is effective in the treatment of tinea capitis in children: an open multi-center study. Br J Dermatol 1997; 137: 251–254.
95. Package insert information—Itraconazole (Sporanox®), Janssen Pharmaceutica, 1995.
96. Lavrijeen A, Balmus K, Nugteren-Huying W, et al. Hepatic injury associated with itraconazole. Lancet 1992; 340: 252–253.
97. Sharkey P, Rinaldi M, Dunn J, et al. High dose itraconazole in the treatment of severe mycosis. Antimicrob Agents Chemother 1991; 35: 707–713.
98. Katz H, Gupta A. Oral antifungal drug interactions. Dermatol Clin 1997; 15: 535–544.
99. de Doncker P, Decroix J, Pierard G, et al. Antifungal pulse therapy in onychomycosis: a pharmacokinetic/pharmacodynamic investigation of monthly cycles on 1 week pulse with itraconazole. Arch Dermatol 1996; 132: 34–41.
100. Hickman J. A double-blind randomized, placebo-controlled evaluation of short term treatment with oral itraconazole in patients with tinea versicolor. J Am Acad Dermatol 1996; 34: 785–787.

5

Nonsteroidal Anti-Inflammatory Drugs and Topical Anti-Inflammatory Agents

Glenn Russo
Tulane University School of Medicine
New Orleans, Louisiana

I. NONSTEROIDAL ANTI-INFLAMMATORY DRUGS

Nonsteroidal anti-inflammatory drugs (NSAIDS) are a group of drugs that inhibit cyclooxygenase and/or lipoxygenase in the metabolic pathway from arachidonic acid to the production of prostaglandins or leukotrienes [1]. Mechanisms in which these agents may decrease inflammation may involve decreasing chemotactic stimuli to leukocytes and stabilizing lysosomes so that there is decreased release of lysosomal enzymes. By inhibiting cyclooxygenase, there may be decreased production of superoxide, which can become an hydroxyl free radical. Both superoxide and hydroxyl free radicals are oxidizing agents that can easily produce tissue damage [2]. Some NSAIDS, such as indomethacin, inhibit phosphodiesterase, which produces an increase in intracellular cAMP. Increased cAMP is known to stabilize cellular lysosomal membranes and thus causes a decrease in the release of tissue-damaging lysosomal enzymes [2].

A. Aspirin (Acetylsalicylic Acid)

Aspirin is still the most widely used NSAID. It irreversibly inhibits the production of prostaglandins by inactivating cyclooxygenase [2]. Aspirin is an acetylated salicylate, which is rapidly absorbed from the upper small intestine. A peak serum value is reached in about 2 h, with a plasma half-life of 15 min. Aspirin is distributed in most body tissues and crosses both the blood–brain and placental barriers [3]. Aspirin in itself is biologically active and does not have to be hydrolyzed to salicylic acid to be effective. It is excreted by the kidney.

Aspirin is 80 to 90% bound to plasma proteins, especially albumin. Therefore, it competes with other substances for binding sites on albumin. Some of these competitors include phenytoin, penicillin, bilirubin, tryptophan, sulfampyrazone, thiopental, and thyroxine [3].

Symptoms of salicylism or aspirin toxicity include headache, tinnitus, dimmed vision, sweating, thirst, nausea, vomiting, and, occasionally, diarrhea. Central nervous system symptoms also occur, including: drowsiness, lassitude, and confusion. Aspirin hypersensitivity syndrome is a severe and sometimes fatal disorder that usually occurs in middle-aged females with a history of asthma and nasal polyps. This reaction occurs within minutes of oral aspirin ingestion and presents with vasomotor rhinitis, urticaria, angioedema, asthmatic attack, and even shock with vasomotor collapse. It should be treated immediately with epinephrine and other well-known medications used for anaphylactic shock [3]. Patients allergic to aspirin may also have hypersensitivity to the food additive tartrazine.

1. Dermatologic Uses

Aspirin, along with bedrest, has long been used in the treatment of erythema nodosum. The usual dosage is two enterically coated aspirin tablets p.o. t.i.d. If no response, dosage may be increased to two tablets p.o. q.i.d. Erythromelalgia can also be treated with aspirin with relief of the burning sensation occurring with as little as one 325-mg tablet per day. This effect has been reported to last sometimes as long as several days from just one tablet [4]. The flushing and warmth sensations that occur while taking niacin can often be curtailed by taking one 325-mg aspirin tablet 30 min before ingesting niacin [5]. Aspirin has also been reported to be effective in the treatment of atrophie blanche. As little as 80 mg of aspirin p.o. b.i.d. and 25 mg dipyridamole p.o. t.i.d. has been successful in treating childhood atrophie blanche [6].

Aspirin has long been known to be effective in reducing the erythema associated with UVB exposure [7]. It should generally be taken several hours before the UVB exposure at a dosage of three to four tablets with food. In patients with polycythemia vera, it has been demonstrated that aspirin in a dosage of 300 mg p.o. b.i.d. or 300 mg 1 h before bath may relieve the pruritus that is characteristically associated with this disorder [8]. It is believed that aspirin reduces the production of prostaglandins in the mast cells which are increased in number in polycythemia vera [8].

Pressure urticaria has also been reported to be improved by aspirin. When patients were given 3900 mg of aspirin in four divided doses for 3 days, the painful pressure lesions were relieved, but not the urticaria [9]. Nonimmunological contact urticaria has also shown improvement when two doses of 1000 mg of aspirin were given a few hours before exposure to contactants. However, dimethylsulfoxide (DMSO) contact urticaria is not affected by aspirin [10].

Table 1 Dermatologic Uses of Aspirin

Erythema nodosum
Erythromelalgia
Niacin-induced flushing
Atrophie blanche
Inflammatory response from UV light
Polycythemia-vera-induced pruritus
Nonimmunological contact urticaria
Necrobiosis lipoidica
Systemic lupus erythematosus
Relapsing polychondritis

Aspirin has also been advocated as therapy for cases of necrobiosis lipoidica [11]. The recommended dosage ranges from 1.5 to 4.5 g per day over a period of a few months. Some systemic lupus erythematosus patients with fatigue, skin eruption, arthritis, fever, or sinusitis have benefited by the use of aspirin in a dosage ranging from 3 to 6 g per day [12]. A few cases of relapsing polychondritis have shown a good response to aspirin [13] (Table 1).

B. Indomethacin

Indomethacin is a NSAID of the indolacetate class. It is a very potent inhibitor of cyclooxygenase and also inhibits neutrophil motility. Indomethacin also decreases the biosynthesis of mucopolysaccharides by uncoupling oxidative phosphorylation [3]. It is rapidly absorbed in the upper gastrointestinal tract. It is metabolized in the liver through demethylation and deacetylation [2]. Ten to twenty percent of the oral dose is excreted unchanged in the urine.

It should be kept in mind that persons who are allergic to aspirin may exhibit cross-reactivity with indomethacin. Indomethacin should be avoided in patients who have a history of gastrointestinal ulceration, since gastrointestinal upset is one of its main side effects [3,2]. Indomethacin can antagonize the naturetic effect of furosemide. Therefore, concominant administration of both of these drugs should be avoided [3]. Probenecid can inhibit the renal excretion of indomethacin and thus increase its serum levels [14].

Indomethacin should be avoided during pregnancy and nursing. It should also be avoided by patients with a history of epilepsy, parkinsonism, or other neurological disorders, as well as in patients who work with machinery [3].

1. Side Effects

The most prominent side effect of indomethacin is gastrointestional upset. Headaches, dizziness, depression, psychosis, hallucinations, and suicide have been reported with indomethacin use [3]. Corneal deposits and toxically induced hepatitis have also been reported [15,16]. Transient elevation in BUN and creatinine with acute oliguric renal failure may also occur [17]. There have also been reports in the literature of neutropenia, thrombocytopenia, and, very rarely, aplastic anemia. Hypersensitivity reactions ranging from skin eruption, urticaria, and asthmatic attack have also been associated with indomethacin use [3].

2. Dermatologic Uses

Indomethacin is considered a first-line therapy, like aspirin, in the treatment of erythema nodosum. The usual recommended dosage ranges from 100 to 150 mg per day. It has also been reported to be of benefit in urticarial vasculitis and delayed pressure urticaria [18,9]. In urticarial vasculitis, indomethacin can be given 25 mg p.o. t.i.d. or 50 mg p.o. q.i.d. for 17 days [18]. As with aspirin, indomethacin has been demonstrated to be effective in reducing the burning effects of UVB, UVA, and PUVA [19–21].

Recently, indomethacin has been shown to be very effective in the treatment of Sweet's syndrome. In a study of 18 patients, 17 were successfully treated with indomethacin [22]. The regimen consisted of an initial week of 150 mg indomethacin p.o. per day, followed by 2 weeks of 100 mg per day. Within 48 h, fever and arthralgia were markedly decreased and skin lesions cleared within 1 to 2 weeks of therapy [22].

Indomethacin farnesil is an ester and prodrug of indomethacin. Indomethacin farnesil releases indomethacin into inflamed tissue. It is currently available in Japan [23], where it has been used in the treatment of recalcitrant angiolymphoid hyperplasia at a dosage of 400 mg p.o. b.i.d. In one report, erythema and itching of lesions began to decrease and lesion size was significantly reduced after just 2 days and peripheral eosinophilia was resolved after 1 month of therapy [24]. After 4 months of therapy the lesions were resolved (Tables 2 and 3).

C. Other Oral NSAIDS

Nimesulide is available in Italy and has been reported to be effective in Hallopeau's acrodermatitis continua of the nail. A dosage of 200 mg p.o. once per day produced significant reduction in inflammation and pain within a few days. If

TABLE 2 Monitoring NSAIDS

1. BUN, creatinine—aspirin, indomethacin
2. Liver function tests—rarely elevated with indomethacin
3. Observe for signs of salicylism with aspirin—headache, tinnitus, CNS symptoms, sweating, thirst

Table 3 Dermatologic Uses of Indomethacin

Erythema nodosum
Urticarial vasculitis
Delayed pressure urticaria
Inflammatory response to UV light
Sweet's syndrome
Indomethacin farnesil:
Angiolymphoid hyperplasia with eosinophilia

nimesulide is used for a long period of time, it can produce longer periods of remission [25].

II. TOPICAL ANTI-INFLAMMATORY AGENTS

A. Topical Doxepin (Zonalon cream)

One of the newest topical agents indicated for pruritus in some eczematous skin conditions is doxepin 5% cream. Doxepin hydrochloride is a dibenzoxepin tricyclic antidepressant with potent H_1 and H_2 antihistamine effects [26], as well as anticholinergic effects [27]. Doxepin is hepatically metabolized to its active form desmethyldoxepin. It then undergoes further glucuronidation and is excreted in the urine [27].

Zonalon cream is contraindicated in patients with narrow angle glaucoma and urinary retention because of its anticholinergic effects. Patients taking monoamine oxidase inhibitors should not use Zonalon cream because of its possible systemic antidepressant effects. Cimetidine should also be avoided because it has been reported to cause wide fluctuations in the serum concentration of tricyclic antidepressants [27]. Alcohol intake while using Zonalon cream can create possible additive sedation. Doxepin is metabolized by the hepatic P450 enzyme system; therefore, dosage of other drugs metabolized by that system, if given concomitantly, may need to be lowered [27].

1. Side Effects

The most common side effects of Zonalon cream include stinging at application site (21%), drowsiness (16%), and dry mouth (5%) [28]. Drowsiness is seen especially in patients covering more than 10% of their body surface area with Zonalon cream [27].

2. Dermatologic Uses

A recent study has demonstrated that Zonalon cream can significantly reduce the pruritus seen in nummular eczema, lichen simplex chronicus, and contact dermatitis. It was well tolerated and produced a significant decrease in pruritus within 24 h after beginning use [28]. A thin layer should be applied to affected areas four times daily, with at least 3 to 4 h between each application; however, most patients generally get relief with just b.i.d. application [27,28].

B. Coal Tar

An old topical agent for anti-inflammatory use in dermatoses is crude coal tar, a compound of over 10,000 different hydrocarbons [29]. Some studies propose that it has an inhibitory effect on DNA synthesis, which would explain its effect in psoriasis [30]. One of its main adverse reactions is that it is known to cause phototoxic reactions [31].

Coal tar can be mixed with petrolatum in various concentrations, mainly 1 to 5% for topical therapy of psoriasis plaques. It is commonly applied before bedtime and washed off in the morning or 1 h before UVB treatment of psoriasis plaques. Over-the-counter tar preparations are in the form of gels, creams, and bath solutions. Coal tar in very high concentrations, such as technical grade crude, can be obtained from chemical companies. It can be applied to the palmar and plantar surfaces in patients with severe keratoderma. One can occlude the tar with Telfa pads and gauze dressings overnight and wash it off in the morning.

C. Ichthammol (Shale Tar)

Ichthammol is a type of shale oil that is rich in sulfur. It has been used for severe eczema in the past and is still in use today. The exact mechanism of action is unknown. However, it is hypothesized that ichthammol has both anti-inflammatory and vasoactive properties. In comparison to coal tar, ichthammol is less irritating and less photosensitizing [31].

Ichthammol 5% in Lassar's paste (a mixture of salicylic acid, zinc oxide, starch, and white soft paraffin) can be applied to severely pruritic areas of the body that are very lichenified or to very thick, indurated plaques of psoriasis. Since this mixture is very thick it is applied and wrapped with gauze and left in place for 2 to 3 days. If the plaques are weeping, the dressing and paste can be changed every day. In essence, this ichthammol mixture can be thought of as an ''Unna boot'' for the treatment of very pruritic plaques of chronic eczema, lichen simplex chronicus, and recalcitrant thickened plaques of psoriasis (Table 4).

D. Bufexamac (Parfenac)

In Europe, bufexamac (*p*-butoxcyphenylacethydroxine acid) is a topical NSAID, licensed for use in ezcema, dermatitis, and perianal pruritus [32]. Bufexamac has some UVA protection properties [33].

TABLE 4 Dermatologic Uses for Topical NSAIDS

Doxepin (Zonalon cream)
Pruritus of nummular eczema, contact dermatitis, and lichen simplex chronicus
Coal tar
Plaque-type psoriasis
Severe palmar–plantar keratoderma
Ichthammol
Pruritus of chronic eczema, lichen simplex chronicus, recalcitrant psoriasis plaques

REFERENCES

1. Greaves MW. Pharmacology and significance of non-steroidal anti-inflammatory drugs in the treatment of skin diseases. J Am Acad Dermatol 1987;16:751–764.
2. Simon LS, Mills JA. Non-steroidal antiinflammatory drugs (Part 1 of 2). N Engl J Med 1980;302(21):1179–1185.
3. Flowers RJ, Moncada S, Vane JR. Analgesic-antipyretic anti-inflammatory agents. In: Goodman LS and Gilman A, eds. The Pharmacologic Basis of Therapeutics, 6th ed. New York: Macmillan, 1980: 688–697.
4. Kurzrock R, Cohen PR. Erythromelalgia and myeloproliferative disorders. Arch Intern Med 1989;149:105–109.
5. Whelan AM, Price SO, Fowler SF, Hainar BL. The effect of aspirin on niacin-induced cutaneous reactions. J Fam Med 1992;34(2):165–168.
6. Suarez SM, Paller AS. Atrophie blanche onset in childhood. J Ped 1993;123:753–755.
7. Miller WS, Ruderman FR, Smith JG. Aspirin and ultraviolet light induced erythema in man. Arch Dermatol 1967;95:357–358.
8. Jackson N, Burt D, Croches J, et al. Skin mast cells in polycythemia vera: Relationship to the pathogenesis and treatment of pruritus. Br J Dermatol 1987;116:21–29.
9. Sussman GL, Harvey RP, Schocket AL. Delayed pressure urticaria. J Allergy Clin Immunol 1982;70:337–342.
10. Lahti A, Väänänen A, Kokkonen EL, Hannuksela M. Acetylsalicylic acid inhibits nonimmunologic contact urticaria. Contact Dermatitis 1987;16:133–135.
11. Unge G, Tornline G: Treatment of diabetic necrobiosis with aspirin or dipyridamole. N Engl J Med 1978;299:1366.
12. Schur PH. The clinical management of systemic lupus erythematosus. In: Decker JL, ed. Systemic Lupus Erythematosus Management. New York: Grune and Stratton, 1983:259–281.
13. McAdam LP, O'Hanlan MA, Bluestone R, Pearson CM. Relapsing polychondritis: Prospective study of 23 patients and a review of the literature. Medicine 1976;55: 193–215.
14. Brooks PM, Bell MA, Sturock RD, Famaey JP, et al. The clinical significance of indomethacin-probenecid interaction. Br J Clin Pharmacol 1974;1:287–288.

15. Burns CA. Indomethacin reduced retinal sensitivity, and corneal deposits. Am J Ophthalmol 1968;66:825–835.
16. Huskissa EC. Antiiinflammatory drugs. Semin Arthritis Rheum 1977;7:1–20.
17. Walshe JJ, Venuto RC. Acute oliguric renal failure induced by indomethacin: possible mechanism. Ann Intern Med 1979;91:47–49.
18. Millns JL, Randle HW, Solley GO, Dicken CH. The therapeutic response of urticarial vasculitis to indomethacin. J Am Acad Dermatol 1983;3:349–355.
19. Kobra-Black A, Greaves MV, Hensly CN, et al. Effects of indomethacin on prostaglandins E_2, F_2 alpha and arachidonic acid in human skin 24 hours after UV-B and UV-C irradiation. Br J Clin Pharmacol 1978;6:261–266.
20. Sondergaard J, Bisgaard H, Thossen S. Eicosanoids in skin UV inflammation. Photo Dermatol 1985;3:359–366.
21. Imodaka G, Tejima T. A possible role of prostaglandins in PUVA-induced inflammation: Implication by organ cultured skin. J Invest Dermatol 1989;92:296–300.
22. Jeanfils S, Joly P, Young P, Le-Corvaisier-Pieto C, Thormine E, et al. Indomethacin treatment of eighteen patients with Sweet's syndrome. J Am Acad Dermatol 1997; 36:436–439.
23. Kobayashi S, Hashida R, Shirota H, et al. Effect of E-0710, a farnesyl ester of indomethacin, on rat synovial cell prostaglandin production in culture. Drug Exp Clin Res 1984;10:845–851.
24. Nomura K, Sasaki C, Murai T, Mitsuhashi Y, et al. Angiolymphoid hyperplasia with eosinophilia: successful treatment with indomethacin farnesil. Br J Dermatol 1996; 134:189–190.
25. Piraccini BM, Fanti PA, Morelli R, Tosti A. Hallopeau's acrodermatitis continua of the nail apparatus: A clinical and pathological study of 20 patients. Acta Dermatol Venereol (Stockh) 1994;74:65–67.
26. Richelson E. Tricyclic antidepressants and histamine H_1 receptors. Mayo Clin Proc 1979;54:669–674.
27. Arkey R, ed. Physicians Desk Reference, 51st ed. Montvale, NJ: Medical Economics Company, Inc., 1997:1042–1043.
28. Drake LA, Millikan LE, and the Doxepin Study Group. The antipruritic effect of 5% doxepin cream in patients with eczematous dermatitis. Arch Dermatol 1995;131: 1403–1408.
29. Frank HG. Coal tar constituents. Indus Eng Chem 1963;55:38.
30. Lowe NL, Breeding JH, Wortzman MS. New coal tar extract and coal tar shampoos: Evaluation by epidermal cell DNA synthesis suppression assay. Arch Dermatol 1982;118:487–489.
31. Kaidby KH, Kligman AM. Clinical and histological study of coal tar photosensitivity in humans. Arch Dermatol 1977;113:592–593.
32. Brogden RN, Pinder RM, Sawyer PR, Speight TM et al. Bufexamac: A review of its pharmacological properties and therapeutic efficacy in inflammatory dermatoses. Drugs 1975;10:351–356.
33. Tong AKF, Vickers CFH. Topical Noncosticorteroid Therapy. In: Fitzpatrick TB, ed. *Dermatology in General Medicine*, 4th ed. New York: McGraw-Hill, Inc., 1993: 2852.

6

Cytotoxic and Immunosuppressive Drugs in Dermatology

Giuseppe Hautmann, Grazia Campanile, Ilaria Ghersetich, and Torello Lotti
University of Florence
Florence, Italy

Chemotherapeutic agents of various origins that inhibit the proliferation of cells are called cytostatics. Depending on their point of attack, they may either selectively block individual phases of the cell cycle or disturb cell metabolism in a nonspecific manner. All cytostatics are toxic to healthy body cells, especially to rapidly proliferating tissues (e.g., bone marrow, the epithelium of the small intestine, hair matrix, and testicular tubules). Consequently, the physician must be well aware of the actions and side effects of the individual preparations and dosages must be established case by case and adjusted according to circumstances.

Cytostatics are usually classified according to their method of action and/or origin: (1) alkylating agents; (2) antimetabolites; (3) vinca alkaloids; (4) antibiotics; (5) other.

The active groups of *alkylating agents* react with (alkylate) DNA and disturb its replication in the S-phase of the cell cycle long term. These cytotoxic drugs include cyclophosphamide, chlorambucil, busulfan, and melphalan, and are used, often in combination with other cytostatics and glucocorticosteroids, for malignant cutaneous lymphomas (mycosis fungoides), hystiocytosis X, and autoimmune diseases such as pemphigus vulgaris, bullous pemphigoid, Wegener's granulomatosis, and systemic lupus erythematosus.

Antimetabolites selectively inhibit DNA synthesis in the S-phase by blocking the binding sites of normal metabolites and causing the formation of defective molecules. One of the most commonly administered metabolites, methotrexate, acts as an antagonist to folic acid, which is necessary for DNA synthesis and cannot be processed further when displaced from its enzyme dehydrofolate reductase. Until just a few years ago, it was widely used in bullous dermatoses, dermatomyositis, Reiter's disease, and, with restrictions, in severe forms of psoriasis and psoriatic arthritis. Another important antimetabolite is azathioprine, a mercaptopurine that is incorporated as a false purine base in DNA which is then inactivated. Cytosine arabinoside and 5-fluorouracil also belong to the antimetabolite group.

The group of *vinca alkaloids* includes vincristine and vinblastine, which act in the metaphase of mitosis, disturbing spindle formation. They are indicated mainly for malignant lymphomas, Kaposi's sarcoma, and histiocytosis X.

Certain *antibiotics* may also exercise powerful cytostatic action, e.g., actinomycin D, bleomycin, and adriamycin, which block the synthesis of DNA, RNA, or protein in different phases. Cyclosporin A belongs to this group.

Finally, the *other* important cytostatic agents include cisplatin, hydroxyurea, hydroxycarbamide, DTIC, procarbazine, and ifosfamide.

As a result of their effects on proliferation and/or protein synthesis, all cytostatics also have immunosuppressive effects. In cytostatic tumor therapy, this leads to the unwanted side effect of weakening the patient's defense against infectious microorganisms and probably also to the development of additional malignant tumors or systemic diseases. On the other hand, immunosuppression can be usefully employed in the treatment of autoimmune diseases. Azathioprine, cyclophosphamide, and methotrexate are particularly useful in the treatment of certain recalcitrant dermatoses. Cyclosporin A is one of the most important immunosuppressive agents.

Dermatologists are often required to prescribe cytotoxic/cytostatic and immunosuppressive agents for the treatment of serious or recalcitrant dermatoses. The most common cytotoxic/cytostatic and immunosuppressive agents currently used in dermatology are: cyclosporin A, azathioprine, cyclophosphamide, chlorambucil, methotrexate, hydroxyurea, 5-fluorouracil, and interferons.

I. CYCLOSPORINE

Cyclosporin A (CsA) was introduced for clinical use in 1978, primarily for the prevention and treatment of organ transplant reaction and graft-versus-host disease, but it has been shown to be useful in the treatment of many dermatological and autoimmune diseases. CsA is a cyclic polypeptide made up of 11 amino acids. It mainly acts on T helper cells by blocking the cell cycle in phase G0 or early G1 and inhibits production of several lymphokines, particularly interleukin-2 and interferon-γ, which are known to be important in the activation of T cells, macrophages, monocytes, and keratinocytes. It has little effect on T suppressor cells, but it does have some effects on T-cell–dependent B-cell function. CsA may also exercise some direct effects on DNA synthesis and proliferation of keratinocytes [1].

CsA is usually administered orally and it is employed primarily as an immunosuppressive agent. About 30% of the ingested drug is adsorbed slowly from the gut. CsA is metabolized in the liver by the cytochrome P-450 system and its metabolites are excreted in the bile. Therefore, dosage adjustments are required within the presence of hepatic failure or with drugs interfering with cytochrome P-450 system activity. The newer formulation (Neoval®) has a more consistent and better absorption profit.

CsA can cause functional and structural changes in the kidneys that are believed to be related to dose and duration of therapy [2,3]. At high doses (>8 mg/kg/day), acute renal failure, acute tubular necrosis, or a hemolytic–uremic syndrome may occur. At the low doses generally used in dermatology, CsA may cause chronic progressive renal insufficiency manifested by a gradual elevation of serum creatinine and blood urea nitrogen. The impairment of renal function is usually reversible with dose reduction or cessation of therapy. In approximately 10% of patients, arterial hypertension may occur; this is dose-related and more common in older subjects and in those with preexisting hypertension or renal disease. Persistent hypertension can increase the nephrotoxic risk of CsA and should be managed by dose reduction or the use of calcium channel blockers. As mentioned above, the effects of CsA on renal tubules may also lead to electrolyte and metabolic disturbances, with hyperkalemia, hypomagnesemia, and hyperuricemia; with low-dose CsA therapy, these abnormalities are usually mild and do not require treatment, but patients should avoid the use of potassium-sparing diuretics.

Finally, hand tremors, paresthesias, gingival hyperplasia, hypertrichosis, and elevation of bilirubin and liver transminases with malaise, fatigue, and myalgia have been reported during the early stages of CsA therapy [4]. Thus patients with renal insufficiency, active severe infection, primary or secondary immunodeficiency, previous or concomitant malignancies, uncontrolled hypertension, or drug or alcohol abuse are not candidates for CsA therapy unless the presumed benefit outweighs the potential risks. Caution should be exercised in subjects exposed to concomitant nephrotoxic drugs, cytotoxic-immunosuppressive drugs, or drugs that may interact with CsA (Table 1).

CsA has been used to treat a variety of dermatoses and autoimmune diseases. The efficacy of this drug in the treatment of psoriasis is well established by several studies [5–7]; it is effective in plaque-type as well as erythrodermic [8] and pustular psoriasis [9,10]. It is also beneficial in cases of psoriatic arthritis [11]. Response is usually seen within 1 month of treatment at recommended doses of 3 to 5 mg/kg/day. The starting dose is usually 3 mg/kg/day, taken either as a single daily dose or as two divided doses. If improvement of disease does not occur within 2 to 4 weeks, the CsA can be increased by 0.5 to 1.0 mg/kg/day,

Table 1 Drug Interactions with Cyclosporine

Drugs that increase CsA concentration
Antibiotics (erythromycin, doxycycline)
Antifungals (ketoconazole, itraconazole, fluconazole)
Calcium-channel blockers (nicardipine, verapamil, diltiazem)
Diuretics (furosemide, thiazides)
Steroid hormones (oral contraceptives, corticosteroids)
Drugs that increase CsA concentration (clinical significance unknown)
Acetazolamide
Colchicine
Ethanol
H_2-antihistamines
Quinolones
Warfarin
Drugs that decrease CsA concentration
Antibiotics (rifampin, iv sulphonamide/trimethoprim)
Anticonvulsants (carbamazepine, phenobarbital, phenytoin)
Drugs that enhance nephrotoxicity
Aminoglycosides
Amphotericin B
Cotrimoxazole/trimethoprim
Nonsteroidal anti-inflammatory drugs

but should not exceed 5 mg/kg/day. With improvement in the skin condition, the dose should be reduced by 0.5 to 1.0 mg/kg/day until the patient's minimum dose requirement is attained. The therapeutic goal is to reach a relatively disease-free state (not necessarily total clearing) with the minimum effective dose of CsA. When the disease is well controlled, discontinuation of CsA treatment should be attempted [12]. Intermittent CsA therapy and adjunctive treatment with other agents (i.e., topical therapy) should be done whenever possible. CsA has also been reported to be helpful in clearing the lesions of recalcitrant generalized *lichen planus* at a dose of 6 mg/kg/day [13–15].

There are several reports on CsA therapy for *alopecia areata*. Cosmetically acceptable regrowth has been obtained in many cases of patchy area clesi and in subjects with severe or total alopecia areata. However, hair loss may resume after discontinuation of therapy [8,16].

This immunosuppressive drug has also been administered in some cases of *pemphigus* and *pemphigoid* as a steroid-sparing agent [17–19]. Several recent studies have demonstrated the efficacy of CsA in atopic dermatitis [20,21] and in atopic dermatitis–related itch. Most cases relapse promptly when CsA is discontinued, and some relapse despite continued treatment. CsA is also effective in other chronic eczematous dermatoses, such as persistent actinic dermatitis and actinic reticuloid [22,23].

Finally, there are several reports of the efficacy of this agent in the treatment of epidermolysis bullosa acquisita, pyoderma gangrenosum (6 to 10 mg/kg/day), cutaneous and systemic lupus erythematosus, systemic sclerosis, morphea, and dermatomyositis [24–30]. Obviously, CsA must be used with extreme caution in subjects with systemic lupus erythematosus and systemic sclerosis because they may have preexisting renal dysfunction.

II. AZATHIOPRINE

Azathioprine is a purine antimetabolite that is formed by attaching an imidazole ring to 6-mercaptopurine. It has been available for nearly 40 years and is widely used in organ transplantation because of its immunosuppressive effects. Before the arrival of cyclosporine, azathioprine and prednisolone were mainstay treatments against organ graft rejection. In most cases, azathioprine is used as a steroid-sparing agent. Its major clinical application is in preventing graft rejection in kidney transplantation. This drug has a favorable therapeutic/adverse reaction ratio and it is very popular in dermatology.

Azathioprine is converted to its active metabolite, 6-mercaptopurine, which acts as a "false precursor," inhibiting purine biosynthesis and hence cell division. It is metabolized by three competing enzymes—hypoxanthine–guanine phosphoribosyltransferase, xanthine oxidase, and thiopurine methyltransferase (TPMT) [31,32]. Hypoxanthine–guanine phosphoribosyltransferase converts azathioprine to a 6-thioguanine nucleotide that is responsible for its cytotoxicity [33]. TPMT is one of the major catabolic pathways and converts azathioprine to inactive metabolites that are excreted by the kidneys. TPMT activity is genetically polymorphic, with 89% of a normal population homozygous for a high-activity allele ($TPMT^H$) and 0–3% homozygous for a low-activity allele ($TPMT^L$) [34]. Subjects with low TPMT activity are at risk for profound myelotoxicity from azathioprine, while those with high TPMT activity can be underdosed with standard empirical administration schedules. It is possible to predict the therapeutic/adverse reactions, thus enabling safer dosage prescription [35,36].

There have been reports of an inhibition of T-cell function, cell-mediated immunity and B-cell function, and antibody production at therapeutic dosages. Natural killer cells, leukocytes, and monocytes may also be affected [37,38]. It has been suggested that azathioprine inhibits the effector phase of the immune response, but has no effect on the induction phase.

Azathioprine is rapidly absorbed after oral administration and is widely distributed to all tissues except the central nervous system.

This drug has important dose-related adverse effects on bone marrow: leukopenia and, less commonly, thrombocytopenia or pancytopenia. There are reports of chromosome aberrations at pharmacological but not therapeutic doses, and increased incidence of malignancies, mainly in transplant recipients [39–41]. In dermatology, azathioprine is an important drug for the treatment of many inflammatory dermatoses, in particular immunobullous disorders (Table 2). Pemphigus generally requires long-term therapy with high doses of steroids, with well-known and severe adverse effects. Azathioprine can be successfully used as a steroid-sparing agent and/or as monotherapy for chronic maintenance treatment [42,43]. Therapy usually is initiated with corticosteroids (100 to 200 mg/day prednisone or equivalent) to control the acute phase of the disease. Nevertheless, many dermatologists prefer to start azathioprine (1 to 3 mg/kg/day) concurrently because the effect of this drug is delayed by 4 to 6 weeks. Others start azathioprine only when it appears that chronic high-dose corticosteroid therapy is necessary. When clinical remission is achieved, first the dose of steroid and then the dose of azathioprine are slowly tapered, depending on the clinical status.

In the treatment of bullous pemphigoid, azathioprine is reserved for resistant cases or for patients who tolerate corticosteroids poorly [44,45]. It has been shown that in cicatricial pemphigoid, azathioprine is comparable to prednisone or cyclophosphamide alone in controlling eye involvement [46].

Numerous experiences suggest that azathioprine may be beneficial in chronic eczematous dermatoses, such as atopic dermatitis, nummular eczema,

Table 2 Azathioprine: Main Indications in Dermatology

Bullous diseases
Bullous pemphigoid
Herpes gestationis
Pemphigus
Connective tissue diseases
Dermatomyositis/polymyositis
Lupus erythematosus
Relapsing polychondritis
Scleroderma
Vasculitis
Miscellaneous
Acne fulminans
Behçet's disease
Erythema multiforme
Pityriasis rubra pilaris
Psoriasis
Pyoderma gangrenosum
Sarcoidosis

exudative discoid, and lichenoid dermatoses of Sulzberger and Garbe [47–49]. Furthermore, azathioprine has been shown to be effective against chronic actinic dermatitis (100 to 200 mg daily for a mean of 11.5 months) [50].

In patients with severe systemic lupus erythematosus complicated by nephritis, cerebritis, and vascular and/or visceral involvement, the addition of azathioprine has significantly reduced morbidity during treatment, and its use should be considered in patients who require a chronic maintenance dose of prednisone greater than 15 mg/day. Other investigators have reported improvement in patients with refractory subacute or chronic cutaneous lupus erthematosus [51–53].

Azathioprine is occasionally given as a steroid-sparing agent in dermatomyositis and polymyositis [54,55]; it is effective in controlling the ocular and extraocular manifestations of Behçet's disease [56]; and it has also been used for rheumatoid ''malignant'' vasculitis and other severe forms of necrotizing vasculitides [57,58].

Azathioprine is contraindicated in subjects with known hypersensitivity to the drug, and reduced dosage may be necessary in cases with hepatic and renal insufficiency. There is no increase in incidence of congenital abnormalities associated with azathioprine (which crosses the placenta), but since hematological abnormalities, reduced levels of immunoglobulins, and increased risk of infection have been reported [59], it should not be administered to pregnant women and nursing mothers.

Dose reduction to 25 to 30% of normal is necessary if the drug is used concurrently with allopurinol, which inhibits the metabolism of azathioprine. The usual starting dose is 1 to 2 mg/kg/day in a single dose. Two divided doses are associated with a lower incidence of gastrointestinal effects. The peak therapeutic response usually occurs at about 8 weeks. If no beneficial response is seen after 6 to 8 weeks, the dose can be increased by 0.5 mg/kg at 4-week intervals to a maximum of 3 mg/kg/day. When the disease is well controlled, the dose should be gradually reduced by 0.5 mg/kg every 2 to 4 weeks until the lowest effective maintenance dose is attained.

III. CYCLOPHOSPHAMIDE

Cyclophosphamide is a cytotoxic agent of the alkylating class that is administered orally or intravenously. After oral administration, the drug is widely distributed throughout the body (including the CNS). The plasma half-life is about 5 to 6 h [60]. Clearance of the drug is predominantly by hepatic degradation; only 10 to 20% of cyclophosphamide is excreted unchanged in urine. Phosphoramide mustard, the active metabolite into which cyclophosphamide is converted by hepatic P-450 microsomal enzymes, alkylates or irreversibly binds to DNA, causing inhibition of DNA replication. Both mitotically active and resting cells can be affected, although the effect is more pronounced on rapidly dividing cells. Cyclo-

Table 3 Cyclophosphamide: Main Indications in Dermatology

Bullous diseases
Pemphigus
Bullous pemphigoid
Connective tissue diseases
Lupus erythematosus
Dermatomyositis
Relapsing polychondritis
Vasculitides
Lymphomatoid granulomatosis
Polyarteritis nodosa
Rheumatoid vasculitis
Severe necrotizing vasculitides
Wegener's granulomatosis
Miscellaneous
Behçet's disease
Cytophagic histiocytic panniculitis
Histiocytosis X
Lichen myxedematosus
Multicentric reticulohistiocytosis
Mycosis fungoides
Pyoderma gangrenosum
Scleromyxedema
Severe atopic dermatitis

phosphamide is able to inhibit both the induction and effector phases of the immune response; it suppresses B cells more than T cells and T suppressor cells more than T helper cells.

The most important side effects are urological, ranging from urinary frequency, dysuria, microscopic hematuria to life-threatening hemorrhagic cystitis. Bladder fibrosis, necrosis, contracture, and vesicouretheral reflux have been reported [61]. At the doses commonly used in dermatology, the average risk of hemorrhagic cystitis is about 5 to 10% [62]; this may occur any time during therapy or may even begin several months after discontinuation of cyclophosphamide. High fluid intake and concurrent administration of mensa, which binds acrolein in urine, may reduce the risk of this complication. Subjects on long-term cyclophosphamide treatment have a 45-fold increase in the incidence of bladder cancer; the cumulative dose appears to be the most important factor.

Leukopenia is a common adverse effect and may be dose-limiting. Thrombocytopenia and anemia occur mainly with higher doses. With high-dose therapy, anagen effluvium, hyperpigmentation of skin and nails, and mucositis may occur. Gastrointestinal adverse effects (anorexia, nausea, vomiting, etc.) are usually dose-related. Cyclophosphamide is also associated with a significantly increased risk of leukemia, lymphoma, and cutaneous squamous cell carcinoma [63].

Cyclophosphamide is the drug of choice for the treatment of severe systemic vasculitides; it is also beneficial for lymphomatoid granulomatosis, rheumatoid vasculitis, polyarteritis nodosa, and other severe necrotizing vasculitides [64–66]. Table 3 presents some uses of cyclophosphamide in dermatology. Cyclophosphamide is administered in combination with corticosteroids to control acute pemphigus and to maintain remission; it is also effective as a steroid-sparing agent in the treatment of pemphigoid [67,68].

Cyclophosphamide was administered with beneficial results in a small series of patients with discoid and subacute lupus erythematosus refractory to conventional therapies [69]. Moreover, cyclophosphamide plus prednisone appears to reduce the rate of progression of lupus nephritis [70].

Cyclophosphamide is contraindicated in patients with known hypersensitivity to the drug. It should not be used during pregnancy because of its teratogenicity. For dermatological afflictions, the recommended oral dose is 1 to 3 mg/kg/day taken in the morning, and the patient should drink plenty of fluids throughout the day to avoid build-up of toxic concentrations of drug metabolites in the bladder. The clinical response becomes evident after 4 to 6 weeks of treatment.

IV. CHLORAMBUCIL

This is an alkylating agent that inhibits DNA synthesis. The most important side effects of this cytotoxic agent are lymphopenia and neutropenia. Its clinical indications in dermatology are mainly vasculitis, neutrophilic dermatoses (including Sweet's syndrome), histiocytosis X, mycosis fungoides, sarcoidoses, and connective tissue diseases. The dosage guidelines are 0.05–0.2 mg/kg/day, with monitoring of blood cell count and platelets every week and serum chemistry every month.

V. METHOTREXATE

Methotrexate (MTX) was one of the most frequently used chemotherapeutic agents in dermatology. It is an analogue of folic acid and inhibits the enzyme dihydrofolate reductase. Reduced folate is required for the synthesis of thymidine and purines, and DNA synthesis is inhibited following the depletion in intracellular pool of these substances [72–74]. The binding of this inhibitor to the enzyme is extremely tight, with virtually complete inhibition of DNA synthesis occurring in normal bone marrow when drug concentrations in the extracellular fluid exceed levels of 10^{-8} M. MTX, therefore, tends to act during the S-phase of the cell cycle.

The cytotoxicity of MTX is largely influenced by pharmacokinetic factors, principally the duration of exposure and the drug concentration reached. The minimum cytotoxic concentration present in the plasma is approximately 10^{-8} M, although cytotoxicity is also proportional to the duration of exposure [75]. The effects of MTX can be aborted by the administration of a rescue agent, leucovorin (5-formotetrahydrofolate), which can be interconverted to the other reduced folates and bypass the block in folate reduction caused by MTX [76]. Interestingly, the administration of leucovorin does not interfere with the antipsoriatic effect of MTX and the adjunctive immunological effect in pemphigus and may be useful in limiting other toxicities of methotrexate as well [77].

Methotrexate can be administered intramuscularly, intravenously, or orally, and 100% of the oral dose is absorbed. However, small alterations in renal function can have profound effects on the duration of the plasma levels, leading to toxicity. Another important aspect of MTX pharmacokinetics is the variability of excretion from subject to subject. This is especially true in the presence of significant third spaces; for example, malignant effusions. Effusions apparently concentrate the drug and can act as a reservoir for later drug release, especially in the presence of diminished renal function [74,78]. Finally, because MTX is bound to plasma proteins, concomitant administration of a drug such as aspirin, which may displace it, can also have a profound enhancing effect [79]. In conventional regimens, peak plasma concentrations of about 10^{-6} M to 10^{-5} M are achieved.

Methotrexate has demonstrated a beneficial effect in a variety of benign and malignant dermatological disorders. Its effects can be classified as either antimitotic (like in the treatment of benign proliferative keratinizing disorders such as psoriasis, pityriasis rubra pilaris, severe cases of epidermolytic ichthyosis, or mycosis fungoides) or immunosuppressive, as in the treatment of pemphigus or pemphigoid. In addition to its use in psoriasis, MTX has also been used to treat dermatomyositis and polymyositis [80], Wegener's granulomatosis [81], Reiter's disease [82], mycosis fungoides [83], pityriasis lichenoides and lymphomatoid papulosis [84], pustular psoriasis [85], congenital ichthyosiform erythroderma [86], and pityriasis rubra pilaris [87]. MTX is also useful in the treatment of pemphigus vulgaris [88]. Like azathioprine, MTX tends to reduce the dose of prednisone required to moderate and maintain remissions.

A large pool of experiences indicates that this is generally a safe drug when given carefully and does not appear to be mutagenic, as it acts primarily by metabolic inhibition [89]. The major use of MTX in dermatology has been in the treatment of psoriasis. Its utility has been established in multiple noncontrolled and controlled trials [74,90–92]. In general, MTX is capable of inducing remissions in 80 to 90% of patients treated and of maintaining these remissions for long periods with continued therapy. A large variety of schedules have been utilized, with weekly administration as a single or divided dose, ranging from 25 to 50 mg/mL and 2.5 to 7.5 mg every 12 h for three doses, respectively. In general, the daily schedules have fallen into disfavor, as they appear to be related to a higher incidence of hepatic toxicity. During therapy, it is important to monitor blood cell count with platelets, serum chemistry, and, in the elderly, creatinine clearance [74].

The major long-term concern regarding MTX in dermatology has been the development of chronic hepatic toxicity, so that it may be useful to take a liver biopsy when the cumulative dose is about 2 g. In fact, because liver function tests can be normal in the presence of hepatic toxicity, a repeat liver biopsy is strongly recommended in subjects with total doses of more than 2000 mg. There is a report regarding a long experience with the effects and side effects of MTX [93]. In a 10-year therapeutic trial with 248 patients, the major risks of hepatic toxicity appeared to be related to the total cumulative dose of MTX, with total cumulative doses of 2000 to 4000 mg correlating with a high percentage of patients in whom fibrosis/cirrhosis developed. Other risk factors appeared to be age, obesity, and, possibly, intercurrent alcohol consumption during MTX therapy.

The second major concern regarding MTX has been the possibility of carcinogenesis, teratogenicity, and pulmonary toxicity. There is no clinical or experimental evidence suggesting that MTX has a carcinogenic effect. Bailin et al. [94] were unable to show an increased rate of malignancy. Although MTX is teratogenic in pregnant females [95], there is no evidence that MTX taken by males or nonpregnant females has any effect on fertility or offspring. Methotrexate does occasionally cause oligospermia, which is reversible. Pulmonary toxicity is related to a hypersensitivity syndrome that rapidly reverses on discontinuance of MTX and treatment with systemic steroids.

Although stomatitis is the most frequently reported side effect of MTX therapy, other cutaneous side effects have been observed, including alopecia, photoreactivity, acneiform lesions, macular and papular exanthems, ulcerations, erythema, hyperpigmentation, and exfoliated dermatitis limited to the hands and feet [96,97]. These side effects appear to be related to the dose and schedule of administration, in addition to being idiosyncratic. In view of the severity of the underlying disease for which MTX is generally used, side effects, unless severe, do not warrant either a decrease in dosage or a change in treatment schedule.

VI. 5-FLUOROURACIL

5-Fluorouracil (5-FU) is largely used as an anticancer chemotherapeutic agent in dermatology. The mechanism of action of 5-FU inhibition involves at least two pathways. The first is through the formation of 5-fluoro-2′-deoxyuridine 5′-monophosphate, a tight-binding inhibitor of thymidylate synthetase capable of inhibiting the synthesis of thymidine [74,98]. There are studies supporting the concept that 5-FU may have an alternative mechanism of action that is preferential in tumor cells. Specifically, 5-FU may be incorporated into RNA, thereby rendering the RNA molecule defective [99]. Because RNA synthesis generally occurs throughout the cell cycle, whereas DNA synthesis is restricted to the S-phase, this alternative mechanism may be of relevance to dermatology. This is true because the growth rate of the lesions for which 5-FU is used is generally not much greater than that of surrounding skin. Therefore, an alternative mechanism must be invoked in order to explain the relative selectivity observed with this agent.

5-Fluorouracil is an excellent example of the potentially unique application of cancer chemotherapeutic agents in dermatology; it is administered principally via topical application (in 1% and 5% concentrations), which permits its use with a minimum of adverse side effects. Topical 5-FU is used extensively for the treatment of superficial basal and squamous cell carcinomas [100] as well as actinic keratoses [74,101,102]. We note that the original enthusiasm for this agent in the treatment of basal and squamous cell carcinomas has been blunted somewhat by apparently high recurrence rates [103]. Furthermore, the treatment of actinic keratoses is complicated by a marked irritant reaction [104], as well as the potential for subsequent permanent scarring, alopecia, and hypo- and hyperpigmentation. 5-FU has also been used in the treatment of porokeratosis [105], keratoacanthomas (intralesional) [106], facial warts [107], and, inadvisably, lentigo maligna [108], with varying success. 5-FU has the added advantage of exposing clinically undetectable keratoses, as well as malignant epitheliomas.

Stomatitis and alopecia are the most common side effects of systemic treatment. Systemic 5-FU therapy has also been associated with nail changes, hyperpigmentation of skin, and phototoxicity. Patients receiving 5-FU at a dose of 15 mg/kg once weekly have noted severe xeroderma, involving especially the palms and soles, often progressing to fissuring. The specific toxic effects following topical administration may include irritation, scarring, alopecia, and hyper- and hypopigmentation.

VII. HYDROXYUREA

Hydroxyurea is a simple compound that exerts a marked cytotoxic effect both in vitro and in vivo. The major biochemical action causes an immediate inhibition of DNA synthesis [74,109]. Biochemical evidence shows inhibition of the enzyme ribonucleotide diphosphate reductase as the principal site of action. This enzyme is critically important for converting ribonucleotides to deoxyribonucleotides and is most active during the S-phase of the cell cycle. The rate of DNA synthesis in mammalian cells is controlled by the supply of deoxyribonucleotides, which in turn is controlled by production through the enzyme ribonucleotide diphosphate reductase. Therefore, even minor inhibition of this enzyme results in a marked decrease in the rate of DNA synthesis.

The principal use of hydroxyurea in dermatology has been for the treatment of psoriasis vulgaris. This use is based on observations of a large number of adverse cutaneous reactions in patients with chronic lymphocytic leukemia undergoing maintenance therapy with hydroxyurea. In 7 of 28 patients, partial alopecia, increased pigmentation, skin atrophy, nail changes, and erythema were noted [110]. Subsequent controlled and uncontrolled studies have indicated response rates of 50 to 60% [111]. The drug has also been used in pustular psoriasis without relevant results.

Although hydroxyurea is not a first-choice drug for the systemic treatment of psoriasis, it remains a possible alternative for those patients with underlying liver disease who do not tolerate MTX. The usual maintenance doses are 1 to 2 g per day in divided doses.

Cutaneous side effects occur in 25 to 35% of subjects treated with hydroxyurea. A variety of cutaneous reactions have been described, including cutaneous vasculitis, macular and papular eruptions, alopecia, stomatitis, and xeroderma. Fixed drug eruptions and nail changes, as well as increased erythema in previously irradiated sites, have also been described [96].

VIII. INTERFERONS

The interferon (IFN) multigene family consists of IFN-α, IFN-β, and IFN-γ. IFNs are an integral part of the cytokine network and exert an important role in the host defense against viral infections, resistance to different kinds of tumors, control of cell growth and differentiation, expression of cell surface molecules and immune system and lymphocyte proliferation, maturation, and circulation. In fact, interferons have antiviral, antiproliferative, and immunomodulatory activities. In the past few years, natural, but mostly recombinant, IFNs have become available for clinical studies. Although most studies have focused on cancer therapy, other indications include infections and immune-mediated diseases.

A. IFN-α

The main functions of IFN-α are antiviral, antiproliferative, and antitumoral, but not truly immunomodulative. It affects cellular metabolism via nuclear alterations and alters cellular transcription, translation, and protein synthesis. Table 4 summarizes the clinical studies performed with recombinant IFN-α (rIFN-α). The subcutaneous administration of rIFN-α (5×10^5 IU/kg/day for about 2 weeks) resulted in suppression and decreased duration of *herpes simplex virus* infection in patients with frequent recurrences [112]. Recombinant IFN-α has been shown to exert a beneficial influence on the clinical course and subjective symptoms of

TABLE 4 Use of Interferon-α in Dermatology

Viral infections
Herpes simplex virus
Herpes zoster
HIV infection
Human papillomavirus infection
Skin tumors
Basal cell carcinoma
Cutaneous T-cell lymphoma
Kaposi's sarcoma (HIV-associated)
Malignant melanoma
Squamous cell carcinoma
Inflammatory skin disorders
Atopic dermatitis
Behçet's disease
Psoriasis

herpes zoster at the dose of 1.7 to 5.1 $\times$ 10^5 IU/kg/day [113]. No significant differences have been shown between rIFN-α and acyclovir in a comparative study [114]. In extensive studies using 10^6 IU/day subcutaneously or intralesionally three times a week for 3 weeks, complete remission was observed in 30 to 80% of rIFN-α–treated patients with *human papilloma virus*–induced wartlike lesions versus 15 to 30% in the placebo-treated group [115]. No recurrences were observed in the IFN-α–treated group during the follow-up period of at least 12 months. The results of studies using IFN-α for the treatment of common warts are controversial [116].

IFN-α produces partial or complete response rates with *cutaneous T-cell lymphoma* (CTCL) in 40 to 85% of patients [117]. The therapy regimens depend on the stage of the disease and the condition of the patient. Using a high-dose rIFN-α treatment (up to 5 $\times$ 10^7 IU/m^2 three times a week for a long, not clearly defined, period) provoked severe toxic reactions in all patients and required at least a 50% dose reduction. To avoid severe side effects, a different approach has been proposed, consisting of intralesional low-dose rIFN-α using 10^6 IU per week for 4 weeks in the plaque stage of CTCL [118]. Treatment with rIFN-α during early stages of Kaposi's sarcoma in AIDS (18 $\times$ 10^6 IU subcutaneously each day for 3 months followed by the same dose three times weekly for another 3 months over a total period of 2 to 2.5 years) could lead to long-term remission and stabilization of the overall clinical picture [119]. Some recent studies indicate that in early stages of malignant melanoma (clinical stage IIa or IIb) systemic treatment with rIFN-α may increase disease-free intervals and quality of life of the patients [120]. However, most promising seems to be the combination of interferons with other agents, such as dacarbazine. Finally, several clinical trials suggest that IFN-α is effective in the intralesional treatment of basal and squamous cell carcinoma [121,122].

IFN-α has been found to improve the clinical condition of patients with discoid lupus erythematosus and subacute cutaneous lupus erythematosus (18 to 120×10^6 IU weekly), but rapid relapse has been reported after discontinuation of this treatment [123]. The efficacy of IFN-α therapy in the management of Behçet's disease, psoriasis, and atopic dermatitis is still controversial [124–126]. Recently, it has been proposed that this drug be used in the treatment of severe photoaging, given its ability to restore the levels of $CD1a^+$ cells in the skin after UV radiation.

B. IFN-β

Table 5 shows the main applications of this type of interferon in dermatology. IFN-β has not demonstrated better results than acyclovir in the local treatment of herpes simplex virus, but it has shown good results in the local, perilesional, and intralesional treatment of HPV-mediated diseases [127,128]. Some data report that IFN-β has a dose-dependent antitumoral effect on malignant melanoma that may be due to the high tissue affinity of this interferon as compared with IFN-α. Use of natural and rIFN-β as an adjuvant therapy appears more promising in patients with stage I malignant melanoma after complete tumor excision [129].

IFN-β seems to be a good alternative (palliative treatment) agent and can be combined with many other cytostatic drugs in the treatment of squamous cell carcinomas of the skin and mucosa and of solid tumors and metastases of the skin and subcutis [130].

C. IFN-γ

There are many applications for IFN-γ in therapy (for details see Table 6). In regard to infectious diseases, there are many contradictory studies on the treat-

Table 5 Use of Interferon-β in Dermatology

Viral diseases
Herpes simplex virus infections
Human papillomavirus infections
Skin tumors
Malignant melanoma
Cutaneous metastatic tumor (breast and bronchial carcinoma)
Squamous cell carcinoma

Table 6 Use of Interferon-γ in Dermatology

Inflammatory diseases
Atopic dermatitis
Psoriatic arthritis
Psoriasis vulgaris
Diseases of rheumatological interest
Behçet's disease
Chronic polyarthritis
Systemic scleroderma
Virus-related diseases
Bowenoid papulosis
Common warts
Condylomata acuminata
Genital warts
Herpes zoster
Nonviral infections
Leishmaniasis
Leprosy
Skin tumors
Basal cell carcinoma

ment of viral skin diseases with IFN-γ; generally, the mean response rate achieved in the treatment of genital warts is 10 to 50% (50 to 400 μg/day subcutis over a total period of 4 weeks). The therapy should last much longer, and cyclic therapy should provide the best results. IFN-γ was seen to have a good therapeutic effect in bowenoid papulosis and herpes zoster, where the drug does not prevent spread of lesions but reduces subjective symptoms, such as acute pain and postherpetic neuralgia [131–133].

In addition to direct antiviral effects, it has been demonstrated that rIFN-γ stimulates in vitro monocyte/macrophages, granulocytes, and natural killer cells. This proved to be useful for the treatment of bacterial, protozoal, and fungal infections. In leprosy and leishmaniasis, intracutaneous injections of 1 to 10 μg of IFN-γ stabilized an infection-dependent downregulation of free-radical production by peripheral blood monocytes and significantly reduced the number of *Mycobacterium leprae* in an infiltrated lesion [134].

In certain patients with basal cell carcinoma for whom surgery presents significant functional and/or technical risks, intralesional rIFN-γ (as well as rIFN-α) injection may be a valuable alternative [121]. No data are yet available on the influence of IFN-γ on squamous cell carcinoma, while there are studies that suggest that IFN-γ is not the appropriate cytokine to be used in malignant lymphoproliferative diseases [135]. Its use is controversial in malignant melanoma [135].

Further clinical studies are necessary to define the exact role of IFN-γ in psoriasis vulgaris as well as in psoriasis arthropathica, where the results are controversial [136]. Behçet's disease seems to respond well to rIFN-γ; only ocular involvement shows lower response [133]. In patients with scleroderma, this drug showed an improvement of the functional activity of the patients and complete remission of fibrotic changes in an early stage of the disease, while no influence of IFN-γ has been found in advanced phases [137].

Promising preliminary results have been achieved with subcutaneous injections of rIFN-γ, including rapid improvement of skin lesions, reduction of subjective symptoms, and partial decrease of total IgE serum concentration in patients with severe atopic dermatitis. The combination of rIFN-γ and low-dose oral steroids remarkably improved the results [138,139].

REFERENCES

1. Furue M, Gaspari AH, Katz SI. Effect of cyclosporin A on epidermal cells. II. Cyclosporin A inhibits proliferation of normal and transformed keratinocytes. J Invest Dermatol 1988; 90: 796–800.
2. Mason J. Renal side-effects of cyclosporin A. Br J Dermatol 1990; 122 (suppl 36): 71–77.
3. Mihatsch MJ, Beelghiti D, Bohman SO, et al. Kidney biopsies in control of cyclosporin A-treated psoriatic patients. Br J Dermatol 1990; 122 (suppl 36): 95–100.
4. Fradin MS, Ellis CN, Voorhees JJ. Management of patients and side effects during cyclosporine therapy for cutaneous disorders. J Am Acad Dermatol 1990; 23: 1265–1275.
5. Ellis CN, Fradin MS, Messana JM, et al. Cyclosporine for plaque-type psoriasis. N Engl J Med 1991; 324: 277–284.
6. Ellis CN, Gorsulowsky DC, Hamilton TA, et al. Cyclosporine improves psoriasis in a double-blind study. JAMA 1986; 256: 3110–3116.
7. Griffiths CEM, Powles AV, Leonard JN, et al. Clearance of psoriasis with low dose cyclosporin. Br Med J 1986; 293: 731–732.
8. Picascia DD, Roenigk HH Jr. Effects of oral and topical cyclosporine in male pattern alopecia. Transplant Proc 1988; 3: 109–111.
9. Meinardi MM, Westerhof W, Bos JD. Generalized pustular psoriasis (von Zumbusch) responding to cyclosporine A. Br J Dermatol 1987; 116: 269–270.
10. Zachariae H, Thestrup-Pedersen K. Cyclosporine A in acrodermatitis continua. Dermatologica 1987; 175: 29–32.
11. Steinsson K, Jonsdottir I, Valdimarsson H. Cyclosporin A in psoriatic arthritis: an open study. Ann Rheum Dis 1990; 5: 284–294.
12. Abeywickrama K, Baker BS, Barnes A, et al. A consensus report: cyclosporin A therapy for psoriasis. Br J Dermatol 1990; 122 (suppl 36): 1–3.

13. Ho VC, Conklin RJ. Effect of topical cyclosporine rinse on oral planus (letter). N Engl J Med 1981; 325: 435.
14. Ho VC, Gupta AK, Ellis CN, et al. Treatment of severe lichen planus with cyclosporine. J Am Acad Dermatol 1990; 22: 94–100.
15. Levell NJ, MacLeod RI, Marks JM. Lack of effect of cyclosporine mouthwash in oral lichen planus (letter). Lancet 1991; 337: 796–797.
16. Gupta AK, Ellis CN, Cooper KD, et al. Oral cyclosporine A for the treatment of alopecia areata: a clinical and immunohistochemical analysis. J Am Acad Dermatol 1990; 22: 242–250.
17. Campolmi P, Bonan P, Lotti T, Palleschi GM, Fabbri P, Panconesi E. The role of cyclosporine A in the treatment of pemphigus erythematosus. Int J Dermatol 1991; 30 (2): 890–892.
18. Cunliffe WJ. Bullous pemphigoid and response to cyclosporin. Br J Dermatol 1987; 117: 113–114.
19. Thivolet J, Barthelemy H, Rigot-Muller G, et al. Effects of cyclosporin on bullous pemphigoid and pemphigus. Lancet 1985; 1: 334–335.
20. Munro CS, Higgins EM, Marks JM, et al. Cyclosporin A in atopic dermatitis: therapeutic response is dissociated from effects on allergic reactions. Br J Dermatol 1991; 124: 43–48.
21. Wahlgren CF, Scheynius A, Hagermark O. Antipruritic effect of oral cyclosporin A in atopic dermatitis. Acta Dermatol Venereol (Stockh) 1990; 70: 323–329.
22. Duschet P, Schwarz T, Oppolzer G, et al. Persistent light reaction: successful treatment with cyclosporin A. Acta Dermatol Venereol (Stockh) 1988; 68: 176–178.
23. Norris PG, Camp RDR, Hawk JLM. Actinic reticuloid: response to cyclosporine. J Am Acad Dermatol 1989; 21: 307–309.
24. Crow LL, Finkle JP, Gammon WR, et al. Clearing of epidermolysis bullosa acquisita with cyclosporine. J Am Acad Dermatol 1988; 19: 937–942.
25. Merle C, Blanc D, Zultak M, et al. Intractable epidermolysis bullosa acquisita: efficacy of cyclosporin A. Dermatologica 1990; 181: 44–47.
26. Penmetcha M, Navaratnam A. Pyoderma gangrenosum: response to cyclosporin A. Int J Dermatol 1988; 27: 253.
27. Feutren G, Querin S, Tron F, et al. The effects of cyclosporine in patients with systemic lupus. Transplant Proc 1986; 4: 643–644.
28. Appelboom T, Itzkowitch D. Cyclosporine in successful control of rapidly progressive scleroderma. Am J Med 1987; 82: 866–867.
29. Ghersetich I, Matucci-Cerinic M, Lotti T. A pathogenetic approach to the management of systemic sclerosis. Int J Dermatol 1990; 29 (9): 616–622.
30. Teofoli P, Mancini A, Lotti T. Cyclospine A inhibits tPA mRNA transcription in A431 cell line 29. Skin Pharmacol 1996; 9: 137–140.
31. Anstey A. Azathioprine in dermatology: a review in the light of advances in understanding methylation pharmacogenetics. J R Soc Med 1995; 88: 155–160.
32. Snow JL, Gibson LE. A pharmacogenetic basis for the safe and effective use of azathioprine and other thiopurine drugs in dermatologic patients. J Am Acad Dermatol 1995; 32: 114–115.
33. Tidd DM, Patterson ARP. A biochemical mechanism for the delayed cytotoxic reaction of a 6-mercaptopurine. Cancer 1974; 34: 738–746.

34. Weinshilboum RM, Sladek SL. Mercaptopurine pharmacogenetics: monogenic inheritance of erythrocyte thiopurine methyltransferase activity. Am J Hum Genet 1980; 32: 651–662.
35. Snow JL, Gibson LE. The role of genetic variation in thiopurine methyltransferase activity and the efficacy and/or side effects of azathioprine therapy in dermatologic patients. Arch Dermatol 1995; 131: 193–197.
36. Tan BB, Lear JT, Gawkrodger DJ, English JSC. Azathiprine in dermatology: a survey of current practice in the U.K. Br J Dermatol 1997; 136: 351–355.
37. Cseuz R, Panayi GS. The inhibition of NK cell function by azathioprine during the treatment of patients with rheumatoid arthritis. Br J Rheum 1990; 29: 358–362.
38. Stevens JE, Villoughly DA. The anti-inflammatory effect of some immunosuppressive agents. J Pathol 1968; 97: 367–373.
39. Voogd CE. Azathioprine, a genotoxic agent to be considered non-genotoxic in man. Mutation Res 1989; 221: 133–152.
40. Penn I. Cancer in immunosuppressed patients. Transplant Proc 1984; 16: 492–494.
41. Penn I. Depressed immunity and the development of cancer. Clin Exp Immunol 1981; 46: 459–475.
42. Burton JL, Greaves MW. Azathioprine for pemphigus and pemphigoid. A 4-year follow-up. Br J Dermatol 1974; 91: 103–109.
43. Roenigk HH, Deodhar S. Pemphigus treatment with azathioprine. Clinical and immunologic correlation. Arch Dermatol 1973; 107: 353–357.
44. Ahmed AR, Maize JC, Provost TT. Bullous pemphigoid. Clinical and immunologic follow-up after successful therapy. Arch Dermatol 1977; 113: 1043–1046.
45. Burton JL, Harman RMM, Peachey RDG, et al. A controlled study of azathioprine in the treatment of pemphigoid. Br J Dermatol 1978; 99 (suppl 16): 14.
46. Mondino BJ, Brown SI. Immunosuppressive therapy in ocular cicatricial pemphigoid. Am J Ophthalmol 1983; 96: 453–459.
47. Freeman K, Hewitt M, Warin AP. Two cases of distinctive exudative discoid and lichenoid chronic dermatosis of Sulzberger and Garbe responding to azathioprine. Br J Dermatol 1984; 111: 215–220.
48. Morrison JGL, Schultz EJ. Treatment of eczema with cyclophosphamide and azathioprine. Br J Dermatol 1978; 98: 203–207.
49. Younger IR, Harris DWS, Colver GB. Azathioprine in dermatology. J Am Acad Dermatol 1991; 25: 281–286.
50. Leigh IM, Hawk JL. Treatment of chronic actinic dermatitis with azathioprine. Br J Dermatol 1984; 110: 691–695.
51. Callen JP, Spencer LV, Burruss JB, et al. Azathioprine: an effective, corticosteroid-sparing therapy for patients with recalcitrant cutaneous lupus erythematosus or with recalcitrant cutaneous leukocytoclastic vasculitis. Arch Dermatol 1991; 127: 515–522.
52. Ashinoff R, Werth VP, Franks AG Jr. Resistant discoid lupus erythematosus of palms and soles: successful treatment with azathioprine. J Am Acad Dermatol 1988; 19: 961–964.
53. Lotti T, Matucci-Cerinic M, Fattorini L, Fabbri P. Immunosuppressive effects of

antimalaric drugs in discoid lupus erythematosus. Ital Gentile Rev Dermatol 1988; 25(3): 257–259.
54. Benson MD, Aldo MA. Azathioprine therapy in polymyositis. Arch Intern Med 1973; 132: 447–451.
55. Bradley WG, Walton JN. Treatment of dermatomyositis (letter). Br Med J 1976; 2: 43.
56. Yazici H, Pazarli H, Barnes CG, et al. A controlled trial of azathyoprine in Behcet's syndrome. N Engl J Med 1990; 322: 281–285.
57. Callen JP, af Ekenstam E. Cutaneous leukocytoclastic vasculitis. Clinical experience in forty-four patients. South Med J 1987; 80: 848–851.
58. Leib ES, Restivo C, Paulus HE. Immunosuppressive and corticosteroid therapy for polyarteritis nodosa. Am J Med 1979; 67: 941–947.
59. Davidson JM, Lindheimer MD. Pregnancy in women with renal allografts. Semin Nephrol 1984; 4: 240–251.
60. Moore MJ. Clinical pharmacokinetics of cyclophosphamide. Clin Pharmacokinet 1991; 20: 194–208.
61. Levine LA, Richie JP. Urologic complications of cyclophosphamide. J Urol 1989; 141: 1063–1069.
62. Stillwell TJ, Benson RC Jr. Cyclophosphamide-induced haemorrhagic cystitis–a review of 100 patients. Cancer 1988; 61: 451.
63. Kovarsky J. Clinical pharmacology and toxicology of cyclophosphamide: emphasis on use in rheumatic diseases. Semin Arthritis Rheum 1983; 12: 359–368.
64. Brodell RT, Miller W, Eisen AZ. Cutaneous lesions of lymphomatoid granulomatosis. Arch Dermatol 1986; 122: 303–306.
65. Panconesi E, Lotti T. Steroids versus nonsteroids in the treatment of cutaneous inflammation. Therapeutic modalities of office use. Arch Dermatol Res 1992; 284: 537–541.
66. Fauci AS, Katz P, Haynes BF, et al. Cyclophosphamide therapy of severe systemic necrotizing vasculitis. N Engl J Med 1979; 301: 235–238.
67. Ebringer A, McKay IR. Pemphigus vulgaris successfully treated with cyclophosphamide. Ann Intern Med 1969; 71: 125–127.
68. Brody HJ, Pirozzi DJ. Benign mucous memebrane pemphigoid. Response to therapy with cyclophosphamide. Arch Dermatol 1977; 113: 1598–1599.
69. Schulz EJ, Menter MA. Treatment of discoid and subacute lupus erythematosus with cyclophosphamide. Br J Dermatol 1971; 85 (suppl 7): 60–65.
70. McCune WJ, Golbus J, Zeldes W, et al. Clinical and immunological effects of monthly administration of intravenous cyclophosphamide in severe systemic lupus erythematosus. N Engl J Med 1988; 318: 1423–1431.
71. Bender RA, Zwelling LA, Doroshow JH, et al. Antineoplastic drugs: clinical pharmacology and therapeutic use. Drugs 1978; 16: 47–56.
72. Goldman ID. The mechanism of action of methotrexate. I. Interaction with a low-affinity, intracellular site required for maximum inhibition of deoxyribonucleic acid synthesis in L-cell mouse fibroblast. Mol Pharmacol 1974; 10: 257–265.
73. Goldman ID. Analysis of the cytotoxic determinants for methotrexate. A role for "free" extracellular drug. Cancer Treat Rep 1975; 6: 51–59.
74. Wick MM. Cytotoxic agents in dermatology. In: Fitzpatrick TB, Eisen AZ, Wolff K,

et al., eds. Dermatology in General Medicine, 3rd ed. New York: McGraw-Hill, 1987: 2577–2582.
75. Pinedo HM, Chabner BA. The role of drug concentration, duration of exposure, and endogenous metabolites in determining MTX cytotoxicity. Cancer Treat Rep 1977; 61: 709–714.
76. Nixon PF, Bertino JR. Effective absorption and utilization of oral formyltetrahydrofolate in man. N Engl J Med 1972; 286: 175–179.
77. Hanno R. Methotrexate in psoriasis. J Am Acad Dermatol 1980; 2: 171–180.
78. Wan SH. Effect of route of administration and effusions on methotrexate pharmacokinetics. Cancer Res 1974; 34: 3487–3493.
79. Taylor JR, Halprin KM. Effect of sodium salicylate on methotrexate-serum albumin binding. Arch Dermatol 1977; 113: 588–591.
80. Giannini M, Callen JP. Treatment of dermatomyositis with methotrexate and prednisone. Arch Dermatol 1979; 115: 1251–1256.
81. Capizzi RL, Bertino JR. Methotrexate therapy of Wegener's granulomatosis. Ann Intern Med 1971; 74: 74–78.
82. Jetton RL, Duncan WC. Treatment of Reiter's syndrome with methotrexate. Ann Intern Med 1969; 70: 349–351.
83. Groth O. Tumor stage of mycosis fungoides treated with bleomycin and methotrexate: report from the Scandinavian Mycosis Fungoides Study Group. Acta Dermatol Venereol (Stockh) 1979; 59: 59–64.
84. Lynch PJ, Saied NK. Methotrexate treatment of pityriasis lichenoides and lymphomatoid papulosis. Cutis 1979; 23: 634–636.
85. Hoffman TE, Watson W. Methotrexate toxicity in the treatment of generalized pustular psoriasis. Cutus 1978; 21: 68–73.
86. Herskowitz LJ. Acute pancreatitis associated with long-term azathioprine therapy in patients with systemic lupus erythematosus. Arch Dermatol 1979; 115: 179–182.
87. Knowles WR, Chernosky ME. Pityriasis rubra pilaris prolonged treatment with methotrexate. Arch Dermatol 1970; 102: 603–609.
88. Lever WF, Schaumburg-Lever G. Immunosuppressants and prednisone in pemphigus vulgaris. Arch Dermatol 1977; 113. 1236–1242.
89. Newberger AE. Biologic and biochemical actions of methotrexate in psoriasis. J Invest Dermatol 1976; 70: 183–187.
90. Roenigk HH Jr. Methotrexate therapy for psoriasis. Arch Dermatol 1973; 108: 35–38.
91. Weinstein GD. Methotrexate. Ann Intern Med 1977; 86: 199–208.
92. Weinstein GD, Frost P. Methotrexate for psoriasis. Arch Dermatol 1971; 103: 33–37.
93. Nyfors A. Methotrexate Therapy for Psoriasis: Effect and Side Effects with Particular Reference to Hepatic Changes. A Survey. Aarhus, Denmark: Laegeforeningens Forlag, 1980.
94. Bailin PL. Is methotrexate therapy for psoriasis carcinogenic? A modified retrospective-prospective analysis. JAMA 1975; 232: 359–364.
95. Carless RG. Methotrexate in young females with psoriasis. N Engl J Med 1971; 285: 296–300.

96. Adrian RM. Mucocutaneous reactions to antineoplastic agents. Cancer 1980; 30: 143–149.
97. Levine N, Greenwald ES. Mucocutaneous side effects of cancer chemotherapy. Cancer Treat Rep 1978; 5: 67–74.
98. Santi DV. Mechanism of interaction of thymidylate synthetase with 5-fluorodeoxyuridylate. Biochemistry 1974; 13: 471–476.
99. Carrico CK, Glazer RI. Effect of 5-fluorouracil on the synthesis and translation of polyadenylic acid-containing RNA from regenerating rat liver. Cancer Res 1969; 39: 3694–3699.
100. Reymann F. Treatment of basal cell carcinoma of the skin with 5-fluorouracil ointment, a 10-year follow-up study. Dermatologica 1979; 158: 368–375.
101. Breza T. Non-inflammatory destruction of actinic keratoses by fluorouracil. Arch Dermatol 1976; 112: 1258–1264.
102. Epstein E. Treatment of lip keratosis (actinic chelitis) with topical 5-fluorouracil. Arch Dermatol 1977; 113: 906–910.
103. Mohs FE. Tendency of fluorouracil to conceal deep foci of invasive basal cell carcinoma. Arch Dermatol 1978; 114: 1021–1024.
104. Kaplan LA. Hypertrophic scarring as a complication of fluorouracil Rx. Arch Dermatol 1979; 115: 1452–1453.
105. Dupre A, Cristoi B. Mibelli's porokeratosis of the lips. Arch Dermatol 1978; 114: 1841–1843.
106. Odom RB, Goette DK. Treatment of keratoacanthomas with intralesional fluorouracil. Arch Dermatol 1978; 114: 1779–1780.
107. Lockshin NA. Flat facial warts treated with 5-fluorouracil. Arch Dermatol 1979; 115: 929–932.
108. Gromet MA. Treatment of lentigo maligna with 5-FU. Arch Dermatol 1977; 113: 1128–1131.
109. Timson J. Hydroxyurea. Mutat Res 1975; 32: 115–123.
110. Kennedy BJ. Skin changes secondary to hydroxyurea therapy. Arch Dermatol 1975; 111: 183–186.
111. Moschella SL, Greenwald MA. Psoriasis with hydroxyurea. An 18-month study of 60 patients. Arch Dermatol 1963; 107: 363–368.
112. Pazin GJ, Harger JH, Armstrong JA, et al. Leukocyte interferon for treating first episodes of genital herpes in women. J Infect Dis 1987; 156: 891–897.
113. Jordan JW, Fired RP, Merigan TC, et al. Administration of human leukocyte interferon in herpes zoster. J Infect Dis 1974; 130: 56–62.
114. Duchet P, Schwarz T, Soyer P, et al. Treatment of herpes zoster. Recombinant alpha-interferon versus acyclovir. Int J Dermatol 1988; 27: 4–9.
115. Reichman RC, Oakes D, Bonnez M, et al. Treatment of condyloma acuminatum with three different interferons administrated intralesionally. Ann Intern Med 1988; 108: 675–678.
116. Androphy EJ, Dvoretzky I, Maluish AE, et al. Response of warts in epidermodysplasia verruciformis to treatment of systemic and intralesional alpha-interferon. J Am Acad Dermatol 1984; 11: 197–201.
117. Bunn PA, Ihde DC, Foon KA. Recombinant interferon alpha 2a, an active agent in advanced cutaneous T cell lymphomas. Int J Cancer 1987; 1: 9–13.

118. Vonderheid EC, Thomson R, Smiles KA, et al. Recombinant interferon alpha 2b in plaque-phase mycosis fungoides-intralesional and low dose intramuscular therapy. Arch Dermatol 1987; 123: 757–761.
119. Bratzke B, Stadler R, Eichhorn R, et al. Disseminiertes mukokutanes Kaposi-Sarkom bei AIDS. Klinische Und Therapeutische Erfahrungen an 13 patienten. Hautarzt 1987; 38: 286–290.
120. Creagan ET, Ahmann DL, Frytak S. Three consecutive phase II studies of recombinant interferon alpha 2a in the advanced malignant melanoma. Cancer 1987; 59: 638–645.
121. Edwards L, Tucker SB, Perednia D, et al. The effect of an intralesional sustained-release formulation of interferon alpha 2b on basal cell carcinoma. Arch Dermatol 1990; 126: 1029–1032.
122. Ikic D, Padovan I, Pipic N, et al. Treatment of squamous carcinoma with interferon. Int J Dermatol 1991; 30: 58–63.
123. Nicolas JF, Tivolet J, Kanitakis J, et al. Response of discoid and subacute cutaneous lupus erythematosus to recombinant interferon alpha 2a. J Invest Dermatol 1990; 95 (suppl): 142s–147s.
124. Stadler R, Bratzke B, Baumann I. Morbus Behcet und exogenes Interferon. Hautarzt 1987; 38: 97–101.
125. Neumann R, Pohl-Markl H, Aberer E. Parenteral interferon alpha treatment of psoriasis. Dermatologica 1987; 175: 23–29.
126. MacKie RM. Interferon alpha for atopic dermatitis. Lancet 1990; 1: 1282.
127. Uyeno K, Yasuno H, Niimura M. Clinical trial of huIFN-beta on herpes zoster in immunocompromised patients. J Invest Dermatol 1989; 93: 583–587.
128. Schoefer H, Sollberg S. Systemische Behandlung vulgaerer Warzen mit beta-interferon. Hautarzt 1991; 42: 396–398.
129. Fierlbeck G, D'Hoedt B, Stroebel W, et al. Intrelaesionale therapie von melanom-metastasen mit rekombinantem interferon beta. Hautarzt 1992; 43: 16–19.
130. Wildfang I, Rathmann R, Schmoll HJ. Lokale therapie mit interferon beta bei therapierefraktaeren metastasen solider tumoren. In: Schmoll HJ, Schoepfe E, eds. Lokale und Systemische Therapie Mit Interferonen. 1990: 127–135.
131. Gross G, Degan W, Hilgrath M, et al. Recombinant interferon gamma in genital warts: results of multicenter placebo-controlled clinical trials. J Invest Dermatol 1989; 93: 553–558.
132. Gross G, Roussaki A, Papendick U. Efficiency of interferons on Bowenoid papulosis and other precancerous lesions. J Invest Dermatol 1990; 95 (suppl): 152s–156s.
133. Mahrle G, Schultze HJ. Recombinant interferon gamma in dermatology. J Invest Dermatol 1990; 95 (suppl): 132s–139s.
134. Kaplan G, Marthur NK, Job CK, et al. The effect of IFN-gamma injection on the disposal of M. leprae. J Interf Res 1989; 9 (suppl 2): 135–139.
135. Legha SS. Interferons in the treatment of malignant melanoma. A review of recent trials. Cancer 1986; 57: 1675–1678.
136. Morhenn VB, Pregerson-Rodan K, Henzl-Mullen R, et al. Use of recombinant interferon gamma administered intramuscularly for the treatment of psoriasis. Arch Dermatol 1987; 123: 1633–1637.

137. Tulli A, Capazzi G, Petitti G, et al. Interferons in scleroderma: clinical use. J Invest Dermatol 1989; 93: 582–585.
138. Pene J, Russet F, Briere F, et al. IgE production by normal human B cells induced by alloreactive T cells clones is mediated by Il-4 and suppressed by IFN-gamma. J Immunol 1988; 141: 1218–1221.
139. Reinhold U, Wehrmann W, Kukel S, et al. Recombinant interferon gamma in atopic dermatitis (letter). Lancet 1990; 1: 1282.

7

Synthetic Antimalarial Drugs in the Therapy of Skin Diseases

Kyrill Pramatarov and Snejina Vassileva
Medical University
Sofia, Bulgaria

Synthetic antimalarials (SAM) are a family of drugs whose origins can be traced to the cinchona tree. The parent compound, quinine, is derived from the bark of this tree. Currently, SAMs are used instead of quinine. The most important agents in this group are chloroquine, hydroxychloroquine, and quinacrine, which were synthesized during the first half of the twentieth century and introduced as antimalarial drugs in 1930. Today, the therapeutic indications of SAM are much wider; aside from their antiprotozoan activity, these agents are well known for their therapeutic effect as first-line or adjuvant drugs in the treatment of several inflammatory dermatoses and connective tissue diseases. For almost 60 years, a great deal of knowledge has been accumulated in the application of SAM in dermatological practice. Additionally, several dermatological and systemic side effects of SAM treatment have emerged and should be considered.

I. PHARMACOKINETICS

Chloroquine (CQ) and hydroxychloroquine (HCQ) share a common active radical—4-aminoquinoline. These compounds are water soluble and are rapidly absorbed from the gastrointestinal tract, reaching peak plasma concentrations 4 to 8 h after an individual dose [1]. The level of absorption of CQ is 90%. Most of it is bound to blood cells, while 60% is bound to plasma proteins. CQ uptake in organs and tissues is extremely high, with increased affinity for the liver, spleen, kidneys, lungs, adrenals, skin [2], and semen [3]. In these organs, concentrations severalfold higher than those in plasma are reached. CQ is mainly excreted via the kidney with 40 to 70% unchanged. Liver metabolites, mainly desethyl-chloroquin, are also excreted. Due to the large amount of stored CQ, blood concentration declines very slowly. Elimination half-lives of CQ and HCQ are greater than 1 month [4]; therefore, a weekly dose of CQ is sufficient for the control of malaria [2]. Body weight and age are important factors for disposition of CQ [5].

II. MECHANISM OF ACTION

The exact mechanism of action of SAM is complex and not yet completely understood [6]. Alteration of absorption of ultraviolet (UV) light, anti-inflammatory activity, DNA binding, as well as immunosuppression, all seem to play a role in the therapeutic action of SAM. As anti-inflammatory agents, they stabilize lysosomal membranes and inhibit the hydrolytic enzymes. They antagonize inflammatory mediators in tissues and also bind to various biochemical compounds such as nucleoproteins, melanin, and porphyrins.

The effects of 3-day oral CQ treatment administered at a dosage of 250 mg four times daily reduce the fasting serum concentration of total cholesterol, low-density lipoprotein, and apolipoprotein. HQ also caused a decrease in fasting plasma glucose levels and an increase in fasting plasma insulin levels [7].

The photoprotective nature of SAM is not entirely understood, but seems related to their ability to bind to DNA and RNA rather than to a direct sunscreening effect. The triplet state of DNA can transfer energy to the triplet state of CQ, thereby interfering with UV-induced thymine dimer formation. CQ may be intercalated between base pairs, serving as a kind of photon sink. This property of nucleoprotein binding may also be important in the inhibition of in vitro immune complex formation as demonstrated by reduced formation of LE-cells, antinuclear antibodies (ANA), and rheumatoid factor (RF), and the decreased Arthus reaction. The anti-inflammatory properties of SAM may be closely related to their affinity for lysosomal structures [6]. Once taken up by lysosomes, in vitro stabilization of the membranes occurs and proteolysis is inhibited. The latter effect may be partially due to inhibition of cathepsin B-1.

Lysosomal alteration interferes with both cellular and humoral immune responses. Inhibition of macrophage, eosinophil, and neutrophil chemotaxis contributes to the anti-inflammatory effect and the mild immunosuppression produced by SAM. In addition, SAM inhibit human mitogen responsiveness in vitro via a selective influence on monocyte capability to secrete interleukin-1 (IL-1). A disruption of intracellular processing of antigen presentation by macrophages might also play a role in the mechanism of action of SAM. Lymphocyte responsiveness is inhibited and lymphocyte blast transformation is suppressed. Nonlysosomal phagocytic functions, including neutrophil and monocyte superoxide anion generation, are altered. Suppression of prostaglandin synthesis also occurs.

Quinacrine (Q) has a quite different chemical structure from that of CQ and HCQ [1]. Today its use is restricted to a few conditions in which these latter are not active, and occasionally, it is used as a temporary substitute for CQ and HCQ.

III. THERAPEUTIC USE OF ANTIMALARIALS

A. Discoid Lupus Erythematosus

Antimalarials were introduced in the treatment of discoid lupus erythematosus (DLE) in the 1940s by the Bulgarian dermatologists Ljuben Popov and Mikhail Kutinchev and the Ukrainian physician Prockopchuk [8].

The exact mechanism of action of SAM in LE is still to be clarified. Their probable therapeutic efficacy is related to their action on nucleic acids, melanin, porphyrins, and immune reactants and cells [9]. A clearing of the immune products from the dermo-epidermal junction is thought to be an important result of antimalarial treatment. This might occur through three basic mechanisms: (1) immunosuppressive action; (2) inhibition of formation and/or tissue binding of immune complexes; (3) increased removal of these complexes by tissue macrophages.

In spite of the fact that HCQ is the only antimalarial drug approved by the Food and Drug Administration for the treatment of LE, CQ and Q are still used for this purpose [6].

The dosage for controling DLE with antimalarials is vague, but the recommended doses are (CQ—125 to 375 mg/day (max 3, 5–4 mg/kg); HCQ—100 to 400 mg/day (max 3–6, 5 mg/kg).

Some patients show either minor or no improvement following antimalarial monotherapy. In patients with refractory DLE, a chloroquine-quinacrine association in a daily dose as low as possible for a few months might be beneficial [11].

The antimalarials have a good effect not only in DLE, but in lupus profundus as well.

B. Subacute Cutaneous Lupus Erythematosus

Antimalarials are first-line treatment for subacute cutaneous LE (SCLE). If patients with SCLE respond poorly to antimalarial monotherapy the association of CQ and Q is recommended. The dosage in such cases is HQ—100 mg t.i.d.; Q—65 mg t.i.d. [12].

C. Systemic Lupus Erythematosus

The mechanism of action of antimalarials in systemic lupus erythematosus (SLE) is similar to that in DLE. They can control the discoid lesions in SLE and the photosensitivity skin changes.

SAM can be applied for 1 to 2 months using CQ and up to 6 months using HCQ. They can promote a remission in nonorgan-threatening SLE and decrease the risk for systemic involvement. Antimalarials are especially useful for cutaneous and inflammatory joint disease, but their action on serositis is modest. Since antimalarials do not depress the bone marrow and do not promote opportunistic infections, they can be combined with other antilupus medications [13].

In mild SLE, antimalarials are capable of relieving subjective symptoms such as joint pains, as has been demonstrated in a double-blind multicenter randomized study of HCQ versus placebo [14]. Significant relief of articular pains was found in the group of SLE patients treated with HCQ.

In SLE patients, HCQ given in addition to corticosteroid therapy is useful in ameliorating the primary symptoms of the disease, but may also be useful in alleviating the adverse effects of the corticosteroid therapy on triglyceride-rich lipoprotein metabolism [15].

Antimalarials can control some additional clinical symptoms of SLE. HCQ is reported to control hypergammaglobulinemic purpura in patients with SLE [16]. HCQ has also been shown to induce simultaneous resolution of SLE and angioneurotic edema due to acquired C1-inhibitor deficiency [17]. In a case of SLE complicated by transverse myelitis, HCQ administered in combination with methylprednisolone and pulse cyclophosphamide produced significant improvement after 1 month of treatment [18].

HCQ has a possible antithrombotic action [19]. It is a platelet inhibitor and appears to decrease the risk of thromboembolism. HCQ is associated with lower serum cholesterol and low-density lipoprotein levels compared to those present in patients treated with corticosteroids, but not antimalarials [15,19].

HCQ may also decrease abnormal cytokine levels. IL-6, soluble suppressor/cytotoxic cells $CD8^-$, and soluble IL-2 receptors are lower in patients taking antimalarials compared to those on corticosteroids alone or without medication. Serum levels of CD8 and soluble IL-2 receptors decrease after 6 weeks of HCQ treatment. This could partly explain the favorable response of SLE patients treated with antimalarials [19].

D. Photodermatoses

Antimalarials can be used in the treatment of some photodermatoses, such as polymorphous light eruption, actinic prurigo, and solar urticaria [20]. Since various immunological processes are involved in these diseases, antimalarials are not first-line drugs and should be restricted to patients who fail to respond to photoprotective measures such as sunscreens and protective clothing. In polymorphous light eruption, actinic prurigo, and solar urticaria, the recommended therapeutic doses are CQ—250 to 500 mg/day for 3 to 5 weeks; HCQ—200 to 400 mg/day for 3 to 5 weeks.

E. Primary Sjögren's Syndrome

Successful treatment of primary Sjögren's syndrome was reported in two small open studies [21]. The results of a 2-year double-blind crossover study of HCQ versus placebo on 19 patients with primary Sjögren's syndrome showed a significant decrease in IgG and IgM and a tendency for a decrease in the erythrocyte sedimentation rate. However, no beneficial clinical effect was found with regard to the symptoms and signs of primary Sjögren's syndrome. In another case, a significant clinical improvement was found in a patient treated with HCQ and corticosteroids for primary Sjögren's syndrome with astasia–abasia [22].

F. Scleroderma

Antimalarials are of limited benefit in scleroderma [23]. Twenty-five patients with systemic sclerosis were treated with CQ in daily doses of 500 mg for 2 weeks and 250 mg subsequently. In a few patients with acrosclerosis, the vasomotor manifestations decreased, but, on the whole, the results were doubtful.

The application of antimalarials in morphea must be documented by well-controlled studies. After administration of antimalarials, in some cases the lilac ring diminished or resolved after several months of treatment and induration decreased. Irregular improvement is probably due to spontaneous regression of the disease. SAM might be recommended for the treatment of more disseminated and generalized forms of the disease. A daily dose of 250 mg CQ for a few months might be tried [24].

There are isolated reports of satisfactory therapeutic results in childhood cases of morphea treated with HCQ. CQ and HCQ have been applied to in doses 200 to 300 mg/day without any side effects [1]. Both CQ and HCQ were applied in combination with penicillin in children with morphea with very good effect [25].

G. Dermatomyositis

The application of antimalarials in dermatomyositis is motivated by the clinical and histological similarities of its dermatological manifestations and those of LE.

Since 1984 [26], it is well known that cutaneous lesions of dermatomyositis are improved by HCQ. Although some dermatologists are skeptical about the results of this therapy, patients with dermatomyositis show photosensitivity and application of antimalarials may be useful [27]. HCQ is the first-line agent, in a dose of 200 to 400 mg/day [28]. Antimalarials can be applied in some milder forms of dermatomyositis, especially in those without muscle weakness or in amyopathic dermatomyositis. In such cases, antimalarials such as HCQ have been applied in a daily dose of 400 mg for 3 months [29]. Sometimes the skin lesions in severe dermatomyositis are not controlled by systemic and local steroid therapy and improve after the administration of antimalarials. In patients treated with HCQ, beneficial response has been noted on both the skin eruption and the accompanying myositis [30]. A reduction of the dose of prednisone and improvement of associated arthralgias have also been documented. HCQ exerts a moderate immunosuppressive action by acting on the efferent arm of the immune reaction. It may stabilize lysosome membranes and inhibit activation of complement. It may also impair chemotaxis of formed elements such as eosinophils, neutrophils, and macrophages. The drug is deposited in the muscle as well as in the skin. The adult dose is 200 mg b.i.d.; children are usually dosed at 2 to 5 mg/kg/day [30]. There is, however, a single report on worsening of the rash in a case of juvenile dermatomyositis after HCQ treatment [31].

H. Pemphigus Foliaceus

Therapy with antimalarial drugs for pemphigus foliaceus has been known since 1965 [32]. Applied alone or as an adjuvant therapy, antimalarials have been reported to control cases with pronounced photosensitivity. This beneficial effect could be explained by the mild immunosuppressive capacity of the antimalarial agents, which minimizes immune complex formation, subsequent epithelial injury, and the inflammatory response.

Three out of 7 patients benefited from SAM treatment, one with complete clearing on HCQ alone. CQ has been applied in two patients with pemphigus erythematosus, one of which was controlled by CQ alone. HCQ is an effective adjuvant therapy in persistent and widespread disease not responsive to corticosteroid therapy alone. This seems especially suitable in patients with pronounced photosensitivity [33].

I. Lichen Planus

In the 1960s, SAM were applied for the treatment of lichen planus, but the results were not promising [34]. A combination of SAM and steroids, in low daily doses for 10 days, might be more effective.

Better results from the treatment with SAM have been obtained in patients with oral lichen planus. Patients received 200 to 400 mg daily as a monotherapy for 6 months. Nine of ten patients had an excellent response. Three of six patients with erosions had complete healing. Pain relief and reduced erythema have been observed after 1 to 2 months of therapy, but erosions required 3 to 6 months of treatment [35].

In a patient with lichen planus of the oral mucosa and the nails, HCQ applied at a dose 500 mg/day for 30 weeks resulted in a normal nail growth, but the lesions reappeared 10 weeks after the withdrawal of the drug [36].

Lichen planus subtropicus, which is a variant of lichen planus, is believed to be induced by sun exposure and antimalarials have been used for treatment since 1976 [37]. The recommended daily dose is 400 mg daily, with improvement occurring in 3 to 4 weeks.

J. Porphyria Cutanea Tarda

The mechanism of action of antimalarials in porphyria cutanea tarda (PCT) is due to the fact that they easily form water-soluble complexes with porphyrins, which leads to their rapid excretion from the hepatocytes. This effect of CQ on urinary porphyrin excretion was first recognized more than 20 years ago. CQ is applied in PCT in low doses, for instance 25 mg daily, 100 mg every other day, or 3 times weekly for 1 month. The dosage can then be increased to 200 mg every other day for another month [38].

In an open trial with a median follow-up of 3 years, 53 patients were treated with 250 mg CQ twice weekly until remission or failure to respond. All patients have had low-to-moderate iron overload or intolerance to phlebotomies. The results confirmed that low-dose CQ is a safe therapy that promotes a high proportion of remissions and sustains the control of PCT associated with low-to-moderate iron overload [39].

High doses of HCQ have also been applied in PCT in an open trial where patients were treated with 250 mg three times daily for 3 days. However, long-term follow-up data showed an overall relapse rate of 33%; furthermore, a transient hepatotoxic reaction occurred in the majority of patients [40]. The reaction was more severe among phlebotomized female patients.

Low doses of CQ (125 mg twice weekly) are used in the treatment of congenital erythropoietic porphyria, but the results are not encouraging. CQ can be used in low doses in infantile PCT. The recommended dose is 100 mg twice weekly for 4 to 5 months in combination with S-adenosyl-L-methionine [41].

K. Rosacea

The actinic damage is one of the possible mechanisms for the development of rosacea. CQ has been applied in daily doses of 500 to 750 mg for 10 to 20 days and then 250 mg/day for 4 weeks. Nevertheless, SAM are no longer popular for the modern treatment of rosacea [42].

L. Granuloma Annulare

Both CQ and HCQ have been reported to be of help in the treatment of childhood cases of disseminated granuloma annulare. The recommended dose of CQ is 3 mg/kg/day for 3 weeks. Doses are then reduced to 1.5 mg/kg/day. HCQ is recommended in a dose of 6 mg/kg/day; after 3 weeks, the dose is reduced to

3 mg/kg/day. The treatment is discontinued 2 weeks after complete healing is achieved [43].

M. Lichen Sclerosus et Atrophicus

A 55-year-old woman with a history of lichen sclerosus et atrophicus with extensive blistering and ulceration was treated with HCQ, which led to clinical improvement. Although SAM may be of therapeutic benefit in cutaneous lichen sclerosus, additional clinical observations are needed to confirm these results [44].

N. Erythema Nodosum Chronicum

Antimalarials may be applied in erythema nodosum chronicum because of their anti-inflammatory action. In a few reports, positive results have been observed from treatment with SAM alone or in combination with potassium jodide. The recommended doses of HCQ are 200 mg twice daily for 2 to 3 months [45].

O. Hypercalcemia

CQ has been applied in a dosage of 500 mg twice daily to a patient with hypercalcemia associated with Wegener's granulomatosis and hyperparathyroidism. Treatment significantly decreased calcium levels. A similar effect has been reported in hypercalcemic patients with sarcoidosis [46].

P. Human Immunodeficiency Virus Type 1

HCQ has been shown to suppress human immunodeficiency virus type 1 (HIV-1) replication in vitro in T cells and monocytes by inhibiting post-transcriptional modification of the virus. A randomized, double-blind, placebo-controlled clinical trial was conducted in 40 asymptomatic HIV-1-infected patients. They received either 800 mg/day HCQ or placebo for 8 weeks. The laboratory and immunological tests confirmed that HCQ might be useful in the treatment of patients with HIV-1-infection [47]. The antiviral effects of HCQ have been confirmed in two patients with AIDS and inflammatory arthritis. HCQ may exert simultaneous anti-inflammatory and antiviral effects in patients with HIV infection and it may be the drug of choice in this population of patients [48].

IV. INTERACTION WITH OTHER DRUGS

The combination of SAM with steroids is suitable for the treatment of several diseases, especially connective tissue disorders. On the other hand, reports on the interaction of antimalarials with drugs other than steroids are sparse. CQ reduces the bioavailability of methotrexate [49]. This has been confirmed in a trial of 11 patients with rheumatoid arthritis who were taking oral doses of 15 mg/week methotrexate plus 250 mg CQ. This combination caused a reduction in the area under the plasma methotrexate concentration versus time curve (AUC). Most probably CQ reduces the bioavailability of methotrexate and this is the possible explanation for a reduction in methotrexate-associated liver toxicity by coadministration of CQ.

CQ enhancement of C_{max} by paracetamol and analgin has been reported, while aspirin does not alter these kinetic parameters [50]. Eighty patients with active rheumatoid arthritis were studied for 24 weeks to compare the efficacy and toxicity of HCQ, dapsone, and the combination of both drugs. The findings suggest that HCQ in combination with dapsone is more effective and less tolerated than the respective therapies alone [51].

V. SIDE EFFECTS OF ANTIMALARIALS

Ocular toxicity is the main side effect of SAM treatment. It is not established yet if this side effect depends on the weight, age, total or daily dose of antimalarials. The main targets of SAM ocular toxicity are the cornea, ciliary body, and retina. It has been accepted that retinopathy is the most important side effect; it is, however, unlikely to occur with HCQ dosages of up to 6.5 mg/kg body weight during a treatment period less than 10 years [52]. At the same time, patients who had received daily doses of 200 mg CQ for periods ranging from 3 to 11 months show a minimal risk for retinal toxicity [53]; the ocular risk is almost negligible at a dosage of less then 6 mg/kg/day. At a daily dosage of 400 mg or more, the risk/benefit ratio is acceptable for a person of average weight, provided that adequate ophthalmological monitoring is ensured. The risk of retinal toxicity is then proportional to the duration of therapy and the cumulative dose. Ophthalmoscopic examinations at 6-month intervals are sufficient to detect occasional side effects [6]. The visual prognosis of retinopathy is excellent if the diagnosis is made at an early stage of the disease [54]. However, ocular toxicity has been reported in an elderly patient on a normal dose of HCQ, so special attention should be given to elderly patients [55]. Keratopathy has been found in 73% of patients treated with CQ; its clinical features and course suggest, however, that this side effect is not a contraindication for treatment with SAM [56].

Several cutaneous, gastrointestinal, hematological, auditory, and central nervous system (CNS) side effects of SAM should also be considered [1,57]. Adverse effects of SAM on the skin include exacerbation of psoriasis (58), a case of acute generalized exanthematous pustulosis [59], pruritus, lichenoid eruption, erythroderma, discolorations, hair bleaching, alopecia [1]. CQ stimulates the mitogen-induced lymphocyte proliferation in psoriasis patients [58]. Among antimalarial-induced CNS complications, headache, seizures, neuromyopathy, confusion, toxic psychoses, and mood disorders should be mentioned [1,60].

REFERENCES

1. Ziering CL, Rabinowitz LG, Esterly NB. Antimalarials for children: indications, toxicities, and guidelines. J Am Acad Dermatol 1993; 28:764–770.
2. Mohr K. Chloroquine. Dtsch Med Wochenschr 1994; 119:273–274.
3. Adeeko AO, Dada OA. Chloroquine excretion in semen following antimalarial-drug administration. Andrologia 1994; 26:165–166.
4. Tett SE. Clinical pharmacokinetics of slow-acting antirheumatic drugs. Clin Pharmacokinet 1993; 25:392–407.
5. Hellgren U, Alvan G, Jerling M. On the question of interindividual variations in chloroquine concentrations. Eur J Clin Pharmacol 1993; 45:383–385.
6. Potter B. Hydroxychloroquine. Cutis 1993; 52:229–231.
7. Powrie JK, Shojaee-Moradie F, Watts GF, et al. Metabolism 1993; 42:415–419.
8. Hauser W. Lupus erythematodes chronicus. In: Gottron HA, Schoenefeld W, eds. Dermatologie and Venerologie. Stuttgart: G. Thieme, 1958, Bd II, teil I:587–592.
9. Chieregato G, Peroni A, Castellani L, et al. Effects of hydroxychloroquine on ''band test'' in discoid lupus erythematosus. Dermatologica 1990; 180:130–132.
10. Tappeiner G. Therapie des Lupus Erythematodes 1994. Z Hautkr 1994; 69:816–822.
11. Lipsker D, Piette JC, Cacoub P, et al. Chloroquine-quinacrine association in resistent cutaneous lupus. Dermatology 1995; 190:257–258.
12. Feldmann R, Salomon D, Saurat JH. The association of the two antimalarials chloroquine and quinacrine for treatment-resistent chronic and subacute cutaneous lupus erythematosus. Dermatology 1994; 189:425–427.
13. Wallace DJ. Antimalarial agents and lupus. Rheum Dis Clin North Am 1994; 20: 243–263.
14. Williams HJ, Egger MJ, Singer JZ, et al. Comparison of hydroxychloroquine and placebo in the treatment of the arthropathy of mild systemic lupus erythematosus. J Rheumatol 1994; 21:1457–1463.
15. Hodis HN, Quismorio FP Jr, Wickham E, et al. The lipid, lipoprotein, and apolipoprotein effects of hydroxychloroquine in patients with systemic lupus erythematosus. J Rheumatol 1993; 20:661–665.
16. Senecal JL, Chartier S, Rothfield N. Hypergammaglobulinemic purpura in systemic autoimmune rheumatic diseases: predictive value of anti-Ro (SSA) and anti-La (SSB) antibodies and treatment with indomethacin and hydroxychloroquine. J Rheumatol 1995; 22:868–875.
17. Ochonisky S, Intrator L, Wechsler J, et al. Acquired C1 inhibitor deficiency revealing systemic lupus erythematosus. Dermatology 1993; 186:261–263.
18. Klaiman MD, Miller SD. Transverse myelitis complicated systemic lupus erythematosus: treatment including hydroxychloroquine. Case report. Am J Phys Med Rehabil 1993; 72:158–161.
19. Wallace DJ, Linker-Israeli M, Metzger AL, et al. The relevance of antimalarial therapy with regard to thrombosis. Lupus 1993; 2 (suppl 1):13s–15s.
20. Maddin S. Current Dermatological Therapy, 2nd ed., Philadelphia: WB Saunders Company, 1991:156–158.

21. Kruize AA, Hene RJ, Kallenberg CG, et al. Hydroxychloroquine treatment for primary Sjogren's syndrome: a two year double blind crossover trial. Ann Rheum Dis 1993; 52:360–364.
22. Lafforgue P, Toussirot E, Bille F, et al. Astasia-abasia revealing a primary Sjogren's syndrome. Clin Rheumatol 1993; 12:261–264.
23. Jablonska S. Scleroderma and Pseudoscleroderma, 2nd ed. Warsaw: Polish Medical Publishers, 1975:618.
24. Mensing H. Therapie der zirkumskripten Sklerodermie. Dermatologie. Stuttgart. Thieme Verlag, 1995:161–162.
25. Nagy E, Ladanyi E. Behandlung der umschriebenen Sklerodermie im Kindesalter. Z Hautkr 1987; 62:547–549.
26. Woo TY, Callen JP, Voorhees JJ, et al. Cutaneous lesions of dermatomyositis are improved by hydroxychloroquine. J Am Acad Dermatol 1984; 10:592–600.
27. Cheong WK, Hughes GRV, Norris PG, et al. Cutaneous photosensitivity in dermatomyositis. Br J Dermatol 1994; 131:205–208.
28. Avgerinou G. Treatment of dermatomyositis. Proc Int Meeting Clin Dermatol, Athens, 1996:58–60.
29. Cosnes A, Amaudric F, Gherardi R, et al. Dermatomyositis without muscle weakness. Long-term follow-up of 12 patients without systemic corticosteroids. Arch Dermatol 1995; 131:1381–1385.
30. Boyd AS, Neldner KH. Therapeutic options in dermatomyositis/polymyositis. Int J Dermatol 1994; 33:240–250.
31. Bloom BJ, Tucker LE, Klein-Gitelman M, et al. Worsening of the rash of juvenile dermatomyositis with hydroxychloroquine therapy. J Rheumatol 1994; 21:2171–2172.
32. Perry HO, Brunsting LA. Pemphigus foliaceus: further observations. Arch Dermatol 1965; 91:10–23.
33. Hymes S, Jordon R. Pemphigus foliaceus: use of antimalarial agents as adjuvant therapy. Arch Dermatol 1992; 128:1462–1464.
34. Dowjanski SI, Slesarenko NA. Lichen ruber planus. Saratow: Saratow University Publishers, 1990:146–147 (Russian).
35. Eisen D. Hydroxychloroquine sulfate (plaquenil) improves oral lichen planus: an open trial. J Am Acad Dermatol 1993; 28:609–612.
36. Mostafa WZ. Lichen planus of the nails: treatment with antimalarials. J Am Acad Dermatol 1989; 20:289.
37. Albers SE, Glass LF, Fenske NA. Lichen planus subtropicus: direct immunofluorescence findings and therapeutic response to hydroxychloroquine. Int J Dermatol 1994; 33:645–647.
38. Malkinson FD. Hydroxychloroquine treatment of porphyria cutanea tarda. Arch Dermatol 1980; 116:1147–1150.
39. Valls V, Ena J, Enriquez de Salamanca R. Low-dose oral chloroquine in patients with porphyria cutanea tarda and low-moderate iron overload. J Dermatol Sci 1994; 7:169–175.
40. Petersen CS, Thomsen K. High-dose hydrochloroquine treatment of porphyria cutanea tarda. J Am Acad Dermatol 1992; 26:614–615.
41. Del C, Battle AM, Stella AM, De Kaminsky AR, et al. Two cases of infantile

porphyria cutanea tarda: successful treatment with oral S-adenosyl-L-methionine and low-dose oral chloroquine. Br J Dermatol 1987; 116:407–415.

42. Yansen T, Plewig G. Klinik und Therapie der Rosazea. Z Hautkr 1996; 71:88–95.
43. Simon M Jr, Von den Driesch P. Antimalarials for control of disseminated granuloma annulare in children. J Am Acad Dermatol 1994; 31:1064–1065.
44. Wakelin SH, Jams MP. Extensive lichen sclerosus et atrophicus with bullae and ulceration—improvement with hydroxychloroquine. Clin Exp Dermatol 1994; 19: 332–334.
45. Alloway JA, Franks LK. Hydroxychloroquine in the treatment of chronic erythema nodosum. Br J Dermatol 1995; 132:661–673.
46. Edelson GW, Talpos GB, None HG. Hypercalcemia associated with Wegener's granulomatosis and hyperparathyroidism: etiology and management. Am J Nephrol 1993; 13:275–277.
47. Sperber K, Louie M, Kraus T, et al. Hydroxychloroquine treatment of patients with human immunodeficiency virus type 1. Clin Ther 1995; 17:622–636.
48. Ornstein MH, Sperber K. The antiinflammatory and antiviral effects of hydroxychloroquine in two patients with acquired immunodeficiency syndrome and active inflammatory arthritis. Arthr Rheum 1996; 39:157–161.
49. Seideman P, Albertioni F, Beck O, et al. Chloroquine reduces the bioavailability of methotrexate in patients with rheumatoid arthritis. A possible mechanism of reduced hepatotoxicity. Arthr Rheum 1994; 37:830–833.
50. Raina RK, Bano G, Amla V, et al. The effect of aspirin, paracetamol, and analgin on pharmacokinetics of chloroquine. Ind J Physiol Pharmacol 1993; 37:229–231.
51. Haar D, Solvkjaer M, Unger B, et al. A double-blind comparative study of hydroxychloroquine and dapsone, alone and combination, in rheumatoid arthritis. Scand J Rheumatol 1993; 22:113–118.
52. Spalton DJ, Verdon-Roe GM, Hughes GR. Hydroxychloroquine, dosage parameters and retinopathy. Lupus 1993; 2:355–358.
53. Bartel PR, Roux P, Robinson E, et al. Visual function and long-term chloroquine treatment. South Afr Med J 1994; 84:32–34.
54. Easterbrook M. The ocular safety of hydroxychloroquine. Semin Arthritis Rheum 1993; 23(2 suppl 1):62s–67s.
55. Falcone PM, Paolini L, Lou PL. Hydroxychloroquine toxicity despite normal dose therapy. Ann Ophthalmol 1993; 25:385–388.
56. Jeddi A, Ben Osman N, Daghfous F, et al. Cornée et antipaludéens de synthèse. J Fr Ophthalmol 1994; 17:36–38.
57. Caminal-Montero L, Gonzalez-Marroquin A, Ferro-Mosquera J, et al. Thrombopenia secondary to hydroxychloroquine. Ann Med Interna 1994; 11:310.
58. Schipfs RE, Ockenfels HM, Schultewolter T, et al. Chloroquine stimulates the mitogen-driven lymphocyte proliferation in patients with psoriasis. Dermatology 1993; 187:100–103.
59. Assier H, Auffret N, Beltzer-Garelly E, et al. Pustuleuse exanthématique aigue genéralisée à l'hydroxychloroquine. Ann Dermatol Venereol 1993; 120:848–850.
60. Akhtar S, Mukherjee S. Chloroquine induced mania. Int J Psychiatry Med 1993; 23:349–356.

8

Cyclosporin A

John Berth-Jones
Walsgrave Hospital
University of Warwick
Coventry, United Kingdom

Cyclosporin A is a noncytotoxic immunosuppressant that was first discovered in 1970. It has had a remarkable impact on modern medicine. Its initial use was for immunosuppression following organ and marrow transplantation and without this drug these procedures would not have become possible on anything approaching the scale on which they are currently undertaken. Subsequently, cyclosporin A has found applications in virtually all branches of medicine where autoimmune or inflammatory processes play a role in the pathology. Dermatologists, being somewhat conservative by nature, have not been quick to jump on this bandwagon. Although reports that cyclosporin A was effective in psoriasis began to appear in 1979, the first controlled trial was not published until 1986.

I. PHARMACOLOGY

Cyclosporin A is an antibiotic produced by the fungus Tolypocladium inflatum Gams. Despite many years of sustained effort, it has not proved possible to obtain the benefits of cyclosporin A by topical application. This is probably due to the large molecular weight of this compound. Since systemic administration is required, the use of this drug in dermatology has been constrained by concern over potential toxicity. Nevertheless it has found a number of applications within the specialty and is most frequently used in psoriasis and atopic dermatitis.

A. Structure

Cyclosporin A is a cyclic undecapeptide with molecular weight 1203.

B. Mechanism of Action

Cyclosporin A inhibits lymphocyte activation. This is effected by blocking transduction of the signal from the lymphocyte receptor that induces transcription of lymphokines. The drug requires a cyclophilin for activity and is only active when bound to a member of this family of enzymes, which are cis-trans isomerases abundant in the cytoplasm of most types of cell. The cyclosporin/cyclophilin complex binds to and inhibits a cytoplasmic enzyme—calcineurin phosphatase. Calcineurin is a calcium–calmodulin-dependent serine–threonine phosphatase. Among the substrates of this enzyme are transcription activating factors [e.g., nuclear factor of activated T cells (NFAT)], which enter the nucleus and ''activate'' the lymphocyte by promoting transcription of lymphokines such as IL-2, interferon-γ, granulocyte macrophage-colony stimulating factor (GM-CSF), IL-3, IL-4, TNF-α and others. Activation of T4 lymphocytes with both Th1 and Th2 lymphokine profiles can be inhibited in this way.

In vitro studies have demonstrated numerous other properties of cyclosporin A, including inhibition of the function of antigen presenting cells as well as of the release of mast-cell mediators, including histamine and leukotrienes, and actions on keratinocytes, including inhibition of proliferation and cytokine secretion. However, at least in vitro, much higher concentrations of the drug are usually required to produce these effects than are required to inhibit lymphocyte activation.

C. Absorption

Cyclosporin A is a lipid-soluble drug. It is somewhat unpredictably absorbed when given orally. Until recently, the only formulation available was a solution in olive oil. Absorption of the drug in this formulation was highly dependent on the presence of lipid and bile in the gut. This formulation has now been superseded by a microemulsion. The small particle size allows greater predictability and consistency of absorption, but even with this formulation about half of the drug is not absorbed.

D. Metabolism

Cyclosporin A undergoes metabolism to inactive products by cytochrome P-450 type 3A isoenzymes (especially isoenzyme 3A4). It is therefore subject to numerous metabolic interactions with other drugs that can significantly alter the blood levels of the drug.

II. DRUG INTERACTIONS

Cyclosporin A is a drug with a narrow therapeutic index. Relatively small changes in blood levels can markedly influence efficacy and toxicity. Drug interactions are therefore an important consideration. Numerous drugs affect the hepatic metabolism of cyclosporin A. Important examples of drugs inhibiting cyclosporin A metabolism are erythromycin, itraconazole, diltiazem, and verapamil. Drugs that may accelerate cyclosporin A metabolism include phenytoin, rifampicin, and carbamazepine. New drug interactions are frequently reported and it is essential to consult an up-to-date reference list of drug interactions whenever other drugs are prescribed for patients taking cyclosporin A.

It is best to avoid cyclosporin A, if possible, in patients requiring any other potentially nephrotoxic drugs, including nonsteroidal anti-inflammatory agents. Cyclosporin A is also generally best avoided in patients taking additional immunosuppressant or carcinogenic therapies. Concomitant treatment with PUVA is therefore undesirable since this is both carcinogenic and immunosuppressive.

III. CONTRAINDICATIONS

There are a number of situations in which cyclosporin A should be avoided if possible. These include patients with renal disease; hypertension; hyperlipidemia; active chronic infection or evidence of previous infection with hepatitis B or C; and any history of malignancy. Cyclosporin A is not known to be teratogenic. Although its use cannot be recommended in pregnancy, it would seem preferable to using cytotoxic drugs, retinoids, and perhaps PUVA. In the elderly, the usefulness of cyclosporin A tends to be restricted by a lower renal reserve.

IV. TOXICITY

The most frequent problem requiring withdrawal of cyclosporin A is renal impairment that is related to dose and duration of treatment [1]. Even short courses of treatment at a dose of 5 mg/kg/day may produce a measurable effect on renal function [2]. This appears to be reversible provided that the recommended dose rate of 5 mg/kg/day is not exceeded and that the dose is reduced, or even stopped, if required, to prevent the serum creatinine rising to more than 130% of baseline. However, even when these guidelines are followed, it cannot be stated that renal impairment is 100% reversible. In a series of eight patients with psoriasis treated by Korstanje et al. for an average of 12 months, glomerular filtration rate (GFR) had fallen by 17.8% and remained 9.8% below baseline even 4 months after stopping cyclosporin A [3]. Zachariae et al. have reported histological changes in the kidney in a group of 30 psoriasis patients treated with doses of up to 6 mg/kg/day for 6 months to 8 years [4]. Changes became pronounced after 2 years and the authors considered that if cyclosporin A therapy was to be continued, estimations of GFR and renal biopsies should be performed. Powles et al. have reported on the renal function of 29 patients with psoriasis treated with cyclosporin A for between 5 and 11 years, who were monitored using a combination of serum creatinine, isotope GFR estimations, and renal biopsies [5]. In the worst case, histology revealed 25% glomerular obsolescence after 10 years of treatment. The higher the dose and the longer the duration of treatment the less reversible the renal changes are likely to be; however, most importantly, renal impairment generally recovers at least partially and does not seem to become progressive after treatment is discontinued [5].

Additional manifestations of nephrotoxicity are the increases in serum potassium and urate observed during treatment. Although these are rarely severe enough to require dose adjustment, it is sometimes necessary to monitor serum potassium and urate in conjunction with the creatinine level.

Treatment with cyclosporin A results in an increase in blood pressure that can be detected even in the short term. Significant hypertension may develop at any time during treatment and this is probably a dose-dependent effect. Hypertension resulting from cyclosporin A therapy can either be treated along conventional lines or the dose of cyclosporin A can be reduced. Nifedipine appears to have a protective effect on renal function during cyclosporin A treatment. Thus this is a particularly useful drug if it is considered necessary to treat hypertension.

An increase in serum bilirubin is often observed during cyclosporin A treatment. In the author's experience, the largest rises have occurred in subjects who already had an elevated bilirubin prior to treatment (Gilbert's syndrome). Isolated increases in serum bilirubin do not usually require cyclosporin A dose adjustment. Rises in transaminases appear to be relatively rare and should prompt screening for occult viral hepatitis.

Other side effects include arthralgia, gastrointestinal disorders (nausea, abdominal pain, diarrhea), gingival hyperplasia, headache, hypertrichosis, paraesthesias, and tremor. Nausea is most frequently encountered after the first few doses and usually resolves. Gum hypertrophy may respond to improved dental hygiene or a reduction in dose. Hypertrichosis is often seen to some degree and may be a particular problem in female patients with dark hair. Cyclosporin A is known to raise serum cholesterol and triglyceride levels.

Infections, including herpes simplex, have not been a prominent problem during treatment of psoriasis or atopic dermatitis. However, cyclosporin A can be hazardous in patients who have suffered from hepatitis B or C.

The risk of malignancy developing as a result of immunosuppression is difficult to quantify at present, but appears to be small. Although there is no doubt that the risk of diverse malignancies, including cutaneous tumors and lymphomas, is increased in transplant patients, this group undergo immunosuppression of a different order of magnitude than dermatological patients. Cutaneous malignancy is a particular hazard in patients with psoriasis who have received significant doses of therapeutic ultraviolet irradiation. Squamous cell carcinomas have been reported in these circumstances.

V. MONITORING

Before starting cyclosporin A it is important to assess the suitability of the patients by carefully assessing any of the contraindications and risk factors discussed above. Blood pressure should be recorded and examination performed for any evidence of lymphadenopathy, malignancy, or infection. Female patients should be encouraged to comply with routine screening for cervical neoplasia.

Serum creatinine should be measured to establish a baseline. It is often surprising how much this varies from day to day, so three estimations should be performed, at intervals of a few days, and the mean should be used as the baseline value. Other potentially useful investigations at baseline are liver function tests, fasting serum lipids, and urinalysis to detect proteinuria or hematuria which may be indicative of preexisting renal disease.

Patients should be reviewed after 2 and 4 weeks on cyclosporin A and then monthly, or at 2-week intervals if there is any cause for concern. During long-term maintenance therapy, if the treatment has been well tolerated for 6 months, it is possible to extend the review interval to 6 or 8 weeks in some patients.

Serum creatinine should be checked at each visit. Small reductions in GFR in the normal kidney are not detected by monitoring serum creatinine because tubular secretion increases to compensate. However, in subjects in whom renal function is already impaired, the creatinine rises much more promptly with small changes in the GFR. This investigation is therefore most sensitive in the circumstances where it is most important. As discussed above, published experience suggests that changes in renal function are largely reversible after stopping treatment provided that the dose is reduced as required to prevent a sustained rise in serum creatinine of more than 30%.

Blood pressure should also be monitored at each review. If hypertension develops, it can either be treated or the dose of cyclosporin A can be reduced.

Plasma trough levels of cyclosporin A have not proved a useful means of predicting the risk of nephrotoxicity during the treatment of skin disease.

VI. SPECIFIC INDICATIONS FOR CYCLOSPORIN A IN DERMATOLOGY

Approved indications vary from country to country. The most frequent applications for the use of cyclosporin A are severe psoriasis and atopic dermatitis and there is a good deal of published experience in these diseases. In addition, cyclosporin A appears to be effective in a very large number of indications which span virtually the whole range of inflammatory dermatoses and connective tissue diseases. Efficacy has been demonstrated in some indications that are quite difficult to explain, since they are not generally considered as lymphocyte-mediated.

Examples include the responses seen in chronic idiopathic urticaria and in Hailey–Hailey disease.

A. Alopecia Areata

The frequent development of hypertrichosis in patients receiving cyclosporin A and the fact that this is believed to be an autoimmune disease have led to several attempts to treat alopecia areata with cyclosporin A. The results have generally been disappointing. Although the disease can sometimes respond, high doses of the drug seem to be required and the condition relapses on discontinuation. There is clearly quite a risk of psychological dependence developing to cyclosporin A when it is used to treat alopecia areata, since this disease is associated with such intense emotional distress. Since the disease itself does not even slightly harm or incapacitate patients physically, extremely careful consideration is required before initiating a drug that is potentially toxic.

B. Atopic Eczema

It is paradoxical that cyclosporin A was used initially in psoriasis, which had not previously been considered an autoimmune disease, well before it was used in atopic dermatitis, which has always been regarded as a disorder involving the immune system. A sizable volume of research has now been published on the use of cyclosporin A in this indication. This began with a series of uncontrolled observations [6] that were followed by controlled trials of cross-over [7–9] and parallel group design [10] to confirm the efficacy and tolerability of the drug. More recent research has examined long-term treatment, compared different treatment regimens, and, perhaps most importantly, examined the efficacy and tolerability of cyclosporin A in childhood atopic dermatitis.

It is quite clear that cyclosporin A is highly effective in atopic dermatitis. The pruritus can be improved within 24 h of starting treatment. The signs and symptoms of the disease and also the quality of life for patients have all been shown to improve during treatment. The requirement for topical steroids is also reduced by this treatment and this can be useful in circumstances where the use of large quantities of topical corticosteroids is causing concern.

Children respond well and seem to tolerate cyclosporin A at least as well as adults [11,12]. Changes in renal function and blood pressure have been less than those seen in adults when children are treated with doses of up to 5 mg/kg/day, although it is possible that this simply reflects the fact that children metabolize the drug more rapidly.

Long-term studies of up to 12 months duration indicate that the response can be maintained without tachyphylaxis and that the drug is well tolerated over this period of time [13,14]. Initial anxiety that herpes simplex and other infections might be increased has proved largely unfounded. In some individuals, treatment has apparently induced prolonged remissions after treatment was discontinued but it is difficult to be certain whether this merely represents the natural history of the disease.

Prompt relapse often occurs after the drug is discontinued. After treatment is stopped, pruritus may return as rapidly as it resolved when the treatment commenced, and this can be distressing, especially to children. For this reason, cyclosporin A should not be stopped abruptly when treating atopic dermatitis. It should be tapered off gradually over a period of at least 1 month, either by gradually reducing the daily dose or by giving the drug once daily and then gradually increasing the number of days between doses. An interesting study by Munro et al. [9] compared a reducing dosage (1 mg/kg/day steps) and a reducing frequency of treatment (1 day decrements; intermittent full-dose therapy). Dose or frequency were reduced every 2 weeks. Improvement was maintained by both regimens; however, cyclosporin A 5 mg/kg once every 5 days was more effective than 1 mg/kg/day.

Intermittent short courses of cyclosporin A are probably more difficult to use in atopic dermatitis than in psoriasis due to the greater speed of relapse in atopic dermatitis. This approach has been investigated both in adults [15] and in children [16] and may be somewhat better tolerated by adults. Even short courses of treatment should be tapered off and not stopped abruptly.

The dose required is usually about 3 mg/kg day and even severe cases usually respond well to this dose. A more rapid improvement is seen if treatment is started at a higher dose and then reduced, but a lower cumulative exposure can be achieved by starting with a lower dose and increasing this until control is achieved.

C. Behçet's Disease

The efficacy of cyclosporin A in Behçet's disease has been confirmed by numerous reports, including a trial in which cyclosporin A compared favorably to colchicine. The orogenital ulceration and also uveitis seem to respond well.

D. Benign Familial Pemphigus and Darier's Disease

Reports suggest that cyclosporin A may play a role in the management of these diseases, particularly during acute inflammatory episodes.

E. Connective Tissue Disease

The treatment of rheumatoid disease has tended to become more aggressive in recent years in an attempt to limit joint damage during the early phase of the illness. There is now an extensive literature on the use of cyclosporin A in rheumatoid disease and it is generally considered to be helpful. There is currently a trend to combine cyclosporin A with methotrexate in order to reduce the doses required and minimize the side effects of each drug.

Encouraging, but somewhat inconsistent, results have been reported in adult and juvenile cases of dermatomyositis and polymyositis. In systemic sclerosis, the results have also been mixed. The risks of renal toxicity and hypertension are clearly significant but the drug can be beneficial, especially in patients without hypertension or renal involvement. Benefit has been reported in systemic lupus erythematosus (SLE) and lupus nephritis may also respond. Several cases of relapsing polychondritis have been reported to respond. Improvement has been reported in morphea, including a case secondary to porphyria cutanea tarda. Results in discoid lupus erythematosus have been disappointing.

F. Eczematous Dermatoses

Response to cyclosporin A has been reported in virtually all types of eczema, including contact allergic dermatitis, chronic actinic dermatitis, pompholyx, and even nodular prurigo.

G. Granulomatous Disorders

More evidence is needed regarding the efficacy of cyclosporin A in this group of disorders. Improvement has been reported in one case of sarcoidosis treated with cyclosporin A alone and in a series of 11 in which sarcoid was treated with cyclosporin A (5 mg/kg/day) combined with corticosteroid and methotrexate. There are reports of sarcoidosis worsening during treatment with cyclosporin A and it has been suggested that this may sometimes be caused by the drug. Overall, the literature does not indicate that sarcoidosis will prove highly responsive to this treatment.

Convincing responses have been reported in granuloma annulare, but not in all cases and in the author's experience the drug has been ineffective in two cases of disseminated disease. Necrobiosis lipoidica diabeticorum has been reported to respond in one case.

H. Immunobullous Disease

In immunobullous dermatoses, cyclosporin A has most often been used concurrently with corticosteroids and has demonstrated a useful steroid-sparing effect as well as improvement in disease control. Fairly consistent benefit has been seen in bullous pemphigoid and pemphigus vulgaris and responses are reported in isolated cases of pemphigus foliaceous and erythematosus, epidermolysis bullosa acquisita, and dermatitis herpetiformis. The use of cyclosporin A in bullous pemphigoid is constrained in some cases by the relatively low renal reserve in this largely elderly population, but sometimes the drug is tolerated surprisingly well.

I. Lichen Planus

Cyclosporin A is highly effective in lichen planus. The symptoms rapidly improve and papules and even hypertrophic lesions resolve. Unfortunately, the disease often relapses fairly promptly when the drug is discontinued. The efficacy of topical cyclosporin A in oral lesions may be due to systemic absorption.

J. Psoriasis

Cyclosporin A is a highly effective and rapidly acting systemic treatment for psoriasis. Reports of chronic plaque psoriasis responding to cyclosporin A began to appear in 1979 [17]. The first controlled trial in psoriasis was published in 1986 [18]. The efficacy of this treatment has been confirmed in double-blind, placebo-controlled trials [19,20] and a much larger volume of open trials. Virtually all patients seem to respond, although the dose required depends on the level of disease activity and occasional patients will not respond to doses within the recommended maximum. It is also established that the effect of the cyclosporin A can be maintained by long-term treatment.

Response to cyclosporin A is not confined to chronic plaque psoriasis and extends to virtually all the clinical variants and manifestations of the disease. It is effective in erythrodermic psoriasis and generalized pustular psoriasis. Benefit has also been reported in the localized forms of pustular psoriasis, palmo-plantar pustulosis [21], and acrodermatitis continua of Hallopeau [22]. Nail dystrophy and scalp involvement also respond. There are numerous reports of improvement in psoriatic arthropathy. Cyclosporin A can also be useful in moderate forms of chronic plaque psoriasis [23,24]. Bullous pemphigoid seems to occur more frequently in patients with psoriasis and cyclosporin A can be useful in some patients with this disease combination, since it can be effective in both conditions.

For treatment of psoriasis, the dose should not exceed a maximum of 5 mg/kg/day and this is usually divided into two equal morning and evening doses. Cyclosporin A may either be employed as a maintenance treatment, using long-term continuous therapy, or as a short course of treatment for 4 to 12 weeks to induce remission, which might then be repeated later following relapse. It seems likely that less severe cases may best be treated with intermittent therapy, while patients with the most active disease require maintenance therapy.

The starting dose ranges from 2.5 to 5 mg/kg/day. Higher doses produce a more rapid response. If improvement is not apparent after 2 weeks, the dose can be increased by 0.5 to 1 mg/kg/day at 2-week intervals, provided that the maximum dose rate of 5 mg/kg/day is not exceeded. Once adequate improvement has occurred, either the drug can be stopped in less severe cases or the dose can be reduced in steps of 0.5 to 1 mg/kg day, at 2-week intervals to determine the lowest dose at which adequate control of the psoriasis can be maintained. Small changes in dose often make a considerable difference in the response. The maintenance dose required may vary over time with disease activity. The aim of maintenance treatment should not be to maintain the patient completely clear of psoriasis, but rather to keep the disease activity at a level tolerable for the patient. Topical treatment probably has a useful dose-sparing action and should therefore be continued.

Consensus guidelines have recently been published on the use of cyclosporin A in psoriasis [25].

K. Pyoderma Gangrenosum and "Neutrophilic Dermatoses"

Cyclosporin A is probably now the drug of first choice in severe cases of pyoderma gangrenosum. Reported responses have been consistent and unequivocal. Improvement is usually apparent within 3 weeks and complete healing takes a few weeks or months. Some patients require maintenance treatment, but in others treatment has been discontinued without relapse during reported follow-up for up to 3 years. High doses of up to 10 mg/kg/day have been required in some cases.

Improvement has been reported in cases of Sweet's syndrome, hidradenitis suppurativa, and leukocytoclastic vasculitis.

L. Toxic Epidermal Necrolysis

There are several reports of successful outcomes following the use of cyclosporin A in drug induced toxic epidermal necrolysis. It is clearly important to start treatment as soon as the diagnosis has been made and it seems likely that cyclosporin A can arrest the progression of the disease.

M. Urticaria

Chronic idiopathic urticaria has been reported to be responsive to cyclosporin A by several investigators. The onset of action is prompt, so the mechanism probably involves a direct inhibition of mast-cell activation.

N. Vitiligo

Results from the use of cyclosporin A in vitiligo have been rather disappointing. Although some cases have responded, the disease does not seem very sensitive to cyclosporin A and it is unlikely that advanced cases can be improved. There is no reason to suppose that the natural history of the disease will be changed and, as in the case of alopecia areata, there is a danger of developing psychological dependence on the drug, which could make it difficult to discontinue if it appears to have been effective.

O. Miscellaneous Dermatoses

Additional dermatoses reported to respond in small numbers of cases or single reports have included eosinophilic pustular folliculitis, epidermolysis bullosa dystrophica, erythema multiforme, hydroa vacciniforme, lichen sclerosus, panniculitis (including Weber-Christian and histiocytic cytophagic types), and pityriasis lichenoides chronica. The author has observed a prompt improvement in distressing pruritus in a patient with papuloerythroderma of Ofuji. Cyclosporin A has been reported to improve symptoms of senile pruritus in an open study performed on 10 cases.

P. Diseases Not Responding to Cyclosporin A

Pityriasis rubra pilaris usually does not seem to respond, although there are isolated reports of benefit. In cutaneous T-cell lymphoma, initial improvement of symptoms is usually followed by rapid deterioration, suggesting that immunosuppression may worsen the prognosis. Cases of lamellar ichthyosis have shown no response. A case of Nekam's disease treated by the author showed no response.

REFERENCES

1. Young EW, Ellis CN, Messana SM, Johnson KJ, Leichtman A, Mihatsch MJ, Hamilton TA, Groisser DS, Fradin NS, Voorhees JJ. A prospective study of renal structure and function in psoriasis patients treated with cyclosporin. Kidney Int 1994; 46: 1216–1222.
2. Berth-Jones J, Sowden JM, Feehally J, Graham-Brown RAC. Treatment of severe refractory atopic dermatitis with cyclosporin. Lancet 1991; 338:643.
3. Korstanje MJ, Bilo HJ, Stoof TJ. Sustained renal function loss in psoriasis patients after withdrawal of low-dose cyclosporin therapy. Br J Dermatol 1992; 127:501–504.
4. Zachariae H, Kragballe K, Hansen HE, Marcussen N, Olsen S. Renal biopsy findings in long-term cyclosporin treatment of psoriasis. Br J Dermatol 1997; 136:531–535.
5. Powles AV, Hardman CM, Porter WM, Cook T, Hulme B, Fry L. Renal function after 10 years' treatment with cyclosporin for psoriasis. Br J Dermatol 1998; 138: 443–449.
6. Van Joost T, Stolz E, Heule F. Efficacy of low-dose cyclosporine in severe atopic skin disease. Arch Dermatol 1987; 123:166–167.
7. Sowden JM, Berth-Jones J, Ross JS, Motley RJ, Marks R, Finlay AY, Salek MS, Graham-Brown RAC, Allen BR, Camp RDR. Double-blind, controlled, crossover study of cyclosporin in adults with severe refractory atopic dermatitis. Lancet 1991; 338:137–140.

8. Wahlgren CF, Scheynius A, Hagermark O. Antipruritic effect of oral cyclosporin A in atopic dermatitis. Acta Derm Venereol (Stockh) 1990; 70:323–329.
9. Munro CS, Levell N, Friedmann P, Shuster S. Low dose or intermittent cyclosporin maintains remission in atopic eczema. Br J Dermatol 1992; 127(suppl 40):13–14.
10. Van Joost T, Heule F, Korstanje M, Van-den-Broek MJTB, Stenveld HJ, Van-Vloten WA. Cyclosporin in atopic dermatitis: a multicentre placebo-controlled study. Br J Dermatol 1994; 130:634–640.
11. Berth-Jones J, Finlay AY, Zaki I, Tan B, Goodyear H, Lewis-Jones S, Cork MJ, Bleehen SS, Salek MS, Allen BR, Friedmann P, Harper J, Camp RDR, Smith S, Graham-Brown RAC. Cyclosporin in severe childhood atopic dermatitis: a multicentre study. J Am Acad Dermatol 1996; 34:1016–1021.
12. Zaki I, Emerson R, Allen BR. Treatment of severe atopic dermatitis in childhood with cyclosporin. Br J Dermatol 1996; 135(suppl 48):21–24.
13. Berth-Jones J, Graham-Brown RAC, Marks R, Camp RDR, English JSC, Freeman K, Holden CA, Rogers SCF, Oliwiecki S, Friedmann PS, Lewis-Jones MS, Archer CB, Adriaans B, Douglas WS, Allen BR. Long-term efficacy and safety of cyclosporin in severe adult atopic dermatitis. Br J Dermatol 1997; 136:76–81.
14. Zonneveld IM, MA De Rie MA, Beljaards RC, Van Der Rhee HJ, Wuite J, Zeegelaar J, Bos JD. The long term safety and efficacy of cyclosporin in severe refractory atopic dermatitis: a comparison of two dosage regimens. Br J Dermatol 1996; 135(suppl 48):15–20.
15. Granlund H, Erkko P, Sinisalo M, Reitamo S. Cyclosporin A in atopic dermatitis: Time to relapse and effect of intermittent therapy. Br J Dermatol 1995; 132:106–112.
16. Ahmed I, Berth-Jones J, Friedmann PS, Graham-Brown RAC, Cork M, Sowden J, Finlay AY, Beard A, Sumner M, Harper JI. Short course versus continuous therapy with cyclosporin in severe childhood atopic dermatitis. Br J Dermatol 1998; 139(suppl 51):22.
17. Mueller W, Herrmann B. Cyclosporin A for psoriasis. New Engl J Med 1979; 301: 555.
18. Ellis CN, Gorsulowsky DC, Hamilton TA, Billings JK, Brown MD, Headington JT, Cooper KD, Baadsgaard O, Duell EA, Annesley TM, Turcotte JG, Voorhees JJ. Cyclosporin improves psoriasis in a double-blind study. JAMA 1986; 256:3110–3116.
19. Van Joost T, Bos JD, Heule F, Meinardi MM. Low-dose cyclosporin A in severe psoriasis. A double-blind study. Br J Dermatol 1988; 118:183–190.
20. Ellis CN, Fradin MS, Messana JM, Brown MD, Siegel MT, Hartley AH, Rocher LL, Wheeler S, Hamilton TA, Parish TG, Ellis-Madu M, Duel E, Annesley TM, Cooper KD, Voorhees JJ. Cyclosporine for plaque-type psoriasis. Results of a multidose, double-blind trial. N Engl J Med 1991; 324:277–284.
21. Reitamo S, Puska P, Lassus A. Cyclosporin in the treatment of palmo-plantar pustulosis. Br J Dermatol 1989; 120:857.
22. Gupta AK, Ellis CN, Nickoloff BJ, Goldfarb MT, Ho VC, Rocher LL, Griffiths CEM, Cooper KD, Voorhees JJ. Oral cyclosporine in the treatment of inflammatory and noninflammatory dermatoses. A clinical and immunopathologic analysis. Arch Dermatol 1990; 126:339–350.

23. Higgins E, Munro CS, Marks J, Friedmann PS, Shuster S. Relapse rates in moderately severe chronic psoriasis treated with cyclosporin A. Br J Dermatol 1989; 121: 71–74.
24. Levell NJ, Shuster S, Munro CS, Friedmann PS. Remission of ordinary psoriasis following a short clearance course of cyclosporin. Acta Derm Venereol 1995; 75: 65–69.
25. Berth-Jones J, Voorhees JJ. Consensus conference on cyclosporin A microemulsion for psoriasis, June 1996. Br J Dermatol 1996; 135:775–777.

9

Tacrolimus (FK-506)

Jose Contreras-Ruiz
National Institute of Pediatrics
Mexico City, Mexico

Francisco A. Kerdel
University of Miami School of Medicine
Miami, Florida

Tacrolimus, a drug originally known as FK-506, is a relatively new immunosuppressant grouped in the same family as cyclosporin A. It was initially used orally and intravenously as an agent for prophylaxis of organ transplant rejection. It later has become of interest to dermatologists because the topical form has proven to be effective in atopic dermatitis with very few, if any, side effects. In recent times, multiple trials, especially in its topical form, are being carried out for diseases where immunosuppression could be beneficial.

I. DRUG (TOPICAL VS. SYSTEMIC)

Tacrolimus is available in oral and intravenous forms. Topical use is limited to the research field. However, in centers where ointments and creams are being studied, they have been prepared using the 1- or 5-mg capsules.

Topically applied tacrolimus has been studied in humans in atopic dermatitis and acute contact dermatitis with good results [1,2]. Topical use in alopecia areata has been limited to animal studies, but there is one case report of tacrolimus solution used for pyoderma gangrenosum, which showed a good response [3].

The advantages of topical over systemic tacrolimus are clear. The drug is minimally absorbed through intact skin [4], and its only reported side effects are a burning or stinging sensation when applied on inflamed skin [5,6]. Another important characteristic is that absorption occurs only through inflamed skin, and is decreased as the skin heals [4]. No serious systemic effects have been reported so far.

Systemic tacrolimus has been used for psoriasis with better results than placebo [7,8]. Unfortunately, this drug does not appear to be effective in psoriasis when used topically [9]. Systemic tacrolimus has also been used in uncontrolled trials in pyoderma gangrenosum [10] with good results. The drug is also effective in suppressing skin graft rejection in experimental animals [11–13].

Although similar to cyclosporin A, tacrolimus lacks some of the side effects associated with cyclosporine such as hirsutism and gingival hyperplasia. Hypertension is seen less frequently and hyperlipidemia is seldom reported.

II. PHARMACOLOGY

A. Structure

Tacrolimus is an 822-kDa immunosuppressant of the macrolide family. It was isolated from a product of *Streptomyces tsukabensis* in 1987 [14]. Tacrolimus appears as white crystals or powder with the molecular formula $C_{44}H_{69}NO_{12}$. Its chemical structure is depicted in Figure 1.

B. Mechanism of Action

The exact mechanism by which tacrolimus exerts its effects is not fully understood. However, it has been shown that tacrolimus achieves immunosuppression

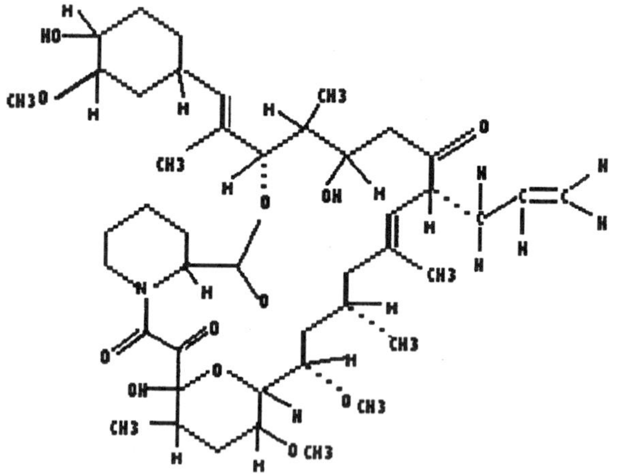

FIGURE 1 Structure of tacrolimus.

by inhibiting T-lymphocyte activation. Evidence suggests that it does so through calcineurin which is a calcium-dependent serine/threonine phosphatase that dephosphorilates NF-ATp (Nuclear Factor of Activated T Cells Protein) and OAP (Octamer Activating Protein). Both of these proteins are important molecules in the regulation of gene transcription that code for several inflammatory mediators such as IL-2, GM-CSF, TNF-α, IFN-γ and other interleukins, necessary for the correct development of the immune response.

The complex formed by tacrolimus and its binding protein, FKBP (FK-506 Binding Protein), associates with calcineurin as a stable compound. The complex acts by inhibiting calcineurin action at a position distant from its active site. This physically blocks the approach of transcription factors to the active site and therefore interfering with the transcription of the genes. The early phase of T-cell activation is thus blocked without impairing the response to exogenously administered cytokines [15,16].

C. Absorption

1. Topical Application

Tacrolimus is not readily absorbed through the intact skin when applied topically. Nevertheless when the skin is inflamed it is sufficiently absorbed to be active [17]. Blood levels of tacrolimus reach 0.05 to 0.25 ng/mL when a concentration of 0.03 to 0.3% is used. The highest levels are reached after 3 to 6 h of application [5].

In a patient with erythroderma, detectable blood levels of 20 ng/mL were reached 6 h after the application of 10 g of a 0.1% ointment. This extremely high concentration decreased to 2.9 ng/mL after 72 h and no side effects were noted. It has been noted that tacrolimus absorption decreases as the skin heals [4].

2. Oral Use

After oral administration, absorption of tacrolimus from the gastrointestinal tract is incomplete, poor, and very erratic. Peak concentrations are reached after 1 to 4 h of ingestion, and the bioavailability of tacrolimus is around 7 to 27% in adult kidney transplant patients, 16 to 28% in adult liver transplant patients, and 13 to 23% in healthy individuals.

The rate and extent of tacrolimus absorption are greatest under fasting conditions, but the variation may be as high as 6 to 56%. This wide range may be due to the poor aqueous solubility of tacrolimus in gastric secretions [18].

D. Metabolism

Tacrolimus is mainly metabolized in the liver by the cytochrome P-450 enzyme system (CYP3A). Less than 1% is excreted unchanged in the urine. In the liver biotransformation occurs via monodemethylation and hydroxylation or a combination of both [19].

E. Excretion

Tacrolimus is excreted through the bile where most of its metabolites are present. In healthy individuals, the mean clearance is 0.04 L/h/kg and the elimination half-life is approximately 8.7 h. In liver-transplanted patients, it is 11.7 ± 3.9 h, the variation depending mostly on hepatic function [19].

III. DRUG INTERACTIONS/CONTRAINDICATIONS

A. Drug Interactions

Since cyclosporin A impairs renal function similarly to tacrolimus, they should not be used together. Tacrolimus and cyclosporin A have shown potential for synergistic and additive impairment of renal function. For the same reason, drugs that alter renal function such as aminoglycosides, amphotericin B, cysplatinum, etc, should be avoided or used with caution.

Drugs metabolized by cytochrome P-450 (CYP3A), either by inhibiting or inducing these enzyme systems, may produce increased or decreased whole blood or plasma levels of tacrolimus (Table 1).

Table 1 Drugs That May Alter Tacrolimus Metabolism

Drugs that may decrease tacrolimus drug levels	
Anticonvulsants	Antibiotics
carbamazepine phenobarbital phenytoin	rifabutin rifampin

Drugs that may increase tacrolimus drug levels				
Macrolides	Antifungals	Ca^{++} Channel Blockers	Prokinetics	Other
clarithromycin erythromycin troleandomycin	clotrimazole fluconazole itraconazole ketoconazole	diltiazem nicardipine nifedipine verapamil	cisapride metoclopramide	bromocriptine cimetidine cyclosporine danazol methylprednisolone protease inhibitors

Since tacrolimus produces immunosuppression, the use of live vaccines should be avoided [18,20].

B. Contraindications

Tacrolimus is contraindicated in patients that have shown allergy to the compound or its vehicle (polyoxyl 60 hydrogenated castor oil).

IV. CURRENT APPROVED INDICATIONS

The only approved indication of tacrolimus in the United States is for the prophylaxis of organ rejection in patients receiving allogenic kidney or liver transplants. In some countries, it is also approved for graft-versus-host disease. Other uses further reviewed in this chapter are currently undergoing investigation. Preliminary results appear promising.

V. OTHER USES FROM USUAL PRACTICE AND LITERATURE

In transplantation medicine, tacrolimus is also used systemically as prophylaxis for rejection of heart, pancreas, and small bowel.

In dermatology, tacrolimus may be helpful in the following conditions.

A. ATOPIC DERMATITIS

An open trial with 50 patients diagnosed with atopic dermatitis using the criteria of Hanifin and Rajka was conducted. Pruritus, erythema, vesicles/papules, and edema were assessed. They showed that face and neck atopic dermatitis significantly improved after twice-daily topical application of 0.03, 0.1, and 0.3% tacrolimus ointment. Pruritus decreased dramatically in the first 3 days. When the dermatitis was lichenified, it took longer for the patients to respond [21].

Three cases of lichenified facial lesions were also successfully treated using 0.1% tacrolimus in petrolatum ointment. Improvement was noted to be significant after a week and complete remission was achieved in 2 weeks and lasted for approximately 2 to 3 months. Two cases relapsed but were easily controlled with conventional treatment [6].

A phase I study in 39 children and adults with moderate-to-severe atopic dermatitis was conducted to evaluate response, pharmacokinetics, and safety of a 0.03% ointment. Ninety-five percent of the patients showed at least good improvement based on signs/symptoms ratings. Burning and vasodilatation were again the most common adverse events. The authors concluded that 0.3% ointment is a safe and effective therapy for atopic dermatitis [1].

A short-term, phase II, randomized, double-blind, multicentric study that compared tacrolimus ointment with vehicle alone was also reported. The authors treated close to 50 patients in each group with moderate-to-severe atopic dermatitis. A 3-week course of topical tacrolimus at a dose of 0.03%, 0.1%, and 0.3% significantly decreased the severity scores in 66.7%, 83.3%, and 75%, respectively, of the cases treated in comparison to placebo (no statistical difference was noted among the three groups) [5].

In conclusion, several forms of topical tacrolimus therapy for atopic dermatitis have demonstrated its efficacy and safety. Lichenified lesions appear to take longer to respond, but even then the response has been good after treatment with topical tacrolimus.

B. Acute Contact Dermatitis

The first studies on acute contact dermatitis were conducted in pigs, comparing tacrolimus, dexamethasone, clobetasol, and cyclosporin A. It was shown that topical application of 0.04, 0.13, and 0.4% tacrolimus produced significant inhibition (51%, 68%, and 77%, respectively) of contact hypersensitivity to 10% dinitrofluorobenzene (DNFB) compared to placebo. Tacrolimus at a concentration of 0.4% was as active as 0.13% clobetasol in blocking the hypersensitivity response [17].

In a study with human volunteers, 0.01 to 0.1% tacrolimus also suppressed the allergic reaction to DNCB in all subjects compared to placebo. Biopsies showed no inflammation in the tacrolimus group, whereas there were severe inflammatory changes in the placebo-treated group [2].

Another study using oral tacrolimus in mice focused on the mechanism by which tacrolimus acts in contact dermatitis. The study demonstrated that tacrolimus and cyclosporin A suppressed the expression of IFN-γ mRNA in the skin. Using RT-PCR, the authors demonstrated that contact dermatitis was induced by the activation of Th1 cells. Tacrolimus and cyclosporin A inhibited the Th1 cell response but they also increased IgE production due to the shift toward a Th2 response [22].

C. Psoriasis

A short-term therapeutic trial on the metabolic effects of tacrolimus in seven patients with severe, chronic plaque-type psoriasis reported complete remission in all of them [8].

Subsequently, in a phase II, multicenter, randomized, double-blind, placebo-controlled study, 50 patients were treated with either oral tacrolimus 0.05 mg/kg per day or placebo. The dose was increased to a maximum of 0.15 mg/kg if no improvement was noted at 6 weeks. Improvement was scored using the Psoriasis Area and Severity Index. At the end of the ninth week, tacrolimus proved to be better in treating recalcitrant plaque-type psoriasis than placebo.

The adverse effects most commonly reported were diarrhea, paresthesia, and insomnia [7].

In a pilot study, topical tacrolimus has been tried recently, but unfortunately it was not effective in treating chronic plaque psoriasis [9].

D. Hair Growth and Alopecia Areata

Studies on the use of tacrolimus on hair growth and in alopecia areata in humans have not been reported. However, topical tacrolimus (0.03–1 μmol) diluted in acetone stimulates hair growth in mice, rats, and Syrian golden hamsters. The same effects have been observed in SCID (C.B-17 scid/scid) mice that lack B- and T-cell immunity, so its immunosuppressive effect is unlikely to be the responsible mechanism. Interestingly enough, oral administration in the same kind of mice of up to 30 mg/kg does not stimulate hair growth [23].

Preliminary reports show that topical tacrolimus (25–125 μg/kg) is effective in promoting hair growth in the Dundee experimental bald rat (DEBR), a model that closely resembles human alopecia areata. In this study, oral use did not yield the same response. There also was no penetration through, or lateral diffusion of, the drug to untreated areas. This was evidenced as the untreated areas continued to loose hair.

Biopsies showed a decrease in the perifollicular mononuclear infiltrate as compared with the untreated animals and also increased the size of the hair follicles [24].

E. Skin Transplantation

The use of topical and IM tacrolimus for skin transplant in mice and rats has proved efficacious. Furthermore, a study in rats using tacrolimus ointment showed that tacrolimus is useful and effective in the suppression of allograft skin rejection. However, the use of tacrolimus for skin transplantation in humans (i.e., burn patients) has not been reported [11–13].

F. Pyoderma Gangrenosum

The systemic use of tacrolimus for recalcitrant pyoderma gangrenosum (PG) was first studied in four patients. In these cases, the associated diseases included ulcerative colitis and arthritis for patient one, Crohn's disease with perianal fistulae, polyarthritis, and Sjögren's syndrome for the second patient, ankylosing spondylitis and scleritis for the third patient, and erosive polyarthritis and streaking leukocyte factor syndrome for the fourth patient. All four patients had a dramatic initial response with decrease in pain, erythema, and drainage. Four to 8 weeks later, three of the four patients had complete healing of the lesions. One patient, however, was dropped from the study because of his refusal to undergo rehabilitation for drug addiction. Attempts at dose reduction in one patient resulted in reactivation but responded to reinstatement of full dose. Of note in this study was that tacrolimus also caused remission of the inflammatory bowel disease, scleritis, and healing of the perianal fistulae in these patients [10].

Recently, another case of PG resistant to cyclosporine was treated effectively with oral tacrolimus (0.1 mg/kg per day). The patient had Crohn's disease complicated by perianal fistulae and an ulcer over the whole circumference of one leg. After tacrolimus was started, the patient improved remarkably and reepithelialization was complete in 1 month. Tacrolimus was discontinued after 3 months and the patient has remained in remission for 10 months with azathioprine maintenance therapy [25].

Topical application of tacrolimus has also been used in pyoderma gangrenosum. Based on clinical diagnosis, with no other concomitant diseases noted, and still on oral prednisone, the patient was started on tacrolimus 0.5% solution with improvement after 2 weeks. Prednisone was then tapered and the patient was continued on tacrolimus alone under hydrocolloidal dressings. Complete resolution was noted after 12 weeks. Only a burning sensation on application was noted as an adverse effect [3].

VI. THERAPEUTIC PROTOCOLS

A. Dosage

The therapeutic effect of tacrolimus can be achieved with concentrations 10 to 100 times lower than those needed for cyclosporine [26,27].

Tacrolimus can be used intravenously, orally, or topically. The route and dose depend on the indication, the severity of the disease, the patient's age and patient's tolerance. Tacrolimus is typically dosed as follows:

1. IV dose for adults is 25 to 50 μg/kg per day. In pediatric patients, the rapid metabolism of the drug requires higher doses to be administered (50–100 μg/kg per day). These doses have been recommended to achieve immunosuppression in transplanted patients and correlate with whole blood levels of 5 to 20 ng/mL [28,29].
2. Oral dose for adults is 150 to 200 μg/kg per day (200–300 μg/kg per day in pediatric patients).

The minimal effective oral dose for psoriasis has been established at 0.1 mg/kg per day. The plasma levels effective in inducing and maintaining complete remission of psoriasis range from 0.5–1.4 ng/mL [7,8].

Topically, several dose regimens have been tried for atopic dermatitis ranging from 0.03 to 0.3% in ointment form. All of them appeared to be effective. The most accepted dosage is 0.1% ointment applied twice daily [4,5].

B. Drug Level Monitoring

Due to the nephrotoxicity and other side effects related to the use of tacrolimus, and to the fact that it is absorbed in such a capricious manner, its levels should be monitored. Tacrolimus can be analyzed in plasma at 37°C because of its temperature-dependent distribution between red blood cells and plasma. The analysis has demonstrated that the therapeutic levels recommended for transplanted patients using whole blood measurements is 5 to 20 ng/mL [29].

REFERENCES

1. Alaiti S, Kang S, Fiedler VC, et al. Tacrolimus (FK 506) ointment for atopic dermatitis: a phase I study in adults and children. J Am Acad Dermatol 1998; 38:69–76.
2. Lauerma A, Maibach H, Graunlund H, et al. Inhibition of contact allergy reactions by topical FK506. Lancet 1992; 340:556.
3. D'Inca R. Tacrolimus to treat pyoderma gangrenosum resistant to cyclosporin. Ann Intern Med 1998; 128:783–4.
4. Kawashima M, Nakagawa H, Ohtsuki, et al. Tacrolimus concentrations in blood during topical treatment of atopic dermatitis. Lancet 1996; 348:1240–1241.
5. Ruzika T, Bieber T, Erwin Schöpf, et al. A short-term trial of tacrolimus ointment for atopic dermatitis. N Engl J Med 1997; 337(12):816–821.
6. Aoyama H, Tabata N, Tanaka M, et al. Successful treatment of resistant facial lesions of atopic dermatitis with 0.1% FK506 ointment. Br J Dermatol 1995; 133:492–500.
7. The European FK506 Multicentre Psoriasis Study Group. Systemic tacrolimus (FK506) is effective for the treatment of psoriasis in a double blind, placebo-controlled study. Arch Dermatol 1996; 132:419–423.
8. Nikolaidis N, Abu-Elmagd K, Thomson H, et al. Metabolic effects of FK506 in patients with severe psoriasis: short-term follow-up of seven cases. Transplant Proc 1991; 23:3325–3327.
9. Zonneveld I, Rubins A, Jablonska S, et al. Topical tacrolimus is not effective in chronic-plaque psoriasis. A pilot study. Arch Dermatol 1998; 134:1101–1102.
10. Abu-Elmagd K, Jegasothy B, Ackerman A, et al. Efficacy of FK 506 in the treatment of recalcitrant pyoderma gangrenosum. Transplant Proc 1991; 23:3328–3329.
11. Fujita T, Takahashi S, Yagihashi A, et al. Prolonged survival of rat skin allograft by treatment with FK506 ointment. Transplantation 1997; 64:922–925.
12. Inamura N, Nakahara K, Kino T, et al. Prolongation of skin allograft survival in rats by a novel immunosuppressive agent, FK506. Transplantation 1988; 45:206.
13. Wada H, Monden M, Gotoh M, et al. An attempt to induce tolerance to skin grafts in congenic mice with FK506. Transplant Proc 1991; 23:3280.
14. Kino T, Hatanaka H, Miyata S, et al. FK506, a novel immunosuppressant isolated from a Streptomyces. II. Immunosuppressive effects of FK506 in vitro. J Antibiot 1987; 40:1256–1265.
15. Sawada S, Suzuki G, Kawase Y, et al. Novel immunosuppressive agent, FK 506: in vitro effects on the cloned T cell activation. J Immunol 1987; 139:1797–1803.

16. Griffith J, Kim J, Kim E, et al. X-ray structure of calcineurin inhibited by the immunophilin-immunosuppressant FKBP12-FK506 complex. Cell 1995; 82:507–522.
17. Meingassner J and Stütz A. Immunosuppressive Macrolides of the Type FK 506: A Novel Class of Topical Agents for Treatment of Skin Diseases? J Invest Dermatol 1992; 98:851–855.
18. Hooks M. Tacrolimus, a new immunosuppressant-a review of the literature. Ann Pharmacother 1994; 28:501–510.
19. Venkataramanan R, Jain A, Warty K, et al. Pharmacokinetics of FK506 in transplant patients. Transplant Proc 1991; 23:2736–2740.
20. Fung J, Alessiani M, Abu-Elmagd K, et al. Adverse effects associated with the use of FK506. Transplant Proc 1991; 23:14–21.
21. Nakagawa H, Etoh T, Ishibashi Y, et al. Tacrolimus ointment for atopic dermatitis. Lancet 1994; 344:883.
22. Nagai H, Hiyama H, Matsuo A, et al. FK-506 and cyclosporin-A potentiate the IgE antibody production by contact sensitization with hapten in mice. J Pharmacol Exp Ther 1997; 283:321–327.
23. Yamamoto S, Hong J, and Ryuchi K. Stimulation of hair growth by topical application of FK506, a potent immunosuppressive agent. J Invest Dermatol 1994; 102: 160–164.
24. McElwee K, Rushton D, Trachy R, et al. Topical FK506: a potent immunotherapy for alopecia areata? Studies using the Dundee experimental bald rat model. Br J Dermatol 1997; 137:491–497.
25. Schuppe H. Topical tacrolimus for pyoderma gangrenosum. Lancet 1998; 352:832.
26. Thomson A. FK 506-how much potential? Immunol Today 1989; 10:6–9.
27. Yoshimura N, Matsui S, Hamashima T, et al. Effect of a new immunosuppressive agent, FK 506, on human lymphocyte responses in vitro. I. Inhibition of expression of alloantigen-activated suppressor cells as well as induction of alloreactivity. Transplantation 1989; 47:351–356.
28. Jain A, Fung J, Tzakis A, et al. Comparative study of cyclosporin and FK506 dosage requirements in adult and pediatric orthotopic liver transplant patients. Transplant Proc 1991; 23:2763–2766.
29. Kershner R and Fitzsimmons W. Relationship of FK506 whole blood concentrations and efficacy and toxicity after liver and kidney transplantation. Transplantation 1996; 62:920–926.

10

Retinoids

Christos C. Zouboulis and Constantin E. Orfanos
University Medical Center Benjamin Franklin
The Free University of Berlin
Berlin, Germany

I. RETINOIDS

The term ''retinoids'' includes both naturally occurring molecules and also synthetic compounds showing biological activities that are characteristic for vitamin A. The current definition of retinoids does not require a chemical analogy to vitamin A (i.e., the ''four isoprenoid units joined in a head-to-tail manner'' structure), as it was defined by the IUPAC-IUB Joint Commission on Biochemical Nomenclature in 1982. In general, retinoids bind and activate specific nuclear receptors, although this may not be a necessary precondition for their action.

Retinoids mainly influence proliferation and differentiation of epithelial cells and a few selected compounds also exert sebosuppressive effects. Because of these properties, they were introduced to dermatology during 1977–1978 [1] and their spectrum has been broadened during the 1980s [2,3]. During the last two decades, retinoids have also been shown to modulate the synthetic activity in cells of mesenchymal origin, exhibit immunomodulatory effects, stimulate angiogenesis, and downregulate carcinogenesis. Therefore, they have been increasingly used for: (1) treatment of hyperkeratotic and parakeratotic skin diseases, with or without dermal inflammation, and for a series of genokeratoses; (2) therapy of severe acne and acne-related dermatoses; and (3) treatment and/or chemoprevention of skin cancer and other neoplasia.

The widening of the therapeutic spectrum of retinoids over the range of dermatological disorders; the identification of the retinoid-binding proteins in the 1980s and, especially, of the nuclear retinoid receptors at the late 1980s to early

1990s leading to a better understanding of the retinoid function at the molecular level; and the current introduction of compounds with selective retinoid receptor agonistic activity in the topical treatment of dermatological diseases underline the impressive development in this area of medical treatment. On the other hand, the unsuccessful efforts in limiting the teratogenic potential of systemic retinoids represent a major drawback.

A. Natural Retinoids

Vitamin A (retinol) and its important derivatives, retinaldehyde and retinoic acid, are fat-soluble unsaturated isoprenoids necessary for growth, differentiation, and maintainance of epithelial tissues, and also for reproduction. In a reversible process, retinol is oxidized in vivo to yield retinaldehyde, which is important for vision. The normal plasma concentration of vitamin A in humans is 0.40 ± 0.13 μg/mL [4].

Retinoic acid is a major oxidative metabolite of retinol and can substitute for retinol in vitamin-A–deficient animals in growth promotion and epithelial differentiation. However, it cannot substitute for retinol in completely maintaining reproduction. The stereoisomers all-*trans*-retinoic acid and 13-*cis*-retinoic acid are both normal constituents of human serum [5]. Unlike the retinol esters that are stored in the liver, retinoic acid is not stored but is rapidly excreted. The normal levels in human plasma are 0.88 ± 0.32 ng/mL for all-*trans*-retinoic acid and 1.63 ± 0.80 ng/mL for 13-*cis*-retinoic acid [6]. Natural retinoic acids can exert serum levels up to 5 ng/mL [7].

Endogenous metabolites of vitamin A are unlikely to be involved in the pathogenesis of skin diseases [4,6]. In contrast, hypervitaminosis A is associated with manifestations resembling the mucocutaneous side effects of oral treatment with synthetic retinoids. Humans require 0.8 to 1 mg or 2400 to 3000 I.U. of vitamin A per day (1 I.U. = 0.3 mg). Vitamin A intoxication only occurs when daily dietary intake of vitamin A exceeds 18,000 to 60,000 I.U. per day in children and 50,000 to 100,000 I.U. per day in adults, given over a period of several months [8]. With restricted liver metabolic capacity, signs of intoxication may appear much earlier—within a few months—as well as when smaller doses are taken (10,000 I.U. per day). Hypervitaminosis A is signaled by increased retinol esters in serum. The normal levels of retinol esters represent 5 to 8% of retinol levels. The latter rarely increase. Pregnant women and women of child-bearing age should not exceed oral intake of 8000 to 10,000 I.U. of vitamin A per day.

B. Synthetic Retinoids

All-*trans*-retinoic acid (tretinoin) was the first retinoid to be synthesized. Although this compound is now established for topical therapy (Table 1), its sys-

TABLE 1 Topical and Systemic Retinoids in Clinical Use

Systemic retinoids Substance	Preparations	Major indications
Isotretinoin	2.5-, 5-, 10-, 20-mg capsules	Severe acne and acne-related dermatoses
Etretinate	10-mg, 25-mg capsules	Psoriasis, disorders of keratinization
Acitretin	10-mg, 25-mg capsules	Psoriasis, disorders of keratinization
Tretinoin	10-mg capsules	Acute promyelocytic leukemia

Topical retinoids Substance	Concentration-basis	Major indications
Tretinoin	0.025, 0.01, 0.05, 0.1, 0.4% cream, 0.025% gel, 0.05, 0.1, 0.2% solution, 0.1% lotion, 0.05% ointment, 0.05% in compresses	Mild/moderate acne, photoaging and biological skin aging
Isotretinoin	0.05% gel	Mild/moderate acne
Alitretinoin (9-*cis*-retinoic acid)	0.1% gel	AIDS-related Kaposi's sarcoma
Motretinide	0.1% cream, solution	Mild/moderate acne
Adapalene	0.1% gel, solution	Mild/moderate acne
Tazarotene	0.05, 0.1% gel	Psoriasis, mild/moderate acne
Retinol (Retinol Actif Pur®)	0.01–0.015% cream	Cosmetic indications
(Retinol Concentré Pur®)	0.1% cream	
Retinol palmitate	0.5–5% lotion, cream	Cosmetic indications
Retinaldehyde (Ystheal®)	0.05% cream, gel, lotion	Cosmetic indications

The major worldwide registration of the drugs is shown in Addendum 1.

temic use did not reveal significant advantages over vitamin A until recently, when the drug showed beneficial effects on acute promyelocytic leukemia.

13-*cis*-Retinoic acid (isotretinoin) is an extremely effective drug if given systemically in severe forms of acne. It is the only retinoid with marked sebostatic activity after oral intake; its topical use diminishes or cancels out sebosuppression [9,10].

Etretinate achieved a breakthrough in the treatment of severe psoriasis and other dermatoses; its widespread clinical use resulted from the good ratio between therapeutic efficacy and adverse effects. The free acid metabolite of etretinate, acitretin, was found to be clinically as effective as etretinate with a much shorter

TABLE 2 Retinoids in Clinical Trials

Substance	Concentration-basis	Major indications
all-*trans*-Retinoyl β-glucuronide (T)	1.2% cream	Mild/moderate acne
11-*cis*, 13-*cis*-12-hydroxymethyl retinoic acid, δ-lactone (T)		Mild/moderate acne
Isotretinoin (T)	0.1% cream	Skin aging, actinic keratoses
Retinol (T)	0.4–1.6% solution	Skin aging
Tamibarotene (Am-80) (T)	0.005–0.008% ointment	Psoriasis
Retinaldehyde (T)	0.5–1% cream	Psoriasis
Arotinoid methyl sulfone (Ro 14-9706) (T)	cream	Actinic keratoses
Fenretinide [N-(4-hydroxyphenyl)-retinamide] (T, S)		Actinic keratoses, chemoprevention trials
Alitretinoin (9-*cis* retinoic acid (S)		Kaposi sarcoma, cutaneous T-cell lymphoma
LGD 1069 (T, S)		Kaposi sarcoma
E 5166 (polyprenoic acid) (S)		Chemoprevention trials
CD 2398 (S)		Chemoprevention trials
Mefarotene (Ro 40-8757) (S)		Used in chemotherapy studies; enhances the activity of adriamycin, cyclophosphamide, 5-fluorouracil, interleukins
2-Trifluororetinin (Ro 23-6457) (S)		Immunosuppressive properties

Abbreviations: T = topical; S = systemic.

elimination half-life, advantageous for clinical use. However, the fact that reesterification in vivo may convert acitretin into etretinate canceled out its major advantage when compared to its precursor [11]. This can be avoided when appropriate precautions are taken.

Receptor-selective retinoids were currently introduced for topical treatment of acne (adapalene and tazarotene) [12] as well as psoriasis (tazarotene) [13]. In addition, 9-*cis*-retinoic acid (alitretinoin) has currently been approved for the topical treatment of AIDS-related Kaposi's sarcoma. Further retinoids in clinical use and retinoids currently examined for their clinical efficacy are shown in Tables 1 and 2.

II. PHARMACOLOGY

A. Structure

The search for more biologically active and less toxic compounds led to the chemical modification of all three portions of the vitamin A molecule, the ring, the polyene chain, and the carboxylic end group [14] (Fig. 1). It was found early on that alterations of the polyene chain may diminish retinoid activity, whereas modifications of the carboxylic end group are often associated with reduced toxicity and maintained or even enhanced biological activity. Substitutions for the ring were found to yield less toxicity with marked increase of the biological activity of the molecule. In further developmental work, additional aromatic rings were introduced; some new retinoids are barely reminiscent of the original retinol molecule, such as the naphthalene carboxylic acid derivatives adapalene and tazarotene [15,16].

Today, retinoids are classified in three generations, according to their chemical structure: nonaromatic, monoaromatic, and polyaromatic (arotinoids) (Fig. 1).

B. Mechanisms of Action

Factors influencing retinoid activity in vivo are cellular uptake and binding to cytosolic proteins, intracellular metabolism, and binding to nuclear receptors. Although retinol is assumed to enter the cells by nonreceptor-mediated endocytosis [17], the exact mechanism of retinoid-induced membrane-associated signal transduction needs to be elucidated. Intracellularly, retinoids interact with cyto-

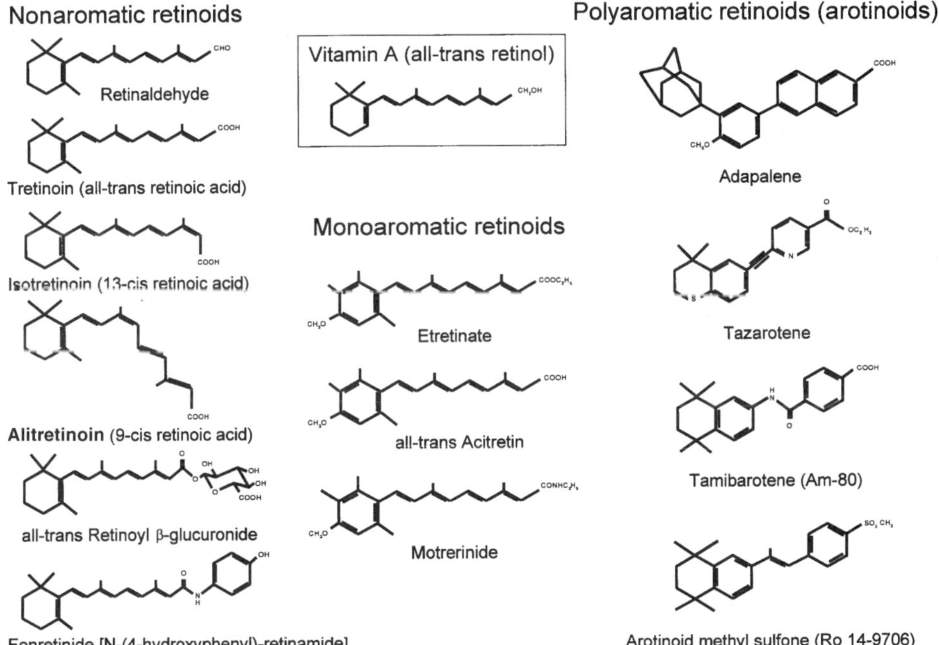

FIGURE 1 Chemical structure of natural and synthetic retinoids.

solic proteins and nuclear receptors in order to induce expression of genes that bear specific DNA sequences recognizing the retinoid/receptor complex [18,19]. These pathways have been well investigated for all-*trans*-retinoic acid, but they may not be valid for all retinoid compounds.

1. Molecular Mechanisms

The discovery of the specific cellular retinoid binding proteins and the nuclear retinoid receptors has extended the understanding for the broad spectrum of the biological activity of retinoids [20]. These observations have also thrown light on the complex interactions between retinoids and further hormonal signal transduction molecules. All-*trans*-retinoic acid is transported by the cellular retinoic acid-binding protein (CRABP) from the cytoplasm to the nucleus (Fig. 2). The dominant CRABP in the skin is CRABP II, whereas expression of low quantities of CRABP I was also found. The expression of CRABP II is modulated by the local use of all-*trans*-retinoic acid. CRABP II is considered an early marker of retinoid activity on the skin and probably can control the bioavailability of retinoids.

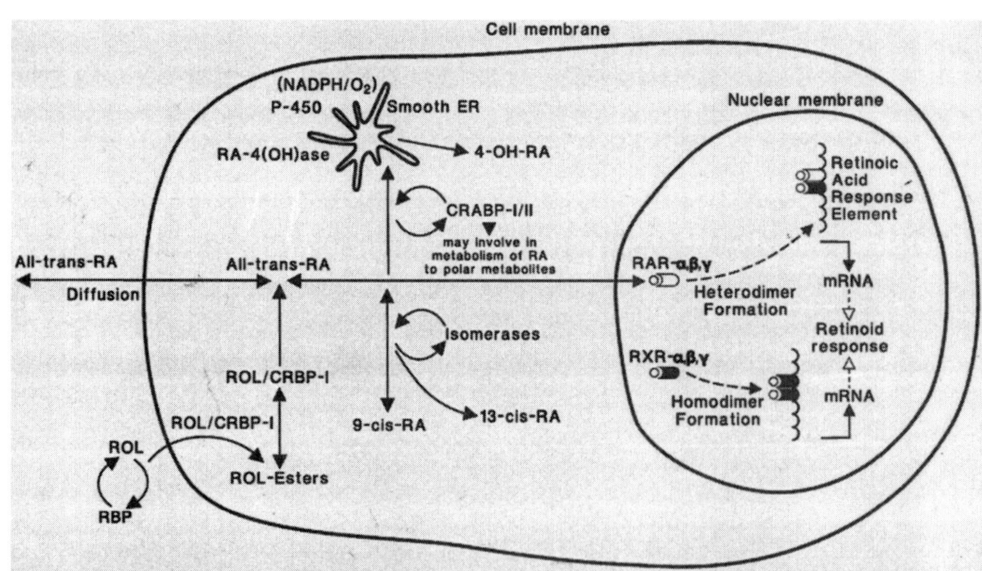

FIGURE 2 Intracellular metabolism and activation of retinoids. ROL = retinol; RBP = retinol-binding protein; RA = retinoic acid; CRBP = cellular retinol-binding protein; CRABP = cellular retinoic acid-binding protein; ER = endoplasmatic reticulum; RAR = retinoic acid receptor; RXR = retinoid X receptor.

In the nucleus, a complex of the retinoid with specific receptor proteins, the retinoid receptor is constructed. Retinoids are thought to exert their effects on the target cells by activating the retinoid receptors. Retinoid receptors are members of the steroid–thyroid hormone superfamily. Two receptor families have been suggested to mediate retinoid activity at the molecular level—the retinoic acid receptors (RARs) and the retinoid X receptors (RXRs). They act as ligand-dependent transcriptional factors (e.g., RARs can bind both all-*trans* and 9-*cis*-retinoic acid with high affinity, while RXRs selectively interact with 9-*cis*-retinoic acid). Retinoid receptors exist as α, β, and γ types, whereby each type includes a number of isoforms. They usually bind retinoids in the form of dimers, as homodimers (RAR/RAR, RXR/RXR) or heterodimers (RAR/RXR), which present higher binding efficiency than the individual receptors [21]. In the heterodimer formation, RXR takes over the gene regulation and can also form heterodimers with receptors of other hormones (e.g., with the thyroid hormone receptor and the vitamin D3 receptor). The retinoid molecule/retinoid receptor dimer complex activates genes that possess specific short DNA sequences in their promoter regions, known as retinoid-responsive elements (RAREs and RXREs). Thus it comes to transcription and translation of these genes followed by the biological retinoid effect. All-*trans* retinoic acid has been shown to induce several genes, in vivo and/or in vitro, bearing retinoid-responsive elements. Three retinoid receptor/target gene interactions are of particular interest.

1. *Positive feedback mechanism.* All three RAR genes contain a retinoid-responsive element and the autoinduction of RARs expression in some tissues could lead to a potential amplification of retinoid effects [22].
2. *Negative feedback mechanism.* RA-induced overexpression of CRABP I in F9 mouse teratocarcinoma cells led to reduction of a certain subset of RA-responsive genes; this finding indicates that retinoid-binding proteins may antagonize retinoid interaction with nuclear receptors [23].
3. *Interaction with other signal transduction mechanisms.* Interaction of retinoid receptors with transcriptional factors activated by other signal transduction mechanisms (e.g., AP-1 [24]), may produce specific retinoid effects. Retinoids with selective inhibition of AP-1 were shown to reduce F9 teratocarcinoma cell proliferation without influencing cell differentiation [25].

Recently, RARs and RXRs have been identified to be encoded by distinct genes that are mapped on chromosomes 17q21.1 (RARα), 3p24 (RARβ), 12q13 (RARγ), 9q34.3 (RXRα), 6p21.3 (RXRβ), and 1q22-23 (RXRγ). The expression of RARs is tissue-specific. Abundant expression of RARγ and RXRα, low amounts of RARα, and no RARβ were shown in normal and psoriatic human epidermis [26,27]. In contrast, 13-*cis*-retinoic acid shows low affinity for RARs;

14-hydroxy-*retro*-retinol, which specifically induces lymphocyte proliferation, does not bind to or activate retinoid receptors [22]; acitretin does not bind to but activates RARs; and Ro 40-1349 binds but does not activate RARs [28]. These controversial data indicate the existence of other additional, unknown retinoid signaling pathways.

A target of current retinoid research is to synthesize substances that, as specifically as possible, bind the retinoid receptors. The receptor-binding retinoids can be divided in three groups according to their function characteristics.

1. Agonists, the classical synthetic retinoids, which stimulate the basal transcriptional activity of the retinoid receptors.
2. Neutral antagonists, which bind the receptors without influencing their activity; they are, however, able to neutralize the influence of both the agonists and the inverse agonists.
3. Inverse agonists, which bind the receptors and restrain their basal transcriptional activity. The last group of substances includes a completely new group of retinoids that may be effective for the topical treatment of cutaneous diseases and also as antidote for the mucocutaneous adverse effects of systemic retinoids.

2. Cellular Mechanisms

The cellular mechanisms of action of the natural and the synthetic retinoids are based on the time- and dose-dependent influence of morphogenesis, epithelial cell proliferation and differentiation, epithelial and mesenchymal synthetic performance, immune modulation, stimulation of angiogenesis, and inhibition of carcinogenesis. The dramatic effects of retinoids on embryogenesis were studied by animal experiments; the clinical malformation pattern in humans is known [29,30].

Retinoids promote cell proliferation in normal epidermis by shortening the mitotic phase of the cell cycle, but act toward normalization in hyperproliferative epithelia. Proliferation of psoriatic keratinocytes is downregulated by retinoids. In vitro, all-*trans*-retinoic acid was shown to either stimulate or inhibit epidermal keratinocyte proliferation, depending on the growth-culture conditions. Possibly, retinoids induce and modulate the expression of growth as well as transcriptional factors and their receptors. Stimulation of keratinocyte proliferation is associated with induction of cAMP, EGF-receptor binding, PKC, and TGF-α [31,32]. Epidermal thickening with voluminous stratum spinosum and stratum granulosum is the histological correlate. On the other hand, TGF-β_2-regulated inhibition of EGF-binding to its receptor leads to downregulation of cell growth. The effect of all-*trans*-retinoic acid on EGF receptor-binding is on a region of the EGF promoter regulated by RARγ.

Parallel to these effects, retinoids alter terminal keratinocyte differentiation toward a metaplastic, nonkeratinizing, mucosalike epithelium. The glycosylation pattern of normal skin treated with all-*trans*-retinoic acid resembles that of a mucosal epithelium, with reduction of tonofilaments, decreased cohesiveness of the stratum corneum, impaired function of the permeability barrier, and increased transepidermal water loss, causing the keratolytic effect of retinoids in hyperkeratotic disorders. In contrast, oral and topical retinoids stimulate terminal differentiation of human epidermal cells, with abnormal differentiation as in the psoriatic plaquc.

In vitro, most markers of terminal differentiation (loricrin, transglutaminase, involucrin, filaggrin, and keratins 1 and 10) are downregulated by all-*trans*-retinoic acid in a dose-dependent manner and keratins 19 and 13, markers of nonstratified and wet stratified epithelia, respectively, are induced by all-*trans*-retinoic acid [33]. In contrast, natural all-*trans*-retinoic acid restored the architecture of the epidermis at the air–medium interface model, which exhibited excessive hyperkeratosis in vitamin-A–depleted medium [34]. Adapalene induced similar effects to all-*trans*-retinoic acid on keratinocytes at the air–medium interface model, despite its different receptor affinity and its inability to bind to CRABP [35].

Isotretinoin is the most effective retinoid in reducing sebaceous gland size (up to 90%); it decreases proliferation of basal sebocytes and suppresses sebum production in vivo. Marked decrease of wax esters, light decrease of squalene, and relative increase of cholesterol concentration has been detected in skin surface lipids. Oral isotretinoin was also shown to decrease glyceride fraction, whereas free sterols and total ceramides were increased in comedonal lipids [36]. 9-*cis*-retinoic acid was recently found inferior to isotretinoin in sebum suppression [37]. Current in vitro studies confirmed the pronounced, direct inhibitory effects of isotretinoin on proliferation, lipid synthesis, and differentiation of human sebocytes in vitro [38–41].

All-*trans*- and 13-*cis*-retinoic acid downregulate collagen degradation by reducing collagenase amounts in tissue and stimulating collagen synthesis (collagen I and III) in dermal fibroblasts of the photodamaged skin. Beyond that, treatment with all-*trans*-retinoic acid over 4 months induced the number of anchoring fibrils (collagen VII) [42]. Moreover, contradictory results have been reported concerning the effects of retinoids on melanocytes. On the one hand, they stimulate the tyrosinase activity and melanogenesis, in particular, in combination with UV light; on the other hand, they inhibit the transport of melanosomes to keratinocytes and thus they decrease epidermal pigmentation.

There are multiple effects of retinoids on the cellular and humoral immunity. Most likely, activating the phospholipase Cγ and the phosphokinase C as well as stimulating the antigen-presenting capacity of the Langerhans cells and inducing ICAM-1 expression on keratinocytes lead to immune-modulating effects. 14-hydroxy-*retro*-Retinol, a natural retinoid, was identified as an essential growth factor for lymphoblastoid cells [43]. Retinoids can enhance antibody production, increasing peripheral blood T helper cells, but not natural killer cells. On the other hand, retinoids can inhibit the antigen-presenting properties of epidermal cells in vitro and, therefore, the mixed epidermal cell–lymphocyte reaction [44]. Topically applied tretinoin was shown to prevent Langerhans cell depletion in human epidermis due to UV light [45], suggesting that normalization of Langerhans cell distribution in psoriatic skin under systemic etretinate treatment may be a direct retinoid effect. In vitro, cell-surface antigens of T- and natural killer cells have been reported to increase after retinoid exposure [46]. Interaction of retinoids and cytokines has been suggested due to the stronger differentiation response of HL-60 cells to combined tretinoin and cytokines, especially IFN-γ, as compared to the single compounds [47]. At the molecular level, the modulation of RARα gene expression in chicken T lymphocytes by retinol and tretinoin indicates that antigen-specific proliferative responses of T lymphocytes may be directly influenced by tretinoin via modulation of RARα expression [48].

Retinoids also exhibit anti-inflammatory activities. The loss of neutrophil migration from dermal capillaries to the epidermis in psoriatic skin under oral etretinate/acitretin or topical retinoid therapy is well documented. In addition, topical isotretinoin was found to be more potent in inhibiting leukotriene B_4-induced migration of neutrophils into human skin than tretinoin and arotinoids [49]. Isotretinoin and tretinoin inhibited nitride oxide and TNF-α production by human keratinocytes and reduced inducible nitride oxide synthase mRNA levels [50].

There is some early information concerning the activity of retinoids on the endothelium. Retinoids are probably able to induce angiogenesis and increase skin blood flow. In contrast, isotretinoin, etretinate, and acitretin were shown to inhibit the proliferation of microvascular endothelial cells growing in vitro, without influencing the expression of HLA-DR and ICAM-1 [51].

Retinoids exhibit a direct protective effect toward cutaneous tumors [52]. The example of tumor cell differentiation in the translocation-associated acute promyelocytic leukemia of mature neutrophils under the influence of all-*trans*-retinoic acid makes possible that retinoids may modulate gene expression. As other possible mechanisms of the antitumor effect of retinoids can be discussed, the inhibition of ornithine decarboxylase and of the expression of cytochrome P-450 1A1.

3. Absorption

Transport mechanisms and pharmacokinetics of vitamin A are known to a large extent [53]. Vitamin A (retinol) is transported in plasma by the specific retinol-binding protein (RBP) to the peripheral tissues. The intracellular absorption of retinol takes place via diffusion without the assistance of receptors. Intracellularly, cellular retinol-binding proteins (CRBP) take over the function of the RBP.

The bioavailability of oral isotretinoin is approximately 25% and can be increased by food 1.5 to 2 times; after 30 min, the drug is detectable in the blood and maximum concentrations are reached 2 to 4 h after oral intake [54]. In some cases, secondary and tertiary concentration maxima consistent with an enterohepatic circulation may occur. The main metabolite, 4-oxo-isotretinoin is present in plasma in a two- to fourfold higher concentration 6 h after a single dose. Steady-state concentrations appear after 1 week of dosing. Isotretinoin is transferred across the placenta [55].

The aromatic retinoid ethylester etretinate is hydrolyzed after oral intake to its free carboxylic acid acitretin in a *cis-trans*-isomeric form. Its bioavailability is approximately 40% with large interindividual variations, since retinoid absorption from the gut is enhanced by fat-rich food. In plasma, most synthetic retinoids are bound to lipoproteins; only <2% of etretinate circulates as free drug. One hour after oral administration, etretinate, all-*trans*-acitretin and 13-*cis*-acitretin can be detected in plasma reaching maximum levels in 2 to 4 h. Remaining amounts of the parent compound are stored in the subcutaneous fat compartment with slow elimination characteristics and terminal elimination half-life of 80 to 175 days after multiple doses. The plasma levels during a long-term washout period (more than 2 years) are extremely low; they are most likely therapeutically ineffective, but may still be teratogenic. Interestingly, overweight patients tend to have slower elimination rates, maintain higher serum concentrations, and clear etretinate later [56]. From the clinical point of view, teratogenicity is the major issue in retinoid treatment because nearly all known retinoid compounds will be transferred through the placenta and be secreted in breast milk, as shown in animal studies [57–60].

All-*trans*-acitretin has a much shorter terminal elimination half-life than etretinate, about 2 to 3 days following cessation of treatment. Similar to other retinoids, all-*trans*-acitretin is incompletely absorbed, and its oral bioavailability ranges from 36 to 95%. Absorption increases when the drug is administered with food [61] and more than 99% of the absorbed drug binds to plasma proteins [62]. All-*trans*-acitretin and its metabolite 13-*cis*-acitretin are interconverted, whereby the individual role of the two compounds in the overall therapeutic effect has not been fully clarified. Steady-state plasma concentrations of all-*trans*-acitretin are reached within 1 to 2 weeks. One month after cessation of a 2- to 7-month treatment period, the residual plasma levels of all-*trans*- and 13-*cis*-acitretin remain below the detection limit and the risk for teratogenicity appears minimal [11].

All-*trans*-retinoic acid is photochemically unstable. With topical application it comes to a partial isomerization into 13-*cis*- and 9-*cis*-retinoic acid as well as to a number of further retinoid metabolites in the epidermis. Approximately

80% of the substance remains at the skin surface. Topically applied retinoids penetrate the epidermis by the stratum corneum and the follicular epithelium, whereby their penetration index is dependent on the basis of the preparation used. The diffusion of retinoids in the stratum corneum is quick; within a few minutes they form a substance reserve in the horny layer. Penetration into the deeper epidermis and into the dermis is usually slower. The percutaneous absorption of tretinoin occurs with amounts between 0.1 and 7.2%. Adapalene probably enters through the follicular channel; however, it is not yet clear whether sufficient quantities can reach the sebaceous gland [63]. With topical use of adapalene once daily over 12 weeks, neither the compound nor its metabolites were detectable in the plasma [12]. When applied twice daily over 14 days (six patients), adapalene plasma levels were detected at 0.38 mg/mL. The highest blood concentration of tazarotene after topical application was 2.0 ± 0.4 ng/mL. With a unique application tazarotene was not detectable in the blood. In psoriatic patients tazarotene concentration in blood was ≤0.15 ng/mL and that of tazarotenic acid was ≤6.1 ng/mL after a single daily application [16]. After topical application of fenretinide, no fenretinide concentration in patients' plasma was found.

4. Metabolism and Excretion

Retinol is naturally oxidized to retinaldehyde by CRBP I and the $NADP^+$-dependent retinol dehydrogenase. Beta-carotenes, which are also taken up by food, can be converted to retinaldehyde. Retinaldehyde is further oxidized with the help of the NAD^+-dependent retinal dehydrogenase to all-*trans*-retinoic acid, which is the most active natural retinoid. All-*trans*-retinoic acid is partially isomerized to 13-*cis*- and 9-*cis*-retinoic acid. Several molecules are generated by metabolic sideways from retinol, retinaldehyde, and retinoic acid. Excessive retinol is converted intracellularly with the help of the enzyme lecithine retinol acetyl transferase to retinyl esters, which can be oxidized with the help of the retinyl ester hydrolase backward to retinol. In contrast to retinol, which binds to retinol-binding protein, synthetic retinoids generally bind to serum lipoproteins and albumins.

The major metabolites of isotretinoin in the blood are 4-hydroxy- and 4-oxo-isotretinoin, while several glucuronide conjugates are detectable in the bile [64]. The half-life elimination rate of isotretinoin ranges from 7 to 37 h while that of its metabolites from 11 to 50 h (Table 3). Since in vivo there is an interconversion between the two stereoisomers—isotretinoin and tretinoin—about 10 to 30% of the drug is metabolized via tretinoin. Excretion of isotretinoin occurs after conjugation with the feces or after metabolization with the urine. The potential clinical activity of the isotretinoin metabolites, including the glucuronides, is under ongoing research. The transport of isotretinoin in plasma occurs almost entirely through binding to albumin. Its epidermal levels are rather low, with no progressive accumulation either in the serum or in the epidermis or subcutis.

TABLE 3 Pharmacokinetic Properties of Isotretinoin, Etretinate and All-*Trans*-Acitretin

	Isotretinoin	Etretinate	All-*trans* acitretin
Bioavailability	25%	40% (30–70%)	20–90%
C_{max}	366 ± 159 mg/mL Dose 80 mg	237–1403 ng/mL Dose 50–70 mg	196–728 ng/mL Dose 50 mg
T_{max}	3 h (1–4 h)	2–3 h	1–4 h
Elimination half-time	7–37 h	80–175 days	2–3 days
Metabolites	4-oxo-isotretinoin	all-*trans*-acitretin, 13-*cis*-acitretin	13-*cis*-acitretin, etretinate

Abbreviations: C_{max} = maximum plasma concentration; T_{max} = time to C_{max}.

After discontinuation of therapy, isotretinoin disappears from serum and skin within 2 to 4 weeks. It seems likely that isotretinoin therapy interferes with the endogenous metabolism of vitamin A in the skin because retinol levels increased by about 50% and dehydroretinol levels decreased by about 80% in some patients [54].

The metabolism of etretinate includes its hydrolysis to all-*trans*-acitretin, isomerization to 13-*cis*-acitretin, oxidation to more water-soluble compounds and conjugation to glucuronides, followed by biliary excretion; only a small part is excreted via the urine. Pharmacological studies indicate that etretinate may be acting as a prodrug for all-*trans*-acitretin, but when esterase is added to an in vitro system the two compounds are equipotent. While etretinate has a half-life of 80 to 175 days, all-*trans*-acitretin has an elimination half-life of only 2 to 3 days [62] (Table 3). It is metabolized into at least four compounds [65], one of which is the presumably inactive 13-*cis*-acitretin. Recent studies have clearly shown that all-*trans*- and 13-*cis*-acitretin are reesterified to their parent compound etretinate [66]. Due to their polar carboxylic acid group, all-*trans*- and 13-*cis*-acitretin are less likely than etretinate to accumulate in the subcutaneous tissue. Both are widely distributed throughout the organism and are excreted with feces and urine. Administration of all-*trans*-acitretin instead of etretinate was therefore considered a preferable therapeutic alternative with comparable efficacy in psoriasis [67,68], based on the assumption that a shorter period of contraception would be advantageous for females. However, partial in vivo conversion of all-*trans*-acitretin into etretinate has been described in vivo and circulating quantities of 5 to 100 ng/mL etretinate were detected in patients treated with oral all-*trans*-acitretin [69,70]. Reesterification does take place under varying conditions in healthy volunteers and patients with psoriasis, as well in animal models and in vitro [66]. Consumption of alcoholic drinks appears to be an important contributing factor for the formation of etretinate, but oral intake of alcohol is not a necessary precondition for reesterification [71–73]. Etretinate appears in human epidermis shortly after its oral administration. Therapeutic levels are reached within 7 to 10 days, with no evidence of accumulation even after further oral intake. The concentration levels are similar in lesional and in nonlesional skin and also in the plasma of patients with psoriasis. The amount of etretinate and all-*trans*-acitretin has little effect on the endogenous vitamin A metabolism in skin [74]. When treatment is discontinued, the epidermal values decrease rapidly and the mucocutaneous side effects associated with high maxima of circulating blood levels disappear in a few days. The drug, however, accumulates in the subcutaneous fat tissue, and reaches levels 20- to 30-fold higher than those in the epidermis. The tissue distribution of etretinate is widespread, including the adrenals and several other organs in low levels; interestingly, the fat tissue contains etretinate almost exclusively whereas in the liver all-*trans*-acitretin predominates. All-*trans*-acitretin concentrations in the subcutaneous fat can vary. Relatively low levels of both drugs were detected in suction blister fluid at steady state, indicating that only minor proportions are free to diffuse outside the vascular space [71].

The effect of a retinoid topically applied on the skin is dependent on (1) the stability of the substance; (2) its ability for tissue penetration; (3) the cellular uptake; and (4) the intracellular metabolism.

Topical retinoids do not usually influence the concentration of natural retinoids in the plasma. Inactivation of topical all-*trans*-retinoic acid takes place via the induction of cytochrome P-450-retinoic acid hydroxylase activity, which catalyzes the metabolism to the inactive 4-hydroxy-retinoic acid. Other inactivation products represent the 4-oxo-retinoic acid and the 5,6-epoxy-retinoic acid. The metabolic pathways of 13-*cis*- and 9-*cis*-retinoic acid in vivo are still unclear. Topically applied 13-*cis*-retinoic acid is partially converted by UV light to all-*trans*-retinoic acid. Adapalene is predominantly eliminated in feces as well as in the urine [12]. Twenty days after the last application no adapalene was detectable in feces. After a 3-month application (six women), adapalene concentrations of 1.1 to 5.5 ng/g fatty tissue were detected, whereby the substance was eliminated from fatty tissue 1 month after discontinuation of the treatment. Tazarotene applied topically is converted to the active tazarotenic acid in the skin [13,16]. Both substances are stable to light. Tazarotenic acid is inactivated to tazaroten sulfoxide and tazarotene sulfone by oxidation. Tazarotene and tazarotenic acid remain in the skin with minimum accumulation. Less than 6% of the applied tazarotene quantity under occlusion for 10 h were found in blood. The compound is eliminated with feces and urine, with an elimination half-time of 17 to 18 h. Tazarotenic acid came to a highest concentration of <0.5 ng/mL 14 to 15 h after the application of the preparation of the skin with an elimination half-time of 20 h [75,76].

III. RETINOID CONTRAINDICATIONS/INTERACTIONS/ ADVERSE EFFECTS

A. Contraindications and Interactions

The adverse effects of oral retinoids are closely associated with those of hypervitaminosis A [77,78]. A most characteristic symptomatology, namely, alopecia, elevation of serum triglycerides, hyperostosis, and extraskeletal calcification indicate retinoid toxicity. Given orally during embryogenesis, retinoids are highly teratogenic [79,80]. Because of these adverse effects, several contraindications for retinoid treatment should be considered. Oral retinoid treatment appears today strictly contraindicated in pregnancy [80,81], during lactation, and in severe hepatic and renal dysfunction [82]. Hyperlipidemia, diabetes mellitus, and severe osteoporosis are relative contraindications. Limiting conditions for retinoids are gastrointestinal diseases and patient noncompliance. Comedication with vitamin A (increased toxicity), tetracyclines (cranial hypertension), and high doses of aspirin (potentiation of mucosal damage) should be avoided. If retinoid therapy is necessary in women of child-bearing age, pregnancy tests have to be performed before and during treatment [81]. Oral contraceptives are recommended since the common retinoids applied for therapy do not interfere with the antiovulatory activity even after prolonged intake [83]. Before drug administration, it is strictly recommended to explain the risk of fetal malformations and information inserts should be signed prior to treatment by females of child-bearing age. Despite some experimental and animal data that retinoids may influence spermatogenesis, no impairment of male reproductive capacity has been documented. Only in one case has it been reported that ejaculatory failure may occur due to isotretinoin [84].

B. Adverse Effects of Systemic Retinoids

1. *Mucocutaneous*

The mucocutaneous adverse effects of oral retinoids include skin and mucosal dryness (xerosis, cheilitis, conjuctivitis, urethritis), skin fragility and/or stickiness, retinoid dermatitis, palmoplantar desquamation, pruritus, and hair loss [75,82]. The incidence and severity of nearly all these symptoms are dose-dependent; they are fully reversible upon drug withdrawal. The incidence may differ slightly depending on the type of retinoid given and the initial dose used. Since the frequency of cheilitis is nearly 100%, its appearance 2 to 3 weeks after initition of treatment can be regarded as a clinical maker for sufficient absorption.

2. *Ocular*

With or without conjuctivitis, eye dryness due to retinoid treatment may cause considerable discomfort in patients wearing contact lenses, and proper administration of artificial tears may be required [75]. Hemeralopia may occur, possibly due to some antagonism of retinoids with 11-*cis*-retinal formation. Also, papillary edema, corneal abnormalities with opacities and cataract, transient acute myopia, and abnormal electroretinogram have been described under retinoid treatment.

3. Pseudotumor Cerebri

Pseudotumor cerebri has been initially documented in patients receiving higher doses of isotretinoin (≥1 mg/kg body weight/day), particularly in combination with tetracyclines/minocyclin. No reports were published by using etretinate/acitretin in the recommended dose levels, but papilledema should be considered in cases with preexistent intraocular hypertension (glaucoma).

4. Hyperlipidemia

Hyperlipidemia during retinoid treatment occurs with increased serum triglycerides (20–40%) and/or with cholesterol increase (10–30%) [85–87]. It is possible that retinoids enhance lipoprotein synthesis decreasing elimination of blood lipids. Increased apoprotein B and to a lesser extent increased total apoprotein A under retinoid treatment support this hypothesis. The influence on serum triglyceride and cholesterol levels is dose-dependent and reverses within 4 to 8 weeks after discontinuation of treatment [86]. In less than 5% of the patients, hyperlipidemia leads to cessation of treatment [85]. Hyperlipidemia is likely to occur in patients with predisposing factors, such as obesity, alcoholism, nicotine abuse, diabetes, familial hyperlipidemia, and users of β-blockers, contraceptives, and thiazides [88]. The greatest increase in triglycerides is associated with the very-low-density lipoprotein fraction (VLDL; under isoterinoin and etretinate) and in cholesterol with the LDL fraction (isotretinoin) and the VLDL and/or LDL fractions (etretinate), with a parallel decrease of the HDL fraction [87,89]. Hyperlipidemia during retinoid treatment can be partially managed by an appropriate diet low in fat. Fish oil diet was found effective in partially reducing hypertriglyceridemia (27%) and inducing the HDL cholesterin fraction (11%) in patients treated with etretinate or acitretin [90]. Lipid-lowering drugs taken orally are also effective, if required [91].

5. Liver Toxicity

Synthetic retinoids have much less affinity to the liver than vitamin A. Most reported retinoid-induced hepatotoxic reactions have occurred under etretinate treatment, probably due to its high tissue-to-blood ratio, but isotretinoin may also be associated with such reactions [82,86,87]. Liver damage is a result of acute toxic reaction. Acute changes in liver enzymes have been documented in 20 to 30% of patients usually within 2 months after commencing therapy, but it has been confirmed that marked alterations are rare [86]. Chronic toxicity due to retinoid treatment is rather a rare event and long-term etretinate treatment is not associated with increased liver toxicity, despite the fact that cases of biopsy-proven hepatitis have been documented under retinoid treatment [92].

6. Bone Changes

Changes of bone formation are a well-recognized, common adverse reaction seen in chronic vitamin A intoxication [8,93]. These changes include hyperostosis, periostosis, demineralization, thinning of the bones, and premature closure of the epiphyses. Short-term retinoid therapy in children (≤2 years) seems to be safe. Data concerning long-term retinoid treatment are conflicting. Recent studies of etretinate treatment in large series of children and adolescents at an initial dose of 1 mg/kg/day for up to 11 years did not register significant bone abnormalities [77,94,95], disputing earlier case reports that suggested chronic bone toxicity in children. Bone abnormalities in children, particularly premature closure of the epiphyses, are indeed associated with high retinoid doses (>1 mg/kg/day), vitamin A supplementation, and treatment for more than 5 years. Should bone abnormalities occur, they may not resolve upon cessation of treatment. In adult patients, chronic retinoid toxicity confined to bones is commonly assumed to be due to isotretinoin than to acitretin/etretinate treatment. The effects of acitretin on the skeletal system are not yet well documented; however, available data suggest similarities to etretinate [96]. In a large prospective study, very low doses of isotretinoin (0.14 mg/kg) were compared with placebo for 3 years in the prevention of basal cell carcinoma; radiographic evidence for significant progression of preexisting hyperostotic anomalies (40% with isotretinoin vs. 18% with placebo) were found [97]. High-dose isotretinoin for ≥2 years seem to induce skeletal hyperostoses and anterior spinal ligament calcification, similar to that seen in diffuse idiopathic skeletal hyperostosis (DISH). Changes occur in cervical spine more often than in the thoracic and lumbal spine. Some patients have shown extraspinal calcification (ankles, pelvis, knees). Small, asymptomatic changes can be detected as early as after 1 year after treatment. Long-term etretinate treatment is known to induce extraspinal tendon and ligament calcification and DISH-like involvement. About 5% of patients treated with acitretin for 1 to 2 years present with changes of the bones. While a definite relationship between hyperostoses and cumulative dosage of isotretinoin could not be established, they are likely to occur at etretinate cumulative doses of >30 g [98]. Osteoporosis seems to be a toxic effect of long-term etretinate, but not isotretinoin, therapy [99]. Since about 50% of patients with skeletal bone changes are asymptomatic, a single radiograph of the ankle, the most common site of involvement, should be performed before treatment and then yearly in long-term and/or high-dose retinoid treatment. In addition, growth measurements are required in children.

7. Arthralgias and Myalgias

Arthralgias and myalgias may occur in up to 2 to 5% of individuals receiving oral retinoids in higher doses (>0.5 mg/kg/day), with or without calcification of ligaments. Their appearance seems more common in adolescents and young adults, particularly those treated with isotretinoin [89,100]. In some cases, severe muscle pain and temporary disability with early morning arthralgias were seen. Occasionally, concomitant malaise and fever may occur. Increase of serum enzymes, including creatine phosphokinase, have also been found. In some rare cases, retinoid hypersensitivity reaction with myoarthralgias has been suspected.

8. *Teratogenicity*

All known biologically active retinoids are highly teratogenic, both in animals and in humans [75,77,78]. Their biological action, beneficial for skin disease, seems related to the teratogenic risk, which is particularly high for females who are exposed to treatment during the first trimester of pregnancy [79,80]. The indiscriminate transfer of retinoids through the placenta leads to similar concentrations of the drug and its isomers both on the maternal and the fetal site [59]. Therefore, systemic teratogenicity of retinoids has remained the major concern today. The clinical pattern of congenital abnormalities induced by retinoids is rather characteristic:

1. CNS and craniofacial abnormalities with internal ear and eye malformations and facial dysmorphia.
2. Bone abnormalities with skeletal malformations, occasionally leading to limb defects.
3. Cardiovascular disorders.

These major birth defect phenotypes can be associated in some cases with lethal outcome. In addition, general retardation, thymus hormone abnormalities, parathyroid hormone deficiency, colobomas, and choanal atresia have been described.

C. Adverse Effects of Topical Retinoids

Topical retinoids applied twice daily have shown no mutagenicity, carcinogenesis, and teratogenicity in animals. Also in pregnant animals no influence of topical retinoids on the fetus could be observed. There are no confirmed observations proving a teratogenic effect of topical retinoids [101–103]. Despite three case reports on a possible retinoid-induced embryopathy under topical application of tretinoin, a current epidemiological study assessed no increased embryopathy risk under topical tretinoin application during pregnancy [101]. Moreover, the daily variation of natural retinoid plasma levels is larger than the plasma levels occurring under topical retinoid application for the treatment of skin diseases [102,104]. However, an individual embryopathy risk under topical application cannot be definitively excluded; therefore, all investigators agree today that the topical application of retinoids should be strictly avoided during the first trimester of pregnancy. In Germany, contraception during administration of topical retinoids is not required, but the administration of topical retinoids is not permitted during the entire period of pregnancy; in the United States, an effective contraception during topical retinoid treatment is recommended.

Skin irritation, xerosis, scaling, and itching of the skin are characteristic adverse effects of topical retinoids [76,105] that occur during the first month of treatment and spontaneously vanish under continuing application. The adverse effects depend on the retinoid and the retinoid concentration as well as the basis used. Skin irritation by tretinoin 0.1% often leads to discontinuation of treatment. Low concentrations of tretinoin (0.025–0.05%) produce similar biological effects as tretinoin 0.1%, but induce less skin irritation. Cream as a basis is less toxic than other bases during the initial phase of treatment. A new preparation of tretinoin 0.1% gel in microspheres was effective in two randomized, double-blind studies with 142 and 138 patients, respectively, with mild-to-moderate acne showing significant less toxicity than the classical tretinoin preparations (Table 1). In 162 patients evaluated, 50% presented no adverse effects, while approximately 35% showed mild irritation. Topical isotretinoin, motretinide (0.1%), and adapalene are less toxic than topical tazarotene (0.1%) and tretinoin (0.05%) [13,88,106,107]. The toxicity of these topical retinoids at concentrations exhibiting similar biological activity can be classified as follows: Adapalene < isotretinoin = motretinide < tazarotene < tretinoin [12,13]. Among the topical retinoids currently tested in clinical studies, retinaldehyde was shown to be less toxic than tretinoin [108], while all-*trans*-retinoyl β-glucuronide, fenretinide, and retinol did not exhibit any adverse effects [109–111].

IV. CURRENT APPROVED INDICATIONS

The current approved indications of systemic and topical retinoids are shown in Table 1.

A. Psoriasis and Related Disorders

The topical and systemic application of retinoids in the treatment of psoriasis has been reported as early as in 1972 [112–114]. Today, the oral retinoids etretinate and acitretin represent the mainstream of systemic antipsoriatic treatment, particularly in severe pustular and erythrodermic types of the disease [53,82,115]. It is well accepted that retinoids work slowly, but reliably, in psoriasis if the dosage is correct and the patient remains under careful supervision. Systemic retinoids are usually administered in combination with other modalities (mild corticosteroids, dithranol, tar) and/or with phototherapy (UVB or PUVA) [88,116–118]. In plaque-type psoriasis, the lesions slowly flatten and gradually disappear under oral etretinate/acitretin treatment (Fig. 3). The drug seems appropriate both for initial treatment and for maintenance in low dose. In pustular types (type Zumbusch, psoriasis inversa, acrolocalized suppurative psoriasis pustulosa Hallopeau), it was recognized that oral etretinate/acitretin is the treatment of choice [119], including palmoplantar pustulosis as a variant [120] (Fig. 4). Also psoriasis of the nails significantly improves under systemic etretinate/acitretin therapy (Fig. 5). In pityriasis rubra pilaris, clinical experiences have somehow been contradictory, but overall there is a beneficial effect, particularly in juvenile types of the disease [121]. In a recent review, the early use of oral retinoids was seen as the best available regimen for clearing [122].

The application of topical retinoids in the treatment of stationary, plaque-type psoriasis is a current development [75,76]. Tazarotene is an acetylenic retinoid of the third generation [13,16]. It is a poorly absorbed, nonisomerizable arotinoid that is rapidly metabolized to its free carboxylic acid, tazarotenic acid. The latter selectively binds to RARβ > RARγ ≫ RARα, without any affinity for RXRs. Tazarotene was found to normalize acanthosis by inhibiting the proliferation of psoriatic keratinocytes. It downregulates the expression of the proliferation-associated gene TIG 1, of the hyperproliferative keratins CK 6/CK 16, and of the EGF receptor. It normalizes the expression of the differentiation markers transglutaminase K, filaggrin, and involucrin. It has mild anti-inflammatory prop-

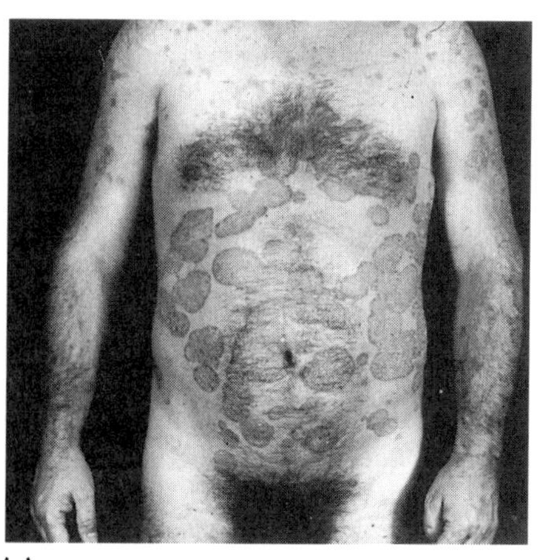

(a)

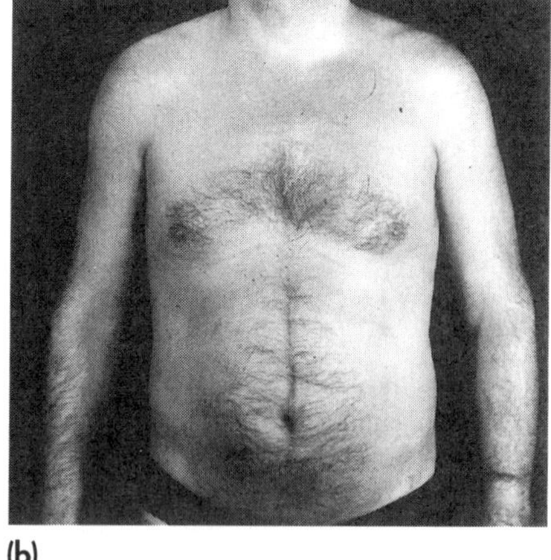

(b)

FIGURE 3 Plaque-type psoriasis (a) before and (b) after a 2½-month course with etretinate 1.0 mg/kg/day (initial dosage). (From Zouboulis ChC, Orfanos CE. Retinoide–Zwölf Jahre Wirksamkeit und Verträglichkeit der systemischen Therapie. In: Tebbe B, Goerdt S, Orfanos CE, eds. Dermatologie. Heutiger Stand. Stuttgart: Thieme, 1995: 301–308.)

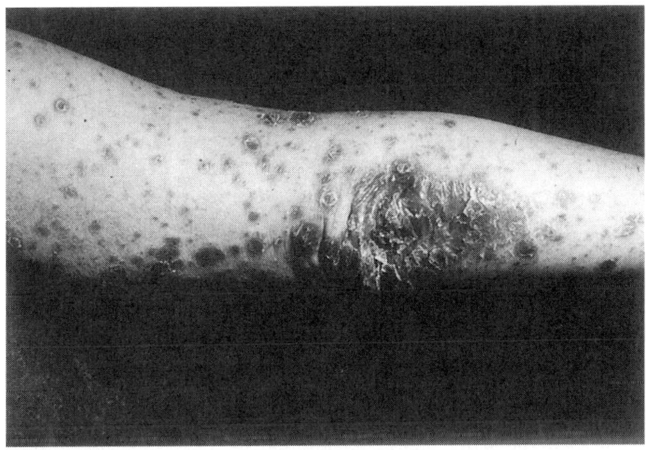

(a)

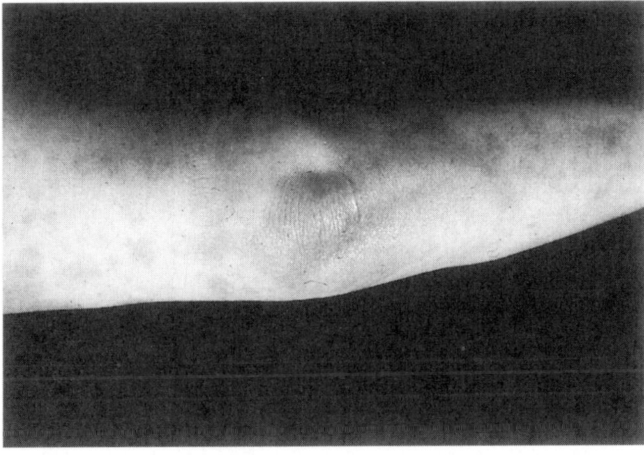

(b)

FIGURE 4 Exanthematic psoriasis (a) before and (b) after a 2-month course with acitretin 0.5 mg/kg/day (initial dosage).

erties probably due to inhibition of the expression of the migration factor MRP-8, of anti-leukoproteinase SKALP, and of the inflammation markers ICAM 1 and HLA-DR, but is also an irritant in high topical doses. Tazarotene was currently released in several European countries and in the United States and Canada as a topical antipsoriatic agent (0.05–0.1% gel) [13,123]. Clinical responses are seen after 2 weeks, with significant clearing after 6 to 12 weeks of treatment. Topically

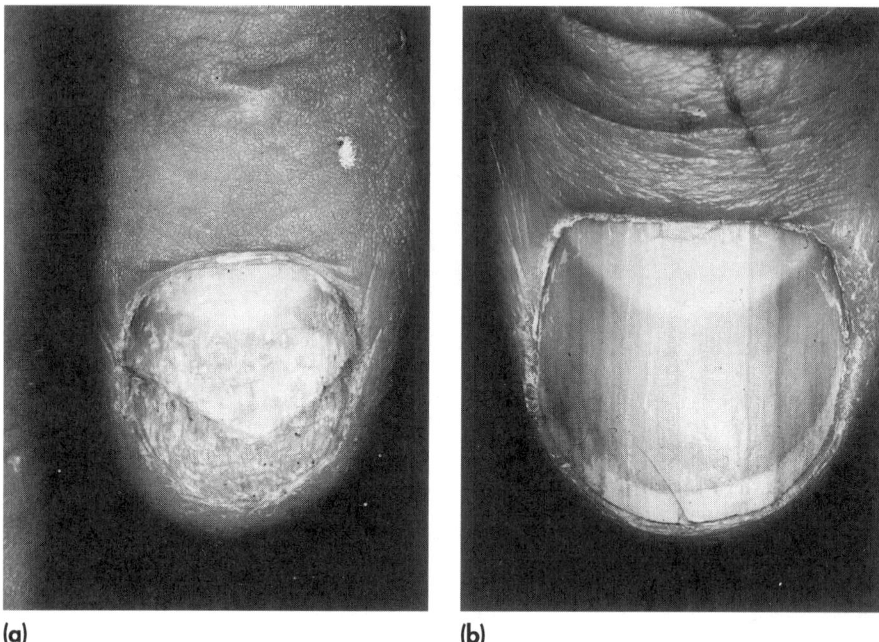

(a) (b)

FIGURE 5 Nail psoriasis (a) before and (b) after a 4-month therapy with etretinate 1.0 mg/kg/day (initial dosage).

applied tazarotene has a low potential for systemic adverse effects. Combination of tazarotene with corticosteroids of low potency seems to increase the overall therapeutic potential and reduce local irritation. The new topical retinoid tamibarotene (Am-80), an arotinoid benzoic ester, has been found effective in improving hyperkeratinization and inflammation in a pilot study with 20 psoriatic patients and is now under clinical investigation [76].

B. Congenital Disorders of Keratinization

Systemic treatment with etretinate, acitretin, and isotretinoin is effective in several disorders of keratinization since their action in promoting keratinocyte differentiation is not specific for psoriasis [53,88,124–127]. Oral retinoids were shown to normalize hyperkeratotic and dyskeratotic conditions and to reduce scaling in keratotic genodermatoses. Clearing is not complete, but the overall improvement of skin appearance and function justifies their use. Darier's disease (Fig. 6), ichthyosis vulgaris, congenital ichthyosis (particularly the dry lamellar type), various types of palmoplantar keratodermas, and also erythrokeratodermia figurata var-

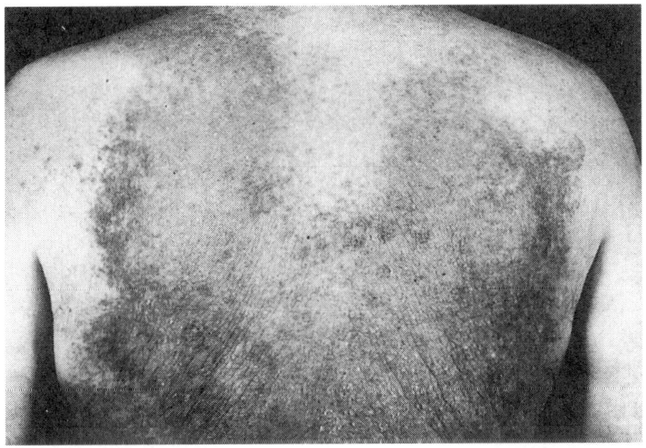

(a)

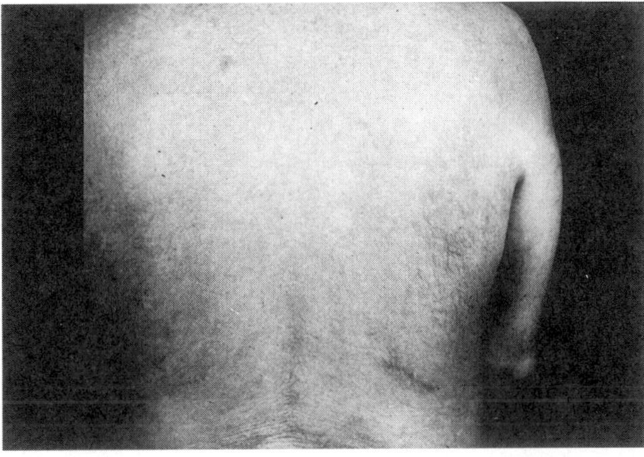

(b)

FIGURE 6 Darier's disease (a) before and (b) after a 3-month treatment with 0.4 mg/kg/day acitretin.

iabilis (Mendes da Costa) respond well or very well to etretinate/acitretin and represent standard indications for oral retinoid treatment [126–129]. Isotretinoin appears inferior to the aromatic compounds because its strong sebostatic action may dry out the skin and cause physical discomfort. Other rare keratotic diseases such as ichthyosis hystrix, hyperkeratotic verrucous naevi, keratosis lichenoides chronica, etc., may respond to oral retinoids to some degree, showing reduction of hyperkeratosis and skin smoothening. Because of the rarity of such entities, however, overall experiences are limited. Finally, in porokeratosis Mibelli of the classical type, in ILVEN naevus, pachyonychia congenita, Netherton's syndrome and monilethrix, the retinoid effect appears to be unsatisfactory.

C. Acne

Systemic application of isotretinoin has revolutionized the treatment of severe acne [130] (Fig. 7). Isotretinoin is the only drug currently available that affects all four pathogenic factors for acne, directly suppressing abnormal desquamation of sebaceous follicle epithelium and sebum production, and diminishing growth of *P. acnes* and its ability to cause inflammation [131]. In contrast, oral 9-*cis*-retinoic acid (0.3–1 mg/kg/day) [132], etretinate (1 mg/kg/day) [133], acitretin (0.3–1 mg/kg/day), as well as arotinoid ethylester (1 μg/kg/day) [134], esarotene (100 mg/day) [135], and temarotene (1 mg–2 g/day) [136] were practically inac-

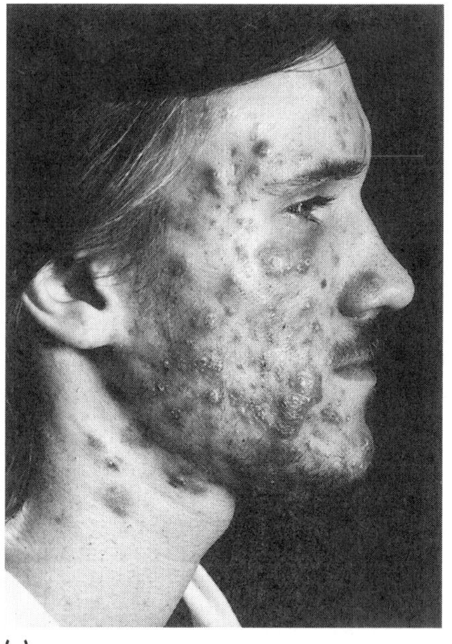

(a)

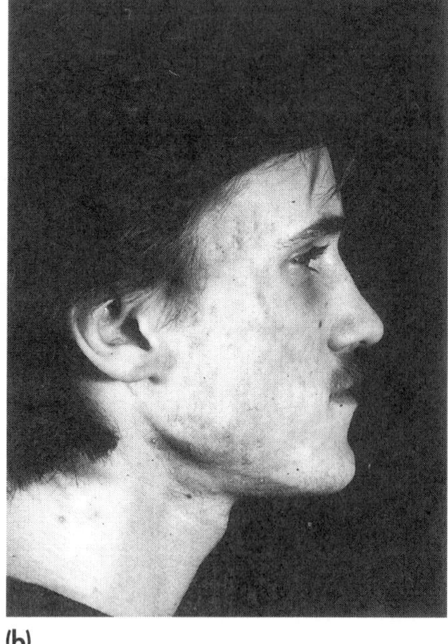

(b)

FIGURE 7 Nodulocystic acne (acne conglobata) (a) before and (b) after 9 months of isotretinoin 1 mg/kg/day (initial dosage) treatment. (Figure 6a from Zouboulis ChC, Orfanos CE. Retinoide–Zwölf Jahre Wirksamkeit and Verträglichkeit der systemischen Therapie. In: Tebbe B, Goerdt S, Orfanos CE, eds. Dermatologie. Heutiger Stand. Stuttgart: Thieme, 1995:301–308.)

tive. The clinical course of isotretinoin therapy shows more rapid improvement of inflammatory lesions as compared to comedones. Pustules are cleared earlier than papules or nodules, and lesions localized on the face, upper arms, and legs tend to clear more rapidly than trunk lesions.

In addition to the fact that contraception is essential in women of childbearing age during isotretinoin treatment [79], estrogens, antiandrogens, and their combinations inhibit sebum production by 12.5–65%. A combination of isotretinoin with systemic corticosteroids may be initially required in acne fulminans [137].

Topical tretinoin, isotretinoin, adapalene, and tazarotene [9,10,13,138,139] are effective comedolytic agents (Fig. 8). They normalize desquamation of the follicular epithelium, promote drainage of preexisting comedones, and inhibit the formation of new lesions. The restored follicular environment impedes the growth of *P. acnes* and minimizes the rupturing of comedones into the surrounding tissue. The efficacy of topical isotretinoin 0.05% versus vehicle for 14 weeks was examined in randomized studies of 268 as well as 313 patients with acne [9,53]. Isotretinoin significantly reduced the inflammatory lesions after 5 and the noninflammatory lesions after 8 weeks, compared to the vehicle. In another double-blind randomized study of 77 patients isotretinoin gel was compared with benzoyl peroxide gel 5% and vehicle [10]. Benzoyl peroxide had a more rapid effect on inflammatory lesions, but both active treatments were efficacious. Adapalene was found in randomized studies of 1114 patients with 0.1% gel preparations to be better or at least equal to 0.025% tretinoin in reducing total or noninflammatory lesions after 12 weeks of treatment [12,138,139]. Tazarotene 0.1% gel significantly reduced lesion counts in patients with mild-to-moderate facial acne [13]. Motretinide, the ethylamide of all-*trans*-retinoic acid, was found effective on acne in a controlled study of 287 patients [88], with a stronger effect that tretinoin 0.05% on inflammatory lesions and a weaker one on comedones. The preparation is approved in Switzerland. All-*trans*-retinoyl β-glucuronide was successfully used in the treatment of mild acne in a placebo-controlled study with 15 patients for 4 months, exhibiting therapeutic results similar to tretinoin 0.1% but significantly less toxicity [109]. Since topical retinoids normalize desquamation of the follicular epithelium and topical antibiotics inhibit *P. acnes*, neutrophil hemotaxis, and the production of free fatty acids, the concomitant use of a retinoid with an antibiotic is recommended. Summarizing, topical retinoids alone or in combinations are regarded today as first-line treatment for both comedogenic and mild inflammatory acne.

D. Skin Photoaging

Well-controlled studies attest to the efficacy of topical tretinoin in improving the features of photoaging [140–143]. It induces epidermal hyperproliferation and a

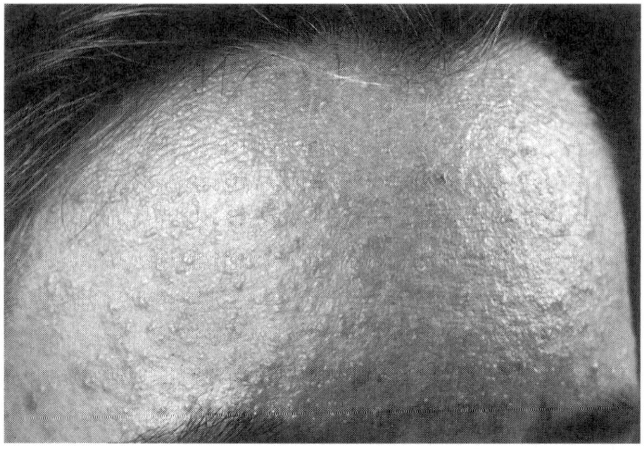

(a)

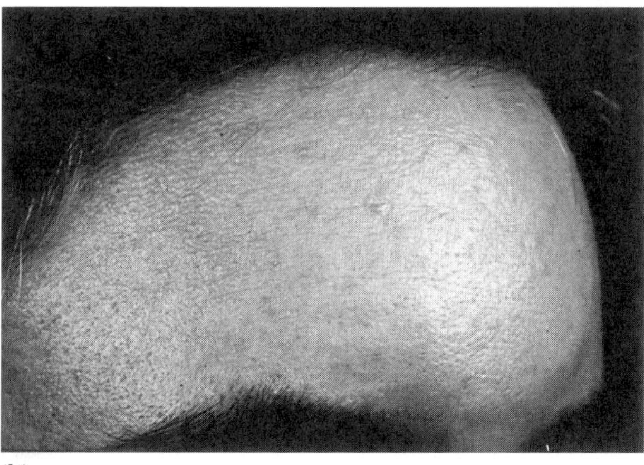

(b)

FIGURE 8 Comedogenic acne (a) before and (b) after a 3-month treatment with topical tretinoin 0.05%.

compact stratum corneum, deposition of glycosaminoglycans in the epidermis, and of collagen in the immediate subepidermal region [42,144]. Epidermal melanin is reduced because of decreased rate of melanosomes transferred from melanocytes to keratinocytes secondary to the increased epidermal proliferation. In addition to tretinoin, isotretinoin was also found to improve photoaging skin changes [145]. Tretinoin has also been shown to improve aging features of sun unexposed skin [146].

E. Retinoids in Cosmetics

Retinol palmitate, one of the major retinyl esters, is used mostly in cosmetics in lotion form at concentrations of 0.5 to 0.6% because of its stability. Like other retinoids administered topically on a long-term basis, it penetrates in the skin and induces epidermal thickening as well as increased collagen accumulation in the dermis. The use of preparations including retinol palmitate is especially advisable after discontinuation of tretinoin treatment for skin photoaging. Retinaldehyde and retinol, which are also used in cosmetics, have been shown to exhibit biological activity on the skin, namely, CRABP II induction, epidermal thickening, and relevant molecular effects [108,111]. Interestingly, retinaldehyde and retinol may act on the epidermis in a similar manner to tretinoin (0.025%), but induce significantly less irritation.

V. OTHER USES

A. Seborrhea

Systemic isotretinoin is the regimen of choice in severe seborrhea, since it specifically affects sebocyte lipid synthesis, decreasing sebum excretion rates by 75% with daily doses as low as 0.1 mg/kg and by 90% with 0.3 to 0.5 mg/kg after 4 weeks [37,147,148]. No other known agent reduces sebum production in this magnitude. In addition, the number of proliferating sebocytes and the size of sebaceous glands decreases by 90% of the pretreatment values. In a recent study, oral 9-*cis*-retinoic acid was found inferior to isotretinoin at the same dosage (20 mg/day) on 26 seborrheic patients after 4 weeks (37% reduction with 9-*cis*-retinoic acid versus 91% with isotretinoin) [37]. In another trial involving 12 healthy volunteers, oral tretinoin (20 mg/day) did not affect sebum excretion rates [149]. Current in vitro studies confirmed the pronounced, direct inhibitory effects of isotretinoin on proliferation, lipid synthesis, and differentiation of human sebocytes [38–41], as well as on reduction of sebaceous gland volume [150]. Inhibition of sebocyte proliferation and lipid synthesis were found to be independent of mechanisms of isotretinoin action. Other nonaromatic retinoids, like tretinoin and 4-hydroxy-tretinoin, also inhibited cell proliferation and lipid synthesis but to a lower extent than isotretinoin, while didehydro-retinoic acid and 9-*cis*-retinoic acid were as active as isotretinoin in suppressing proliferation of human sebocytes in vitro [39,64].

In contrast, aromatic retinoids did not significantly reduce sebum synthesis in several clinical studies. Etretinate (1 mg/kg/day, 8 weeks) [133], acitretin (0.3–1 mg/kg/day), and arotinoid ethylester (1 μg/kg/day, 6 weeks) [134], esarotene (100 mg/day, 6 weeks) [135], and temarotene (1 mg–2 g/day, 8–12 weeks) [136,151] did not reveal notable sebosuppressive activity. Arotinoic acid, a most potent inhibitor of sebocyte differentiation in animal models, was found inferior to isotretinoin in a few patients tested [152]. These retinoids were not sebosuppressive when applied topically.

B. Acneiform Dermatoses

The efficacy of oral isotretinoin in severe or recalcitrant rosacea has been well documented [88,153–155]. Marked regression of skin lesions and recession of concomitant erythema and edema are seen within 4 to 8 weeks (Fig. 9). Also, topical tretinoin has been shown to improve inflammation in severe rosacea [155]. The anti-inflammatory action of retinoids must be considered a candidate mechanism for their efficacy in rosacea, since there is no evidence for a follicular disorder, and sebum synthesis is normal.

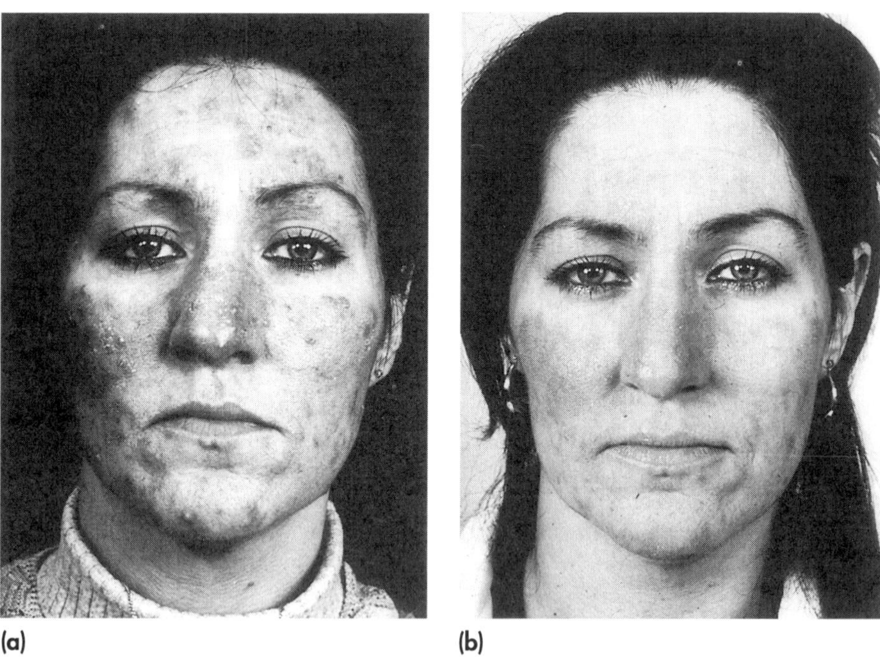

(a) (b)

FIGURE 9 Recalcitrant rosacea (a) before and (b) after 2 months of isotretinoin 1 mg/kg/day (initial dosage).

Rhinophyma responds to systemic isotretinoin preferably at its early inflammatory stages. Improvement of early rhinophyma probably occurs because of diminution of the sebaceous glands, while fibrotic changes are resistant. Teleangiectasia responds only partially because of the recession of general inflammation [154].

Familial nevoid sebaceous hyperplasia was reported to markedly respond to oral isotretinoin; however, the disease relapsed 2 months after discontinuation of treatment [156] (Fig. 10).

Gram-negative folliculitis responds well to oral isotretinoin, which usually induces long-term remissions. The efficacy of isotretinoin is probably a result of a reduction of the sebaceous gland volume, sebostasis, and skin "drying," which impair the growth conditions of *Klebsiella, Enterobacter, Citrobacter, Escherichia coli*, and *Pseudomonas aeruginosa* (Gram-negative folliculitis type I) as well as of *Proteus mirabilis* (type II).

Acneiform dermatoses of the elderly, such as sebaceous gland hyperplasia, actinic elastosis with comedone formation (Favre-Rachouchot disease), and demodex folliculitis can improve by a long-term isotretinoin treatment. Acne ne-

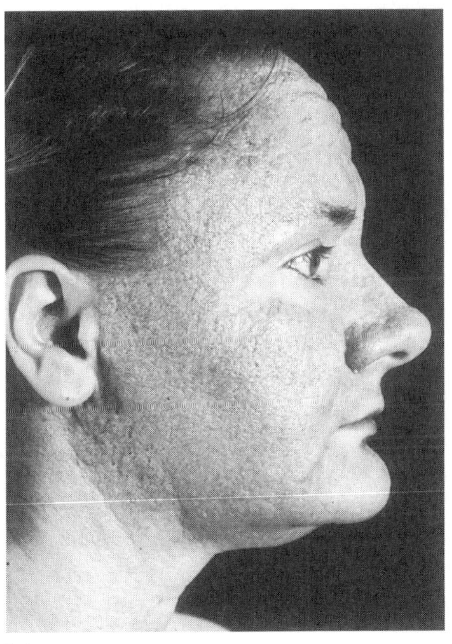

(a)

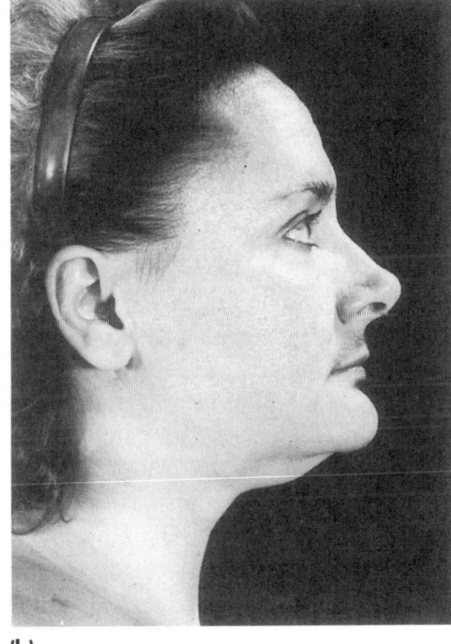

(b)

FIGURE 10 Familial nevoid sebaceous hyperplasia (a) before and (b) after 4 months therapy with 0.7 to 0.5 mg/kg/day isotretinoin.

croticans [157] and recalcitrant oil acne [158] may respond to treatment followed by long-term remission, but halogen acne seems resistant [159].

Preoperative isotretinoin treatment of hidradenitis suppurativa and a maintenance postoperative treatment has been recommended in some cases [160]. Surgical intervention is required in inverse acne, because isotretinoin is by itself, with rare exceptions, insufficient to stop the disease. The overall inflammation responds to isotretinoin but the noninflammatory or cystic lesions remain relatively uninfluenced.

C. Disorders of Pigmentation

Epidermal melasma, actinic lentigines, and superficial postinflammatory hyperpigmentation respond to topical tretinoin, either alone or in combination with hydroquinone and hydrocortisone, in conjunction with a broad-spectrum sunscreen [161]. Epidermal melanin is reduced by retinoic acid. Possible mechanisms include reduction in the transfer rate of melanosomes to keratinocytes and inhibition of tyrosinase activity leading to reduction of melanogenesis [162].

D. Retinoids in Prevention and Treatment of Skin Cancer

The exact mechanisms by which oral retinoids act beneficially in precancerous skin conditions and prevent skin cancer is still largely unknown, but their ability to promote terminal epithelial cell differentiation and induce apoptosis as well as to control cell growth may be involved. Retinoids can mediate relevant signals by interacting with the transcription factor AP-1. This complex of the two protooncogenes c-fos and c-jun plays a crucial role in cell cycle progression [163]. Inhibition of the AP-1 complex by retinoids may decrease the rate of cell proliferation [25]. Recently, the significance of the sphingomyelin cycle as a growth and differentiation control mechanism in human skin has been demonstrated [164]. This mechanism leads to elevation of intracellular ceramide levels and, as shown in hematopoietic cell lines, ceramides may represent a new second messenger, leading to inhibition of cell growth, induction of differentiation, and apoptosis [165]. In this context, retinoic acid was shown to elevate intracellular ceramide levels while inhibiting cell proliferation [166].

Synthetic retinoids have been administered in several randomized chemoprevention trials. The data collected suggest that topical or oral administration of synthetic retinoids have a significant effect in reversing premalignant skin lesions and maintaining normal differentiation [52,167,168]. Successful prevention of basal cell carcinoma and squamous cell carcinoma in patients with xeroderma pigmentosum has been described under oral isotretinoin [169] and oral etretinate [170]. Isotretinoin was shown to reduce the occurrence of basal cell carcinomas by 80% and of squamous cell carcinomas by 60% over a period of

2 years; etretinate was found to reduce the rate of squamous cell carcinoma by 75%. Furthermore, both retinoids have been shown to be beneficial in preventing the appearance of cutaneous tumors in the nevoid basal cell carcinoma syndrome [171]. Etretinate has been advocated for chemoprevention in renal transplant recipients [172]. Transplant recipients show a more than 20-fold increased risk to develop skin cancer and an increased metastatic potential leading to a 10-fold higher mortality rate due to skin cancer.

Keratoses were the first skin alterations to be topically treated with tretinoin [173]. Treatment of actinic keratoses, bowenoid epithelial precanceroses, actinic cheilitis [174], etc., with various retinoids seems well established today; marked response of actinic keratoses to topical tretinoin and isotretinoin has been described [175]. Interestingly, arotinoid methyl sulfone cream was found to be more effective than tretinoin cream in actinic keratoses in a double-blind study [176]. Furthermore, less local adverse effects were seen under application of the potent arotinoid ester. Also fenretinide treatment exhibited complete (56%) or partial remissions (44%) in 18 patients with facial actinic keratoses tested [110]. Systemic administration of etretinate has been shown to reduce actinic keratoses by 90% [177], but oral intake seemed inferior in comparison to topical treatment in this indication.

Oral leukoplakia was shown to be sensitive to oral retinoids (etretinate and isotretinoin); regressions between 61% (isotretinoin) and 92% (etretinate) have been reported [75]. In contrast, leukoplakia does not respond to topical retinoids. Keratoacanthoma has been described to respond in nearly all patients given oral isotretinoin [178] and etretinate [179]. However, relapses may occur after therapy. As a rule, oral retinoids are not recommended as first-line treatment for this condition, but postsurgical retinoid administration may prevent relapse in multiple tumors.

In contrast to the benefits of chemoprevention, no satisfactory therapeutic results have been obtained in basal cell carcinomas that show minor response to oral retinoid treatment. The retinoid effect is particularly unsatisfactory in nodular, ulcerous, and/or sclerodermiform tumors [75]. Also, squamous cell carcinomas respond neither to etretinate nor to isotretinoin monotherapy. Recently, however, effective combinations of isotretinoin with interferon-α 2a were reported in advanced disease [180–182]. Melanomas are not sensitive to retinoids [75]. Monotherapy with isotretinoin, etretinate, tretinoin, and fenretinide, as well as a combination of isotretinoin with interferon α-2a has been shown to be ineffective. Also, vitamin A does not seem to prevent the development of melanoma if used as an adjuvant.

In contrast, successful monotherapy of cutaneous T-cell lymphoma has been early reported with etretinate, isotretinoin [183,184] as well as with the potent arotinoid Ro 13-6298 [185]. The combination of etretinate and PUVA appears to be superior to etretinate alone [88]. The combination of etretinate and electron beam therapy provided no additional benefit for the course of the disease, as compared to monotherapy with electron beam alone [75]. Some synergistic effect was found with the combination of retinoids and chemotherapy in advanced mycosis fungoides. A new promising approach for oral treatment of cutaneous T-cell lymphoma is the combined administration of etretinate or isotretinoin and interferon-α-2b or interferon-α-2a [186–190]. Remission rates between 53% and 77% have been reported. Retinoids and interferons may act synergistically: interferons are thought to enhance the expression of RARs and, vice versa, retinoids may increase the expression of interferon receptors.

Some beneficial effect of oral tretinoin has been reported in patients with HIV-related Kaposi's sarcoma [75]. In a phase II study utilizing tretinoin 100 mg/m^2/day stable disease was found in two of eight patients; in another preliminary study with seven patients, thrcc partial remissions and three stable disease courses were obtained with tretinoin 2 mg/kg/day. Possibly, systemic retinoids

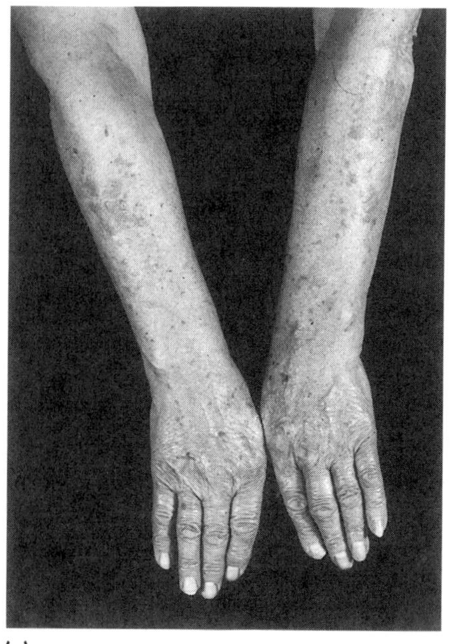

(a)

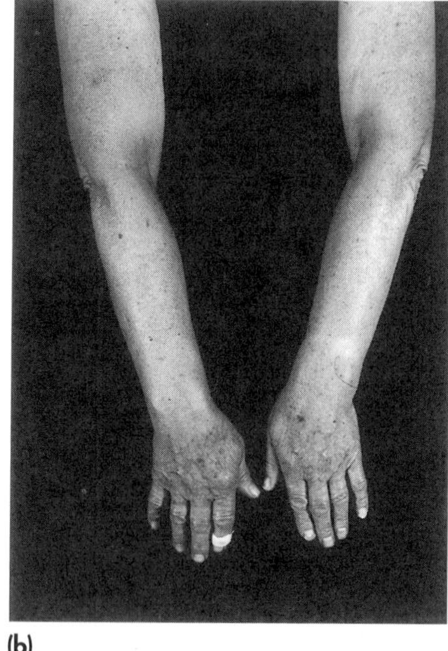

(b)

FIGURE 11 Disseminated lichen planus (a) before and (b) after 6 months of treatment with acitretin 0.5 mg/kg/day.

may inhibit or reduce endothelial cell proliferation in vivo, as they do in vitro [51].

E. Miscellaneous Disorders

Oral retinoids have been successfully used in several other dermatoses. In particular, oral etretinate/acitretin was found to be effective in three entities of different pathogenic backgrounds.

1. Lichen planus (Fig. 11), including oral manifestations of lichen mucosae oris with papillomatous and erosive/bullous lesions [191]. Low-dose oral tretinoin was also found to be effective in both oral and skin lesions [192] as well as topical tretinoin in oral lesions; however, the latter often recur [88].
2. Cutaneous variants of lupus erythematosus, particularly the hyperkeratotic lesions of chronic-discoid lupus erythematosus.

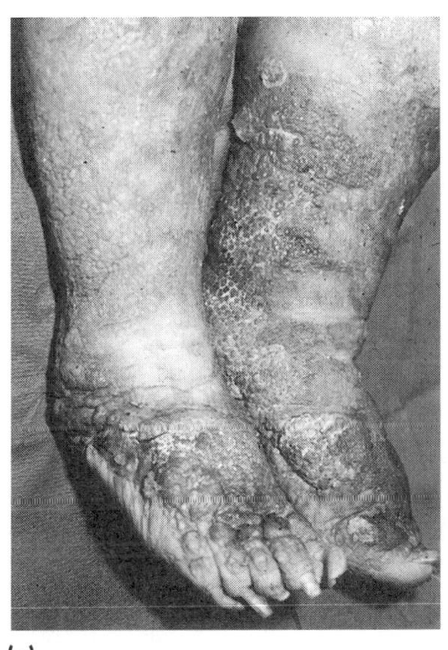

(a)

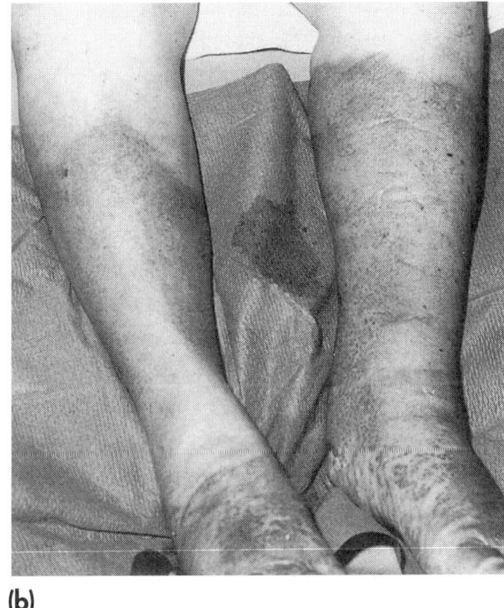

(b)

FIGURE 12 Elephantiasis nostras verrucosa (a) before and (b) after 5 weeks of treatment with etretinate 0.75 mg/kg/day (initial dosage for 3 weeks, followed by 0.5 and 0.25 mg/kg/day). (From Zouboulis ChC, Biczó S, Gollnick H, Reupke H-J, Rinck G, Szabó M, Fekete J, Orfanos CE. Elephantiasis nostras verrucosa: beneficial effect of oral etretinate therapy. Br J Dermatol 1992;127:411–416.)

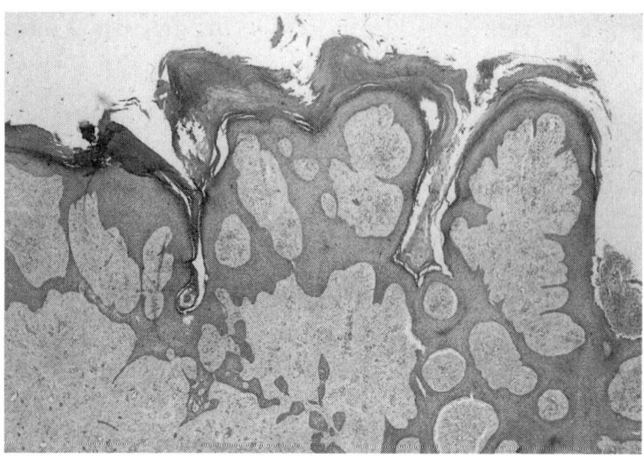

(a)

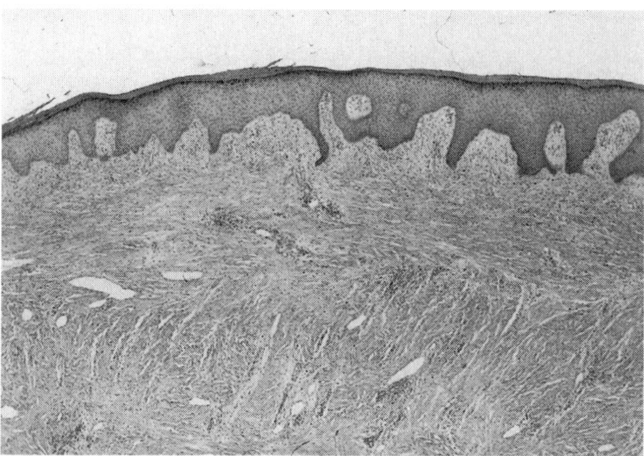

(b)

FIGURE 13 (a) The histology of patient in Figure 12 shows irregular acanthosis with focal hypergranulosis, marked orthohyperkeratosis and elongated rete ridges. Little dysplasia or mitotic activity is seen and the basal cell layer appears intact. The dermis shows chronic inflammatory infiltrate with dilated capillaries (H & E, × 23). (b) After treatment marked improvement with acanthotic epidermis, absence of hyperkeratosis and shortened rete ridges can be seen. Dermal inflammation and number of capillaries are reduced (× 34). (From Zouboulis ChC, Biczó S, Gollnick H, Reupke H-J, Rinck G, Szabó M, Fekete J, Orfanos CE. Elephantiasis nostras verrucosa: beneficial effect of oral etretinate therapy. Br J Dermatol 1992;127:411–416.)

3. Lichen sclerosus et atrophicus mostly localized in the anogenital area in females (kraurosis vulvae) [193].

Sometimes oral retinoids are helpful in reducing the dose of a topical or systemic corticosteroid regimen (e.g., in lichen planus, lupus erythematosus). The beneficial effect of retinoids in these entities underlines their immunomodulatory dermal action. A marked improvement of the epidermal and dermal changes in elephantiasis nostras verrucosa was demonstrated under etretinate treatment [194] (Figs. 12, 13). Prurigo nodularis is another entity that seems to respond well to oral retinoid treatment. The use of oral retinoids in bullous diseases, and also in pyoderma vegetans, Kyrle's disease, etc., remains unsatisfactory. Some effects have been detected in sarcoidosis or sarcoid granulomas and in granuloma annulare disseminatum [75,88], but randomized trials or case series are lacking. Topical tretinoin was found effective on plane warts [195] as well as mollusca contagiosa in children, and early erythematous stretch marks [196]. Topical retinoids can also be considered as alternative treatment in palmoplantar keratosis, nevus comedonicus, seborrheic warts and miliaria, while common warts of the elderly are rather resistant.

VI. THERAPEUTIC PROTOCOLS

A. Dosage

1. Psoriasis

The dose required for antipsoriatic treatment is 0.3 to 1.0 mg/kg body weight/day etretinate/acitretin, administered in 1 to 2 daily doses with meals (morning, noon) [82,115,197]. There are some differences concerning drug dosage information in different countries [115]; however the gold standard remains 0.5 to 0.6 mg/kg body weight/day to be given over a period of 6 to 12 weeks. Drug absorption is increased two- to fivefold and is more consistent if taken with fatty foods. The initial dose level may vary individually according to the needs of the patient, type of the disease, previous treatments, and concomitant drug administration. Retinoid monotherapy is preferred because of various interactions of retinoids (e.g., with ketoconazole, phenytoin, carbamazepine, barbiturates, tetracyclines, aspirin, and most likely with other nonsteroidal antiinflammatory drugs). No interaction of acitretin with phenprocumon has been detected [198]. Also, retinoids do not interfere with oral contraceptive efficacy [83].

A major advantage of retinoids in psoriasis is that they act synergistically with other common treatments such as topical corticosteroids, dithranol, tar, and also UVA/UVB phototherapies. In combined regimens, the oral dose of etretinate or acitretin can be reduced to 0.3 to 0.5 mg/kg body weight/day, thus minimizing their adverse effects. The retinoid and PUVA regimen is considered today as a

TABLE 4 Established Treatment of Psoriasis with Etretinate/Acitretin Alone or in Combination with Other Modalities

	Dosage	Duration
I. Plaque-type psoriasis		
Monotherapy (or with topical dithranol)	0.3 to 1.0 mg/kg/day	4 to 12 weeks
Combination with UVB (ReUVB, ReSUP)	0.3 to 0.5 mg/kg/day	6 weeks
Combination with psoralen and UVA (RePUVA)	0.3 to 0.5 mg/kg/day	4 to 6 weeks
II. Erythrodermic psoriasis		
Low initial dosage, slowly increasing up to 0.5 to 0.6 mg/kg/day over 3 months. Maintenance required for 6 months		
III. Pustular psoriasis		
High initial dosage, slowly decreasing to 0.5 to 0.6 mg/kg/day over 3 to 6 months. Maintenance required for 6 to 12 months		

Other combinations of oral etretinate/acitretin with methotrexate, cyclosporin, hydroxyurea, etc., do not seem to apply, even if they are efficient, because of increased toxicity.

most effective treatment for recalcitrant severe psoriasis [199,200]; over 80 to 90% of all cases can be cleared after 20 to 30 UV sessions and response can be maintained on low-dose oral retinoid treatment. However, the rate of relapses after withdrawal of treatment is 20 to 50% during the first 6 months, comparable to dithranol and UVB/SUP treatment (Table 4).

In randomized studies comparing the antipsoriatic potential of etretinate with acitretin, only slight differences concerning efficacy (30 vs. 50% complete remission of moderate-to-severe plaque-type psoriasis within 4 to 8 weeks; 71 vs. 83% marked or complete remission after 12 weeks) and relapse rates (46.7% vs. 40.6%, respectively) were registered [67,68,201]. However, mucocutaneous adverse effects, such as xerosis, palmoplantar desquamation, and hair loss were seen in higher rates with acitretin at dosage levels exceeding 35 to 40 mg/kg body weight/day. Thus, it is recommended to limit the dosage of acitretin to ≤ 40 mg/day and to administer the drug in two daily doses (morning, noon) to avoid maximal peaks of absorption and, therefore, increased toxicity.

Since carboxylic acids are not stored in subcutaneous tissue but are more rapidly metabolized, it was originally thought that acitretin would replace etretinate in clinical practice; however, reesterification does take place in vivo, with or without the presence of alcohol [72,73]. Both drugs are now in clinical use; long-term contraception over 2 years after drug withdrawal for women of child-bearing age is required for both.

2. Other Disorders of Keratinization

In most genokeratoses, treatment with low initial doses of etretinate/acitretin (0.3 to 0.6 mg/kg/day) is preferred for avoiding mucocutaneous adverse effects such as retinoid dermatitis, intertriginous maceration, oozing, and also increased bulla formation (e.g., in epidermolytic hyperkeratosis). Especially in lamellar ichthyosis, a dosage of ≤25 mg/day acitretin has to be administered [202]. Of course, in these disorders treatment with minimal doses is life-long, since the genetic disease itself remains intractable. Therefore, teratogenicity and bone toxicity of oral retinoids should be monitored and controlled carefully mostly in the younger patient group. The major advantage of retinoids, their synergistic activity with other common treatments, has to be considered in the treatment of genokeratoses in order to keep retinoid dosage as low as possible.

3. Acne

There is still debate as to the choice of isotretinoin dose. Some authors favor 0.5 mg/kg/day [134], others advocate a higher dosage of 1 mg/kg/day [203] (Table 5). A 6-month treatment course is sufficient for 99% of patients; it has been documented that an initial dosage of 1 mg/kg/day for 3 months, subsequently reduced to 0.5 and, if possible, to 0.2 mg/kg/day for 3 additional months according to the course of the disease will optimize the therapeutic outcome [131]. However, relapses may occur after a single 6-month course. A 22 to 30% relapse rate was noted in patients followed for 10 years after a single isotretinoin 1 mg/kg/day course (cumulative dose > 120 mg/kg) treatment as compared to 39 to 82% with lower dosage regimens [204]. Today, we recommend a 4- to 10-month course of isotretinoin 0.5 to 1 mg/kg/day in most cases of severe acne, with a

Table 5 Oral Isotretinoin Regimens for the Treatment of Severe Acne

	Duration of therapy	
Daily dose	Cumulative dose 120 mg/kg	Cumulative dose 150 mg/kg
0.5 mg/kg	8 months	10 months
1.0 mg/kg	4 months	5 months
1.0 mg/kg for 3 months, 0.5 mg/kg thereafter	5 months	7 months
1.0 mg/kg for 3 months, reducing 0.2 mg/kg/month thereafter	5 months	7 months

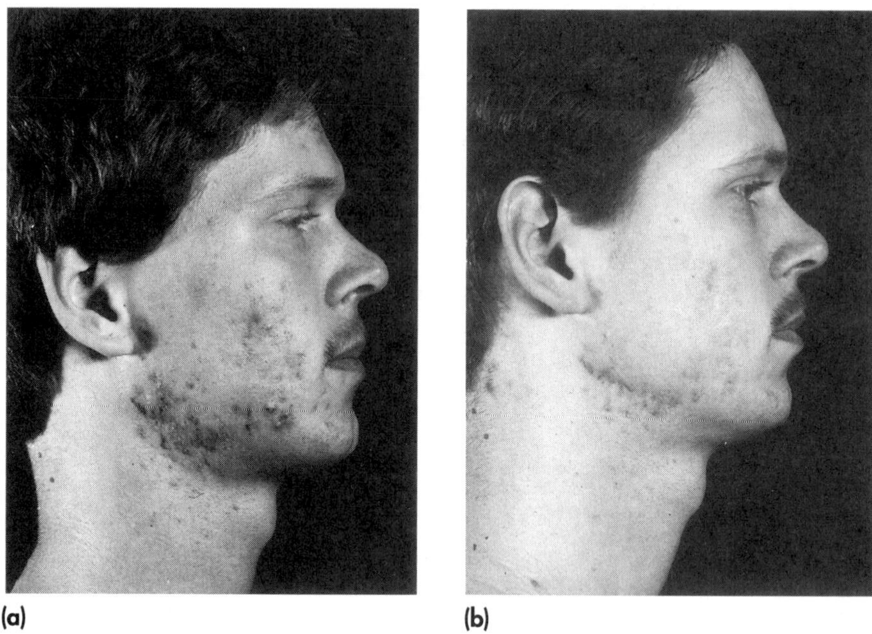

Figure 14 Scarring papulopustular acne (a) before and (b) after 10 months of treatment with isotretinoin 0.5 mg/kg/day (initial dosage).

>120 to 150 mg/kg cumulative dose [205]. Factors contributing to the need of longer treatment include a low-dose regimen (0.1–0.5 mg/kg/day), presence of severe acne lesions, extrafacial involvement, and prolonged history of the disease [205]. Higher dosages are indicated for severe involvement of the chest and back [204]. Although oral isotretinoin is still approved for severe acne only, an international survey has shown that dermatologists also prescribe the compound in less severe cases of acne (Fig. 14) when (1) the disease improves <50% after 6 months of conventional oral antibiotic and topical combination therapy; (2) acne lesions heal with scarring; (3) the disease induces psychological distress; and (4) acne significantly relapses during or quickly after conventional therapy [206].

Topical retinoids (tretinoin, isotretinoin, adapalene, tazarotene, motretinide) substantially improve comedogenic and mild inflammatory acne in 6 weeks, with maximal improvement occurring in 3 to 4 months [53]. Initially (8–10 days), the retinoid preparation has to be administered once daily at night to reduce skin and lesion irritation; given alone, the retinoid can be subsequently applied twice daily. The advantage of tretinoin over the other topically applied retinoids in acne treatment is that the compound is offered in many different concentrations and galenic preparations. To minimize topical discomfort, treatment is usually initiated with a 0.05% tretinoin concentration using a cream as basis, going over to a gel for further treatment. Long-lasting remissions can be maintained with continued application on an infrequent, but regular, basis (twice or thrice per week). Topical retinoids may heighten susceptibility to sunlight; therefore, the use of sunscreens is recommended. Combination therapies utilizing single retinoid and antimicrobial/antibiotic preparations should be sequential (i.e., the antimicrobial/antibiotic preparation being applied in the morning, and tretinoin preferably administered at night). An exception could be made when using the combination benzoyl peroxide with a less irritative retinoid (adapalene, isotretinoin). The retinoid followed by a sunscreen can be administered in the morning and benzoyl peroxide at night. Currently, galenic preparations of a retinoid/antibiotic combination have been successfully tested in topical acne treatment and are approved or going to be approved for a single daily application at night.

4. Skin Photoaging

For treatment with tretinoin, a mild cream formulation (0.025%) is usually prescribed first, increasing to 0.05% or 0.1% depending on the clinical response [53,75]. Creams tend to be nondrying and less irritating; gel and solution formulations are more suitable for individuals with oily skin or those living in humid climates. Compliance may be decreased in women who desire to wear cosmetics, as the polymer in gel formulations may impede their adherence. The preparation has to be administered once daily for 8 to 12 months, and thereafter the treatment must be continued twice or thrice weekly to maintain the therapeutic result.

5. Seborrhea

Taking good tolerance into account, an individual dose of 0.1 to 0.3 mg/kg/day over 4 weeks is sufficient to produce a sebostatic effect for at least 8 weeks after discontinuation of treatment (Table 6). Patients who have received oral isotretinoin therapy for seborrhea do not usually experience rebounds for months or years. However, the duration of the antiseborrheic effect seems to be dose-dependent. In recurrent patients, 5 to 10 mg/day may be sufficient as a maintenance sebosuppressive dose over several years.

6. Acneiform Dermatoses

The efficacy of isotretinoin 0.4 to 1 mg/kg/day for 2 to 6 months in severe or recalcitrant rosacea has been well documented [88,154,155]. Marked regression of skin lesions and recession of concomitant erythema and edema are seen within 4 to 8 weeks. Data on long-term remissions in severe rosacea are contradictory;

Table 6 Recommended Isotretinoin Dosage for Miscellaneous Dermatoses

Disease	Isotretinoin dosage	Duration	Maintenance of the result after discontinuation of treatment
Seborrhea	0.1 to 0.3 mg/kg/day	4 weeks	up to 8 weeks
(recurrent disease	5 to 10 mg/day over months or years)		
Severe rosacea	0.4 to 1 mg/kg/day	2 to 6 months	up to 2 years
	or 10 mg/day	4 months	4 months
Early rhinophyma	0.5 to 1 mg/kg/day	3 to 6 months	
Familial nevoid sebaceous hyperplasia	0.5 to 0.7 mg/kg/day	4 months	2 months
	(maintenance by 20 mg thrice a week)		
Gram-(−) folliculitis	0.5 to 1.0 mg/kg/day	2 to 6 months	long-term remissions
	(in individual cases initially ≤2.0 mg/kg/day)		
Acneiform dermatoses of the elderly	2.5 to 10 mg/day	long-term	
Acne necroticans	1 mg/kg/day	5 weeks	
Recalcitrant oil acne	0.5 mg/kg/day	3 months	
Hydradenitis suppurativa	0.8 to 1 mg/kg/day	4 weeks	
	0.5 to 0.7 mg/kg/day	additional 4- to 8-weeks	
	0.2 to 0.4 mg/kg/day	postoperative treatment	

however, remissions of up to 2 years have been documented. The daytime use of a sunscreen is essential. In a recent, randomized trial, low-dose systemic isotretinoin (10 mg/day) was able to reduce inflammatory papules to 30% and erythema to 60% of the baseline after 16 weeks of treatment. The effect lasted at least 16 weeks after drug withdrawal. Topical tretinoin (0.025% cream once a day at night) also reduced papules to 43% and erythema to 73% of baseline [155].

Early inflammatory rhinophyma responds to systemic isotretinoin 0.5 to 1 mg/kg/day for 3 to 6 months. Rhinophyma treatment with isotretinoin 1 mg/kg/day for up to 18 weeks resulted in 9 to 23% reduction of the nasal volume in nine patients [154].

A patient with familial nevoid sebaceous hyperplasia significantly improved under oral isotretinoin 0.5 to 0.7 mg/kg/day over 4 months, whereas 20 mg thrice a week were sufficient to prevent a relapse [156].

Gram-negative folliculitis responds well to oral isotretinoin 0.5 to 1.0 mg/kg/day (in individual cases initially ≤2.0 mg/kg/day) for 8 to 24 weeks, and usually exhibits long-term remissions [88].

Acneiform dermatoses of the elderly can improve by long-term treatment with 2.5 to 10 mg/day isotretinoin. The recommended dosage and duration of treatment for acne necroticans is 1 mg/kg/day isotretinoin for 5 weeks [157] and for recalcitrant oil acne 0.5 mg/kg/day isotretinoin for 12 weeks [158]. Preoperative isotretinoin treatment of hydradenitis suppurative is recommended with 0.8 to 1 mg/kg/day isotretinoin for at least 4 weeks, reducing to 0.5 to 0.7 mg/kg/day for an additional 4- to 8-week period and 0.2 to 0.4 mg/kg/day as a maintenance postoperative treatment in some cases [160].

A summary of the recommended dosage for acneiform dermatoses is shown in Table 6.

7. Chemoprevention of Skin Cancer

Isotretinoin at a dosage of 0.4 mg/kg/day is shown to be effective for prevention of epithelial skin cancer [207]. In renal transplant recipients, oral intake of 25 to 50 mg/day etretinate has been advocated for chemoprevention [172]. Recently, a combination of topical tretinoin and low-dose etretinate (10 mg/day) has been proposed for chemoprophylaxis [208], also for reducing the adverse effects of oral medication. Good results were obtained in the treatment of actinic keratoses using topical isotretinoin 0.1% gel; 40% of all facial lesions disappeared after 24 weeks [175]. In cutaneous T-cell lymphoma, a dosage of isotretinoin 1 mg/kg/day and interferon-α2a 3 to 6 $\times$ 10^6 IU/day has been recommended [184].

8. Miscellaneous Disorders

A dosage of 10 to 20 mg/day oral isotretinoin administered for up to 2 years has been recommended in the treatment of lichen planus [192]. A topical retinoid gel for the treatment of oral lesions can be prescribed as follows: Rx Retinoid (e.g., tretinoin) 0.1–Glycerini 20.0–Polyacrylati mucilago aquosa ad 100.0.

B. Drug Level Monitoring

Oral retinoid treatment requires clinical experience and regular monitoring (Table 7). Retinoids are not the "easy" drug for the "difficult" patient. Initial high-

Table 7 Clinical Monitoring Under Retinoid Treatment

Short duration of treatment <6 months Once monthly	Long duration of treatment >6 months Before initiation of treatment and once per year during therapy
Pregnancy test (also twice prior to the initiation of treatment)	x-ray of the spine
Blood cell count, BSR	Skelett scintigraphy
Liver enzymes	Eye examination (including fundus)
Serum lipids	
Serum creatinine, urea	
Serum creatine kinase	

dose retinoid therapy may cause physical discomfort, and the large number of undesired potential adverse reactions to be discussed and explained during the first consultation may limit the enthusiasm of the individual to give his or her consent for treatment.

Today, clinical monitoring requires physical examination every 4 weeks to manage mucocutaneous side effects and to ensure compliance. After administration of isotretinoin and etretinate/acitretin, elevations of blood sedimentation rate, transaminases (ALT, AST), γ-glutamyl transferase, plasma urea, and serum lipid levels may occur. Liver enzymes (transaminases, alkaline phosphatase, γ-glutamyl transferase), serum creatinine, and blood glucose should be assessed every 4 to 8 weeks. If elevations appear, the retinoid dose should be reduced to 50% or the treatment must be interrupted. Elevations of serum lipids and, more rarely, of cholesterol were shown to be occasional adverse effects of oral retinoids [82,87,115,209]. Such elevations are more often seen in older patients, particularly in those with familial predisposition or other risk factors such as diabetes, obesity, heavy smoking, hypertension, oral contraceptives, and corticosteroids [210]. Furthermore, it was shown that the amounts of creatine kinase, apolipoprotein B, total cholesterol, and LDL cholesterol increased significantly during therapy with isotretinoin [211]. Triglyceride and cholesterol levels have to be monitored every 4 weeks over a period of 2 to 3 months during the initial phase (12 h after intake of food) and every 8 weeks thereafter. Selection of patients and appropriate diet schedules are recommended as necessary precautions for reducing the risk of hyperlipidemia.

Prior long-term therapy with oral retinoids (e.g., in disorders of keratinization [88,125]), x-rays of the spine and the long bones should be taken, particularly in adolescents and young adults. There are no established regulations for the time intervals of skeletal monitoring; the decision should be made individually for each patient. Particularly in children and adolescents, regular radiological examinations of the skeletal system and the epiphyseal cartilage of tubular bones and measurements of general growth are necessary [212].

Monitoring of retinoid blood concentrations during and after oral retinoid therapy remains of major importance for managing cases of nonresponders or considering recommendations for pregnancy. In some patients showing little clinical response, the retinoid blood concentrations have been extremely low, and only an increase in dosage was followed by target blood concentrations and sufficient clinical response [213–215]. HPLC is the method of choice for highly sensitive and selective retinoid detection and measurements [5,216–218]. Following simultaneous extraction with organic solvent, the compounds can be measured by normal or reverse-phase HPLC [214,215,219], with a detection limit of approximately 2 to 4 ng/mL plasma. If traces of retinoids are detected in the blood of pregnant women, interruption of pregnancy is recommended. It is assumed that plasma levels of isotretinoin below the detection limit of 2 ng/mL are not teratogenic because the natural occurring 13-*cis*-retinoic acid reaches levels between 1.0 and 2.2 ng/mL under fasting conditions [220]. In the absence of these predictors in blood, however, the presence of retinoid traces in fat tissue is not fully excluded: with plasma concentrations of etretinate below the detection limit, etretinate and 13-*cis*-acitretin could be detected in subcutaneous tissue [221]. The prevalence of detectable etretinate concentrations in subcutaneous tissue was found to be higher (83%) than in plasma (45%), both among current acitretin users and also among those who had stopped acitretin therapy. Based on the different pharmacokinetic data mentioned earlier, current guidelines include the use of contraception 1 month before initiation of oral treatment with isotretinoin and etretinate/acitretin and continuation of contraception for 1 to 2 months after isotretinoin and 2 years after etretinate/acitretin treatment. A negative pregnancy test is required in all young females considered for treatment 2 weeks before initiation of treatment, at the second or third day of a normal menstrual cycle. Since traces of etretinate were detected in blood and fat tissue of a woman of child-bearing age 52 months after cessation of acitretin treatment [222], it has been suggested that the recommended contraception period of 2 years should be reconsidered. Nevertheless, in women of child-bearing age receiving oral retinoid treatment, close monitoring is recommended.

Appendix: Major Worldwide Registration of Systemic and Topical Retinoids

Systemic retinoids		
Isotretinoin		
Accutane™	5-, 10-, 20-, 40-mg capsules	USA
	10-, 40-mg capsules	Canada
Roaccutane®/Roaccutan®/Roacutan®	10-, 20-mg capsules	Argentina, Aruba, Australia, Bahrain, Bangladesh, Belgium, Bolivia, Brazil, Bulgaria, Burma, China (incl. Hong Kong), Colombia, Costa Rica, Croatia, Cuba, Curacao, Cyprus, Czech Republic, Denmark, Dominican Republic, El Salvador, Equador, Estonia, Finland, Germany, Ghana, Greece, Guatemala, Honduras, Hungary, Iceland, Iran, Iraq, Ireland, Israel, Italy, Jordan, Kazakhstan, Korea, Kuwait, Latvia, Lebanon, Lithuania, Luxembourg, Malaysia, Malta, Mexico, Moldova, Morocco, Netherlands, New Zealand, Norway, Oman, Panama, Peru, Philippines, Poland, Portugal, Qatar, Romania, Russia, Saudi Arabia, Singapore, Slovakia, Slovenia, South Africa, Spain, Sri Lanka, Sweden, Switzerland, Syria, Taiwan, Thailand, Trinidad/Tobago, Tunisia, Turkey, United Arab Emirates, United Kingdom, Uruguay, Venezuela, Yugoslavia, Zimbabwe
	5-, 10-, 20-mg capsules	France
Roacnetan®	10-, 20-mg capsules	Chile
Etretinate		
Tigason®	10-, 25-mg capsules	Japan

Neotigason®	10-, 25-mg capsules	Argentina, Armenia, Aruba, Australia, Austria, Bahrain, Bangladesh, Belgium, Bjelorussia, Brazil, Bulgaria, Canada, Chile, Colombia, Costa Rica, Croatia, Curacao, Cyprus, Czech Republic, Denmark, Dominican Republic, El Salvador, Estonia, Finland, Germany, Greece, Guatemala, Honduras, Hong Kong, Hungary, Iceland, Iraq, Ireland, Israel, Italy, Jamaica, Jordan, Kazakhstan, Korea, Kuwait, Latvia, Lithuania, Luxembourg, Malaysia, Mexico, Moldova, Netherlands, New Zealand, Nicaragua, Norway, Oman, Pakistan, Panama, Philippines, Poland, Portugal, Qatar, Romania, Russia, Saudi Arabia, Singapore, Slovakia, Slovenia, South Africa, Spain, Sweden, Switzerland, Taiwan, Thailand, Trinidad/Tobago, Tunisia, Turkey, Ukraine, United Arab Emirates, United Kingdom, Uruguay, Uzbekistan, Venezuela, Yugoslavia
Soriatane®, Soriatane™	10-, 25-mg capsules	Algeria, France, United States
Tretinoin		
Vesanoid®	10-mg capsules	Argentina, Australia, Austria, Bahrain, Brazil, Canada, Chile, Colombia, Croatia, Czech Republic, Denmark, Finland, France, Germany, Greece, Hong Kong, India, Israel, Italy, Japan, Korea, Luxembourg, Malaysia, Mexico, Moldova, Netherlands, New Zealand, Norway, Peru, Philippines, Poland, Portugal, Russia, Singapore, Slovakia, South Africa, Sri Lanka, Sweden, Switzerland, Turkey, United Kingdom, United States, Uruguay, Venezuela, Yugoslavia
Topical Retinoids		
Tretinoin		
Aberel®	0.025% gel, 0.2% solution, 0.05% in compresses	France
Aberela®	0.05% cream, 0.025% gel, compresses)	Sweden
Acid A® Vit	0.05% cream, lotion	Belgium, Netherlands
Acnelyse®	0.1% cream	Turkey

Appendix Continued

Airol®	0.05% cream	Czech Republic, Germany, Greece, Italy, Poland, Russia, Saudi Arabia
	0.05% solution	Czech Republic, Austria, Germany, Italy, Russia, Saudi Arabia, Switzerland
Airol® Vanishing	0.05% cream	Switzerland
Aknebon®	0.05% cream, lotion	Turkey
Aknoten®	0.05% cream, 0.025% gel	Croatia, Yugoslavia
Allamatic®	0.05% cream	Greece
A-Vitaminsyre® DAK	0.05% cream	Denmark
Avitcid®	0.025, 0.05, 0.1%, cream, 0.05% solution	Finland
Cordes® VAS	0.05% cream	Germany
Dermairol®	0.05% cream	Sweden
Dermojuventus®	0.4% cream	Spain
Derugin®	0.05% gel	Czech Republic
Effederm®	0.05% cream, lotion	France
Epi-Aberel®	0.05% cream, 0.025% gel, 0.1% solution	Germany
Eudyna®	0.05% cream, gel	Austria, Bolibia, Bolivia, Bulgaria, Colombia, Costa Rica, Cyprus, Czech Republic, Dominican Republic, Egypt, El Salvador, Ecuador, Germany, Guatemala, Honduras, Hong Kong, Indonesia, India, Israel, Korea, Kuwait, Malaysia, Mexico, Netherlands Antilles, Nicaragua, Panama, Philippines, Saudi Arabia, Singapore, Taiwan, Thailand, Venezuela, United Arab Emirates
Locacid®	0.05% cream	Czech Republic, France, Portugal
	0.1% solution	Czech Republic, France
	0.1% lotion	Portugal
Masc® retynowa	0.05% ointment	Poland
Relastef®	0.01, 0.025, 0.05% cream	Italy

Renova™	0.05% cream	Canada, Sweden, United States
Retacnyl®	0.025, 0.05% cream	France
Retin A™	0.01% cream	Canada, Italy
	0.025% cream	Brazil, Canada, Czech Republic, Italy, Switzerland, United Kingdom, United States
	0.05% cream	Austria, Brazil, Canada, Czech Republic, France, Italy, Portugal, Saudi Arabia, Switzerland, United States
	0.1% cream	Canada, United States
	0.01% gel	Canada, United Kingdom, United States
	0.025% gel	Austria, Canada, Czech Republic, Saudi Arabia, Switzerland, United States
	0.025% lotion	United Kingdom
	0.05% solution	United States
	0.1% solution	Czech Republic, Switzerland
	0.05% in compresses	Austria
Retin A® forte	0.05% cream, 0.025% gel	United Kingdom
Retin A ® Garze	0.05% in compresses	Italy
Retin A®-Micro™	0.1% gel in microspheres	United States
Retino® Jel	0.025% gel	Turkey
Retinova™	0.05% cream	France, United Kingdom
Retitop®	0.05% cream	France
Stieva A®	0.01, 0.025, 0.05% cream, 0.01, 0.025, 0.05% gel, 0.025, 0.05% solution	Canada
Stieva A® forte	0.1% cream	Canada
Tretinoina Sarne	0.05% cream	Italy
Tretinoine	0.05% gel	Belgium
Tretinoine Kefrane	0.05% gel	France
Vitacid®	0.025, 0.05, 0.1% cream	Portugal
Vitacid® A	0.05% cream	Yugoslavia

Appendix Continued

Vitamin A acid	0.01, 0.025, 0.05, 0.1% cream, 0.01, 0.025, 0.05% gel	Canada
Vitanol-A®	0.05% cream, 0.01, 0.025, 0.05% gel, 0.05% lotion	Brazil
Isotretinoin		
Isotrex®	0.05% gel	Australia, Austria, Bahrain, Bangladesh, Canada, Colombia, Germany, France, Hong Kong, Ireland, Italy, Jordan, Korea, Lebanon, Luxembourg, Malaysia, Malta, Morocco, Mauritius, Mexico, New Zealand, Pakistan, Philippines, Portugal, Saudi Arabia, Singapore, South Africa, Spain, Sri Lanka, Taiwan, Thailand, Tunisia, United Arab Emirates, United Kingdom, Venezuela, Zimbabwe
Stiefodrex®	0.05% gel	Greece
Alitretinoin		
Panretin™	0.1% gel	Canada, United States
Motretinide		
Tasmaderm®	0.1% cream, solution	Switzerland
Adapalene		
Differin®	0.1% gel, solution	Argentina, Australia, Austria, Belgium, Brazil, Canada, Colombia, Curacao, Finland, Germany, Hong Kong, Ireland, Italy, Lebanon, Luxembourg, New Zealand, Norway, Philippines, Portugal, Singapore, South Africa, Sweden, Switzerland, Trinidad/Tobago, United Kingdom, United States, Uruguay
Differine®	0.1% gel, solution	France, Morocco, Spain
Redap®	0.1% gel	Denmark
Zatop®	0.1% gel	Greece
Adapalene® Gel	0.1% gel	Israel
Adapaleno® Gel Topico	0.1% gel	Chile
Tazarotene		
Zorac®	0.05, 0.1% gel	Argentina, Austria, Belgium, Finland, France, Germany, Greece, Ireland, Italy, Luxembourg, Spain, Sweden, United Kingdom
Tazorac™	0.05, 0.1% gel	Canada, United States
Zorak®	0.05, 0.1% gel	South Africa

REFERENCES

1. Orfanos CE, Schuppli R. Oral retinoids in Dermatology, Proceedings of the Workshop during the XVth World Congress of Dermatology 1977, Mexico City. Dermatologica 1978; 157(suppl 1): 1–64.
2. Orfanos CE. Oral retinoids. Present status. Br J Dermatol 1980; 103:473–481.
3. Voorhees JJ, Orfanos CE. Oral retinoids. Broad spectrum dermatologic therapy for the 1980s. Arch Dermatol 1981; 117:418–421.
4. Safavi K. Serum vitamin A levels in psoriasis: results from the first national health and nutrition examination survey. Arch Dermatol 1992; 128:1130–1131.
5. Tang G, Russel RM. 13-cis-retinoic acid is an endogenous compound in human serum. J Lipid Res 1990; 31:175–182.
6. Matsuoka LY, Wortsman J, Tang G, Russell RM, Parker L, Gelfand R, Mehta RG. Are endogenous retinoids involved in the pathogenesis of acne? Arch Dermatol 1991; 127:1072–1073.
7. Blaner WS, Olson JA. Retinol and retinoic acid metabolism. In: Sporn MB, Roberts AB, Goodman DS, eds. The Retinoids. Biology, Chemistry, and Medicine, 3rd ed. New York: Raven Press, 1994:229–256.
8. Biesalski HK. Comparative assessment of the toxicology of vitamin A and retinoids in man. Toxicology 1989; 57:117–161.
9. Chalker DK, Lesher JL Jr, Smith JG Jr, Klauda HC, Pochi PE, Jacoby WS, Yonkosky DM, Voorhees JJ, Ellis CN, Matsuda-John S, Shalita AR, Smith EB, Raimer SS, Knox JM II, Kantor II. Efficacy of topical isotretinoin 0.05% gel in acne vulgaris: results of a multicenter, double-blind investigation. J Am Acad Dermatol 1987; 17:251–254.
10. Hughes BR, Norris JFB, Cunliffe WJ. A double-blind evaluation of topical isotretinoin 0.05%, benzoyl peroxide gel 5% and placebo in patients with acne. Clin Exp Dermatol 1992; 17:165–168.
11. Pilkington T, Brogden RN. Acitretin—A review of its pharmacology and therapeutic use. Drugs 1992; 43:597–627.
12. Brogden RN, Goa KL. Adapalene—A review of its pharmacological properties and clinical potential in the management of mild to moderate acne. Drugs 1997; 53:511–519.
13. Foster RH, Brogden RN, Benfield P. Tazarotene. Drugs 1998; 55:705–711.
14. Dawson MI, Hobbs PD. The synthetic chemistry of retinoids. In: Sporn MB, Roberts AB, Goodman DS, eds. The Retinoids. Biology, Chemistry, and Medicine, 3rd ed. New York: Raven Press, 1994:5–178.
15. Bernard BA. Adapalene, a new chemical entity with retinoid activity. Skin Pharmacol 1993; 6(suppl 1):61–69.
16. Chandraratna RAS. Tazarotene—first of a new generation of receptor-selective retinoids. Br J Dermatol 1996; 135:18–25.
17. Vieira AV, Schneider WJ, Vieira PM. Retinoids: transport, metabolism, and mechanisms of action. J Endocrinol 1995; 146:201–207.
18. Giguère V. Retinoic acid receptors and cellular retinoid binding proteins: Complex interplay in retinoid signaling. Endocrine Rev 1994; 15:61–79.

19. Ross AC. Cellular metabolism and activation of retinoids: roles of cellular retinoid-binding proteins. FASEB J 1993; 7:317–327.
20. Craven, NM, Griffiths CEM. Topical retinoids and cutaneous biology. Clin Exp Dermatol 1996; 21:1–10.
21. Leid M, Kastner P, Lyons R, Nakshatri H, Saunders M, Zacharewski T, Chen J-Y, Staub A, Garnier J-M, Mader S, Chambon P. Purification, cloning, and RXR identity of the HeLa cell factor with which RAR or TR heterodimerizes to bind target sequences efficiently. Cell 1992; 68:377–395.
22. Mangelsdorf DJ, Umesono K, Evans RM. The retinoid receptors. In: Sporn MB, Roberts AB, Goodman DS, eds. The Retinoids. Biology, Chemistry, and Medicine, 3rd ed. New York: Raven Press, 1994:319–349.
23. Boylan JF, Goudas LJ. Overexpression of the cellular retinoic acid-binding protein-I (CRABP-I) results in a reduction in differentiation-specific gene expression in F9 teratocarcinoma cells. J Cell Biol 1991; 112:965–979.
24. Schüle R, Evans RM. Cross-coupling of signal transduction pathways: zink finger meets leucine zipper. Trends Genet 1991; 7:377–381.
25. Fanjul A, Dawson MI, Hobbs PD, Jong L, Cameron JF, Harlev E, Graupner G, Lu XP, Pfahl M. A new class of retinoids with selective inhibition of AP-1 inhibits proliferation. Nature 1994; 372:107–111.
26. Elder J, Åström A, Pettersson U, Tavakkol A, Griffiths CEM, Krust A, Kastner P, Chambon P, Voorhees JJ. Differential regulation of retinoic acid receptors and binding proteins in human skin. J Invest Dermatol 1992; 98:673–679.
27. Fisher GJ, Talwar HS, Xiao J-H, Datta SC, Reddy AP, Gaub MP, Rochette-Egly C, Chambon P, Voorhees JJ. Immunological identification and functional quantitation of retinoic acid and retinoid X receptor proteins in human skin. J Biol Chemistry 1994; 269:20629–20635.
28. Apfel C, Crettaz M, Siegenthaler G, Hunziker W. Synthetic retinoids: differential binding to retinoic acid receptors. In: Saurat J-H, ed. Retinoids 10 Years On. Basel: Karger, 1991:110–120.
29. Kistler A. Limb bud cell cultures for estimating the teratogenic potential of compounds: validation of the test system with retinoids. Arch Toxicol 1987; 60:403–414.
30. Lammer EJ, Chen DT, Hoar RM, Agnish ND, Benke PJ, Braun JT, Curry CJ, Fernhoff PM, Grix AW Jr, Lott IT, et al. Retinoic acid embryopathy. N Engl J Med 1985; 313:837–841.
31. Tong PS, Horowitz NN, Wheeler LA. Trans-retinoic acid enhances the growth response of epidermal keratinocytes to epidermal growth factor and transforming growth factor beta. J Invest Dermatol 1990; 94:126–131.
32. Zheng Z-S, Polakowska R, Johnson A, Goldsmith LA. Transcriptional control of epidermal growth factor receptor by retinoic acid. Cell Growth Differ 1992; 3:225–232.
33. Asselineau D, Darmon M. Retinoic acid provokes metaplasia of epithelium formed by adult human epidermal keratinocytes. Differentiation 1995; 58:297–306.
34. Asselineau D, Bernard BA, Bailly C, Darmon M. Retinoic acid improves epidermal morphogenesis. Dev Biol 1989; 133:322–335.

35. Asselineau D, Cavey MT, Shroot B, Darmon M. Control of epidermal differentiation by a retinoid analogue unable to bind to cytosolic retinoid acid-binding proteins (CRABP). J Invest Dermatol 1992; 98:128–134.
36. Melnik B, Kinner T, Plewig G. Influence of oral isotretinoin treatment on the composition of comedonal lipids. Implications for comedogenesis in acne vulgaris. Arch Dermatol Res 1988; 280:97–102.
37. Geiger J-M, Hommel L, Harms M, Saurat J-H. Oral 13-cis retinoic acid is superior to 9-cis retinoic acid in sebosuppression in human beings. J Am Acad Dermatol 1996; 34:513–515.
38. Shapiro SS, Hurley J, Vane FM, Doran T. Evaluation of potential therapeutic entities for the treatment of acne. In: Reichert U, Shroot B, eds. Pharmacology of Retinoids in the Skin. Basel: Karger, 1989:104–112.
39. Zouboulis ChC, Korge B, Akamatsu H, Xia L, Schiller S, Gollnick H, Orfanos CE. Effects of 13-cis-retinoic acid, all-trans-retinoic acid, and acitretin on the proliferation, lipid synthesis and keratin expression of cultured human sebocytes in vitro. J Invest Dermatol 1991; 96:792–797.
40. Zouboulis ChC, Xia L, Korge B, Gollnick H, Orfanos CE. Cultivation of human sebocytes in vitro. Cell characterization and influence of synthetic retinoids. In: Saurat J-H, ed. Retinoids 10 years on. Basel: Karger, 1991:254–273.
41. Zouboulis ChC, Krieter A, Gollnick H, Orfanos CE. Progressive differentiation of human sebocytes in vitro is characterized by increased cell size and altered antigenic expression and is regulated by culture duration and retinoids. Exp Dermatol 1994; 3:151–160.
42. Griffiths CEM, Russman AN, Majmudar G, Singer RS, Hamilton TA, Voorhees JJ. Restoration of collagen formation in photodamaged skin by tretinoin (retinoic acid). N Engl J Med 1993; 329:530–535.
43. Buck J, Derguini F, Levi E, Nakanishi K, Hammerling U. Intracellular signaling by 14-hydroxy-4, 14-retro-retinol. Science 1991; 254:1654–1656.
44. Dupuy P, Bagot M, Heslan M, Dubertret L. Synthetic retinoids inhibit the antigen presenting properties of epidermal cells in vitro. J Invest Dermatol 1989; 93:455–459.
45. Halliday GM, Ho KK, Barnetson RS. Regulation of the skin immune system by retinoids during carcinogenesis. J Invest Dermatol 1992; 99:83S–86S.
46. Prabhala RH, Maxey V, Hicks MJ, Watson RR. Enhancement of the expression of activation markers on human peripheral blood mononuclear cells by in vitro culture with retinoids and carotenoids. J Leukocyte Biol 1989; 45:249–254.
47. Bollag W. Retinoid and interferon: a new promising combination? B J Haematol 1991; 79(suppl 1):87–91.
48. Halewy O, Arazi Y, Melamed D, Friedman A, Sklan D. Retinoic acid receptor-alpha gene expression is modulated by dietary vitamin A and by retinoic acid in chicken T lymphocytes. J Nutr 1994; 124:2139–2146.
49. Wozel G, Chang A, Zultak M, Czarnetzki BM, Happle R, Barth J, van de Kerkhof PC. The effect of topical retinoids on the leukotriene-B_4-induced migration of polymorphonuclear leukocytes into human skin. Arch Dermatol Res 1991; 283:158–161.

50. Bécherel P-A, Mossalayi MD, Le Goff L, Francès C, Chosidow O, Debré P, Arock M. Mechanism of anti-inflammatory action of retinoids on keratinocytes. Lancet 1994; 344:1570–1571.
51. Imcke E, Ruszczak Zb, Mayer-da-Silva A, Detmar M, Orfanos CE. Cultivation of human dermal microvascular endothelial cells in vitro: immunocytochemical and ultrastructural characterization and effect of treatment with three synthetic retinoids. Arch Dermatol Res 1991; 283:149–157.
52. Gollnick H, Orfanos CE. Theoretical aspects of the use of retinoids as anticancer drugs. In: Marks R, ed. Retinoids in cutaneous malignancy. Oxford: Blackwell, 1991:41–65.
53. Zouboulis ChC, Orfanos CE. Retinoide–Zwölf Jahre Wirksamkeit und Verträglichkeit der systemischen Therapie. In: Tebbe B, Goerdt S, Orfanos CE, eds. Dermatologie. Heutiger Stand. Stuttgart: Thieme, 1995:301–308.
54. Rollmann O, Vahlquist A. Oral isotretinoin (13-cis-retinoic acid) therapy in severe acne: drug and vitamin A concentrations in serum and skin. J Invest Dermatol 1986; 86:384–389.
55. Benifla JL, Ville Y, Imbert MC, Frydman R, Thomas A, Pons JC. Fetal tissue dosages of retinoids: experimental study concerning a case of isotretinoin (Roaccutan) administration and pregnancy. Fetal Diagn Ther 1995; 10:189–191.
56. Chalmers RJ. Retinoid therapy—a real hazard for the developing embryo. Br J Obstet Gynecol 1992; 99:276–278.
57. DiGiovanna JJ, Zech LA, Ruddel ME, Gantt G, Peck GL. Etretinate. Persistent serum levels after long-term therapy. Arch Dermatol 1989; 125:246–251.
58. Rollmann O, Vahlquist A. Retinoid concentrations in skin, serum and adipose tissue of patients treated with etretinate. Br J Dermatol 1983; 109:439–447.
59. Reiners J, Lofberg B, Kraft JC, Kochhar DM, Nau H. Transplacental pharmacokinetics of teratogenic doses of etretinate and other aromatic retinoids in mice. Reprod Toxicol 1988; 2:19–29.
60. Rollmann O, Phil-Lundin I. Acitretin excretion into human breast milk. Acta Dermatol Venereol (Stockh) 1990; 70:487–490.
61. McNamara PJ, Jewell RC, Jensen BK, Brindley CJ. Food increases the bioavailability of acitretin. J Clin Pharmacol 1988; 28:1051–1055.
62. Brindley C. An overview of recent clinical pharmacokinetic studies with acitretin (Ro 10-1670, etretin). Dermatologica 1989; 178:79–87.
63. Shroot B, Michel S, Allec J, Chatelus A, Wagner N. A new concept of drug delivery for acne. Dermatology 1998; 196:165–170.
64. Vane FM, Buggé CJL, Rodriguez LC, Rosenberger M, Doran TI. Human biliary metabolites of isotretinoin: identification, quantification, sythesis and biological activity. Xenobiotica 1990; 20:193–207.
65. Rubio F, Jensen BK, Henderson L, Garland WA, Szuna A, Town C. Disposition of [^{14}C] acitretin in humans following oral administration. Drug Metab Dispos 1994; 22:211–215.
66. Chou RC, Wyss R, Huselton CA, Wiegand U-W. A potentially new metabolic pathway: ethyl esterification of acitretin. Xenobiotica 1992; 8:993–1002.
67. Gollnick H, Bauer R, Brindley CJ, Orfanos CE, Plewig G, Wokalek H, Hoting E

et al. Acitretin versus etretinate in psoriasis. Clinical and pharmacokinetic results of a German multicenter study. J Am Acad Dermatol 1988; 19:458–468.
68. Gollnick H, Zaun H, Ruzicka T, Sommerburg C, Loew S, Mahrle G, Niedecken H-W, Paul E, Pfister-Wartha A, Reinel D, et al. Relapse rate of severe generalized psoriasis after treatment with acitretin or etretinate. Eur J Dermatol 1993; 3:442–446.
69. Lambert WE, De Leenheer AP, De Bersaques JP, Kint A. Persistent etretinate levels in plasma after changing the therapy to acitretin. Arch Dermatol Res 1990; 282: 343–344.
70. Grønjøj Larsen F, Jakobsen P, Knudsen J, Weismann K, Kragballe K, Nielsen-Kudsk F. Conversion of acitretin to etretinate in psoriatic patients is influenced by ethanol. J Invest Dermatol 1993; 100:623–627.
71. Grønjøj Larsen F. Pharmacokinetics of etretinate and acitretin with special reference to treatment of psoriasis. Acta Dermatol Venereol (Stockh) 1995; 190:1–33.
72. Laugier JP, De Sousa G, Bun H, Geiger J-M, Surber C, Rahmani R. Acitretin biotransformation into etretinate: role of ethanol on in vitro hepatic metabolism. Dermatology 1994; 188:122–125.
73. Almond-Roesler B, Orfanos CE. Trans-Acitretin wird in Etretinat rückmetabolisiert. Bedeutung für die orale Retinoidtherapie. Hautarzt 1996; 47:173–177.
74. Laugier JP, Berbis P, Brindley C, Bun H, Geiger J-M, Privat Y, Durand A. Determination of acitretin and 13-cis acitretin in skin. Skin Pharmacol 1989; 2:181–186.
75. Orfanos CE, Zouboulis ChC, Almond-Roesler B, Geilen CC. Current use and future potential role of retinoids in dermatology. Drugs 1997; 53:358–388.
76. Zouboulis ChC, Orfanos CE. Topische Dermatika: Retinoide. In: Korting HC, Sterry W, eds. Therapeutische Verfahren in der Dermatologie: Dermatika und Kosmetika. Berlin: Springer, in press.
77. Mills CM, Marks R. Adverse reactions to oral retinoids. Drug Safety 1993; 9:280–290.
78. Fritsch P, Sidoroff A. Safety of retinoids and indications for use. Curr Opin Dermatol 1993; 207–213.
79. Dai WS, LaBraiso JM, Stern RS. Epidemiology of isotretinoin exposure during pregnancy. J Am Acad Dermatol 1992; 26:599–606.
80. Geiger J-M, Baudin M, Saurat J-H. Teratogenic risk with etretinate and acitretin treatment. Dermatology 1994; 189:109–116.
81. Mitchell AA, Van Bennekom CM, Louik C. A pregnancy-prevention program in women of childbearing age receiving isotretinoin. N Engl J Med 1995; 333:101–106.
82. Gollnick HPM. Oral retinoids—efficacy and toxicity in psoriasis. Br J Dermatol 1996; 135(suppl 49):6–17.
83. Berbis P, Bun H, Geiger J-M, Rognin C, Durand A, Serradimigni A, Hartmann D, Privat Y. Acitretin (Ro 10-1670) and oral contraceptives: interaction study. Arch Dermatol Res 1988; 280:388–389.
84. Colemann R, MacDonald D. Effects of isotretinoin on male reproductive system. Lancet 1994; 344:198.
85. Olsen EA, Weed WW, Meyer CJ, Cobo LM. A double-blind, placebo-controlled

trial of acitretin for the treatment of psoriasis. J Am Acad Dermatol 1989; 21:681–686.

86. Gupta AK, Goldfarb MT, Ellis CN, Voorhees JJ. Side-effect profile of acitretin therapy in psoriasis. J Am Acad Dermatol 1989; 20:1088–1093.
87. Barth JH, MacDonald-Hull SP, Mark J, Jones RG, Cunliffe WJ. Isotretinoin therapy for acne vulgaris: a re-evaluation of the need for measurements of plasma lipids and liver function tests. Br J Dermatol 1993; 129:704–707.
88. Orfanos CE, Ehlert R, Gollnick H. The retinoids. A review of their clinical pharmacology and therapeutic use. Drugs 1987; 34:459–503.
89. Vahlquist C, Selinus I, Vessby B. Serum lipid changes during acitretin (etretin) treatment of psoriasis and palmo-plantar pustulosis. Acta Dermatol Venereol (Stockh) 1988; 68:300–305.
90. Ashley JM, Lowe NJ, Borok ME, Alfin-Slater RB. Fish oil supplementation results in decreased hypertriglyceridemia in patients with psoriasis undergoing etretinate or acitretin therapy. J Am Acad Dermatol 1988; 19:76–82.
91. Vahlquist C, Olsson AG, Lindholm A, Vahlquist A. Effects of gemfibrozil (Lopid) on hyperlipidemia in acitretin-treated patients: results of a double-blind cross-over study. Acta Dermatol Venereol (Stockh) 1995; 75:377–380.
92. Sanchez MR, Ross B, Rotterdam H, Salik J, Brodie R, Freedberg IM. Retinoid hepatitis. J Am Acad Dermatol 1993; 28:853–858.
93. Silverman AK, Ellis CN, Voorhees JJ. Hypervitaminosis A syndrome: a paradigm of retinoid side effects. J Am Acad Dermatol 1987; 16:1027–1039.
94. Glover MT, Peters AM, Atherton DJ. Surveillance for skeletal toxicity of children treated with etretinate. Br J Dermatol 1987; 116:609–614.
95. Paige DG, Judge MR, Shaw DG, Atherton DJ, Harper JI. Bone changes and their significance in children with ichthyosis on long-term etretinate therapy. Br J Dermatol 1992; 127:387–391.
96. Hohl D, Pelloni F, Sigg C, Gilardi S, Jung T. A prospective study of skeletal changes during short-term acitretin therapy. Dermatology 1992; 185:23–26.
97. Tangrea JA, Kilcoyne RF, Taylor PR, Helsel WE, Adrianza ME, Hartman AM, Edwards BK, Peck GL. Skeletal hyperostosis in patients receiving chronic, very-low-dose isotretinoin. Arch Dermatol 1992; 128:921–925.
98. Simpson KR, Rosenbach A, Lowe NJ. Etretinate for retinoid-responsive dermatoses: further observations of long-term therapy. J Dermatol Treat 1993; 4:179–182.
99. DiGiovanna JJ, Sollitto RB, Abangan DL, Steinberg SM, Reynolds JC. Osteoporosis is a toxic effect of long-term etretinate therapy. Arch Dermatol 1995; 131:1263–1267.
100. Callot V, Ochonisky S, Vabres P, Revuz J. Arthrite aiguë au cours d'un traitment par l'isotrétinoïne. Ann Dermatol Venerol 1994; 121:402–403.
101. Jick SJ, Terris B, Jick H. First trimester topical tretinoin and congenital disorders. Lancet 1993; 341:1181–1182.
102. Nau H. Embryotoxicity and teratogenicity of topical retinoic acid. Skin Pharmacol 1993; 6(suppl 1):35–44.
103. Santana D, Bun H, Joachim J, Durand A, Reynier JP. Plasma concentrations after three different doses of topical isotretinoin. Skin Pharmacol 1994; 7:140–144.
104. Clewell HJ III, Andersen ME, Wills RJ, Latriano L. A physiologically based phar-

macokinetic model for retinoic acid and its metabolites. J Am Acad Dermatol 1997; 36:S77–S85.
105. Griffiths CEM, Voorhees JJ. Human in vivo pharmacology of topical retinoids. Arch Dermatol Res 1994; 287:53–60.
106. Cunningham WJ, Bryce GF, Armstrong RB, Lesiewicz J, Kim H-J, Sendagorta E. Topical isotretinoin and photodamage. In: Saurat J-H, ed. Retinoids: 10 Years On. Basel: Karger, 1991:182–190.
107. Gollnick HP, Dummler U. Retinoids. Clin Dermatol 1997; 15:799–810.
108. Saurat JH, Didierjean L, Masgrau E, Piletta PA, Jaconi S, Chatellard-Gruaz D, Gumowski D, Masouyé I, Salomon D, Siegenthaler G. Topical retinaldehyde on human skin: biologic effects and tolerance. J Invest Dermatol 1994; 103:770–774.
109. Gunning DB, Barua AB, Loyd RA, Olson JA. Retinoyl β-glucuronide: a nontoxic retinoid for the topical treatment of acne. J Dermatol Treat 1994; 5:181–185.
110. Moglia D, Formelli F, Baliva G, Bono A, Accetturi M, Nava M, De Palo G. Effects of topical treatment with fenretinide (4-HPR) and plasma vitamin A levels in patients with actinic keratoses. Cancer Lett 1996; 110:87–91.
111. Kang S, Duell EA, Fisher GJ, Datta SC, Wang Z-Q, Reddy AP, Tavakkol A, Yi JY, Griffiths CEM, Elder JT, Voorhees JJ. Application of retinol to human skin in vivo induces epidermal hyperplasia and cellular retinoid binding proteins characteristic of retinoic acid but without measurable retinoic acid levels or irritation. J Invest Dermatol 1995; 105:549–556.
112. Orfanos CE, Schmidt HW, Mahrle G, Runne U. Die Wirksamkeit von Vitamin-A-Säure bei Psoriasis. Topische Kombinationsbehandlung mit Corticoiden. Zwei neue VAS-Präparate zur peroralen Therapie. Arch Dermatol Forsch 1972; 244: 424–426.
113. Orfanos CE, Schmidt HW, Marhle G, Gartmann H, Lever WF. Retinoic acid in psoriasis: its value for topical therapy with and without corticosteroids. Clinical, histological and electron microscopical studies on forty-four hospitalized patients with extensive psoriasis. Br J Dermatol 1973; 88:167–182.
114. Runne U, Orfanos CE, Gartmann H. Perorale Applikation zweier Derivate der Vitamin A-Säure zur internene Psoriasis-Therapie. 13-cis-beta-Vitamin-A-Säure und Vitamin A-Säure-aethylamid. Arch Derm Forsch 1973; 247:171–180.
115. Geiger J M, Saurat J-H. Acitretin and etretinate. How and when they should be used. Dermatol Clin 1993; 11:117–129.
116. Lauharanta J, Geiger J-M. A double-blind comparison of acitretin and etretinate in combination with bath PUVA in the treatment of extensive psoriasis. Br J Dermatol 1989; 121:107–112.
117. Lowe NJ, Prystowsky JH, Bourget T, Edelstein J, Nychay S, Armstrong R. Acitretin plus UVB therapy for psoriasis. Comparisons with placebo plus UVB and acitretin alone. J Am Acad Dermatol 1991; 24:591–594.
118. Ruzicka T, Sommerburg C, Braun-Falco O, Koster W, Lengen W, Lensing W, Letzel H, Meigel WN, Paul E, Przybilla B, et al. Efficiency of acitretin in combination with UV-B in the treatment of severe psoriasis. Arch Dermatol 1990; 126: 482–486.
119. Orfanos CE, Landes E, Bloch PH. Traitément du psoriasis pustuleux par un nou-

veaux rétinoide aromatique (Ro 10-9359). Ann Dermatol Vénéreol 1978; 103:807–811.
120. Lassus A, Geiger JM. Acitretin and etretinate in the treatment of palmoplantar pustulosis: a double-blind comparative trial. Br J Dermatol 1988; 119:755–759.
121. Borok M, Lowe NJ. Pityriasis rubra pilaris. J Am Acad Dermatol 1990; 22:792–795.
122. Dicken CH. Treatment of classic pityriasis rubra pilaris. J Am Acad Dermatol 1994; 31:997–1001.
123. Krueger GG, Drake LA, Elias PM, Lowe NJ, Guzzo C, Weinstein GD, Lew-Kaya DA, Lue JC, Sefton J, Chandraratna RA. The safety and efficacy of tazarotene gel, a topical acetylenic retinoid, in the treatment of psoriasis. Arch Dermatol 1998; 134:57–60.
124. Peck GL, Yoder FW. Treatment of lamellar ichthyosis and other keratinising disorders with an oral synthetic retinoid. Lancet 1976; 2:1172–1173.
125. Peck GL, Yoder FW, Olsen TG, Pandya MD, Butkus D. Treatment of Darier's disease, lamellar ichthyosis, pityriasis rubra pilaris, cystic acne, and basal cell carcinoma with oral 13-cis retinoic acid. Dermatologica 1978; 157(suppl 1):11–12.
126. Happle R, Van de Kerkhof PCM, Traupe H. Retinoids in disorders of keratinization: Their use in adults. Dermatologica 1987; 175(suppl 1):107–124.
127. Blanchet-Bardon C, Nazzaro V, Rognin C, Geiger J-M, Puissant A. Acitretin in the treatment of severe disorders of keratinization. Results of an open study. J Am Acad Dermatol 1991; 24:982–986.
128. Lauharanta J, Kanerva L, Turjanmaa K, Geiger JM. Clinical and ultrastructural effects of acitretin in Darier's disease. Acta Dermatol Venereol (Stockh) 1988; 68: 492–498.
129. Christophersen J, Geiger J-M, Danneskiold-Samsoe P, Kragballe K, Grønjøj Larsen F, Laurberg G, Serup J, Thomsen K. A double-blind comparison of acitretin and etretinate in the treatment of Darier's disease. Acta Dermatol Venereol (Stockh) 1992; 72:150–152.
130. Peck GL, Olsen TG, Yoder FW, Strauss JS, Downing DT, Pandya M, Butkus D, Arnaud-Battandier J. Prolonged remissions of cystic and conglobate acne with 13-cis retinoic acid. N Engl J Med 1979; 300:329–333.
131. Orfanos CE, Zouboulis ChC. Oral retinoids in the treatment of seborrhoea and acne. Dermatology 1998; 196:140–147.
132. Ott F, Bollag W, Geiger J-M. Oral 9-cis retinoic acid versus 13-cis retinoic acid in acne therapy. Dermatology 1996; 193:124–126.
133. Goldstein JA, Socha-Szott A, Thomsen RJ, Pochi PE, Shalita AR, Strauss JS. Comparative effect of isotretinoin and etretinate on acne and sebaceous gland secretion. J Am Acad Dermatol 1982; 6:760–765.
134. Harms M, Philippe I, Radeff B, Masouyé I, Geiger J-M, Saurat J-H. Arotinoid Ro 13-6298 and etretin: two new retinoids inferior to isotretinoin in sebum suppression and acne treatment. Acta Dermatol Venereol (Stockh) 1986; 66:149–154.
135. Geiger J-M. Retinoids and sebaceous gland activity. Dermatology 1995; 191:305–310.
136. Strauss JS, Davey WP, Denton SJ, Stranieri AM. Effect of an orally administered

arotinoid, Ro 15-0778, on sebum production in man. Arch Dermatol Res 1988; 280:152–154.

137. Karvonen SJ. Acne fulminans. Report of clinical findings and treatment of twenty-four patients. J Am Acad Dermatol 1993; 28:572–579.
138. Verschoore M, Langner A, Wolska H, Jablonska S, Czernielewski J, Schaefer H. Efficacy and safety of CD 271 alcoholic gels in the topical treatment of acne vulgaris. Br J Dermatol 1991; 124:368–371.
139. Shalita A, Weiss JS, Chalker DK, Ellis CN, Greenspan A, Katz HI, Kantor I, Millikan LE, Swinehart T, Swinyer L, Whitemore C, Baker M, Czernielewski J. A comparison of the efficacy and safety of adapalene gel 0.1% and tretinoin gel 0.025% in the treatment of acne vulgaris. A multicenter trial. J Am Acad Dermatol 1996; 34:482–485.
140. Weiss JS, Ellis CN, Headington JT, Tincoff T, Hamilton TA, Voorhees JJ. Topical tretinoin improves photoaged skin: a double-blind, vehicle-controlled study. JAMA 1988; 159:527–532.
141. Weinstein GD, Nigra TP, Pochi PE, Savin RC, Allan A, Benik K, Jeffes E, Lufrano L, Thorne EG. Topical tretinoin for treatment of photoaged skin: a multicenter study. Arch Dermatol 1991; 127:659–665.
142. Olsen EA, Katz HI, Levine N, Shupack J, McCarley Billys M, Prawer S, Gold J, Stiller M, Lufrano L, Thorne EG. Tretinoin emollient cream: a new therapy for photodamaged skin. J Am Acad Dermatol 1992; 26:215–224.
143. Griffiths CEM, Kang S, Ellis CN, Kim KJ, Finkel LJ, Ortiz-Ferrer LC, White GM, Hamilton TA, Voorhees JJ. Two concentrations of topical tretinoin (retinoic acid) cause similar improvement of photoaging but different degrees of irritation. Arch Dermatol 1995; 131:1037–1044.
144. Woodley DT, Zelickson AS, Briggaman RA, Hamilton TA, Weiss JS, Ellis CN, Voorhees JJ. Treatment of photoaged skin with topical tretinoin increases epidermaldermal anchoring fibrils. JAMA 1990; 263:3057–3059.
145. Sendagorta E, Lesiewicz J, Armstrong RB. Topical isotretinoin for photodamaged skin. J Am Acad Dermatol 1992; 27:S15–S18.
146. Kligman AM, Dogadkina D, Lavker RM. Effects of topical tretinoin on non-sun-exposed protected skin of the elderly. J Am Acad Dermatol 1993; 29:25–33.
147. Strauss JS, Stranieri AM. Changes in long term sebum production with 13-cis retinoic acid on skin surface lipid composition. J Invest Dermatol 1980; 74:66–73.
148. King J, Jones DH, Daltrey DC, Cunliffe WJ. A double-blind study of the effect of 13-cis-retinoic acid on acne, sebum excretion rate and microbial population. Br J Dermatol 1982; 107:583–590.
149. Hommel L, Geiger J-M, Harms M, Saurat J-H. Sebum excretion rate in subjects treated with oral all-trans retinoic acid. Dermatology 1996; 193:127–130.
150. Ridden J, Ferguson D, Kealey T. Organ maintenance of human sebaceous glands: in vitro effects of 13-cis retinoic acid and testosterone. J Cell Sci 1990; 95:125–136.
151. Vane FM, Chari SS, Shapiro SS, Nordstrom KM, Leyden JJ. Comparison of the plasma and sebum concentrations of the arotinoid Ro 15-0778 and isotretinoin in acne patients. In: Marks R, Plewig G, eds. Acne and Related Disorders. London: Dunitz, 1989; 183–189.

152. Saurat J-H, Mérot Y, Borsky M. Arotinoid acid (Ro 13-7410): a pilot study in dermatology. Dermatologica 1988; 176:191–199.
153. Schmidt JB, Gebhardt W, Raff M, Spona J. 13-cis-retinoic acid in rosacea. Acta Dermatol Venereol (Stockh) 1984; 64:15–21.
154. Irvine C, Kumar P, Marks R. Isotretinoin in the treatment of rosacea and rhinophyma. In: Marks R, Plewig G, eds. Acne and Related Disorders. London: Dunitz, 1989:301–305.
155. Ertl GA, Levine N, Kligman AM. A comparison of the efficacy of topical tretinoin and low-dose oral isotretinoin in rosacea. Arch Dermatol 1994; 130:319–324.
156. Gollnick H, Orfanos CE. Familial nevoid sebaceous hyperplasia with hyperandrogenism. In: Wilkinson DS, Mscaró JM, Orfanos CE, eds. Clinical Dermatology. The CMD Case Collection. New York: Schattauer, 1987:350–352.
157. Petiau P, Cribier B, Chartier C, Kalinkova L, Heid E, Grosshans E. Acne necrotica varioliformis, resolution with isotretinoin. Eur J Dermatol 1994; 4:608–610.
158. Finkelstein E, Lazarov A, Cagnano M, Halevy S. Oil acne: successful treatment with isotretinoin. J Am Acad Dermatol 1994; 30:491–492.
159. Scerri L, Zaki I, Millard LG. Severe halogen acne due to a trifluoromethylpyrazole derivative and its resistance to isotretinoin. Br J Dermatol 1995; 132:144–148.
160. Plewig G, Steger M. Acne inversa (alias acne triad, acne tetrad or hidradenitis suppurativa). In: Marks R, Plewig G, eds. Acne and Related Disorders. London: Dunitz, 1989:345–357.
161. Griffiths CEM, Finkel LJ, Ditre CM, Hamilton TA, Ellis CN, Voorhees JJ. Topical tretinoin (retinoic acid) improves melasma. A vehicle-controlled clinical trial. Br J Dermatol 1993; 129:415–421.
162. Bulengo-Ransby SM, Griffiths CEM, Kimbrough-Green CK, Finkel LJ, Hamilton TA, Ellis CN, Voorhees JJ. Topical tretinoin (retinoic acid) therapy for hyperpigmented lesions caused by inflammation of the skin of black patients. N Engl J Med 1993; 328:1438–1443.
163. Pfahl M. Nuclear receptor/AP-1 interaction. Endocr Rev 1993; 14:651–658.
164. Geilen CC, Bektas M, Wieder Th, Orfanos CE. The vitamin D_3 analogue, calcipotriol, induces sphingomyelin hydrolysis in human keratinocytes. FEBS Lett 1996; 378:88–92.
165. Hannun YA, Obeid LM. Ceramide: an intracellular signal for apoptosis. Trends Biol Sci 1995; 20:72–77.
166. Kalén A, Borchardt RA, Bell RM. Elevated ceramide levels in GH_4C_1 cells treated with retinoic acid. Biochim Biophys Acta 1992; 1125:90–96.
167. Bollag W, Holdener EE. Retinoids in cancer prevention and therapy. Ann Oncol 1992; 3:513–526.
168. Lippman SM, Brenner SE, Hong WK. Cancer chemoprevention. J Clin Oncol 1994; 12:851–873.
169. Kraemer KH, Di Giovanna JJ, Moshell AN, Tarone RE, Peck GL. Prevention of skin cancer in xeroderma pigmentosum with the use of oral isotretinoin. N Engl J Med 1988; 318:1633–1637.
170. Berth-Jones J, Cole J, Lehmann AR, Arlett CF, Graham-Brown RA. Xeroderma pigmentosum variant: 5 years of tumour suppression by etretinate. J R Soc Med 1993; 86:355–356.

171. Hodak E, Ginzburg A, David M, Sandbank M. Etretinate treatment of the nevoid basal cell carcinoma syndrome. Therapeutic and chemoprevention effect. Int J Dermatol 1987; 26:606–609.
172. Kelly JW, Sabto J, Gurr FW, Bruce F. Retinoids to prevent skin cancer in organ transplant recipients. Lancet 1991; 338:1407.
173. Stüttgen G. Zur Lokalbehandlung von Keratosen mit Vitamin A-Säure. Dermatologica 1962; 124:65–80.
174. Ehlert R, Orfanos CE. Lokale Anwendung von Vitamin-A-Säure bei chronischer aktinischer Cheilitis. Hautarzt 1989; 40:728.
175. Alirezai M, Dupuy P, Amblard P, Kalis B, Souteyrand P, Frappaz A, Sendagorta E. Clinical evaluation of topical isotretinoin in the treatment of actinic keratoses. J Am Acad Dermatol 1994; 30:447–451.
176. Misiewicz J, Sendagorta E, Golebiowska A, Lorenc B, Czarnetzki BM, Jablonska S. Topical treatment of multiple actinic keratoses of the face with arotinoid methyl sulfone (Ro 14-9706) cream versus tretinoin cream: a double blind, comparative study. J Am Acad Dermatol 1991; 24:448–451.
177. Watson AB. Preventive effect of etretinate therapy on multiple actinic keratoses. Cancer Detect Prev 1986; 9:161–165.
178. Shaw JC, White CR. Treatment of multiple keratoacanthomas with oral isotretinoin. J Am Acad Dermatol 1986; 15:1079–1082.
179. Mensing H, Wagner G. Etretinate-Therapie bei solitären Keratoakanthomen. Z Hautkr 1988; 63:234–236.
180. Lippman SM, Parkinson DR, Itri LM, Weber RS, Schantz SP, Ota DM, Schusterman MA, Krakoff IH, Gutterman JU, Hong WK. 13-cis retinoic acid and interferon alpha-2a: effective combination therapy for advanced squamous cell carcinoma of the skin. J Natl Cancer Inst 1992; 84:235–241.
181. Toma S, Palumbo R, Vincenti M, Aitini E, Paganini G, Pronzato P, Grimaldi A, Rosso R. Efficiency of recombinant alpha-interferon 2a and 13-cis retinoic acid in the treatment of squamous cell carcinoma. Ann Oncol 1994; 5:463–465.
182. Eisenhauer EA, Lippman SM, Kavanagh JJ, Parades-Espinoza M, Arnold A, Hong WK, Massimini G, Schleuniger U, Bollag W, Holdener EE, et al. Combination 13-cis retinoic acid and interferon alpha 2a in the therapy of solid tumors. Leukemia 1994; 8:1622–1625.
183. Kessler JF, Jones SE, Levine N, Lynch PJ, Booth AR, Meyskens FL Jr. Isotretinoin and cutaneous helper T-cell lymphoma (mycosis fungoides). Arch Dermatol 1987; 123:201–204.
184. Molin L, Thomsen K, Volden G, Aronsson A, Hammar H, Hellbe L, Wantzin GL, Roupe G. Oral retinoids in mycosis fungoides and Sézary syndrome: a comparison of isotretinoin and etretinate. A study from the Scandinavian mycosis fungoides group. Acta Dermatol Venereol (Stockh) 1987; 67:232–236.
185. Tousignant J, Raymond GP, Light MJ. Treatment of cutaneous T-cell lymphoma with the arotinoid Ro 13-6298. J Am Acad Dermatol 1987; 16:167–171.
186. Braathen LR, McFadden N. Successful treatment of mycosis fungoides with the combination of etretinate and human recombinant interferon alpha-2a. J Dermatol Treat 1989; 1:29–32.
187. Zachariae H, Thestrup-Pedersen K. Interferon alpha and etretinate combination

treatment of cutaneous T-cell lymphoma. J Invest Dermatol 1990; 95(suppl):206–208.

188. Dreno B, Claudy A, Meynadier J, Verret JL, Souteyrand P, Ortonne J-P, Kalis B, Godefroy WY, Beerblock K, Thill L. The treatment of 45 patients with cutaneous T-cell lymphoma with low doses of interferon-alpha 2a and etretinate. Br J Dermatol 1991; 125:456–459.
189. Altomare GF, Capella GL, Pigatto PD, Finzi AF. Intramuscular low dose alpha-2b interferon and etretinate for treatment of mycosis fungoides. Int J Dermatol 1993; 32:138–141.
190. Knobler RM, Trautinger F, Radaszkiewicz T, Kokoschka EM, Micksche M. Treatment of cutaneous T-cell lymphoma with combination of low-dose interferon alpha-2b and retinoids. J Am Acad Dermatol 1991; 24:247–252.
191. Laurberg G, Geiger J-M, Hjorth N, Holm P, Hou-Jensen K, Jacobsen KU, Nielsen AO, Pichard J, Serup J, Sparre-Jorgensen A, et al. Treatment of lichen planus with acitretin. A double-blind placebo controlled study in 65 patients. J Am Acad Dermatol 1991; 24:434–437.
192. Ott F, Bollag W, Geiger J-M. Efficacy of oral low-dose tretinoin (all-trans-retinoic acid) in lichen planus. Dermatology 1996; 192:334–336.
193. Bousema MT, Romppanen U, Geiger J-M, Baudin M, Vaha-Eskeli K, Vartiainen J, Vuopala S. Acitretin in the treatment of severe lichen sclerosus et atrophicus of the vulva: a double-blind, placebo-controlled study. J Am Acad Dermatol 1994; 30:225–231.
194. Zouboulis ChC, Biczó S, Gollnick H, Reupke H-J, Rinck G, Szabó M, Fekete J, Orfanos CE. Elephantiasis nostras verrucosa: beneficial effect of oral etretinate therapy. Br J Dermatol 1992; 127:411–416.
195. Kubeyinje EP. Evaluation of the efficacy and safety of 0.05% tretinoin cream in the treatment of plane warts in Arab children. J Dermatol Treat 1996; 7:21–22.
196. Kang S, Kim KJ, Griffiths CEM, Wong T-Y, Talwar HS, Fisher GJ, Gordon D, Hamilton TA, Ellis CN, Voorhees JJ. Topical tretinoin (retinoic acid) improves early stretch marks. Arch Dermatol 1996; 132:519–526.
197. Gollnick HPM, Orfanos CE. Clinical efficacy of etretinate and acitretin. European experience. In: Roenigk HH, Maibach HI, eds. Psoriasis. New York: Marcel Dekker, 1991:725–748.
198. Hartmann D, Mosberg H, Weber W. Lack of effect of acitretin on the hypoprothrombinemic action of phenprocumon in healthy volunteers. Dermatologica 1989; 178:33–36.
199. Saurat J-H, Geiger J-M, Amblard P, Beani JC, Boulanger A, Claudy A, Frenk E, Guilhou JJ, Grosshans E, Merot Y, et al. Randomized double-blind multicenter study comparing acitretin-PUVA, etretinate-PUVA and placebo-PUVA in the treatment of severe psoriasis. Dermatologica 1988; 177:218–224.
200. Tanew A, Guggenbichler A, Hönigsmann H, Geiger J-M, Fritsch P. Photochemotherapy for severe psoriasis without or in combination with acitretin: a randomized, double-blind comparison study. J Am Acad Dermatol 1991; 25:682–684.
201. Geiger J-M, Czarnetzki BM. Acitretin (Ro 10-1670, etretin): overall evaluation of clinical studies. Dermatologica 1988; 176:182–190.

202. Steijlen PM, Van Dooren-Greebe RJ, van de Kerkhof PCM. Acitretin in the treatment of lamellar ichthyosis. Br J Dermatol 1994; 130:211–214.
203. Goulden V, Layton AM, Cunliffe WJ. Long-term safety of isotretinoin as a treatment for acne vulgaris. Br J Dermatol 1994; 131:360–363.
204. Layton AM, Knaggs H, Taylor J, Cunliffe WJ. Isotretinoin for acne vulgaris–10 years later: a safe and successful treatment. Br J Dermatol 1993; 129:292–296.
205. Cunliffe WJ, van de Kerkhof PCM, Caputo R, Cavicchini S, Cooper A, Fyrand OL, Gollnick H, Layton AM, Leyden JJ, Mascaró J-M, Ortonne J-P, Shalita A. Roaccutane treatment guidelines: results of an international survey. Dermatology 1997; 194:351–357.
206. Stainforth JM, Layton AM, Taylor JP, Cunliffe WJ. Isotretinoin for the treatment of acne vulgaris: which factors may predict the need for more than one course? Br J Dermatol 193; 129:297–301.
207. Goldberg L, Hsu S, Alcalay J. Effectiveness of isotretinoin in preventing the appearance of basal cell carcinomas in basal cell nevus syndrome. J Am Acad Dermatol 1989; 21:144–145.
208. Rook AH, Jaworsky C, Nguyen T, Grossman RA, Wolfe JT, Witmer WK, Kligman AM. Beneficial effect of low-dose systemic retinoid in combination with topical tretinoin for the treatment and prophylaxis of premalignant and malignant skin lesions in renal transplant recipients. Transplantation 1995; 59:714–719.
209. Marsden JR. Lipid metabolism and retinoid therapy. Pharm Ther 1989; 40:55–65.
210. Gollnick H, Tsambaos D, Orfanos CE. Risk factors promote elevations of serum lipids in acne patients under oral 13-cis retinoic acid (isotretinoin). Arch Dermatol Res 1981; 271:189–196.
211. Fex GA, Aronsson A, Andersson A, Larsson K, Nilsson-Ehle P. In vivo effects of 13-cis retinoic acid treatment on the concentration of proteins and lipids in serum. Eur J Clin Chem Clin Biochem 1996; 34:3–7.
212. Halkier-Sörensen L, Laurberg G, Andersen J. Bone changes in children on long-term treatment with etretinate. J Am Acad Dermatol 1987; 16:999–1006.
213. Orfanos CE. Retinoide: der neue Stand. Erhaltungstherapie, Resorptionsstörungen bei ''non-responders'', Interaktionen und Interferenzen mit Medikamenten, Behandlung von Kindern und Knochentoxizität, Acitretin und 13-cis-Acitretin. Hautarzt 1989; 40:123–129.
214. Gollnick H, Rinck G, Bitterling T, Orfanos CE. Pharmakokinetik von Etretinat, Acitretin und 13-cis-Acitretin: neue Ergebnisse und Nutzen der Blutspiegel-orientierten klinischen Anwendung. Z Hautkr 1990; 65:40–50.
215. Almond-Roesler B, Blume-Peytavi U, Bisson S, Krahn M, Rohloff E, Orfanos CE. Monitoring of isotretinoin therapy by measuring the plasma levels of isotretinoin and 4-oxo-isotretinoin. Dermatology 1998; 196:176–181.
216. De Leenheer AP, Lambert WE. High-performance liquid chromatographic determination of etretinate and all-trans and 13-cis acitretin in human plasma. J Chromat 1990; 500:637–642.
217. Decker MA, Zimmermann CL. Simultaneous determination of etretinate, acitretin and their metabolites in perfusate plasma, bile or hepatic tissue with reversed-phase high-performance liquid chromatography. J Chromat B: 1995; 667:105–113.

218. Wyss R. Chromatographic and electrophoretic analysis of biomedically important retinoids. J Chromat B Biomed Appl 1995; 671:381–425.
219. Wyss R, Bucheli F. Quantitative analysis of retinoids in biological fluids by high-performance liquid chromatography using column switching. II. Simultaneous determination of etretinate, acitretin and 13-cis acitretin in plasma. J Chrom B Biomed Appl 1988; 431:297–307.
220. Jakobsen P. Simultaneous determination of the aromatic retinoids etretin and etretinate and their main metabolites by reversed-phase liquid chromatography. J Chromat 1987; 415:413–418.
221. Sturkenboom MCJM, de Jong-Van Den Berg LTW, van Voorst-Vader PC, Cornel MC, Stricker BH, Wesseling H. Inability to detect plasma etretinate and acitretin is a poor predictor of the absence of these teratogens in tissue after stopping acitretin treatment. Br J Clin Pharmacol 1994; 38:229–235.
222. Maier H, Hönigsmann H. Concentration of etretinate in plasma and subcutaneous fat after long-term acitretin. Lancet 1996; 348:1107.

REVIEW ARTICLES, BOOKS, AND BOOK CHAPTERS

Brogden RN, Goa KL. Adapalene. A review of its pharmacological properties and clinical potential in the management of mild to moderate acne. Drugs 1997; 53:511–519.

Craven NM, Griffiths CEM. Topical retinoids and cutaneous biology. Clin Exp Dermatol 1996; 21:1–10.

Foster RH, Brogden RN, Benfield P. Tazarotene. Drugs 1998; 55:705–711.

Fritsch P, Sidoroff A. Safety of retinoids and indications for use. Curr Opin Dermatol 1993; 207–213.

Geiger J-M. Retinoids and sebaceous gland activity. Dermatology 1995; 191:305–310.

Geiger J-M, Saurat J-H. Acitretin and etretinate. How and when they should be used. Dermatol Clin 1993; 11:117–129.

Gollnick HPM. Oral retinoids—efficacy and toxicity in psoriasis. Br J Dermatol 1996; 135(suppl 49):6–17.

Gollnick H, Ehlert R, Rinck G, Orfanos CE. Retinoids: an overview of pharmacokinetics and therapeutic value. Meth Enzymol 1990; 190:291–304.

Gollnick H, Orfanos CE. Theoretical aspects of the use of retinoids as anticancer drugs. In: Marks R, ed. Retinoids in Cutaneous Malignancy. Oxford: Blackwell, 1991; 41–65.

Gollnick HP, Dummler U. Retinoids. Clin Dermatol 1997; 15:799–810.

Griffiths CEM, Voorhees JJ. Human in vivo pharmacology of topical retinoids. Arch Dermatol Res 1994; 287:53–60.

Mahrle G. Retinoids in oncology. In: Mali JWH, ed. Current Problems in Dermatology. Basel: Karger, 1985:128–163.

Mills CM, Marks R. Adverse reactions to oral retinoids. Drug Safety 1993; 9:280–290.

Orfanos CE, Ehlert R, Gollnick H. The retinoids. A review of their clinical pharmacology and therapeutic use. Drugs 1987; 34:459–503.

Orfanos CE, Garbe C. Therapie der Hautkrankheiten. Berlin: Springer Verlag, 1995.

Orfanos CE, Zouboulis ChC, Almond-Roesler B, Geilen CC. Current use and future potential role of retinoids in dermatology. Drugs 1997; 53:358–388.

Orfanos CE, Zouboulis ChC. Oral retinoids in the treatment of seborrhoea and acne. Dermatology 1998; 196:140–147.

Peck GL, Coats-Walton DA. Retinoids in Dermatology. Current usage. Sober AJ, Fitzpatrick ThB, eds. The Year Book of Dermatology. St. Louis: Mosby, 1995; 1–32.

Pilkington T, Brogden RN. Acitretin–a review of its pharmacology and therapeutic use. Drugs 1992; 43:597–627.

Sporn MB, Roberts AB, Goodman DS, eds. The retinoids. Biology, Chemistry, and Medicine, 3rd ed. New York: Raven Press, 1994.

Zouboulis ChC, Orfanos CE. Retinoide—Zwölf Jahre Wirksamkeit und Verträglichkeit der systemischen Therapie. In: Tebbe B, Goerdt S, Orfanos CE, eds. Dermatologie. Heutiger Stand. Stuttgart: Thieme, 1995:301–308.

Zouboulis ChC, Orfanos CE. Topische Dermatika: Retinoide. In: Korting HC, Sterry W, eds. Therapeutische Verfahren in der Dermatologie: Dermatika und Kosmetika. Berlin: Springer, 2000, in press.

11

Nicotinamide and Sulfapyridine

Joel E. Bernstein
Winston Laboratories, Inc.
Vernon Hills, Illinois

I. INTRODUCTION

Nicotinamide and sulfapyridine are vastly different drugs that share some important chemical and pharmacological characteristics and are uniquely effective in a puzzling variety of seemingly unrelated dermatological conditions. What appears to be a significant common feature of this potent, moderately toxic antibiotic (sulfapyridine) and this essential vitamin (nicotinamide, which in activated form plays an important role in a number of key metabolic reactions in the body) is the presence of a pyridine ring (Fig. 1) in both drugs. This pyridine ring has been postulated to be related to the anti-inflammatory properties of both drugs [1]. In fact, it has become clear that the anti-inflammatory actions of both drugs seem to account for their efficacy in certain varied dermatological disorders, rather than their antibacterial or coenzyme properties.

Nicotinamide (also called niacinamide) is a water-soluble component of the vitamin B complex that is found in many foods, including yeast, milk, fish, eggs, whole grains, and green vegetables. In vivo, nicotinamide is formed from niacin and then incorporated into nicotinamide adenine dinucleotide (NAD) and nicotinamide adenine dinucleotide phosphate (NADP). NAD and NADP function as coenzymes for a wide variety of enzymatic oxidation–reduction reactions essential for tissue respiration, lipid metabolism, and glycogenolysis. Sulfapyridine is a derivative of *p*-aminobenzenesulfonamide (sulfanilamide), a compound first shown to have antibacterial properties in 1932. Sulfapyridine was first reported to have therapeutic utility for the treatment of pneumococcal pneumonia in 1938. In 1939, Sulzberger demonstrated that sulfapyridine could be used to treat acro-

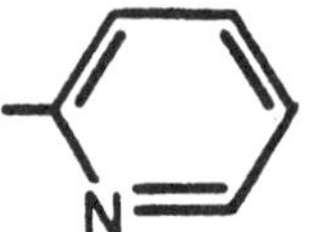

FIGURE 1 Pyridine ring.

dermatitis of Hallopeau, the first successful use of sulfa-based drugs in a noninfectious dermatological process [2]. Shortly thereafter, Costello showed that sulfapyridine was effective in treating patients with dermatitis herpatiformis (DH) [3]. Brewer's yeast, a dried byproduct of the manufacture of some alcoholic beverages, was empirically found in the late 1940s to be useful in the management of inflammatory acne and dermatitis herpetiformis. Brewer's yeast was known to contain a high concentration of nicotinic acid, and, on this basis, in 1950, Johnson and Binkley successfully utilized nicotinic acid for treatment of DH [4]. However, nicotinic acid's modest effectiveness, coupled with its troublesome side effects (particularly flushing and headaches), led to its virtual abandonment from dermatological therapy until several decades later when its congener, nicotinamide [5–8], came into use.

II. CHEMISTRY AND PHARMACOLOGY

A. Chemistry

The structural formulas for nicotinamide and sulfapyridine are provided in Figure 2. Both sulfapyridine and nicotinamide are white crystalline powders that are colorless and tasteless. Nicotinamide is highly water soluble, while sulfapyridine is the least water soluble of the sulfonamides. This latter property probably accounts for the erratic absorption of orally administered sulfapyridine.

B. Pharmacology

1. Mechanism of Action

The principal mode of action of both nicotinamide and sulfapyridine in the treatment of noninfectious dermatological disease remains unknown. However, both compounds have a number of putative anti-inflammatory effects that are thought to be the bases for their therapeutic activity in dermatological disease. Nicotinamide's anti-inflammatory actions include suppression of antigen-induced lymphocyte transformation [9], inhibition of 3′–5′ cyclic AMP phosphodiesterase [10], and considerable histamine-release blocking activity [11]. Topically applied nicotinamide is a potent inhibitor of potassium-iodide-induced inflammation [1].

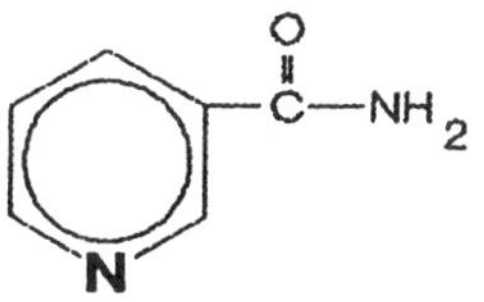

FIGURE 2 Structural formulas of nicotinamide (niacinamide) and sulfapyridine.

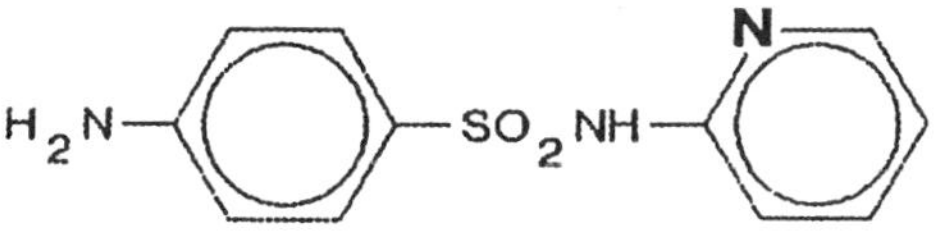

This may be particularly significant to its use in dermatology since iodides are known to precipitate or exacerbate dermatitis herpetiformis, inflammatory acne and pyoderma gangrenoseum [12]. Nicotinamide is also a protease inhibitor [13] and an agent that has been employed to stimulate repair of DNA damaged by chemical and physical means [14].

Evidence for the nonbacterial action of sulfapyridine in dermatological disease consists of the following [12]: (1) sulfapyridine doses that are too small to maintain effective antibacterial blood levels are often effective; (2) prolonged disease suppressive maintenance therapy with sulfapyridine is usually required; (3) some other sulfonamides and antibiotics with similar bacteriostatic or bacteriocidal spectra are not effective; and (4) simultaneous administration of para-aminobenzoic acid does not negate the suppressive effect of sulfapyridine.

Like nicotinamide, sulfapyridine has a variety of anti-inflammatory effects. Sulfapyridine is known to inhibit the febrile response to polysaccharides and to diminish immunological responses to these antigenic substances [12]. Sulfapyridine inhibits the alternate pathway of complement [15], suppresses integrin-mediated neutrophil adherence [16], and interferes with myeloperoxidase iodination [17].

2. Absorption, Metabolism, and Excretion

Nicotinamide is rapidly and almost completely absorbed from all portions of the GI tract. When nicotinamide doses of less than 500 mg are orally administered, only small amounts of the unchanged vitamin are excreted in the urine. When doses above this level are administered, unchanged nicotinamide represents the major urinary component. The principal route of metabolism of nicotinamide is by the formation of *N*-methylnicotinamide, which may in turn be further metabolized. Percutaneous absorption of topically applied nicotinamide is small with approximately 10% of the topically applied drug penetrating the skin [18,19].

Sulfapyridine is absorbed more slowly and erratically than nicotinamide, probably because of its poor water solubility. Absorption takes place mainly in the proximal small intestine and peak serum levels are obtained 12 to 24 h after an oral dose. After absorption, sulfapyridine moves through the portal circulation to the liver where it is acetylated by the enzyme *N*-acetyltransferase. Slow acetylators may have higher serum levels of sulfapyridine and an increase in side effects. Sulfapyridine may be further metabolized by hydroxylation and conjugation with glucuronide in the liver. Thirty to 60% of orally administered sulfapyridine is excreted in the urine, with the bulk of the remainder excreted in the feces.

3. Therapeutic Usage

Oral nicotinamide and oral sulfapyridine have been shown to be beneficial in a number of seemingly unrelated dermatological disorders, including bullous diseases such as dermatitis herpetiformis and bullous pemphigoid, epidermal inflammatory disorders such as subcorneal pustular dermatosis and pustular psoriasis, dermal adnexal inflammatory diseases such as erythema elevatum diutinum and inflammatory acne, as well as other inflammatory disorders such as vasculitis and pyoderma gangrenosum.

Sulfapyridine has been generally replaced in dermatological therapy today by dapsone. This is due to the observations that sulfapyridine is somewhat less effective in managing dermatological disease than dapsone and is associated with a higher incidence of adverse reactions. Sulfapyridine's role (as well as that of dapsone) in the management of inflammatory and nodulocystic acne was virtually eliminated with the introduction of 13-*cis*-retinoic acid. Today, sulfapyridine is utilized primarily as an alternative to corticosteroids or dapsone in the management of bullous disorders, especially dermatitis herpetiformis, bullous and cicatricial pemphigoid, and chronic bullous dermatosis of childhood. While dapsone is the first-line treatment in these disorders, some patients with DH show a superior response to sulfapyridine [20]. Further, sulfapyridine has been successfully substituted for dapsone in patients in whom dapsone had to be discontinued due to a serious side effect [21].

Sulfapyridine is available in 500-mg tablets and therapy is usually initiated in divided doses of 1.5 to 3.0 g daily, with increases of 500 mg daily (up to 6 g daily) if the clinical response is unsatisfactory. Most patients are adequately maintained on 1.5 to 2.0 g daily.

The most common side effects of sulfapyridine are nonspecific complaints involving the nervous system or gastrointestinal tract and include headache, malaise, anorexia, nausea, vomiting, or weakness. These occur in nearly 40% of patients treated with sulfapyridine [22], but in some can be ameliorated by a modest reduction in dosage [12]. More serious side effects include severe hemolytic anemia, methemoglobinemia, agranulocytosis, leukopenia, exfoliative dermatitis, hepatitis, peripheral motor neuropathy, psychosis, and sulfapyridine-induced renal damage. Such adverse reactions can be dangerous or fatal, but can be minimized by careful clinical and laboratory screening of patients while under treatment with the drug.

Nicotinamide has been utilized as a less toxic alternative to corticosteroids, sulfones, and sulfapyridine in the varied conditions known to be responsive to sulfones and sulfonamides, particularly bullous disorders and inflammatory acne. While oral nicotinamide by itself has been reported to be clinically beneficial in polymorphous light eruption [23] and necrobiosis lipoidica [24], the bulk of oral nicotinamide's dermatological use has been as part of a treatment regimen combining it with oral tetracycline. The combination of nicotinamide and tetracycline has been reported to be effective in a variety of dermatological conditions, including erythema elevatum diutinum, dermatitis herpetiformis, bullous pemphigoid, pemphigus, linear IgA dermatosis, and lichen planus pemphigoides [5–8,25–28]. The combination of nicotinamide in a dosage of 1.5 to 3.0 g daily and tetracycline 1.5 to 3.0 g daily in divided doses (three or four times daily) has proved to be an effective alternative to dapsone or corticosteroids, particularly in DH and bullous pemphigoid, and in at least one controlled study was as effective in the treatment of bullous pemphigoid as oral prednisone [7]. Unlike nicotinic acid, which may produce pruritus, flushing, headache, and gastrointestinal distress in therapeutic doses, nicotinamide may be given in doses up to 3 g daily without side effects. Nicotinamide lacks nicotinic acid's vasodilating effects as well as its ability to reduce blood lipid levels.

On account of nicotinamide's anti-inflammatory effects, particularly its effects on suppressing potassium-iodide–induced inflammation, nicotinamide 4% gel has received extensive evaluation in the treatment of inflammatory acne vulgaris [29,30]. These studies demonstrate that nicotinamide gel is a safe and effective treatment for papulopustular acne, is equally effective as clindamycin [29], and is not associated with adverse reactions of any consequence. Consequently, nicotinamide gel therapy for acne provides the therapeutic advantages of topical antibiotics without producing the antibiotic-resistant staphylococci and propionibacteria that use of topical and systemic antibiotics has unfortunately propagated. Nicotinamide gel is marketed in Canada, the United Kingdom, Ireland, and Australia, but has not yet been approved for marketing in the United States.

III. SUMMARY AND CONCLUSIONS

Nicotinamide and sulfapyridine are dissimilar agents that share a characteristic pyridine ring and have similar anti-inflammatory properties. These agents are clinically beneficial in a variety of diverse inflammatory dermatological conditions, particularly the bullous diseases, dermatitis herpetiformis, and bullous pemphigoid. Oral nicotinamide is generally used in combination with tetracycline, and the combination is a useful alternative to sulfapyridine, dapsone, or oral corticosteroids in these disorders. Nicotinamide 4% in a gel vehicle has proved to be a safe and effective alternative to topical and systemic antibotics in the treatment of inflammatory acne vulgaris. Unfortunately, while approved widely in English-speaking countries around the world, this therapeutic modality remains unavailable in the United States.

REFERENCES

1. Bernstein JE, Lorincz AL. The effects of topical nicotinamide, tetracycline and dapsone on potassium iodide-induced inflammation. J Invest Dermatol 1980; 74:257–258.
2. Sultzberger MB. Acrodermatitis continua pustulosa (Hallopeau) treated with sulfapyridine. Arch Dermatol Syph 1939; 40:1019–1021.
3. Costello M. Dermatitis herpetiformis treated with sulfapyridine. Arch Dermatol Syph 1940; 41:134.
4. Johnson HH Jr, Brinkley GW. Nicotinic acid therapy of dermatitis herpetiformis. J Invest Dermatol 1950; 14:233–238.
5. Kohler IK, Lorincz AL. Erythema elevatum diutinum treated with nicotinamide and tetracycline. Arch Dermatol 1980; 116:693–695.
6. Ma A, Medenica M. Response of generalized granuloma annulare to high-dose nicotinamide. Arch Dermatol 1983; 119:836–839.
7. Fivenson DP, Breneman DL, Rosen GB, Hersh CS, Cardone S, Mutasim D. Nicotinamide and tetracycline therapy of bullous pemphigoid. Arch Dermatol 1994; 130: 753–758.
8. Berk MA, Lorincz AL. The treatment of bullous pemphigoid with tetracycline and nicotinamide. Arch Dermatol 1986; 2:318–321.
9. Burger DR, Vandenbark AA, Daves D. Nicotinamide: suppression of lymphocyte transformation with a component identified in human transfer factor. J Immunol 1976; 117:797–801.
10. Shimoyama M, Kawai M, Hoshi Y, Ueda I. Nicotinamide inhibition of 3′ −5′ cAMP phosphodiesterase in vitro. Biochem Biophys Res Commun 1972; 49:1137–1141.
11. Bekier E, Wyczolkowska J, Szyc H, Maslinski CZ. The inhibitory effect of nicotinamide on asthma-like symptoms and eosinophilia in guinea pigs, anaphylactic mast cell degranulation in mice, and histamine release from rat peritoneal mast cells by compound 48/80. Int Arch Allergy Appl Immunol 1974; 47:737–748.
12. Lorincz AL, Pearson RW. Sulfapyridine and sulfone type drugs in dermatology. Arch Dermatol 1962; 85:2–16.
13. Troll W. Anticarcinogenic action of protease inhibitors. Adv Cancer Res 1987; 49: 265–283.
14. Licastro F, Walford RL. Modulatory effect of nicotinamide on unscheduled DNA

synthesis in lymphocytes from young and old mice. Mech Age Devel 1986; 35:123–131.

15. Provost TT, Tomasi TB. Evidence for the activation of complement via the alternative pathway in skin diseases. II. Dermatitis herpetiformis. Clin Immunopathol 1974; 3:178–186.
16. Booth SA, Moody CE, Dahl MV, Herron MJ, Nelson RD. Dapsone suppresses integrin-mediated neutrophil adherence function. J Invest Dermatol 1992; 98:135–140.
17. Kazmierowski JA, Ross JE, Peigner DS, Wuepper KD. Dermatitis herpetiformis: effects of sulfones and sulfonamides on neutrophil myeloperoxidase-mediated iodination and cytotoxicity. J Clin Immunol 1984; 4:55–64.
18. Feldman RJ, Maibach HI. Absorption of some organic compounds through the skin of man. J Invest Dermatol 1970; 54:399–404.
19. Franz TJ. Percutaneous absorption on the relevance of in vitro data. J Invest Dermatol 1975; 64:190–195.
20. Lang PG. Sulfones and sulfonamides in dermatology today. J Am Acad Dermatol 1979; 1:479–492.
21. Ahrens EM, Meckler RJ, Callen JP. Dapsone-induced peripheral neuropathy. Int J Dermatol 1986; 25:314–316.
22. Bernstein JE, Lorincz AL. Sulfonamides and sulfones in dermatologic therapy. Int J Dermatol 1981; 20:81–88.
23. Neuman R, Rappold E, Pohl-Markl H. Treatment of polymorphous light eruption with nicotinamide. Br J Dermatol 1986; 115:77–80.
24. Handfield-Jones S, Jones S, Peachey R. High dose nicotinamide in the treatment of necrobiosis lipoidica. Br J Dermatol 1988; 118:693–696.
25. Kolbach DN, Remme JJ, Bos WH, Jonkman MF, DeJong MC, Pas HH, van der Meer JB. Bullous pemphigoid successfully controlled by tetracycline and nicotinamide. Br J Dermatol 1995; 133:88–90.
26. Zemtsov A, Nelder KH. Successful treatment of dermatitis herpetiformis with tetracycline and nicotinamide in a patient unable to tolerate dapsone. J Am Acad Dermatol 1993; 28:505–506.
27. Chaffins ML, Collison D, Fivenson DP. Treatment of pemphigus and linear IgA dermatosis with nicotinamide and tetracycline: a review of 13 cases. J Am Acad Dermatol 1993; 28:998–1000.
28. Fivenson DP, Kimbrough TL. Lichen planus pemphigoides: combination therapy with tetracycline and nicotinamide. J Am Acad Dermatol 1997; 36:638–640.
29. Shalita AR, Smith JG, Parish LC, Sofman MS, Chalker DK. Topical nicotinamide compared with clindamycin gel in the treatment of inflammatory acne vulgaris. Int J Dermatol 1995; 34:434–437.
30. Griffiths CEM. Nicotinamide 4% gel for the treatment of inflammatory acne vulgaris. J Dermatol Treat 1995; 6:S8–S10.

12

Antihistamines

Andreas D. Katsambas and Maria Goula
University of Athens
A. Syngros Hospital
Athens, Greece

I. GENERAL PRINCIPLES

Histamine, β-imidazolylethylamine, is formed by the enzymatic decarboxylation of the amino acid histidine by histidine decarboxylase. It is present in mast cells, basophils, platelets, and in the stomach. Histamine is stored and bound ionically to a protoglycan-protein complex in mast-cell granules.

Histamine, which is a neurotransmitter, acts as a chemical messenger through three different types of histamine tissue receptors, each with a distinct role [1].

H_1 receptors are found in the skin and brain where they act as an alerting mechanism for the central nervous system. Through the H_1 receptors, the following effects are mediated: vasodilatation of small blood vessels resulting in increased permeability, smooth muscle contraction, and itching. The H_2 receptors are best known for mediating the effects on gastric acid production and secreting various hormones. The H_3 receptors are found in the brain and are responsible for autoregulation of histamine production and release [2]. The H_1-type antihistamines, both the traditional and the low-sedating, and the H_2-type antihistamines to a much lesser extent, are considered first-line medications in dermatological practice. However, inhibitors of the H_3 receptors have not as yet found a role in dermatological treatment.

The histamine receptor antagonists, or antihistamines, first became available for clinical use as therapeutic agents in the 1940s. The antihistamines are classified in three categories [3]: (1) traditional, classic, or first-generation H_1-

type antihistamines; (2) low-sedating or second-generation H_1-type antihistamines; and (3) H_2-type antihistamines.

II. PHARMACOLOGY

A. Structure

First-generation H_1-type antihistamines and histamine have in common a substituted ethylamine moiety as an integral part of their molecule (Fig. 1). The activity of an H_1-type antihistamine is increased if a halogen is substituted in the *para* position of the phenyl or benzyl group of R1. In order to have maximum activity, the terminal nitrogen of the ethylamine group should be a tertiary amine with methyl groups or a cyclic moiety in R2 and R3. First-generation H_1-type antihistamines have been divided into six chemical classes on the basis of substitution at the X position with nitrogen, oxygen, or carbon [3]. The six chemical classes and the most commonly used antihistamines (generic names) that correspond to each chemical class are presented in Table 1.

First-generation H_1-type antihistamines may cause sedation of varying intensity due to the fact that they cross the blood-brain barrier.

Second-generation, or low-sedating H_1-type antihistamines, were developed recently and have replaced to a large extent first-generation antihistamines in dermatological treatment because they lack both sedative and anticholinergic effects. The low sedative effect of second-generation antihistamines is expected because they only minimally cross the blood-brain barrier. Moreover, these agents preferentially bind to peripheral H_1 receptors. Low-sedating H_1-type antihistamines now available in most countries are astemizole, cetirizine, loratadine, terfenadine, and its active metabolite, fexofenadine. There are also a number of low-sedating antihistamines (acrivastine, azelastine, ebastine, temelastine) that are available only in certain countries or awaiting approval. H_2-type antihistamines (cimetidine, ranitidine, famotidine, nizatidine) possess an imidazole ring and lack the aryl ring of H_1-type antihistamines. These therapeutic agents are less lipophilic, which presumably accounts for their lack of CNS effects. Although H_2 antihistamines were developed for use in peptic ulcer disease, the presence of

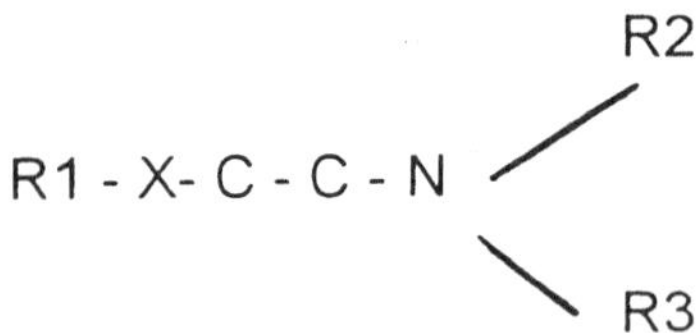

FIGURE 1 Ethylamine moiety of H_1 antihistamines.

Table 1 First-Generation H_1-Type Antihistamines

Chemical class	Generic name
Alkylamine (propylamine)	Brompheniramine maleate
	Chlorpheniramine maleate
	Dexchlorpheniramine maleate
Aminoalkyl ether (ethanolamine)	Clestamine fumarate
	Diphenhydramine hydrochloride
Ethylenediamine	Tripelennamine citrate
	Tripelennamine hydrochloride
Phenothiazine	Methdiliazine
	Methdilazine hydrochloride
	Promethazine hydrochloride
Piperidine	Azatadine meleate
	Cyproheptadine hydrochloride
Piperazine	Hydroxyzine hydrochloride
	Hydroxyzine pamoate

H_2 receptors in the cutaneous microvasculature justifies their use in dermatology [3].

B. Mechanism of Action

Antihistamines do not reverse the effects of histamine. They competitively inhibit the action of histamine by blocking its receptors on the vascular endothelial cell surface. As a result, antihistamines prevent the effects of histamine (i.e., localized vasodilation and transudation of fluid), leading to the formation of the typical wheal [4].

C. Absorption, Metabolism, and Excretion

The majority of H_1-type antihistamines have similar pharmacological properties. These drugs are well absorbed from the gastrointestinal tract after oral administration, and their beneficial effects start from 15 to 30 min after ingestion [5]. Peak serum concentrations are reached within 1 to 3 h, and pharmacological effects are maximal within 1 to 2 h and usually persist for 4 to 6 h [5]. Exceptions to this are hydroxyzine, brompheniramine, chlorpheniramine, which have half-lives of approximately 20 h in adults [6]. Therefore, some of these agents may require administration much less frequently than with conventional antihistamines (divided doses at intervals of 4–6 h).

The half-life of hydroxyzine is prolonged in patients with primary biliary cirrhosis. This fact suggests that its pharmacokinetics may be altered in other hepatic diseases.

The liver is the main site of metabolism of H_1-type antihistamines. The metabolism takes place by the hepatic cytochrome P-450 system in which they are conjugated to form glucuronides. H_1-type antihistamines are almost totally excreted in the urine 24 h after oral administration [6].

The pharmacokinetic characteristics of the new, low-sedating H_1-type antihistamines have been intensively investigated the last few years. The onset of action of terfenadine, loratadine, and cetirizine is reached in approximately 1 to 2 h, and the peak effect is achieved 4–6 h after oral ingestion. Duration of action is, in general, longer than that found in classic H_1-type antihistamines, with a reported elimination half-life of between 6.5 and 10 h for terfenadine, loratadine, and cetirizene, and 104 h for astemizole [4,7]. Astemizole has a slow onset of action (1–3 days) and may take up to 12 days to reach its peak effect [7]. Owing to its metabolites, the plasma half-life of astemizole goes through two phases: the initial phase lasts from 7 to 9 days and the second one lasts 19 days, which is an important consideration in view of its potential for interaction with other agents.

III. DRUG INTERACTIONS/CONTRAINDICATIONS

The most common side effect of first-generation H_1-type antihistamines is drowsiness, which varies from patient to patient. However, not infrequently, drowsiness may be eliminated or completely disappear within a few days of continued use. Moreover, if the classic H_1-type antihistamines are given as a simple dose in the evening, the resulting somnolence can be adequately tolerated. Convulsions, appetite stimulation, weight gain, dry mouth, blurring of vision, difficulty in micturition, and impotence may also occur [8].

The majority of first-generation H_1-type antihistamines show an accentuation of the central depressive effect. Taken in combination with CNS depressants, such as diazepam, or with alcohol, they result in increased drowsiness [1].

Also, these agents should not be administered with the monoamine oxidase inhibitors because their anticholinergic effect may be prolonged and accentuated (dryness of the mucous membranes, urinary retention, increased intravenular pressure). For this reason, classic antihistamines should not be administered to patients with glaucoma. On the contrary, the new-generation H_1-type antihistamines are safe to use in patients taking monoamine oxidase inhibitors and they can be administered without problem to patients with glaucoma or urinary retention [6,9].

Torsade de pointes, a form of potentially lethal venticular tachycardia associated with prolongation of the QT interval, has been reported to occur after terfenadine or astemizole overdose and in patients taking concomitantly itraconazole, ketoconazole, or macrolide antibiotics such as erythromycin [10]. During 1992 to 1993 the first pharmacovigilance inquiries on cardiac adverse effects of terfenadine and astemizole took place in France. In 1997, the FDA recommended the withdrawal of terfenadine-containing products due to mortality from potentially fatal adverse reactions [11].

Relative contraindications to the use of antihistamines include hepatic diseases, epilepsy, prostatic hypertrophy, glaucoma, and porphyria.

Although no relation between the first-generation H_1-type antihistamines and the development of even minor fetal malformations has been established [2], sporadic cases of fetal effects and prenatal death have been reported [13,14]. Teratogenic effects have been observed only in experimental animals after the administration of the piperazine subgroup; however, fetal abnormalities have not been reported in humans [3].

Traditionally, the old compounds, chlorpheniramine, tripelennamine, and diphenydramine are used in pregnancy. Terfenadine, astemisole, and loratadine have all been approved by the FDA for use in pregnancy; however, the first two carry a category C caution and loratadine a category B caution [4]. Cetirizine is not recommended for use in early pregnancy. Extremely small amounts of loratadine are excreted in breast milk [15].

H_1-type antihistamines can cause drug allergies including eczematous dermatitis, urticaria, petechiae, fixed drug eruptions, and photosensitivity. Allergic contact dermatitis may develop after the topical application of some H_1-type antihistamines. It is reported that contact dermatitis has occurred after ingestion of diphenhydramine in patients who had previously applied the drug topically. It is also reported that photosensitivity dermatitis has occurred after ingestion of promethazine and diphenhydramine [16,17].

IV. CURRENT APPROVED INDICATIONS—OTHER USES

Pruritus, urticaria, and angioedema have primarily been relieved and treated with the use of antihistamines in dermatology [3].

Comparative studies of the subgroups of traditional H_1-type antihistamines have shown them to be almost of equal efficacy. If an agent from one therapeutic subgroup is not effective, then an agent from another subgroup should be administered. There are, however, times when H_1-type antihistamines from different subgroups may be combined.

The low-sedating H_1-type antihistamines—terfenadine, astemizole, cetirizine, and loratadine—were found very effective in the treatment of acute and chronic urticaria and angioedema. In comparative studies, in which low-sedating H_1-type antihistamines are compared with each other and with traditional H_1-type antihistamines, no statistically significant differences in efficacy have been proven [18]. There are, however, some important differences between all these agents in terms of dosing, convenience, and side effects.

Tricyclic antidepressant drugs, such as doxepin hydrochloride and ketotifen, have been used with therapeutic benefit in chronic idiopathic urticaria. They act on both H_1 and H_2 receptors [3] and have been used successfully to relieve the symptoms of diffuse cutaneous mastocytosis, urticaria pigmentosa, symptomatic mastocytosis, and bronchial asthma [19]. However, the sedation and other adverse effects are comparable to those of first-generation antihistamines.

Azelastine and oxatamide are antihistaminelike drugs, but they also have other properties somewhat comparable to those of cromoglycate. They have some popularity as treatment for difficult urticaria as well as for asthma.

Traditional and low-sedating H_1 antihistamines may also be used in the treatment of physical urticaria. Doxepin and ketotifen may also be used in patients with various types of physical urticaria [3].

Pruritus of various causes and atopic dermatitis have been treated successfully with H_1-type antihistamines, both traditional and the low-sedating ones. Anticipation of the efficacy in atopic dermatitis is based on the fact that certain antihistamines inhibit the release of mediators other than histamine (leukotrienes, prostaglandins).

V. THERAPEUTIC PROTOCOLS

A. General Guidelines

The dosage and frequency of administration of antihistamines are recommended by the manufacturers and are usually based on the inhibition of experimental histamine weals. However, there are times when dermatologists feel the need to cautiously exceed these doses, beginning with a modest dose and gradually increasing the dose until either the condition is under control or side effects necessitate a lower dose [20].

The combination of H_1- and H_2-type antihistamines is beneficial to patients with acute and chronic idiopathic urticaria and angioedema as well as certain forms of physical urticaria. This combination should be considered in patients with refractory chronic idiopathic urticaria, in whom H_1-type antihistamines alone or in combination are ineffective.

B. Dosage

1. Traditional H_1-Type Antihistamines

a. Alkylamines (Dexchlorpheniramine)
Adults: 4–8 mg every 6 h
Children 2–5 years of age: 2 mg every 6 h
Children 5–11 years of age: 2–4 mg every 6 h

b. Ethanolamines (Diphenydramine Hydrochloride)
Adults: 25–50 mg every 4 h
Children up to 12 years of age: 5 mg/kg/24 h in divided doses

c. Ethylendiamines (Tripelenamine Hydrochloride)
Adults: 25–50 mg every 4 h
Children under 12 years of age: 5 mg/kg/24 h in divided doses

d. Phenothiazines (Promethazine Hydrochloride)
Adults: 25 mg 3 times daily
Children 6.25–12.5 mg 3 times a day and 25 mg at bedtime

e. Piperidines (Cyproheptadine Hydrochloride)
Adults: 4 mg 3 times daily
Children 0.25 mg/kg daily

f. Piperazine (Hydroxyzine Hydrochloride)
Adults: 25 mg 3–4 times daily
Children under 6 years of age: 50 mg/day in divided doses

2. Low-Sedating or Second-Generation Antihistamines

a. Terfenadine
Adults: 60 mg twice daily or 120 mg daily
Children 2–6 years old: 15 mg once or twice daily
Children 6–12 years old: 30 mg once or twice daily

b. Astemizole
Adults: 10 mg once daily
Children 2–6 years old: 0.2 mg/kg/24 h
Children 6–12 years old: 5 mg/day

Astemizole's major metabolite has a half-life of 9.5 days and a steady serum concentration not earlier than after 4 to 6 weeks of ingestion. Astemizole is not ideal for use in acute urticaria.

c. Cetirizine
Adults: 10 mg daily
Children: 6–12 years old: 5 mg daily

d. Loratadine
Adults: 10 mg daily
Children: 6–12 years old: 5 mg once daily

e. Fexofenadine (active metabolite of terfenadine)
Adults: 180 mg once daily (evening)

This drug has been newly marketed to avoid the cardiotoxic effects of terfenadine. No drowsiness has been reported to date.

3. H_2-type Antihistamines

a. Cimetidine
Adults: 300 mg 3 times daily, 400 mg twice daily, or 800 mg once daily
Children: Intramuscularly, 2 mg/kg every 6 h

b. Ranitidine
Adults: 150 mg twice daily or 300 mg at bedtime

c. Famotidine
Adults: 40 mg at bedtime for 1–2 months, and 20 mg at bedtime thereafter

4. Tricyclic Antidepressants

a. Amitriptyline
Adults: 25 mg/day at bedtime

b. Doxepin
Adults 25 mg/day at bedtime or in divided doses
The dose can be increased slowly over a 30-day period, up to 75 mg
Children under 12 years of age: tricyclic antidepressants should not be used

REFERENCES

1. Thiers BH. Current therapy: antihistamines update. Dermatol Clin 1991; 93: 603–609.
2. Hill SJ. Distribution, properties and functional characteristics of three classes of histamine receptors. Pharmacol Rev 1990; 42:45.
3. Soter NA. Antihistamines. In: Fitzpatrick T, Eisen A, Wolf K, Freedberg I, Austen KF, eds. Dermatology in General Medicine, 4th ed. New York: McGraw-Hill Book Company, 1995: 2909–2916.
4. Maddin ST. Efficacy and safety of antihistamines in allergic disorders. J Eur Acad Dermatol Venereol 1997; 8(suppl 1): S18–S23.
5. Douglas WW. Histamine and 5-hydroxytryptamine (serotonin) and their antagonists. In: Gilman AG, Goodman LS, Gilman A, et al., eds. Goodman and Gilman's The Pharmacological Basis of Therapeutics, ed. 7. New York: Macmillan, 1985: 618–627.
6. Drouin MA. H_1 antihistamines: perspective on the use of the conventional and new agents. Ann Allergy 1985; 55: 747–752.
7. Richards DM, et al. Astemizole: a review of its pharmacodynamic properties and therapeutic efficacy. Drugs 1984; 28:38.

8. Pearlman DS. Antihistamines: pharmacology and clinical use. Drugs 1985; 12:258–273.
9. Monroe EW. Chronic urticaria: review of non-sedating H_1 antihistamines in treatment. J Am Acad Dermatol 1988; 19:842–849.
10. Monahan BP, et al. Torsades de pointes occuring in association with terfenadine use. JAMA 1990; 264:2788.
11. FDA Talk paper. T97:3. 13 Jan 1997.
12. Hernonen OP, Sloan D, Shapiro S. Birth Defects and Drugs in Pregnancy. Littleton, MA: Publishing Sciences Group, 1977:323–337.
13. Saxen I. Cleft palate and maternal diphenhydramine intake. Lancet 1974; 1:407–408.
14. Kargas GA, Kargas SA, Bruyere HJ, et al. Perinatal mortality due to interaction of diphenhydramine and temazepam. N Engl J Med 1985; 313:1417.
15. Hilbert J, et al. Excretion of loratadine in human breast milk. J Clin Pharmacol 1988; 28:694.
16. Coskey RJ. Contact dermatitis caused by diphenhydramine hydrochloride. J Am Acad Dermatol 1983, 8:204–206.
17. Takeshi H. Allergic and photoallergic dermatitis from diphenhudramine. Arch Dermatol 1976; 112:1124–1126.
18. Monroe E. Therapy of acute and chronic urticaria. J Eur Acad Dermatol 1997; 8(suppl 1):S11–S17.
19. Shear NH, Krafchik BR, MacLeod SM. Diffuse cutaneous mastocytosis: treatment with Ketotifen and cimetidine. Clin Invest Med 1983; 6:36.
20. Kalogeromitros D, Katsarou-Katsari A. Diagnostic and therapeutic approaches to urticaria and angioedema. Hellen Dermatol Venereol Rev 1995; 6:79–89.

13

Psoralens

Warwick L. Morison
Johns Hopkins University
Baltimore, Maryland

Psoralens are a group of photoactive compounds that absorb photons resulting in photochemical reactions and through this process alter the structure and function of cells and tissues. The "dark" effects of psoralens are minimal and it is only through photosensitization that they produce pharmacological effects. Much is known about the properties of psoralens and the waveband, UVA (320 to 400 nm) radiation, that activates them, but relatively little is known about how the psoralen/UVA interaction influences the function of cells.

Two treatments in dermatology are based upon psoralen photosensitization. Psoralen photochemotherapy is usually referred to by the acronym PUVA therapy (P from psoralen and UVA). This treatment involves topical or oral administration of a psoralen compound and subsequent exposure of the skin to UVA radiation. Extracorporeal photophoresis involves removal of blood from a patient who has ingested psoralen, or direct addition of psoralen to the blood, exposure of the blood to UVA radiation, and subsequent reinfusion of the blood back to the patient. Most of this chapter will be devoted to PUVA therapy with only a brief mention of photophoresis since it is only utilized in a few specialized centers.

There is a long history of use of psoralens for skin disease back to at least 1550 BC when plant extracts combined with exposure to sunlight were used for treatment of vitiligo. This crude form of PUVA therapy is still used today in certain countries in the Middle and Far East. In 1948, Fahmy and his associates at the University of Cairo isolated three compounds from the fruit of Ammi Majus [1] and named them ammoidin (8-methoxypsoralen), ammidin (8-iso-amylinoxypsoralen), and majudin (bergapten or 5-methoxypsoralen). El Mofty, also at the University of Cairo, reported moderate success in using these compounds in the treatment of vitiligo. A synthetic psoralen, trimethylpsoralen, was introduced in 1964 and has also been used to a limited extent for treatment of vitiligo.

I. PHARMACOLOGY

A. Structure

Psoralens belong to the furocoumarin group of compounds derived from the fusion of the furan ring with coumarin. The parent compound psoralen and several dozen other psoralens are naturally occurring compounds found in several groups of plants and some fungi. In addition, many other psoralens have been synthesized with the aim of developing more potent or safer compounds.

The structure of the psoralen compounds used in therapy today are given in Figure 1. 8-Methoxypsoralen or methoxsalen is the main psoralen used in North America. 5-Methoxypsoralen is used widely in Europe. Psoralen is used in India and some other countries.

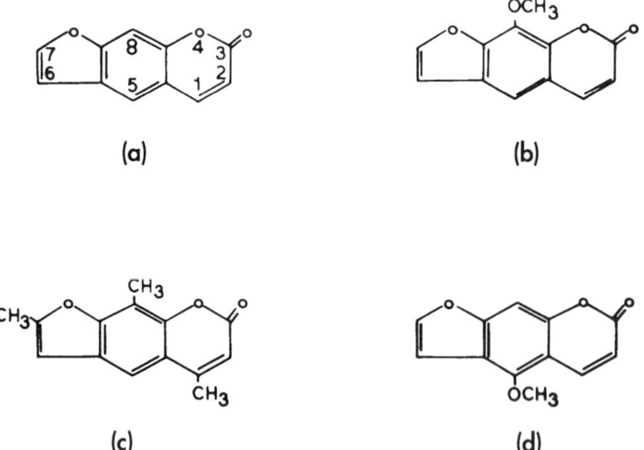

FIGURE 1 Psoralen compounds used in therapy: (a) psoralen, (b) 8-methoxypsoralen, (c) trimethylpsoralen, and (d) 5-methoxypsoralen.

B. Mechanism of Action

Most attention will be focused on methoxsalen since it is most widely used. Methoxsalen is a linear psoralen and is a photoactive compound capable of absorbing ultraviolet radiation in the UVA, UVB, and UVC regions. Cutaneous photosensitization is due to absorption of UVA radiation with maximal effectiveness in the 330- to 340-nm range. Upon absorption of UVA radiation, methoxsalen is raised to an electronically excited state called a singlet excited state ($_1$8-MOP) that is very short-lived. By intersystem crossing $_1$8-MOP is converted to a triplet excited state ($_3$8-MOP), which is longer-lived and responsible for initiating the photochemical reactions of the compound.

The photochemical reactions initiated by 8-MOP are of two types:

1. Type I direct photochemical reactions in which the excited state reacts with biological substances including: (a) pyrimidine bases in DNA to give monofunctional adducts; (b) pyrimidine bases on both strands of DNA to form bifunctional adducts or crosslinks; (c) amino acids of proteins; and (d) lipoproteins of cell membranes.
2. Type II indirect photochemical reactions by formation of reactive oxygen species that then react with substrate molecules such as DNA, proteins, and the cell membrane.

Most interest in the biological activity of methoxsalen has focused on its reaction with DNA, since formation of adducts and crosslinks results in inhibition of DNA synthesis. Such inhibition was at first thought to be the likely mechanism for the therapeutic effect of PUVA therapy in psoriasis, a condition marked by epidermal proliferation. However, the mechanism of this effect is probably more complex and may depend on photochemical changes in other molecules and cells apart from epidermal cells. One theory for the therapeutic action of PUVA therapy is its photoimmunological effect. According to this hypothesis, PUVA therapy alters the function of the immune system by a cytotoxic effect on lymphocytes or other cells or by a change in cytokine profile. A broader hypothesis is that PUVA therapy is cytotoxic for any activated cells responsible for initiating and maintaining a disease process. The main evidence for this theory is that PUVA treatment does appear to be more cytotoxic for activated versus resting cells and, while it can be therapeutic in the inflammatory phase of a disease, this effect is lost in the absence of inflammation. For example, PUVA therapy is therapeutic in the acute inflammatory phase of scleroderma but not in the subsequent fibrotic phase. A better understanding of the mechanism of action of PUVA therapy depends not only on study of the effects of the treatment but also on more complete information about the mechanism of the diseases in which it is therapeutic.

The main adverse effects of psoralens, namely, mutagenesis and carcinogenesis, are likely due to interaction with DNA or inadequacy of the repair systems involved in removing lesions from DNA.

C. Absorption

The psoralens used for therapy are all poorly soluble in water and this is a major limiting factor in their absorption from the gastrointestinal tract. Methoxsalen is the best absorbed compound while absorption of trimethylpsoralen is negligible. Two factors appear to have a marked influence on absorption of methoxsalen: drug formulation and influence of food. In one study, a preparation containing large crystals in a hard-gelatin capsule was slowly and incompletely absorbed with large interindividual variations in serum levels [2]. Twenty-five subjects given 0.6 mg/kg body weight of methoxsalen under fasting conditions had a mean peak concentration of 129 ± 94.1 mg/mL 3 h after administration. In contrast, in the same study, methoxsalen solution in a soft-gelatin capsule was more rapidly and completely absorbed; the mean peak concentration was 242 ± 125 ng/mL reached 1 to 8 h after administration. However, interindividual variation in absorption was still marked. Intake of food with the medication has the effect of slowing and impeding absorption and this has been demonstrated using both photosensitivity [3] and serum levels as endpoints [4]. Absorption of 5-methoxypsoralen is probably influenced by the same factors, although this has not been carefully studied. It is also available in crystalline and soluble formulations. However, overall it is less well absorbed than methoxsalen and, when equal doses of the two compounds are given orally, the serum levels of 5-methoxypsoralen are only about 25% of those reached with methoxsalen [5].

The bioavailability of methoxsalen is also subject to a significant, but saturable, first-pass effect as the drug passes the intestinal membrane and liver on its way to the central compartment. This is clearly demonstrated by a study in which a fourfold increase in methoxsalen dose (from 10 mg to 40 mg) increased the 1-h plasma level by a factor of 25 [6]. This first-pass effect is probably enhanced by slow absorption from the intestine.

D. Distribution

Psoralens appear to be distributed to all organs of the body after oral administration, but photochemical binding probably only occurs in the skin, eyes, and blood. For bioavailability studies, serum levels are usually measured. However, the only concentration of importance is the level at the target site in the skin since it is there that an interaction with UVA radiation will occur, leading to a therapeutic benefit. Direct measurement of the phototoxic response of the skin is the only means of assessing the cutaneous content of psoralens. A greater proportion of 5-methoxypsoralen is bound to serum proteins as compared with methoxsalen

(70% vs. 25%), and this presumably diminishes the photoactivity of that compound [7].

E. Metabolism

Methoxsalen is metabolized rapidly and completely. Most of the metabolites presently known have their origin in a metabolic attack on the furan moiety yielding an aryl-diol and arylacetic-acid and these are excreted as conjugates [8].

F. Excretion

Excretion of metabolites is fairly quick. After administration of radioactive methoxsalen to rats, over 90% of radioactivity is excreted within 24 h [9]. In humans, urinary excretion is 74% and excretion in feces is 14% [8]. Excretion of the parent compound in the urine is negligible.

G. Activation of Psoralens

Psoralens are activated by UVA radiation. Broadband fluorescent bulbs with a peak emission at 350 nm are the most common source of radiation. Treatment is usually given in a whole-body radiator lined with these bulbs or in a hand-and-foot unit equipped with these bulbs for localized disease.

H. Cutaneous Responses

PUVA treatment produces erythema and pigmentation of normal skin. The erythemal response to PUVA treatment differs from sunburn in certain respects. It appears later and lasts longer than a sun-induced erythema. PUVA-induced erythema usually appears 24 to 36 h after exposure and peaks at 48 h, but in some individuals the peak may be delayed to 72 or 96 h. Erythema is usually associated with pruritus and this can persist for weeks. Erythema is followed by pigmentation in all individuals who possess functional melanocytes. Pigmentation from PUVA therapy is usually darker and lasts longer than a sun-induced tan. Treatment with PUVA therapy produces hyperplasia of the epidermis and thickening of the stratum corneum. These changes, together with pigmentation, are effective in raising the threshold for erythema from subsequent exposure to UV radiation with or without psoralens.

Methoxsalen is more phototoxic than 5-methoxypsoralen when both compounds are administered in usual therapeutic doses (0.6 mg/kg of methoxsalen and 1.2 mg/kg 5-methoxypsoralen). This is probably a reflection of the greater bioavailability of methoxsalen with a contribution from higher protein binding of 5-methoxypsoralen.

II. TOXICOLOGY

A. Short-Term Side Effects

Most of the short-term adverse effects of PUVA therapy are mild and readily corrected by changes in the treatment protocol in the individual patient. These effects have been described in detail [10].

1. Adverse Effects Due to Methoxsalen Alone

1. Gastrointestinal disturbances: Nausea, anorexia, and, less commonly, vomiting appear to be due to a central mechanism triggered by high serum levels of the drug. Reduction in dose of methoxsalen or ingestion with food usually overcomes this problem.
2. CNS disturbances: These include headaches, dizziness, light-headedness, depression, insomnia, and a feeling of detachment from the environment. These are the most common adverse effects of PUVA therapy and also appear to be induced by high serum levels of methoxsalen. A reduction in drug dosage is required in some patients to relieve these symptoms.
3. Idiosyncratic reactions: Rare events reported are bronchoconstriction (6 reports), drug fever (3 reports), exanthema (3 reports), and hepatic toxicity and contact allergy (2 reports each).

2. Phototoxic Reactions

1. Erythema: Symptomatic erythema occurs in about 10% of patients and is probably most common in patients who absorb methoxsalen well. It appears about 24 to 36 h after treatment and can be minimized by spacing treatments at least 48 h apart.
2. Pruritus: So-called ''PUVA itch'' develops gradually over a week or more and is probably due to phototoxic damage to cutaneous nerves. This symptom is relieved by interruption of treatment and subsequent resumption at a lower dose.
3. Photo-onycholysis: Occasional patients develop painful discoloration of the nails due to phototoxic injury to the nail bed.
4. Phytophotodermatitis: Blisters, painful erythema, and subsequent hyperpigmentation may result from accidental topical application of

methoxsalen. This most commonly occurs when patients are exposed to leaking capsules of Oxsoralen Ultra.

B. Long-Term Side Effects

The most complete information on the long-term toxic effects of PUVA therapy have been provided by a prospective study of over 1300 patients who were initially treated in 1975–1976 in a 16-center study in the United States [11]. This study has consisted of examination of patients plus telephone interviews.

1. Nonmelanoma Skin Cancer

Methoxsalen combined with exposure to UVA radiation is carcinogenic for skin in mice and therefore is considered a possibility for humans. An increased incidence of squamous cell carcinomas of the skin was first found 2 years after commencement of treatment [12] and this has been followed by subsequent reports [13–16], the results of which can be summarized as follows.

1. The overall incidence is about 12%, which is at least 10 times the frequency in the general population.
2. The incidence is related to total dose, so that more than 260 treatments greatly increased the risk, intensity of treatment, and skin type, with skin types I and II accounting for most of the increased risk.
3. Prior exposure to radiograph and arsenic and a past history of skin cancer may increase the risk.
4. Lesions are mainly on the trunk and lower extremities with a high incidence on male genitalia.

2. Melanoma Skin Cancer

A recent report, again from the same prospective study, suggests there may also be an increased risk of melanoma in this population. The increase is small and first appeared about 15 years after initiation of PUVA therapy.

3. Photoaging of the Skin

Photoaging or actinic damage is seen with 34% of patients having these changes on buttock skin after 5 years [17]. The frequency of these changes is highest in people with fair skin and increases with total exposure dose.

4. Ophthalmologic Changes

PUVA therapy induces cataracts in mice [18], which has prompted use of eye protection in humans exposed to treatment. The prospective study did not find an increased frequency of cataracts after 5 years of exposure to treatment [19].

5. Autoimmune Phenomena

Lupus erythematosus can be induced and exacerbated by exposure to ultraviolet radiation [20]. In the prospective study in 1023 patients who had two or more serum ANA determinations over a 2-year period, a similar incidence of positive tests was found when first and last tests were compared [21]. There have been a few reports of SLE or an SLE-like syndrome occurring in patients on PUVA therapy; this infrequent event probably occurs in people with a predisposition to the disease. There are also two reports of bullous pemphigoid developing in patients on PUVA therapy and, again, a predisposition is likely to be the cause in these patients.

6. Hepatic Function

The 16-center PUVA study did not report any trend for change in liver function tests as a result of exposure to PUVA therapy. Two studies have found no change in liver biopsies performed before and after exposure to PUVA therapy [22,23].

7. Pregnancy

There have been no reports of an adverse effect of PUVA therapy on pregnancy outcome or the occurrence of congenital defects. However, there have been no published studies of the teratogenicity of PUVA therapy.

III. DRUG INTERACTIONS

Drug interactions with psoralen are extremely uncommon and only one has been identified. Compounds that activate the P-450 cytochrome enzyme system in the liver increase the metabolic breakdown of psoralens. These agents include phenytoin and carbamazepine. Patients on these drugs will show a decreased response to PUVA and, in some cases, will lose all effect of the treatment. This problem is rare and difficult to overcome except by carefully increasing the dose of psoralen.

IV. CONTRAINDICATIONS

PUVA therapy is contraindicated in certain situations.

A. Absolute Contraindications

1. Xeroderma pigmentosum should not be treated with UV radiation because patients with this disease have defective repair of UV-induced damage in DNA.

2. Lupus erythematosus is usually exacerbated by UV radiation and this is probably a contraindication to PUVA therapy. Detection of the Ro antibody in serum is a contraindication without other evidence of lupus.
3. Lactation is also a contraindication to PUVA therapy.

B. Relative Contraindications

1. Age, infirmity, lack of motivation, and minimal disease are all relative contraindications to this treatment. The patient must fully understand the nature of the treatment in order to follow the directions provided.
2. Pemphigus and pemphigoid are probably exacerbated in all patients by PUVA therapy.
3. History or family history of melanoma is a contraindication in most patients, although in certain circumstances the treatment may be used.
4. A past history of nonmelanoma skin cancer, previous treatment with ionizing radiation or arsenic, and extensive solar damage are contraindications to PUVA therapy in most patients. The main exception to this is the older patient, but this decision will depend on the need for treatment and other options available.
5. Uremia and severe hepatic failure are usually contraindications to PUVA therapy because drug metabolism and excretion will be disturbed. Careful monitoring of these patients is necessary if the treatment is used.

Some other contraindications are sometimes raised. Cataracts and aphakia are not contraindications but rather a warning that careful attention must be paid to eye protection. Photodermatoses should also be treated with care since they may be exacerbated by treatment. Concomitant cytotoxic therapy or immunosuppressive therapy may also contraindicate PUVA therapy in some patients.

V. INDICATIONS

A. Current Approved Indications

In the United States, PUVA therapy using methoxsalen has been approved by the FDA for use in patients with psoriasis. Trimethylpsoralen is approved for the treatment of vitiligo. Photophoresis is approved for treatment of mycosis fungoides.

B. Other Uses

PUVA has been found to be useful in a wide variety of conditions. Most of the conditions reported to respond to PUVA therapy are listed in Table 1.

TABLE 1 Response of Nonpsoriatic Dermatoses to PUVA Therapy

	Controlled trial	Open trial	Anecdote
Atopic dermatitis	++		
Seborrheic dermatitis		+++	
Hand dermatitis	++		
Allergic contact dermatitis		+	
Nodular prurigo		+++	
Persistent palmoplantar pustulosis	++		
Alopecia areata		+++	
Chronic graft-vs-host disease	++		
Granuloma annulare		+++	
Lichen planus, cutaneous and oral		+++	
Transient acantholytic dermatosis			+++
Pityriasis lichenoides		+++	
Lymphomatoid papulosis		++	
Pigmented purpuric dermatoses		+++	
Scleromyxedema			++
Granuloma faciale			+++
Dermatitis herpetiformis		++	
Histiocytosis X			+++
Acne vulgaris	+		
Sarcoidosis			+++
Ichthyosis linearis circumflexa			+++
Erythrokeratoderma progressiva symmetrica			+++
Impetigo herpetiformis			+++
Twenty-nail dystrophy			++
Papuloerythroderma			+++
Keratosis lichenoides chronica			++
Hypereosinophilic syndrome			+++
Urticaria			
Physical			+++
Dermographism	+		
Idiopathic			++
Urticaria pigmentosa	++		
Pruritus			
Polycythemia vera			+++
Idiopathic			++
Necrobiosis lipoidica diabeticorum			+
Scleroderma			++
Xeroderma pigmentosum		—	

$^{+++}$ Complete response; $^{++}$ partial response; $^{+}$ minimal response; — no response.

VI. THERAPEUTIC PROTOCOLS

A. Methoxsalen

Methoxsalen is available as both a crystalline form in a hard-gelatin capsule and as a liquid in a soft-gelatin capsule. It is mainly used in the latter form under the trade name Oxsoralen Ultra (ICN Pharmaceuticals, Inc.). The recommended dose is 0.6 mg/kg body weight, but this dose usually produces many side effects; thus it is preferable to use a dose of 0.4 mg/kg body weight as outlined by the dose schedule in Table 2. The medication should be taken 1 h before exposure to UVA radiation and it is important to avoid food for 1 h before and after ingestion.

B. UVA Radiation

The starting dose of UVA radiation can be determined by measuring the minimum phototoxic dose or by the use of skin typing as outlined in Table 3. Most physicians find the latter technique preferable. Treatments are given either two or three times a week, with the dose of UVA radiation being increased according to the schedule outlined in Table 4. Suggested final clearing doses of UVA radiation are also determined by skin type.

Additional treatment is required if there is significant disease on limbs or on the hands and feet. In the case of significant disease on the limbs, an extra exposure is given to the limbs only in the whole-body unit while exposure to the hands and feet is most effectively given in a specialized treatment unit designed for this purpose. Clearance of disease is defined as 95% clearance of the original disease and is then followed by a period of maintenance, with decreasing frequency of treatment. A reasonable protocol for this maintenance period is four treatments at weekly intervals, then four treatments every other week, four treatments every third week, and finally four monthly treatments. If the patient has a significant recurrence of disease (>5%), then a clearance schedule should be resumed.

TABLE 2 Dose Schedule for Oxsoralen Ultra

Patient weight		Drug dose
lbs.	kg	(mg)
<66	<30	10
66–143	30–65	20
144–200	65–90	30
>200	>90	40

Table 3 Skin Types

Skin type	History	Examination
I	Always burn, never tan	
II	Always burn, sometimes tan	
III	Sometimes burn, always tan	
IV	Never burn, always tan	
V		Brown[a]
VI		Black

[a] Chinese, Mexican, American Indian.

C. Combination Treatments

PUVA therapy is combined with various other treatments to effect more rapid clearance at a lower exposure dose of therapy. The common combined treatments are PUVA + methotrexate, PUVA + etretinate (which is also called Re-PUVA), and PUVA therapy + UVB phototherapy. Combination treatment is particularly indicated in patients with thick plaques and in patients with high skin types, since reliance on PUVA therapy alone is associated with a high failure rate in these groups of patients.

D. Bath Water PUVA

Topical application of psoralens has the advantages of avoiding gastrointestinal and ocular toxicity. However, using the topical methoxsalen solution available in the United States can result in marked hyperpigmentation, which is almost as unattractive as psoriasis. The European approach of using a very dilute solution of psoralens as a bath can provide a more practical approach to topical therapy.

Table 4 Dose of UVA Radiation for B.I.W. and T.I.W. Schedules

Skin type	UVA radiation dose (J/cm^2)		
	Initial	Increments	Final
I	1.5	0.5	5
II	2.5	0.5	8
III	3.5	0.5–1.0	12
IV	4.5	1.0	14
V	5.5	1.0	16
VI	6.5	1.0–1.5	20

Trioxsalen is dissolved in a bathtub of water (50 mg/150 L); the patient lies in the bath for 15 min and is then exposed to UVA radiation. The pigmentation from this treatment is uniform and photosensitivity to the skin lasts less than 24 h. Several European clinics have reported excellent results treating psoriasis with this approach to therapy [24].

The possibility of using bath water delivery of psoralens in the United States was raised by a recent study that reported favorable results in dissolving 30 mg of 1% methoxsalen in 80 L of water and immersing the patient in it for 15 min, immediately prior to UVA radiation exposure. This treatment was successful in clearing psoriasis in some patients with only a few episodes of phototoxicity [25]. However, it is somewhat impractical since the drug costs $55 to $60 per bath. An alternative is to use the solution from capsules; there is one published study of this approach [26].

The main advantage of using bath water delivery of psoralen is the avoidance of systemic effects of methoxsalen. However, it can be detected in serum and consequently eye protection must be used. The idea of having several bathtubs in an office or clinic may not be an attractive idea for all physicians.

E. Photophoresis

Photophoresis is a term coined to describe extracorporeal photochemotherapy. The patients are given a treatment on each of two consecutive days once a month. Several courses of treatment are required to obtain a remission in the treatment of mycosis fungoides. The patient takes a regular dose of methoxsalen orally and 1 h later is connected to the treatment unit via an indwelling catheter in a vein. One unit of blood is removed and leukophoresed to yield a buffy coat, which is then passed through a plastic channel between two banks of UVA fluorescent bulbs. The irradiation procedure continues for 1 to 2 h and the treated buffy coat is returned to the patient. Variability in absorption of methoxsalen can affect the treatment. This has led to trial of a new approach in which the psoralen is added directly to the buffy coat.

In a cooperative clinical study involving five centers, 27 of 37 patients with cutaneous T-cell lymphoma (CTCL) were considered improved after an average of 22 weeks of treatment [27]. The response was best in Sezary syndrome (82% responders), while patients with less extensive plaques and tumors often failed to respond. In most instances, treatment must be continued on a maintenance basis, although a few patients have stopped treatment.

REFERENCES

1. Fahmy IR, Abu-Shady H. The isolation and properties of ammoidin, ammidin and majudin, and their effect in the treatment of leukodermia. Q J Pharm Pharmacol 1948;2:499–503.

2. Sullivan TJ, Walter JL, Kouba RF, Maiwald DC. Bioavailability of a new oral methoxsalen formulation. Arch Dermatol 1986;122:768–769.
3. Levins PC, Gange RW, Momtaz-T K, Parrish JA, Fitzpatrick TB. A new liquid formulation of 8-methoxypsoralen: bioactivity and effect of diet. J Invest Dermatol 1984;82:185–187.
4. Roelandts R, Van Boven M, Deheyn T, Vander Stichele G, Degreef H, Daenens P. Dietary influences on 8-MOP plasma levels in PUVA patients with psoriasis. Br J Dermatol 1981;105:569–572.
5. Brickl R, Schmid J, Koss FW. Clinical pharmacology of oral psoralen drugs. Photodermatology 1984;1:174–186.
6. Schmid J, Prox A, Zipp H, Koss FW. The use of stable isotopes to prove the saturable first-pass effect of methoxsalen. Biomed Mass Spectrometry 1980;7:560–564.
7. Artuc M, Stuettgen G, Schalla W, Schaefer H, Gazith J. Reversible binding of 5- and 8-methoxypsoralen to human serum proteins (albumin) and to epidermis in vitro. Br J Derm 1979;101:669–683.
8. Schmid J, Prox A, Reuter A, Zipp H, Koss FW. The metabolism of 8-methoxypsoralen in man. Eur J Drug Metab Pharm 1980;5:81–92.
9. Wulf HC, Andreasen MP. Distribution of 3H-8-MOP and its metabolites in rat organs after a single oral administration. J Invest Dermatol 1981;76:252–258.
10. Morison WL. Phototherapy and Photochemotherapy of Skin Disease, vol. 2, 2d ed. New York: Raven Press, 1990.
11. Melski JW, Tanenbaum L, Parrish JA, Fitzpatrick TB, Bleich HL, and 28 Participating Investigators. Oral methoxsalen photochemotherapy for the treatment of psoriasis: a cooperative clinical trial. J Invest Dermatol 1977;68:328–335.
12. Stern RS, Thibodeau LA, Kleinerman RA, Parrish JA, Fitzpatrick TB, and 22 Participating Investigators. Risk of cutaneous carcinoma in patients treated with oral methoxsalen photochemotherapy for psoriasis. N Engl J Med 1979;300:809–813.
13. Roelandts R. Mutagenicity and carcinogenicity of methoxsalen plus UV-A. Arch Dermatol 1984;120:662–669.
14. Stern RS, Laird N, Melski J, Parrish JA, Fitzpatrick TB, Bleich HL. Cutaneous squamous-cell carcinoma in patients treated with PUVA. N Engl J Med 1984;310: 1156–1161.
15. Stern RS, Lange R, and Members of the Photochemotherapy Follow-Up Study. Nonmelanoma skin cancer occurring in patients treated with PUVA five to ten years after first treatment. J Invest Dermatol 1988;91:120–124.
16. Stern RS, and Members of the Photochemotherapy Follow-Up Study. Genital tumors among men with psoriasis exposed to psoralens and ultraviolet A radiation (PUVA) and ultraviolet B radiation. N Engl J Med 1990;322:1093–1097.
17. Stern RS, Parrish JA, Fitzpatrick TB, Bleich HL. Actinic degeneration in association with long-term use of PUVA. J Invest Dermatol 1985;84:135–138.
18. Freeman RG, Troll D. Photosensitization of the eye by 8-methoxypsoralen. J Invest Dermatol 1969;53:449–453.
19. Stern RS, Parrish JA, Fitzpatrick TB. Ocular findings in patients treated with PUVA. J Invest Dermatol 1994;103:534–538.
20. Kind P, Lehmann P, Plewig G. Phototesting in lupus erythematosus. J Invest Dermatol 1993;100:53S–57S.

21. Stern RS, Morison WI, Thibodeau LA, Kleinerman RA, Parrish JA, Geer DE, Fitzpatrick TB. Antinuclear antibodies and oral methoxsalen photochemotherapy (PUVA) for psoriasis. Arch Dermatol 1979;115:1320–1324.
22. Zachariae H, Kragballe K, Sogaard H. Liver biopsy in PUVA-treated patients. Acta Dermatoven 1979;59:268–270.
23. Nyfors A, Dahl-Nyfors B, Hopwood D. Liver biopsies from patients with psoriasis related to photochemotherapy (PUVA): findings before and after 1 year of therapy in twelve patients. J Am Acad Dermatol 1986;14:43–48.
24. Fischer T, Alsins J. Treatment of psoriasis with trioxsalen baths and dysprosium lamps. Acta Derm Venereol (Stockh) 1976;56:383–390.
25. Lowe NJ, Weingarten D, Bourget T, Moy LS. PUVA therapy for psoriasis: comparison of oral and bath-water delivery of 8-methoxypsoralen. J Am Acad Dermatol 1986;14:754–760.
26. Vallat VP, Gilleaudeau P, Battat L, Wolfe J, Heftler N, Gottlieb SL, Hodak E, Gottlieb AB, Krueger JG. PUVA bath therapy with 8-methoxypsoralen. In: Weinstein GD, Gottlieb AB, eds. National Psoriasis Foundation: Therapy of Moderate-to-Severe Psoriasis. Portland: National Psoriasis Foundation, 1993:39–56.
27. Edelson R, Berger C, Gasparro F, Jegasothy BV, Heald PW, Wintroub B, Vonderheid E, Knobler R, Wolff K, Plewig G, McKiernan G, Christensen I, Oster M, Honigsmann H, Wilfore H, Kokoschka E, Rehle T, Perez M, Stingl G, Laroche L. Treatment of cutaneous T-cell lymphoma by extracorporeal photochemotherapy. N Engl J Med 1987;316:297–303.

14

Antiparasitic Therapy

Mohamed Amer
Zagazig University
Zagazig, Egypt

Animal parasites are divided into two groups: (1) protozoa (unicellular); and (2) metazoa (multicellular), which are characterized by segmentation of the ovum. Both groups are divided into phyla, the most important of which are (1) protozoa, (2) nemathelminthes (parasitic worms), and (3) arthropoda.

Each phylum is divided into classes, and further subdivided into orders, families, genera, and species.

In this chapter, the treatment of the most common diseases caused by each phylum is discussed. The prevention of these diseases, when feasible, will be mentioned.

I. TREATMENT OF PROTOZOA OF DERMATOLOGICAL IMPORTANCE

A. Cutaneous Amoebiasis

Cutaneous amoebiasis is caused by *Entamoeba histolytica*; in patients with AIDS, it may be caused by *Acanthamoeba castlani*.

The disease usually presents with deeply invading ulcers or ulcerative granuloma (Amoeboma), which is very painful. The common sites are the perianal region and in or around a surgical wound in the abdomen. This may be the only manifestation of the disease or it may be associated with the involvement of other organs [1]. Treatment varies accordingly.

1. Treatment

Combinations of drugs may be necessary because some are more effective in the gut lumen (e.g., metronidazole, emetine, and dehydroemetine) and others are active systemically [2] (e.g., diloxanide and the tetracyclines). Chloroquine is often given as a supportive treatment for liver abscesses.

1. Metronidazole is given in a dosage of 800 mg three times daily for up to 10 days (35–50 mg/day for children) and is probably safest for treating cutaneous infection.
2. Tinidazole is given as a single daily dose of 2 g for 3 to 5 days (50–60 mg/kg/body weight for children) and may be more effective.
3. Local cleansing of cutaneous ulcer with antiseptic solutions may be necessary.

Cutaneous lesions usually respond rapidly, with improvement occurring in 4 to 5 days.

B. Trypanosomiasis

Two distinct types of infection by protozoan of the genus trypanosoma exist—the African and the American forms. The African form is subdivided into two clinical varieties, gambiense and rhodesiense trypanosomiasis, both transmitted by tsetse flies.

Cutaneous lesions are usually limited to the site of initial fly bite. A chancre develops at the entry site 5 to 10 days after the bite. It is a painful red nodule usually on exposed areas and associated with regional lymphadenopathy. Scratching may lead to secondary infection and ulceration. The secondary or invasive stage usually develops 1 to 3 weeks after the initial bite and is manifested by fever accompanied by or shortly followed by a characteristic eruption [3], which consists of transient erythematous annular or serpiginous plaques. Painful transient edema of the hands, feet, and eyelids usually occurs.

1. Treatment

Treatment of African trypanosomiasis depends on the stage of the disease [3].

In the early stages, suramin is the drug of choice. It is administered intravenously in a freshly prepared solution. The first test dose of 0.1 g is followed by a weekly dose of 1 g for 6 weeks if no renal toxicity develops.

In cases of gambiense infection pentamidine may be given intramuscularly in a freshly prepared solution of 4 mg/kg every other day for a total of 10 injections.

Arsenic preparations such as melasporol and suramin may be given in late stages when CNS involvement occurs.

C. American Trypanosomiasis

American trypanosomiasis, also called Chagas disease, is caused by *Trypanosoma cruzi*. The acute stage of the disease (1–4 months) is the only form associated with cutaneous manifestations.

Chagoma, the most distinctive feature of this stage, is boardlike tender induration associated with regional lymphadenopathy. Unilateral eyelid edema, conjunctivitis, and periauricular adenopathy is known as Romana's sign.

1. Treatment

The treatment of choice in the acute stage depends mainly on two effective specific parasiticidal drugs, namely nifurtimox (Lampit), administered to adults in three divided doses of 8 to 10 mg/kg body weight for 2 to 3 months; in children under 2 years of age, 20 mg/kg body weight; and children over 2 years, 15 mg/kg/day in four divided doses. Side effects such as anorexia, insomnia, and polyneuritis are dose related and often disappear after dose reduction. The second drug of choice, benznidazole (Rochagan), is administered in 5 mg/kg body weight for 2 to 3 months. Photosensitivity, erythema multiforme, and erythroderma are common side effects.

There is no specific effective therapy for the chronic form of the disease and the treatment is usually symptomatic.

Prevention depends chiefly on avoidance and/or irradication of the insect vector. Community public health measures are mandatory to eliminate breeding places.

D. Leishmaniasis

Leishmania is a genus of protozoan parasite that infects a broad range of hosts including insects, amphibians, and mammals. In the human host, leishmania are obligate intracellular parasites, transmitted by the bites of infected female sandflies. Transmission to humans is usually from infected nonmammal reservoirs and, depending upon the parasite species, can result in cutaneous, mucocutaneous, or visceral disease.

1. Classification of the Cutaneous Leishmaniasis [4]:

Old world cutaneous leishmaniasis is caused by the following:

1. *L. tropica minor*. This organism causes the urban, usually anthroponotic, cutaneous leishmaniasis. It is found in the Near East from Turkey to India, North and West Africa, and Mediterranean Europe.
2. *L. tropica major*. This form causes the zoonotic rural cutaneous leishmaniasis in Iran, Pakistan, the Middle East, and North and West Africa. Rodents are the main reservoirs.

3. *L. aethiopica*. This species commonly causes diffuse cutaneous leishmaniasis in the highlands of Ethiopia and Kenya. The hydrax is the reservoir.

New World cutaneous leishmaniasis is found in Central and South America. It is caused by species of *L. mexicana complex* (e.g., *L. mexicana mexicana*) and the *L. braziliensis* complex (e.g., *L. braziliensis panamenesis*).

Mucocutaneous leishmaniasis, found in South America, is caused by *L. braziliensis*, and is a life-threatening disease.

When considering the treatment of cutaneous leishmaniasis, one must keep in mind the wide variety of species/subspecies of the parasite involved. The clinical form taken by the infection depends on the immunological response of the host. The host's defense to these intracellular pathogens largely depends on the cell-mediated immune response.

The most common form of cutaneous leishmaniasis is acute cutaneous leishmaniasis (ACL), also known as Oriental sore or Baghdad boil. This lesion is at the center of the spectrum. The initial nodular erythematous lesion usually breaks down to form an ulcer. Such lesions heal spontaneously in weeks or months but usually leave a scar [4].

At the anergic end of the spectrum is diffuse cutaneous leishmaniasis (DCL). The primary lesion spreads and the parasite is disseminated throughout the whole body surface. The infection is usually very chronic.

The hypernergic end of the spectrum includes the following: (1) chronic cutaneous leishmaniasis (CCL), which follows from ACL that does not heal, and erythematous papules at the edge of the lesion may be evident; and (2) recurrent cutaneous leishmaniasis (RCL), also known as leishmaniasis recidivans, which occurs at or near acute lesions that have completely or partly healed. These lesions can appear months or years after healing of the primary lesion [5].

2. Treatment of Leishmaniasis

Leishmaniasis, like trypanosomiasis and microfilariasis, has not seen major advances in treatment in the last decades. The detection and treatment of human cases are considered very important for controlling cutaneous leishmaniasis. Control of the vector sandfly and the animal reservoir (e.g., rodents and wild hydraxes) is also needed.

Spontaneous healing also occurs. For the first 2 or 3 months, the lesions continue to become progressively worse, then healing begins and is complete within 12 to 15 months. Considering this fact and that recovery is supposed to confer life-long immunity, a pertinent question could be asked: Why treat leishmaniasis [4]?

In New World cases, there is, of course, the fear of the consequences of *L. braziliensis* infections, which are always treated. In Old World ACL, treatment is desired where there are lesions on exposed parts of the body, especially the face. The healed scars and areas of depigmentation are ugly. Another reason to treat is to prevent secondary bacterial infection of the lesions.

Infections with *L. aethiopica* should receive special attention, since they involve large areas of the body surface and tend to have a long course. Healing of these lesions gives rise to severe fibrosis that could restrict the use of fingers.

Another reason for the need to treat is that treatment is one of the most important methods of controlling the disease in the population [6].

a. Traditional Therapies Pentavalent antimonials, such as glucantime (methyl glucamine antimoniate) and pentostam (sodium stiboglyconate), are used most frequently in a dose of 10 mg antimony/kg body weight for adults, 20 mg/kg body weight for children by intravenous or intramuscular injection daily, plus local infiltration with either of the drugs. In chronic leishmaniasis (the hypernergic spectrum), intralesional steriods should be tried in conjunction with antimonials to shift the hypernergic activity toward a normogenic response.

Toxicity includes headache, fainting, muscle and joint pain, ECG changes, and seizures. Antimonials should be avoided in patients with myocarditis, hepatitis, or nephritis. The mechanism of action of antimonials is unclear. Numerous enzymes of the parasites are inhibited selectively. Of significance, phosphofructokinase, which catalyzes a rate-limiting step of glycolysis, is inhibited [7].

Amphotericin B has been used and found effective in the mucocutaneous form. The drug should be diluted in 5% dextrose solution and given 1 mg/kg over 6 h on alternate days. Amphotericin B is very toxic to the kidney. Urea and urine protein levels should be carefully monitored. Decreased serum potassium levels are found in 25% of patients receiving the drug. Infusions of amphotericin B are associated with thrombophlebitis, which can be prevented by adding a small amount of heparin to the infusion.

Details of the mechanism of action of amphotericin B are not clear. In fungal infections, its action is likely to occur through interaction with ergosterol in fungal membranes. The newer preparation of amphotericin B offers promise for future therapy.

b. Other Drugs Metronidazole is used in protozoal infections such as amoebiasis and trichomoniasis. Its selective toxicity is probably due to the reduction of a nitro-group on the drug inside the parasite. It now appears that metronidazole is unlikely to play a primary role in the therapy of leishmaniasis.

Nifurtimox is the drug of choice for American trypanosomiasis (Chagas disease), where it is active against the amastigote phases of the parasite. The dose is 8 to 10 mg/kg/day for 3 to 120 days. However, the dose takes too long to administer.

Rifampicin, as used in one trial 1200 mg/day, elicited clinical cure in 3 to 8 weeks in 41 of 46 cases of cutaneous leishmaniasis. Rifampicin has been tried with other drugs (e.g., with isoniazid, pentamidine, sodium stibogluconate, or amphotericin B).

Antimalarials (e.g., 8-aminoquinoline, quinacrine), 5 to 10% solution, may be administered intralesionally with good anticipated results.

Levamisol has immunopotentiating effect on T cells. Butler [8] observes that even in endemic areas the prevalence of cutaneous leishmaniasis is low. He believes that most local inhabitants are inoculated in early life with the parasite by sandflies and have subclinical infections, which gives long-term immunity. Butler proposes that clinical cutaneous leishmaniasis infections in later life are due to a declining cell-mediated immunity, which can be potentiated by levamisol. In this trial, 28 patients were cured with levamisol without other medication. This interesting proposal requires further investigation.

Phenothiazines, which include chlorpromazine, are psychoactive drugs. Henriksen [9] treated three patients with *L. aethiopica* diffuse cutaneous leishmaniasis with topical chlorpromazine. Inflammation improved and parasite smears were negative after 1 month of treatment.

Allopurinol is used in hyperuricemia. Oral allopurinol (15 mg/kg/day) produced questionable cure in two of five patients with mucocutaneous leishmaniasis. Clinical cure occurred in two patients, 2 months from start of treatment, but a significant fluorescent antibody titre still existed at 1 year [10].

Ketoconazole has been reported to be effective (400 mg/day for 3 months) on six Nicaraguan patients with early skin lesions [11].

c. Rational Approaches Difluoromethylornithine (DFMO) blocks polyamine synthesis (which has an important function in the growth of Leishmania) by inhibiting ornithine decarboxylase (ODC) essential for polyamine synthesis [12].

Antipain and leupeptin are peptide analogues that lead to inhibition of cysteine proteinases and stop the in vitro multiplication of the parasite [13].

Transfer factor is a dialyzable extract of leukocytes obtained from healthy donors who have recovered from cutaneous Leishmaniasis. This factor is injected subcutaneously near the skin lesion.

3. Nonmedical Treatment of Leishmaniasis

1. Plastic surgery has an important role in treating disfiguring scar, especially scars of Leishmania recidivans.
2. Heat treatment: Leishmania organisms are very thermosensitive for both heat and cold. Heat therapy has been used quite often in the past.
3. Cryotherapy with a carbon dioxide cryomachine. Cryotherapy is short and quick and gives little discomfort. Cryotherapy also spares pregnant and weak patients from toxic drug effects.

II. PARASITIC WORMS

Parasitic worms infect humans worldwide and are particularly common in tropical countries. There are two main groups, roundworms (Nemathelminthes) and flatworms (Platyhelminthes). A single class of Nemathelminthes Nematodes, causes disease. There are two important classes of Platyhelminthes, Trematoda (flukes) and Cestoda (tapeworms).

A. Nematodes

Nematodes that are parasitic in humans may be intestinal or tissue roundworms. Enterobiasis (pinworm, oxyuriasis, threadworm infestation) may result, with anal and perianal pruritus at night, especially in children, being the leading symptoms [14].

1. Treatment

1. Mebendazole, given as a single oral dose of 100 mg for all ages, gives a cure rate of 90 to 100%. There is minimal absorption of this drug, which seems to be free of side effects.
2. Levamisol is given as a single oral dose of 3 to 5 mg/kg body weight and provides another alternative. Both drugs should be readministered after 2 weeks.

B. Human Hookworm Disease

The disease occurs in nearly all subtropics and tropics and is caused by two intestinal hookworms, *Necator americanus* (New World hookworms) and *Ancylostoma duodenale* (Old World hookworms).

Larvae penetrating the skin cause ground itch: severe pruritus, erythema, edema, papular, vesicular, or bullous eruptions usually develop on the feet. This is transient and subsides spontaneously in 2 weeks unless complicated by secondary bacterial infection. The rash is more common with *Necator sp.* infections [15].

1. Treatment

1. Topical application of thiabendazole may be helpful.
2. If secondary infection occurs, antibacterials should be administered.
3. The treatment of intestinal disease depends mainly on tetrachloroethylene in cases of *Necator sp.* infections given in a gelatinous capsule on an empty stomach, preceded by a saline purge the day before. The dose is 5 capsules (1 mL each) for adults and 0.1 mg/kg body weight for children. Another saline purgative is given a few hours later. Treatment should be repeated 2 weeks later if three successive stool examinations show eggs still present.

4. For *A. doudenale* infections, pephenium hydroxy naphthoate (Alcopara) is preferable. Two packets of 2.5 g on an empty stomach are given to adults, and half of this dose may be given to children. In heavy infections, this may be repeated in 15 days.
5. Thiabendazole taken orally is also effective.
6. In case of mixed infections with Ascaris, piprazine may be used before the treatment of hookworms.
7. Anemia should be corrected.

C. Strongyloidiasis

Strongyloides stercoralis is a roundworm with a life cycle similar to that of the hookworm, but with a heterogenic nature that yields alternating parasitic and free-living generation.

The skin changes are pronounced and occasionally characteristic. They are caused by penetration of the larvae or allergic reaction. The dermatitis that develops due to penetration of the skin by the larvae is similar to ground itch, but less intensive. Later in the disease urticarial eruption associated with erythema lasting for several days may occur. This may be associated with a peculiar type of creeping eruption, which migrates at a rate of several centimeters per hour in a serpiginous manner. This is called larva currens as opposed to larva migrans, caused by *Ancylostoma braziliensis* (dog hookworms) [16].

1. Treatment

1. Thiabendazole (Mintezole) given orally for 3 days, 25 mg/kg body weight, may be effective.
2. Ivermectin (antiparasitic agent used extensively in veterinary practice) has shown promise for the treatment of strongyloidiasis [17]. The control of the disease depends mainly on improvement of waste disposal facilities.

D. Trichiniasis (Whip Worms)

Trichuris trichura infection is more prevalent in moist and warm tropical regions especially in rural areas. The infection occurs by ingestion of infected ova that originated directly or indirectly from the soil. The only important skin eruption is urticaria, which is probably due to systemic hypersensitivity.

1. Treatment

Mebendazole or thiabendazole may be used.

E. Gnathostomiasis

The characteristic of the infection caused by *Gnathostoma spinigerum* is that it combines features of creeping eruption and myasis. Humans are dead-end hosts;

the parasite fails to mature and wanders in human tissue for as long as 10 years. The usual route for migration leads from stomach to liver, skeletal muscles, and subcutaneous tissues. Intermittent erythematous, edematous, migratory plaques of different sizes appear suddenly; they are pruritic and may be associated with abscess formation or small haemorrhagic spots. On rare occasions, the worms emerge spontaneously from the lesion [18].

1. Treatment

1. Surgical removal of the parasite is the treatment of choice.
2. Freezing the advancing end of the lesion where the parasite is located with ethylchloride or dry ice has been reported to be effective.

F. Creeping Eruption

There is considerable confusion about the disorders included in this category. Several different parasites produce similar clinical pictures. *Ancylostoma braziel-iense, A. caninum, A. doudenale, Necator americanus, Uncinaria stenocephala*, and *Capillaria philippinensis* are some of them. The lesion arises as a result of larvae tunneling in the epidermis.

1. Treatment

The treatment depends on the severity of infection.

1. Oral albendazole is now considered the first-line treatment. It is given 400 mg bid for 1 to 2 weeks. Side effects are absent or minimal.
2. Topical and oral thiabendazole may also be effective.

III. TISSUE ROUNDWORMS

Extraintestinal human nematodes include filarial worms, guinea-worm, *Dracunculus medinensis*, and *Trichinella* sp.

A. Filariasis

Wuchereria bancrofti and *Brugia malayi* cause bancroftian and malayian filariasis, respectively. The latter is more prevalent in South East Asia while bancroftian filariasis is endemic in extensive tropical and subtropical regions; it has been reported in almost every country in these zones. Humans are the only host for *W. bancrofti* while *B. malayi* has been found in primates and felines. The bite of a mosquito of the genera Culex, Aedes, Mansonia, and Anopheles injects larvae of the parasite, which migrate to the lymphatics and lymph nodes and develop within about 1 year into mature worms [19].

Clinical manifestations range from asymptomatic infection to severe elephentiasis.

1. Treatment

1. Diethylcarbamazine has been the drug of choice. It rapidly reduces circulating microfilariae and may affect the adult worm. The drug is given in tablet form, starting with smaller doses: (1) 50 mg for the first day; (2) 50 mg t.d.s the second day; (3) 100 mg t.d.s. the third day; and (4) 2 mg/kg body weight daily to complete a 3-week course of treatment. This course is advocated to minimize the Jarisch–Herxheimer reaction, which develops within 6 h after the first dose and reaches its maximum in 24 to 48 h. It usually subsides in 3 to 6 days, even with continuation of treatment. The reaction usually manifests itself with fever, orchitis, abdominal pain, bone aches, and arthritis. Antihistamines given at the beginning of treatment may help to control the reaction. If clinical response is unsatisfactory, a second course after 3 months may be given. Treatment will not reverse elephantiasis.
2. Recently, ivermectin has been suggested as an effective line of treatment for lymphatic filariasis. A single dose of 100 to 200 μg/kg ivermectin is given. Side effects are similar to those of diethylcarbamazine. The drug is suitable for mass treatment. Its mechanism of action, however, is not well understood [17].
3. Surgical treatment may be needed to correct massive scrotal involvement, hydrocele, and elephantiasis.

B. Loiasis (Loa-loa)

Loiasis is a chronic infection limited to rain forests. It is caused by the filarial worm, Loa-loa and is transmitted by Chrysops flies. The adult, a wide threadlike worm measuring between 25 to 75 mm, migrates continuously through the subcutaneous tissue at a maximum rate of 0.5 to 1 cm. The adult worms appear in the eye, occasionally beneath the skin, and produce Calabar swellings [19].

1. Treatment

1. Diethylcarbamazine is very effective in the treatment of loiasis; it kills the adults and microfilariae. The dose is similar to that used for the treatment of bancroftian filariasis.
2. Low-dose mebendazole has also been used in a dosage of 100 mg t.d.s. for 45 days.

C. Onchocerciasis

Onchocerciasis is a filarial disease caused by *Onchocerca volvulus* and is transmitted by flies of the genus simulium. Twenty to forty million people worldwide are victims of this disease, which may cause blindness; this disease has a negative impact on economic development all over tropical Africa and in some Asian countries as well. There are also foci in Central and South America. The most characteristic lesions are subcutaneous nodules that contain the worms. These may be acute or chronic. Regional lymph node inflammation and ocular damage may also occur.

1. Treatment

Between 1982 to 1984, several reports [20–22] appeared about the effect of treating mildly infected individuals with a single oral dose of ivermectin, ranging from 5 to 200 μg/kg body weight. The drug appeared to be effective, safe, and well tolerated. It was also shown that ivermectin was as effective as diethylcarbamazine in its microfilaricidal effect and was associated with less significant skin reaction.

1. Ivermectin is now the drug of choice for treatment of *O. volvulus* infection in humans. It is administered as a single oral dose of about 150 μg/kg body weight and is an effective microfilaricidal agent that suppresses disease in the skin and eyes and prevents progression of ocular disease. It should be given every 6 months. The mechanism of action of ivermectin is not well understood. It is thought to block the action of the neurotransmitter GABA, as evident by its paralytic action on intesinal nematodes. In mammals, GABA-dependent neuronal transmission only occurs in the central nervous system (CNS) and ivermectin does not enter the CNS. In patients with onchocerciasis, ivermectin was found to decrease the motility of microfilaria and promate cell-mediated cytotoxicity. It also has been shown to inhibit release of microfilaria from the uterus of adult worms, which may affect transmission.
2. Diethylcarbamazine is given in cases of mild-to-moderate onchocercal dermatitis without eye involvement. Several repeated courses over a long period may be needed to destroy the new load of microfilariae. The dosage is the same as for the treatment of filariasis.
3. Suramin, which is a urea derivative, may be used especially in treatment of cases with eye involvement. It is a microfilaricidal and it also kills adult worms. The dosage is the same as for the treatment of trypanosomiasis. Urine examination should be performed before starting treatment and before each weekly injection to detect the possible presence of albumin. Arterial blood pressure should also be checked because the drug is eliminated very slowly through the kidneys. Renal dysfunction, pregnancy, hypertension, and severe anemia are absolute contraindications. Side effects, such as urticaria, edema (especially of the palms and soles), arthritis, and erythroderma may be controlled by

antihistamines or even corticosteroids and treatment may need to be interrupted.

IV. PLATYHELMINTHES

Among platyhelminthes, two types are of medical importance, trematoda and cestoda. The trematodes of cutaneous importance are schistosomes or blood flukes.

Cutaneous manifestations of schistosomes can be divided into four types, depending upon the stage of development of the parasite and the chronicity of systemic disease as well [23].

1. Dermatitis schistosomica (swimmer's itch) is caused by the penetration of the human or nonhuman cercariae through the skin.
2. Bilharzid or schistosomid (Katayama disease) is an allergic anaphylactoid reaction that occurs when a large number of eggs (new antigenic materials) are released and antibodies produced in response to the presence of developing worm crossreact with them.
3. Bilharziasis cutanea tarda is a specific schistosomal skin lesion caused by deposition of eggs in the dermis.
4. Lesions related to complications of schistosomiasis are spider nevi, vulval leukoplakia, and, rarely, carcinoma of the vulva.

A. Treatment

Cercarial dermatitis may be prevented by thorough drying of skin immediately after leaving water; repellants such as citronella oil or protective clothing are also helpful. Antipruritic lotions and antihistamines may reduce itching and thus prevent causing secondary infection from scratching, which may require a course of oral antibiotics. Norfloxacin may be given, 400 mg twice daily, for 5 to 10 days.

Oral preparations for schistosomiasis include lucanthone and niridazole, 25 mg/kg body weight daily for 10 days. Hycenthone is also available in the form of IM injections. It should be noted that treatment of *S. mansoni* must be repeated several times. Antischistosomal treatment must start as early as possible before tissue reaction and fibrosis become irreversible [23].

Praziquantel is the drug of choice for the treatment of infections due to all species of schistosoma. It is given as a single oral dose of 40 mg/kg. Side effects are few and include abdominal distress, with or without nausea, headache, slight drowsiness and, very rarely, itching of the skin and rise in temperature [24].

For schistosomal skin granuloma, the antischistosomal drugs will lead to involution of the lesions usually in 4 to 6 weeks, but larger lesions will respond better to intralesional triamcinalone (4 mg/mL) weekly for 1 month. Surgical excision of large lesions may be necessary.

REFERENCES

1. Fujita WH, Barr RJ, Gottschalk WR. Cutaneous amoebiasis. Arch Dermatol 1981; 117:309–310.
2. Knight R. The chemotherapy of amoebiasis. J Antimicrob Chemother 1980; 6:577–593.
3. Foulkes JR. Human trypanosomiasis in Africa. Br Med J 1981; 283:1172–1174.
4. Chong H. Oriental sore. A look at trends in and approaches to the treatment of leishmaniasis. Int J Dermatol 1986; 25:615–623.
5. Farah F, Malak J. Cutaneous leishmaniasis. Arch Dermatol 1971; 103:467–474.
6. Strick R, Barok M, Gasiorowski H. Recurrent cutaneous leishmaniasis. J Am Acad Dermatol 1983; 9:437–443.
7. Gutteridge W, Coombs G. Biochemistry of parasitic protozoa. London: MacMillan, 1977.
8. Butler P. Levamisole and immune response phenomena in cutaneous leishmaniasis. J Am Acad Dermatol 1982; 6:1070–1077.
9. Henriksen T, Lenden S. Treatment of diffuse cutaneous leishmaniasis with chlorpromazine ointment. Lancet 1983; 1:126.
10. Marsden P, Cuba C, Barretta A. Allopurinol treatment in human leishmania braziliensis infections. Trans R Soc Trop Med Hyg 1984; 78:419–420.
11. Urcayo F, Zaias N. Oral ketoconazole in the treatment of leishmaniasis. Int J Dermatol 1982; 21:414–416.
12. McCann P, Bacchi C, Clarkson A. Further studies on difluoromethylornithine in African trypanosomiasis. Med Biol 1981; 59:434–440.
13. Coombs G, Hart D, Capaldo J. Proteinase inhibitors as antileishmenial agents. Trans R Soc Trop Med Hyg 1982; 76:660–663.
14. Broadbent V. Children's worms. Br Med J 1975; i:89.
15. Gilles HM, Williams EJW, Ball PAJ. Hookworm infection and anaemia. Q Rev Med 1964; 33:1–24.
16. Stone OJ, Newell GB, Mullins JF. Cutaneous strongyloidiasis: larva current. Arch Dermatol 1972; 106:734–736.
17. Campbell WC. Ivermectin: an update. Parasitol Today 1985; 1:10–16.
18. Radomyos P, Daengsvang S. A brief report on Gnathostoma spinigerum specimens obtained from human cases. Southeast Asian J Trop Med Pub Health 1987; 18:215.
19. Davis BR. Filariasis. Dermatol Clin 1989; 7:313–321.
20. Aziz MA, Diallo S, Diop IM, Lariviere M, Porla M. Efficacy and tolerance of ivermectin in human onchocerciasis. Lancet 1982; 2:171–173.
21. Couland JP, Lariviere M, Gervais MC, Gaxotte P, Aziz MA, Delual AM, Cenac J. Treatment of human onchocerciasis with ivermectin. Bull Soc Pathol Exot Filiales 1983; 76:681–688.
22. Awadzi K, Dadzie KY, Schulz-Key H, Haddock DRW, Gilles HM, Aziz MA. Ivermectin in onchocerciasis (letter). Lancet 1984; 2:2921.
23. Amer M. Cutaneous schistosomiasis. Int J Dermatol 1982; 21:44.
24. Mamoud AAF. Praziquantel for the treatment of helminthic infections. In: Stollerman GH, ed. Advances in Internal Medicine. Chicago: Year Book Medical Publishers, 1987:419–434.

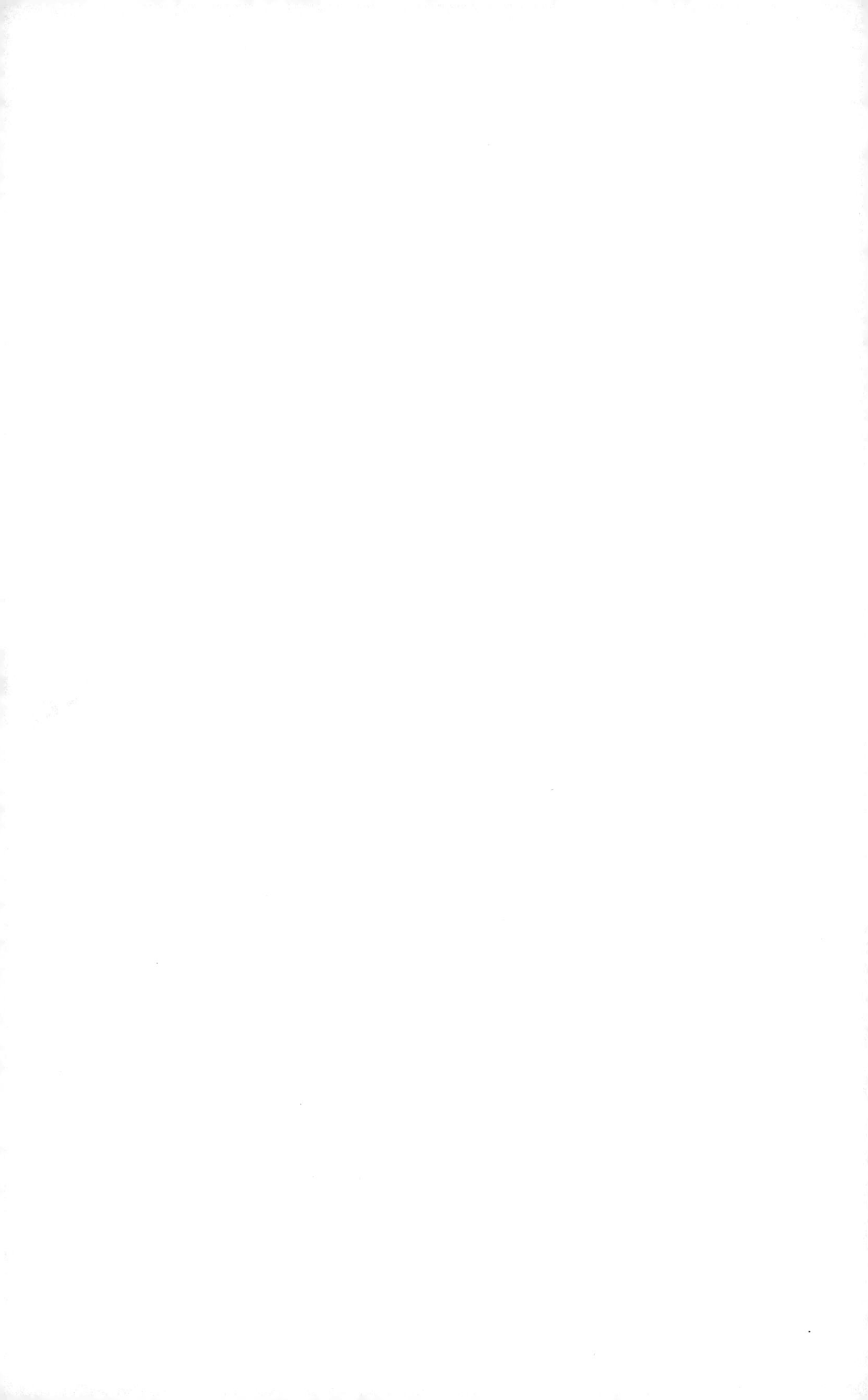

15

Acne

Ranella J. Hirsch and Alan R. Shalita
State University of New York Health Science Center at Brooklyn
Brooklyn, New York

Acne has multifaceted origins with a multitude of therapies addressing each. Optimum treatment is directed at the particular pathophysiology of the individual patient. Several factors contribute to the pathogenesis of acne. The first is an androgen-induced hypertrophy of the sebaceous glands with resultant overproduction of sebum.

The second factor in acne pathogenesis is hyperkeratosis of follicular epithelium and a consequent retention keratosis. Epithelial desquamation is altered and the stratum corneum becomes thicker and more cohesive. The horny cells continue to build up and eventually occlude the follicular canal with a dense keratotic plug [1]. The plugged follicle is termed a microcomedo; this is the earliest of all acne lesions [2].

The third factor in acne pathogenesis is the proliferation of *Propionibactorium acnes*, a normal inhabitant of skin flora. A condition for overgrowth in this medium is an anaerobic site filled with a lipid substrate. *P. acnes* hydrolyzes serum triglycerides to glycerol and free fatty acids as part of its metabolism. It is believed that *P. acnes* thereby sets the stage for the rupture of the comedo by the release of low molecular weight chemotactic factors, which diffuse through the thinned follicular epithelium and attract neutrophils into the comedonal lumen. There, the neutrophils release hydrolytic enzymes that damage the follicle wall and lead to its rupture. When closed comedones rupture and extrude their contents into the dermis instead of onto the surface of the skin, inflamed papules, pustules, and nodules result. Deeper lesions may heal with atrophic or, less commonly, hypertrophic scarring. In the most severe disease, termed acne conglobata, numerous inflamed nodules become confluent and form sinuses, and scarring can be extensive. Each of these causal factors is a potential target for therapy.

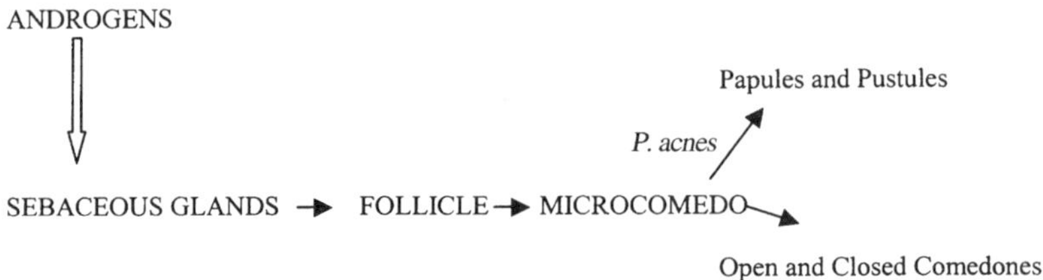

FIGURE 1 Pathogenesis of acne.

The aforementioned sequence of inflammatory events (Fig. 1) is fueled by a variety of pathologic processes. The extruded sebum contains keratin, lipids, and hair, all of which can directly initiate inflammation by means of a nonimmune foreign body reaction. *P. Acnes* activates both complement pathways to produce additional chemotactic factors; this attracts more leukocytes and further exacerbates the inflammation. It is this fact that explains the rationale of antibiotic therapy for acne vulgaris. Antibiotic therapy works in a twofold capacity; it both reduces the absolute number of pathogenic organisms and also inhibits *P. acnes'* metabolic activity. They also exert anti-inflammatory activity by inhibiting leukocyte migration.

Other factors that contribute to acne microcomedo formation are the use of comedogenic substances, most notably halogenated hydrocarbons, certain greasy cosmetics, and exogenous free fatty acids (FFAs). Another factor is the myth among patients that the acne they see is the product of insufficient cleansing, which leads them to scrub their face. This friction can exacerbate acne by causing microcomedones to rupture and thereby initiate an inflammatory reaction [3]. Other myths that need to be corrected include the belief that greasy foods or chocolate contribute to acne flares.

Treatment must consider the whole person ie, one must not underestimate the psychological components of acne care and management. Many patients arrive with incorrect expectations as to the length of time required to see skin improvement after the initiation of therapy [4]. It must be emphasized to patients that acne management requires both time commitment and total compliance.

APPROACH TO THE ACNE PATIENT

Many therapeutic modalities exist. The correct one for each patient is best decided on afer a thorough history and physical examination are performed. Important questions include:

1. Prior treatments tried. What success or failures have you experienced with different therapies?

Table 1 Severity Grading Scale of Acneform Inflammatory Lesions

	Mild	Moderate	Severe
Pustules/Papules	Few to several	Several to many	Numerous and/or extensive
Nodules	None	Few to several	Many
Additional Factors	Psychosocial circumstances	Occupational difficulties	Inadequate therapeutic responsiveness

2. Any family history of acne?
3. Products used (cleansers, soaps, and moisturizers)?
4. Any history of menstrual flares.

They should also be questioned about any past irritation with medications obtained either over the counter or by prescription. Then, after examining the patient, we classify them as described in Table 1.

TOPICAL TREATMENT OF ACNE

Patients with mild acne (few to many comedones) will do well with only topical treatment; those with more severe and recalcitrant acne will require systemic medication. The ideal acne treatment would be entirely topical to avoid systemic effects. It would reduce abnormal keratinization, inhibit sebum production, and limit the production and activity of *P. acnes*. Although there is no topical agent available to do all of this, we have different modalities of treatment for the different pathophysiological components. We use estrogens or isotretinoin to limit sebum production, and Benzoyl peroxide and antibiotics to serve as antibacterials. Tretinoin is an effective medication to reduce hyperkeratosis.

Tretinoin

Subcategories of topical agents are comedolytics and antibactorials. In the comedolytic category, the most effective topical agent is tretinoin. It is agent of choice for noninflammatory acne comprised of open and closed comedones. Since the pioneer study by Kligman et al. in 1969, topical tretinoin has become a standard agent in the treatment of acne. Its efficacy in the reduction of lesions has been shown in multiple investigations [5]. Although the exact mode of action of tretinoin is unknown, current evidence suggests that topical tretinoin decreases cohesiveness of follicular epithelial cells with decreased microcomedo formation. Additionally, tretinoin stimulates mitotic activity and increased turnover of follicular epithelial cells causing extrusion of the comedones. This in turn reduces the number of inflammatory lesions resulting from the eventual rupture of the microcomedones [6]. This correlates with a histologic picture of acantholysis, parakeratosis, and thinning and loosening of the stratum corneum. This antikeratinizing activity of tretinoin has also been investigated [7]. New comedo formation is also prevented with continued use.

Another important consequence of this ''unplugging'' of lesions by tretinoin is that it makes the depths of the involved follicles less anaerobic and more accessible to benzoyl peroxide or topical antibiotics. The enhanced penetration yields a synergistic effect with increased drug efficacy and a faster response to treatment. Tretinoin also has the beneficial effect of lightening postinflammatory hyperpigmentation changes in pigmented patients [8]. With initial dosing, patients should be instructed in the proper application of tretinoin. The face should be washed no more than twice daily with a mild soap using the fingers rather than an abrasive cleanser. Astringents and harsh soaps are to be avoided. To avoid the irritating effects of tretinoin on wet skin, the skin should be permitted to dry over 20 to 30 minutes before application of a thin layer of tretinoin. It is recommended that a pea-sized drop be applied to the entire face, not just the affected area. In patients for whom the tretinoin is too irritating, therapy can be started every other or every third day.

Mild erythema and peeling may occur, but more severe dryness is to be avoided. Topical application of tretinoin can lead to local irritation; the irritancy increases as one progresses from the use of cream preparations to gels to the solution. It is therefore recommended to begin therapy at the lowest strength preparation and titrate to higher strengths as is needed and tolerated by the patient. In order of increasing strength we have 0.025% cream followed by 0.01% gel, then 0.05% cream then 0.025% gel, then 0.01% cream and 0.05% solution. The solution is the strongest and most irritating. The gel is drying and is for use with oily skin. The cream is lubricating and is for use in dry skin. There is also a microencapsulated form of tretinoin that seems to be equally efficacious but is less irritating. Many dermatologists now prefer to initiate treatment with this ''micro'' form of tretinoin.

Continual topical application leads to temporary thinning of the stratum corneum. Hence patients must be carefully instructed regarding their increased susceptibility to sunburn and irritation from cold. Topical astringents will also not be tolerated. The incidence of contact allergy with tretinoin is very small.

During the first few weeks, patients will likely experience redness, burning, and occasionally peeling. Most patients adapt to the medication after 3 to 5 weeks of therapy and are able to manage daily application. If treatment is initiated at a higher concentration, it is common to experience a flare of papules and pustules as the comedones are being extruded after 4 to 6 weeks. It is at this point when patient compliance is most vulnerable. This vulnerability is best managed with early and repeated reminders to patients of the likely sequence of events and reassurance that is a part of therapy. By the tenth week after the initiation of treatment, most patients have begun to improve. For the minority of patients unable to tolerate tretinoin, an alternate agent should be selected. Treatment may be continued for months to prevent recurrence of lesions, and all other topical acne agents should be stopped before the initiation of retinoic acid therapy.

Chemically, tretinoin is all transretinoic acid. Drug interactions are seen with use of concomitant topical medications, medicated or abrasive soaps and cleansers, and soaps and cosmetics that have a strong drying effect. Products with high concentrations of alcohol, astringents, spices, or lime should likewise be used with caution because of possible interaction with tretinoin.

Topical Isotretinoin

Topical isotretinoin was developed as a safer alternative to the oral medication. Although effective in mild to moderate inflammatory and noninflammatory lesions, it works only by affecting abnormal follicular keratinization. It has no effect on sebum production [9]. It is not available for use in the United States.

Adapalene

Adapalene is a synthetic derivative of napthoic acid with retinoid-like activity. Biochemical and pharmacological profile studies have shown that adapalene is a modulator of cellular differentiation, keratinization, and inflammatory processes suggesting that its therapeutic role is both as a comedolytic agent as well as an anti-inflammatory agent. In a randomized trial, adapalene 0.1% gel was more effective than tretinoin 0.025% gel against noninflammatory lesions, and as effective against inflammatory lesions in mild to moderate acne with a lower frequency of local irritation [10]. Volunteers in clinical trials frequently do not show the same response pattern as active patients in physician's offices. Clinically, the results with adapalene have been more erratic.

Tazarotene

The newest topical agent is tazarotene. Although conclusive data have not been submitted, it is assumed to have a similar mechanism of action to other retinoids. It has an irritation profile similar to that of tretinoin. It has been shown to be effective in acne treatment but formal, comparative clinical trials have not been completed. Some experience has shown improvement with inflammatory and noninflammatory lesions and some clinicians report excellent results, especially with stubborn comedones.

Salicylic Acid

Salicylic acid is effective against comedones and inflammatory lesions in acne vulgaris. It represents a useful but less effective option for patients unable to tolerate treatment with tretinoin, because its comedolytic activity is only approximately 25% that of tretinoin [11].

TOPICAL ANTIMICROBIALS

Benzoyl Peroxide

Benzoyl peroxide (BP) is a powerful oxidizing agent and antimicrobial that works by decreasing the population of *P. acnes*. It is most effective for inflammatory acne consisting of papules and pustules. Clinical studies show a modest reduction in comedones, probably as an indirect effect. Benzoyl peroxide has been shown to reduce the concentration of two skin bacteria, *P. acnes* and *S. epidermitis* by two logs [12]. BP has no effect on sebum production or composition [13].

Mild cases of acne often can be treated with BP alone. It is available without prescription in 2.5%, 5%, and 10% lotions, creams, gels, and cleansers. Water-based gels are less irritating, but alcohol in acetone-base gels, if tolerated, may be more effective. It produces a drying effect that varies from mild desquamation to scaliness, peeling, and cracking. It should be applied in a thin layer to the entire affected area. Cleansers should be left on the skin for 4 to 5 minutes before rinsing to achieve maximum benefit. Many patients experience mild erythema and scaling for the first several weeks of use but typically adapt quickly.

Irritation, redness, and scaling are common but generally mild side effects of topical BP use; a lower strength preparation is usually the easiest solution to this problem. Rarely, in 1 to 3% of patients, an allergic contact dermatitis may be seen; this responds to withdrawal of the offending agent [14]. BP can also bleach the color out of clothing.

Topical Antibiotics

Topical antibiotics are most useful in the management of mild inflammatory acne. They can be the initial treatment modality or used as an adjunct to treatment with tretinoin or benzoyl peroxide. Bacteriostatic antibiotics are thought to improve acne by decreasing the formation of by-products, but not necessarily the actual number, of *P. acnes*. Sublethal levels of antibiotic are able to reduce the production of chemotactic factors by *P. acnes* that play an important role in the disruption of microcomedones and the promotion of subsequent inflammation. Papular and pustular acne respond best; the activity of comedonal or cystic acne may not be altered. The topical antibiotics that have been used successfully are erythromycin and clindamycin. Oral agents that have been used include tetracycline, minocycline, doxycycline, erythromycin, clindamycin, and TMP-SMX [15]. Topical antibiotics appear not to be as effective as their systemic counterparts; this is likely a reflection of the drug's distribution into the follicle. However, we recommend starting with the topical antibiotics first, reserving the oral medications for more severe cases that have failed topical therapy. These agents should be applied twice daily to the point of mild dryness and erythema but not discomfort. Clinical experience suggests that clindamycin and erythromycin are easy to use and are equally efficacious. Clindamycin phosphate is available in 1% concentration in a hydroalcoholic vehicle as solutions and as a nonalcoholic lotion. There have been case reports of pseudomembranous colitis on rare occasions; care should be given in prescribing use in patients with a history of inflammatory bowel disease. Erythromycin base applied topically is nonsensitizing and effective. It is available as a 1.5% and 2% solution, 2% pledgets, 2% ointment, or a combination 3% erythromycin and 5% benzoyl peroxide (Benzamycin). Increased levels of *P. acnes* resistance has been reported in patients with patients treated with erythromycin alone. Resistance has not been seen in patients treated with a combination of benzoyl peroxide and erythromycin. Chalker et al. report a double-blind study comparing the effectiveness of 3% erythromycin and 5% benzoyl peroxide each alone and also in combination. The combination product was found to be better than any of the others especially for combined inflammatory lesions. This combination drug is, therefore, preferable [16]. Furthermore, the combination product is less irritating than erythromycin alone.

Xerac

Aluminum chloride hexahydrate (Xerac) is an effective antiperspirant that also has an antibacterial effect. It may be of use in cases of acne in which sweating is prominent or appears to be a contributing factor to the disease. However, its effects are not well studied.

Azelaic Acid

Azelaic acid is a dicarboxylic acid derived from *Pitysporum ovale* that was shown to be as effective as BP, retinoic acid, and tetracycline [17]. The exact mechanism of action of azelaic acid is not known. In vitro, azelaic acid has been shown to possess antimicrobial activity against *Propionibactorium acnes* and *Staphylococcus epidermidis*. The antimicrobial action may be attributable to inhibition of microbial cellular protein synthesis.

A normalization of keratinization leading to an anticomedonal effect of azelaic acid may also contribute to its clinical activity [18]. Electron microscopic and immunohistochemical evaluation of skin biopsies from human subjects treated with azelaic acid showed a reduction in the thickness of the stratum corneum, a reduction in number and size of keratohyalin granules, and a reduction in the amount and distribution of filaggrin (a protein component of keratohyalin) in epidermal layers. This is suggestive of the ability to decrease microcomedo formation [19]. However, clinical experience, to date, with this agent has been disappointing.

MISCELLANEOUS TOPICALS

Nicotinamide

Nicotinamide, which has potent anti-inflammatory activity in vitro, is available in a gel formulation that has more widespread use in Europe. Shalita et al. report a 1995 study on the efficacy of topical Nicotinamide in the management of inflammatory acne vulgaris. They report similar efficacy of 4% nicotinamide gel with 1% clindamycin gel. This is a particularly useful clinical finding inasmuch as there is continuing emergence of resistant micro-organisms with topical antimicrobials [20].

Drying and Peeling Agents

In selected patients, particularly those with pustular acne, agents that induce continuous mild drying and peeling of the skin can produce quick and effective results. Several products are available both over the counter and by prescription. The active ingredients are sulfur, salicylic acid, and resorcinol. The goal of therapy is to induce a continuous mild peel; this is achieved by modifying the strength and frequency of the applied product.

COMBINATION THERAPY

Because of acne's multifactorial origins, most patients respond better if therapy encompasses more than one area of pathophysiology. Combination therapy is therefore rational and effective. Sebaceous follicles undergoing acnegenesis are characterized by abnormal desquamation of the follicular epithelium. This results in the preclinical lesion, the microcomedo, which is the precursor to both inflamed and noninflamed clinical lesions. This suggests that tretinoin, which reduces abnormal desquamation, should be used in all patients unless precluded by skin sensitivity. In patients with comedonal acne, treatment should begin with tretinoin cream 0.05% applied daily. If there is no improvement after 8 weeks of treatment, increase to the 0.1% cream. Refractory cases may require use of the 0.05% liquid. Similarly, one may initiate therapy with the 0.01% gel or the 0.1% microencapsulated gel and progress to the 0.25% or 0.1% cream. Acne surgery may be undertaken after 1 month of tretinoin therapy.

The efficacy of benzoyl peroxide and topical antibiotics may be increased by concurrent therapy with tretinoin, because tretinoin increases the cutaneous penetration of other topically applied agents [3]. Benzoyl peroxide and topical antibiotics may exert a synergistic antimicrobial effect when used together; a preparation consisting of 3% erythromycin and 5% benzoyl peroxide in a gel base is more effective in the improvement of inflammatory acne than either agent alone [16].

We favor treatment of inflammatory acne with a sequential regimen of topical tretinoin and BP/erythromycin. The patient begins therapy with a topical antimicrobial agent such as Benzamycin. This should be used in conjunction with the lowest concentration of tretinoin available in the vehicle selected, usually the 0.01% gel, 0.025% cream, or the microencapsulated gel. If the patient's response is inadequate, we increase the tretinoin concentration. Failing improvement with this combination, an oral antibiotic can be added, either tetracycline 500 mg twice daily, doxycycline 100 mg twice daily, or minocycline 75 to 100 mg twice daily. Judicious use of intralesional corticosteroids and comedo extraction is of benefit during this treament program.

Most topical acne medications are applied twice daily. This can be amended to once daily or alternate-day dosing if a patient experiences irritation. Furthermore, when a patient uses two types of topical medications concomitantly, an alternating schedule of application is recommended to limit irritation.

Both the patient's skin type and his or her preference determine the choice of vehicle in a topical medication. Gels are nongreasy and have a drying effect, which may be a desirable treatment goal for patients with oily skin. Creams and lotions are cosmetically pleasing, moisturizing preparations that most patients find acceptable. Solutions, although drying, may be useful for application in large areas of the skin.

SYSTEMIC THERAPIES

Systemic treatments are indicated in the management of patients with moderate to severe involvement including inflammatory pustules, papules, nodules, and/or scarring. Systemic treatments for acne vulgaris include oral antibiotics, isotretinoin, and hormonal agents. There are strict guidelines for the use of each of these modalities given their propensity to cause side effects. Systemic therapy is, on the whole, more effective than topical treatment; this is presumably because the drugs penetrate the follicle more readily.

Oral Antibiotics

Oral antibiotics are indicated for several groups of patients with inflammatory acne: those with moderate to severe disease; those for whom topical therapy has failed or cannot be tolerated; those with involvement of the shoulders, back, and chest (areas where the application of topical antibiotic might be difficult); and those with mild to moderate acne in whom there is a potential for scarring and/or substantial pigmentary change.

The beneficial effects of antibiotics are multifold. In addition to decreasing the follicular concentration of *P. acnes*, levels of free fatty acid are also decreased. It is known that the bacteria and their FFA by-products secrete several chemotactic factors that cause the inflammatory response. Subacteriocidal levels of antibiotic can cause the decreased production of these inflammatory factors and therefore reduce the inflammatory response.

Patients should be reassured that multiple studies and years of clinical experience have abundantly shown that the long-term use of antibiotics in the management of acne vulgaris is safe and efficacious. Better clinical results and a lower rate of relapse after stopping antibiotics are achieved by starting treatment at higher dosages and tapering off only after control is achieved [21]. Typical starting doses are listed in Table 2. They must be taken for several weeks in order to be effective and are often used for weeks or months to achieve maximum

TABLE 2 Antibiotics Used to Treat Acne

Antibiotic	Usual Dose	Adverse Effects	Comments
Tetracycline	250–500 mg BID	GI upset Photosensitivity Vaginal candidosis	Best taken on empty stomach Highest incidence of GI upset Most widely prescribed antibiotic for ance Inexpensive
Erythromycin	500 mg BID	GI upset Vaginal candidosis	Resistance emerging Safe in pregnancy
Minocycline	50–100 mg BID	Vestibular disturbances Bule-gray pigmentary changes in areas of cutaneous inflammation Vaginal candidosis	Relatively expensive Must take with meals
Doxycycline	100 mg BID	GI upset Photosensitivity Vaginal candidosis	May take with meals Less expensive than Minocycline
Clindamycin	75–150 mg BID	Pseudomembranous colitis	Highly effective
Ampicillin	500 mg BID	Maculopapular rash	TCN alternative Efficacy with gram negative acne Safe in pregnancy
TMP/SMX	One DS tablet BID	Rash, hives Photosensitivity	Consider for resistant pustular acne Efficacy with gram negative acne

benefit. Attempts to control acne with short courses of antibiotics, as has been tried to manage premenstrual flares, are usually not effective and are not recommended [22].

Tetracycline is the most frequently prescribed oral antibiotic for acne. It is least expensive, has few side effects, and is well tolerated for long periods of time. It is effective in low doses because high concentrations are achieved in sebaceous follicles. After a 6-week course of treatment, inflammatory lesions are decreased by 50%. Because absorption is inhibited in the presence of bivalent cations such as present in foods and dairy products, the drugs must be taken on an empty stomach. This restriction can yield poor compliance.

Efficacy and compliance with treatment are obtained by starting tetracycline (TCN) administration at 500 mg BID and continuing at this dosage until a significant decrease in the number of lesions occurs. This usually occurs in 3 to 6 weeks [23]. Thereafter, the dose may be decreased to 250 mg BID or oral therapy may be changed to use of a topical antibiotic. Higher doses (1.5–3 g/day) may be needed for some patients. If there is no response after 6 weeks of treatment, treatment with tetracycline should be re-evaluated.

There are several significant side effects to tetracycline use, particularly GI upset and Candida vaginitis [24]. The incidence of photosensitivity is rare but is increased with the use of higher doses. Due to effects on the p450 system, women on certain oral contraceptives may need increased dosing of the OCP. Pseudotumor cerebri, a rare self-limited disorder, is a rare complication of tetracycline use. Patients should be monitored for the development of headaches and visual changes.

Minocycline is a tetracycline derivative that has been of use in cases of pustular acne that have not responded to other oral antibiotic agents. Rossman et al. reported three times daily 50 mg dosing of Minocycline versus 250 mg four times daily of tetracycline yielded significant improvement in patients to Minocycline who did not respond to tetracycline [25]. Compared with tetracycline, minocycline is more lipid soluble and better absorbed. On a clinical level, this translates to smaller doses. Although it is the most effective antibiotic available to treat acne, its cost may sometimes limit its widespread use. Increased efficacy, however, frequently translates into increased cost effectiveness.

Because its absorption is not significantly inhibited by food, it can be taken with meals; this decreases the frequency of GI upset. Like tetracycline, it significantly decreases the number of inflammatory acne lesions. Although minocycline was equal in efficacy to tetracycline in the quantitative reduction of acne lesions, treatment with minocycline led to a more rapid clinical improvement that treatment with tetracycline [26], as well as a greater and more persistent reduction in facial *P. acnes* counts and inflammatory lesions [27]. Thus, despite its cost, its simpler regime and early onset of clinical improvement justify its position as a first line acne agent.

Minocycline can cause reversible vestibular disturbances; the risk for this can be decreased by starting with low doses and titrating upward. The usual starting dose is 50 to 100mg BID. The dosage is tapered when a significant decrease in the number of lesions is observed, typically in 3 to 6 weeks. Minocycline, like other tetracycline-class antibiotics, can cause fetal harm when administered to a pregnant woman. If any tetracycline is used during pregnancy or if the patient becomes pregnant while taking these drugs, the patient should be apprised of the potential hazard to the fetus. The use of drugs of the tetracycline class during tooth development (last half of pregnancy, infancy, and childhood to the age of 8 years) may cause permanent discoloration of the teeth (yellow-gray-brown). It can also cause a blue discoloration of acne cysts or sites of trauma; this is reversible with discontinuation of the drug. Also, because of its high level of lipid solubility, it readily penetrates the cerebrospinal fluid (CSF). Consequently, in susceptible individuals CNS effects occur and must be carefully watched for. There are also rare reports of serum sickness–like reactions, hepatitis, and lupus.

Erythromycin is as effective as tetracycline at the same dose [15] at a greater cost. However, it is not used much anymore because of growing resistance. Doxycycline is also very effective in the treatment of acne. Doxycycline patients must be warned to avoid excessive exposure to sunlight because of the significant photosensitivity that accompanies its use. In one study, it was shown to be as clinically effective as Minocycline and less expensive [28]. Clindamycin is an extremely effective agent for acne. However, the risk of pseudomembranous colitis limits its systemic use to only very severe cases responsive to nothing else [29].

In certain patients, after long-term use of oral antibiotics for acne there is the development of pustules and cysts that grow gram negative organisms when cultured [2]. For this so-called gram negative acne, Ampicillin and Bactrim are the agents of choice. Ampicillin also has a limited role in pregnant women with acne in whom the use of tetracycline, erythromycin, and minocycline must be avoided. A dosage of 500 mg BID is maintained until satisfactory control is achieved. Bactrim (TMP-SMX) also has been shown to decrease FFA levels and inhibit inflammatory acne. Trimethoprim is very lipophilic, which enhances follicle preparation. Its use is limited by a high percentage of allergic reactions.

The emergence of strains of *P. acnes*, which are less sensitive to antibiotics, is a growing problem. Many strains of *P. acnes* are now resistant to erythromycin and cross-resistance to clindamycin occurs. Decreased sensitivity to tetracycline is also more common. There appears to be less resistance to doxycycline whereas most organisms remain sensitive to minocycline. The combination of BP and erythromycin appears to eliminate the less sensitive strains of *P. acnes*, and it is possible that concomitant use of BP and systemic antibiotics may offer a similar benefit. In the meantime, it is the consensus of most experts in the field that antibiotics should be used for relatively short periods of time as necessary and not for maintaining treatment unless absolutely necessary.

Hormonal Therapy

Hormonal therapy for acne, particularly in the form of oral contraceptives, has provided successful treatment for some 25 years. Although most patients with acne have no serum androgen abnormalities, patients with normal hormone levels may show a response. With the introduction of oral isotretinoin, hormonal therapy use has decreased, but the recent approval of an oral contraceptive for treating acne has renewed physician awareness of the benefits of these drugs in acne therapy. Estrogens given as anovulatory agents may be of use in moderate to severe or otherwise unresponsive cases of acne in young women. It is particularly of value in patients whose acne has characteristics that suggest a hormonal influence: inadequate response to other acne treatments, acne that began or worsened in adulthood, premenstrual flares of acne, patients with excessive facial oiliness, and acne accompanied by mild to moderate hirsuitism [30].

Undesirable antiandrogen side effects such as gynecomastia, impotence, decreased libido, and infertility generally preclude the use of these agents in men. The effect of the estrogen is systemic adrenal and androgen inhibition rather than local suppression at the gland site [1]. This means that small doses of androgen can overcome the sebum suppressive effects of large doses of estrogen in women as well as in men. There is direct correlation between the degree of sebaceous gland inhibition and acne improvement.

There are three options for treatment with hormonal manipulation. Estrogen suppression of ovarian androgen, glucocorticoid suppression of adrenal androgens, and antiandrogens such as spironolactone that work at the peripheral level. Ovarian hypersecretion of androgen production can be suppressed with oral contraceptive therapy. Oral contraceptives with estrogen (ethynyl estradiol) and progestins of low androgenic activity are most useful. In the United States, a triphasic norgestimate plus ethinylestradiol combination pill has lately been approved for the treatment of acne in women, on the basis of placebo-controlled studies showing its efficacy [31]. Improvement has been noted within 3 months of initiation of therapy [1].

Prednisone (5–10 mg) or dexmethasone (0.25–0.5 mg) administered at night are very useful in female patients with severe acne unresponsive to conventional therapy who suffer from adrenal gland overproduction of androgens. Taken at night, it suppresses the AM corticotropin surge and produces clinical improvement in some patients [32]. Concomitant administration of prednisone and estrogen may act synergistically in suppressing sebum production by inhibiting both adrenal and ovarian androgen production.

Spironolactone is, in addition to being a weak diuretic, an antiandrogen that blocks the binding of androgen to its receptor [33]. It has some utility in the treatment of recalcitrant acne in adult women. It must not be used in pregnant women because it can block the development of male genitalia in the developing fetus [34]. Therefore, it is recommended that it be used in conjunction with an oral contraceptive. It can be used when the source of the androgen is either adrenal or ovarian. Treatment should be initiated at 25 to 50 g/day. Many patients achieve satisfactory results at 50 to 100 g/day, but some may require as much as 200 g/day [30].

Indications for Spironolactone Use in Acne Treatment
Adult women with inflammatory facial acne
Presence of coexisting symptoms, such as irregular menses or symptoms of premenstrual syndrome
Inadequate response to standard acne treatment, including topical treatment, systemic antibiotics, or isotretinoin
Hormonal influence as suggested by
• premenstrual flares
• onset after age 25
• distribution on the lower face, including the mandibular line and chin
• coexistent facial hirsutism

Clinically, spironolactone yields a significant reduction in sebum production with a decrease in lesion counts. Side effects are dose related and include menstrual irregularities, breast tenderness, and a decrease in libido. The severity of these side effects is usually mild, and most women tolerate therapy well.

Cyproterone acetate is a potent androgen-receptor blocker and progestational agent. It is available outside the United States in several oral contraceptive products (2 mg cyproterone acetate in combination with 35–50 μg ethinyloestradiol). These preparations are equally effective in the treatment of acne, although treatment with the higher estrogen dose is associated with a greater frequency of estrogen-related side effects [35].

Isotretinoin

In a landmark paper [36], Peck et al. showed that isotretinoin (13-cis retinoic acid) produced profound improvement with prolonged periods of remission from clinical disease in patients with acne conglabata. Many investigators have verified their dramatic results and isotretinoin now stands as the agent of choice in the management of severe nodulocystic acne. Chemically, isotretinoin is 13-cis-retinoic acid and is related to both retinoic acid and retinol. The exact mechanism of action of isotretinoin is unknown [37]. It is, importantly, not suitable for all types of acne.

Indication for Treatment of Acne Patients with Isotretinoin
Severe recalcitrant nodular and cystic acne
Moderate acne unresponsive to conventional therapy
Patients who have scars or tend to scar (psychological or physical)
Severely dysmorphic patients
Acne fulminans (after appropriate pretreatment with antibiotics and glucocorticoids)
Gram negative folliculitis
Pyoderma faciale/rosacea fulminans (after appropriate pretreatment with antibiotics and glucocorticoids)

Proper patient selection is perhaps the most challenging task placed before the isotretinoin-prescribing clinician. A major requirement for the use of isotretinoin is a lack of responsiveness to more conventional therapies. Often patients that are incorrectly included in this group include patients with ''microcysts'', which are old, mature, closed comedones and old sebaceous cysts, and which can periodically become inflamed and thus clinically resemble nodulocystic acne lesions. These lesions will not respond to isotretinoin treatment and will require surgical removal. Similarly, lesions in old sinus tracts and tunnels will also require surgical removal; this is also the case in hidroadenitis suppurativa [3].

A complete medical history must be obtained before isotretinoin therapy. Patients with a history of pancreatitis, coronary artery disease, and/or hepatitis must be carefully monitored while receiving treatment. Importantly, contrary to what many physicians believe, age is not, in itself, a factor in patient selection.

Oral administration of isotretinoin results in a direct or indirect modification of several of the main factors that contribute to the pathogenesis of acne. It causes a rapid reduction in the size and activity of sebaceous glands by inhibiting differentiation of sebocytes; the result is a pronounced decrease in sebum production and a secondary suppression of *P. acnes*, which uses sebum as a nutrient. Isotretinoin also has anti-inflammatory properties and inhibits comedogenesis [38].

These effects are maintained during treatment and persist at various levels after therapy. Clinical improvement in nodular acne patients occurs in associaton with a reduction in sebum secretion. The decrease in sebum secretion is temporary and is related to the dose and duration of treatment with isotretinoin, and reflects a reduction in sebaceous gland size and an inhibition of sebaceous gland differentiation.

The cumulative dose may be more important than the duration of therapy. A cumulative dose of greater than 120 mg/kg is associated with significantly better long-term remission [39]. This dosage level can be achieved by either 1 mg/kg/day for 5 months or at a smaller dosage for a longer period. A standard course of isotretinoin therapy is 16 to 20 weeks. Approximately 85% of patients clear at the end of 16 weeks; 15% require longer treatment. Side effects are related to the dosage. Patients can be treated for a longer duration at a lower dosage if mucocutaneous side effects become a problem.

Strauss et al. reported the result of a double-blind study evaluating the efficacy of three different dosing levels (0.1, 0.5, 1.0 mg/kg/day) in the treatment of 150 patients with nodulocystic acne. A highly significant clinical response was seen in at all doses with no significant difference in the clinical response between doses. However, 42% of the patients who received the low dose required retreatment with isotretinoin after cessation of therapy. This finding, coupled with the lack of significant differences in the clinical side effects and laboratory abnormalities suggest that higher dosing levels be suggested for the treatment of nodulocystic acne [37].

Approximately 39% of patients relapse and require oral antibiotics or additional isotretinoin. Some patients require multiple courses of therapy. The response to repeat therapy is consistently successful, and side effects are similar to previous courses.

Many patients experience a moderate to severe flare of acne during the initial weeks of treatment. Starting at 10 to 20 mg twice daily and gradually increasing the dosage during the first 4 to 6 weeks can minimize this. Treatment is discontinued at the end of 20 to 30 weeks and the patient observed for a period of 2 to 5 months. Those patients with persistently severe acne may receive a second course of treatment after the posttreatment observation period. Truncal acne relapses more than facial acne [40].

Patients on isotretinoin require certain laboratory tests before embarking on a treatment regimen and also during their course on the medication. Before treatment, we recommend a full liver panel, a complete blood count, a triglyceride level, and a pregnancy test. Triglycerides should be rechecked at 2 to 4 week intervals. Blood counts and liver functions should be checked every 6 to 8 weeks. Pregnancy tests should be performed at every visit.

Side effects occur frequently, are dose dependent, and are reversible shortly after discontinuing treatment. The most common side effects are mucous/skin effects, elevated triglyceride levels, musculoskeletal effects, and headaches. The skin of certain sensitive individuals may become excessively red, edematous, blistered, or crusted. These effects are proportional to the strength of the preparation used, ie, the stronger the preparation, the greater the chance for irritation. Thus the recommendations for treatment are to begin at the lowest-dose preparation and increase in strength as tolerated by the patient [36,41]. The most significant effect of isotretinoin is that of teratogenicity. It is a potent teratogen with known involvement of craniofacial, cardiac, thymic, and CNS structures [42]. It is not mutagenic, however; women can safely get pregnant after a course of tretinoin. It is recommended that they should wait for 1 month after stopping isotretinoin treatment and one normal menstrual cycle [43].

Historically, a number of physicians had inadvertently prescribed isotretinoin to pregnant women. For this reason, the manufacturer introduced a pregnancy prevention program. Women must be educated about risks to the fetus and the absolute need for reliable contraception. Our procedure is to perform a pregnancy test on all sexually active women and delay treatment until the third day of their next normal menstrual period. We generally require two forms of contraception and repeat pregnancy tests regularly.

ADJUNCTIVE THERAPY

Acne Surgery

Gentle removal of comedones by pressing over the lesion with a comedo extractor both serves to relieve the patient of unsightly lesions and enhance compliance with treatment. We prefer the key hole extractor (Shalita) and use a # 11 blade to lance closed comedones. One must take caution to avoid overvigorous expression of comedones as this can lead to an increased inflammatory response. Recurrence of comedones after removal is common. Open comedones have been shown to recur within 24 to 40 days and closed comedones within 30 to 50 days. This can be significantly reduced with concomitant use of tretinoin. An alternative method for closed comedones is to use gentle electrodessication with an epilating needle at the lowest setting.

Intralesional Corticosteroids

Intralesional corticosteroids are the therapy of choice for nodular acne lesions. The high local concentration of corticosteroid injected leads to a rapid involution of these nonpyogenic, sterile, inflammatory lesions [44]. Most lesions, especially early ones, will flatten and disappear within 72 hours after injection. Especially purulent nodules can be incised and drained. Care should be taken to insert the needle through the thinnest portion of the cyst roof and deposit into the cyst cavity. Atrophy may occur if steroids are injected into the base of the cyst. Patients can be reassured that if skin depression does occur, in most cases it is temporary. Small lesions are injected with 2.5 to 3 mg/ml of Triamcinolone Acetate and larger ones with 5 mg/ml. Generally the particular concentration used is of less importance than the total amount given.

In the past, superficial radiographic therapy, ultraviolet light therapy, and cryotherapy have been used with some success in acne management. Superficial radiographic therapy worked by temporarily suppressing the sebaceous glands. However, this treatment modality comes with significant side effects including a marked increase in the risk of eventual thyroid carcinoma [45]. For this reason, this therapy is rarely used today. There is no proof that ultraviolet (UV) light therapy is effective and cryosurgery is rarely used anymore. Vleminckx's solution (sulfurated lime) with hot compresses for 10 to 20 minutes twice a day are very useful in very active, nodular disease. Alpha hydroxy acids are available in topical cream or lotion formulations or as a peeling agent. They function by reducing corneocyte cohesion and may have some efficacy in the total management of a patient, although little hard data are available [46].

Scar Revision

Various methods, including dermabrasion, chemical peeling, laser resurfacing, punch grafts, and collagen injections can be used to improve atrophic acne scarring. Consultation with a dermatological or plastic surgeon is often advisable in the management of acne scarring. Generally it is advisable to wait until disease activity has been gone for several months. During dermabrasion the epidermis and part of the dermis is planed away with a high-speed, motor-driven, finely abrasive brush. Re-epithelialization takes 3 to 4 weeks.

Scar excision may be the method of choice for those patients with pitted scars that are too deep to be planed by dermabrasion. These deep or "ice pick" scars may be excised and closed carefully for good cosmetic result. There are also collagen suspensions and implants that are used to correct depressed cutaneous scars.

In summary, acne therapy begins with a thorough evaluation of the patient, including a thorough history. A treatment program can then be designed around the particular pathophysiological components of their presentation. Modifications can be made for the care of each individual. Patients need to have realistic expectations. Although cure is not a goal in acne treatment, current therapies permit excellent control for patients. If patient and physician are able to stay the course of therapy, the management of acne can prove to be a most rewarding experience for both.

REFERENCES

1. Pochi PE. Endocrinology of Acne. *J Invest Dermatol* 1984; 120:351–355.
2. Leyden JJ, EA. Gram negative folliculitis: a complication of antibiotic therapy in acne vulgaris. *Br J Dermatol* 1973; 88:583.

3. Shalita A. Acne vulgaris: pathogenesis and treatment. *Cosmet Toiletries* 1983; 98: 57–60.
4. Drake L, EA. Guidelines for treatment of acne vulgaris. *J Am Acad Dermatol* 1990; 22(4):676–680.
5. Kligman AM, Fulton JE Jr, Plewig G. Topical Vitamin A in acne vulgaris. *Arch Dermatol* 1969; 99:469–476.
6. Leyden JJ, Shalita AR. Rational therapy for acne vulgaris: an update on topical treatment. *J Am Acad Dermatol* 1986; 15:907-914.
7. Eichner R, KM, Capetola RJ, Gendimenico GJ, Mezick JA. Effects of topical retinoids on cytoskeletal proteins: implications for retinoid effects on epidermal differentiation. *J Invest Dermatol* 1992; 98:154–161.
8. Bulengo-Ransby SM, Griffiths CE, Kimbrough-Green CK, et al. Topical tretinoin (retinoic acid) therapy for hyperpigmented lesions caused by inflammation of the skin in black patients. *New Engl J Med* 1993; 328:1438–1443.
9. Chalker DK, Lester JL Jr, Smith JG Jr, et al. Efficacy of a topical isotretinoin 0.05% gel in acne vulgaris: results of a multicenter, double-blind investigation. *J Am Acad Dermatol* 1987; 17:251–254.
10. Shalita AR, WJ, Chalker DK, et al. A comparison of the efficacy and safety of adapalene gel 0.1% and tretinoin gel 0.025% in the treatment of acne vulgaris: a multicenter trial. *J Am Acad Dermatol* 1996; 34:482–485.
11. Shalita A. Treatment of mild and moderate acne vulgaris with salicylic acid in an alcohol-detergent vehicle. *Cutis* 1981; 28:556–561.
12. Mills OH Jr, Marsden JR, Kligman AM. Acne vulgaris: oral therapy with tetracycline and topical therapy with Vitamin A acid. *Arch Dermatol* 1982; 106:200–203.
13. Shalita A. Topical acne therapy. *Dermatol Clin* 1983; 1:399–403.
14. Lever L, MR. Current views on the etiology, pathogenesis, and treatment of acne vulgaris. *Drugs* 1990; 39:681–692.
15. Gammon WR, Meyer C, Lantis S, et al. Comparative efficacy of oral erythromycin versus oral tetracycline in the treatment of acne vulgaris: a double blind study. *J Am Acad Dermatol* 1986; 14:183–186.
16. Chalker DK, Shalita A, Smith JG, Swann RW. A double-blind Study of the effectiveness of a 3% erythromycin and 5% benzoyl peroxide combination in the treatment of acne vulgaris. *J Am Acad Dermatol* 1983; 9:933–936.
17. Mayer da Silva A, Gollnick H, Imcke E, et al. Azelaic acid vs. placebo: effects on normal human keratinocytes and melanocytes. *Acta Dermatol Venereol* 1987; 67: 116–123.
18. Fitton A, Goa KL. Azelaic acid: a review of its pharmacological properties and therapeutic efficacy in acne and hyperpigmentary skin disorders. *Drugs* 1991; 41: 780–798.
19. Bladon PT, BB, Cunliffe WJ, et al. Topical azelaic acid and the treatment of acne: a clinical and laboratory comparison with oral tetracycline. *Br J Dermatol* 1986; 114:493–499.
20. Shalita AR, Smith JG, Parish LC, Sofman MS, Chalker DK. Topical nicotinamide compared with clindamycin gel in the treatment of inflammatory acne vulgaris. *Internat J Dermatol* 1995; 34(6):434–437.
21. Greenwood R, BB, Cunliffe WJ. Evaluation of a therapeutic strategy for the treat-

ment of acne vulgaris with conventional therapy. *Br J Dermatol* 1986; 114:353–358.

22. Rajka G. On therapeutic approaches to some special types of acne. *Acta Dermatovener* 1986; 120(suppl):39–42.
23. Cunliffe W. Evolution of a strategy for the treatment of acne. *J Am Acad Dermatol* 1987; 25:698–705.
24. Reisner R. Anti-biotic and anti-inflammatory therapy of acne. *Dermatol Clin* 1983; 1:385–397.
25. Rossman RE. Minocycline treatment of tetracycline resistant and tetracycline responsive acne vulgaris. *Cutis* 1981; 27:196–197.
26. Hubbell CG, Hobbs ER, Rist T, White JW. Efficacy of minocycline compared with tetracycline in treatment of acne vulgaris. *Arch Dermatol* 1982; 118:989–992.
27. Leyden JJ, McGinley KJ, Kligman AM. Tetracycline and minocycline treatment: effects on skin surface lipid levels and propionibacterium acnes. *Arch Dermatol* 1982; 118:19–22.
28. Laux B. Treatment of acne vulgaris: a comparison of doxycycline versus minocycline. *Hautarzt* 1989; 40:577–581.
29. Christian GL, Krueger GG. Clindamycin versus placebo as adjunctive therapy in moderately severe acne. *Arch Dermatol* 1975; 111:997–1000.
30. Shaw J. Antiandrogen and hormonal treatment of acne. *Dermatol Clin* 1996; 14:803–811.
31. Redmond GP, Olson WH, Lippman JS, et al. Norgestimate and ethinyl estradiol in the treatment of acne vulgaris: a randomized, placebo-controlled trial. *Obstet Gynecol* 1997; 89:615–622.
32. Habif TE. Acne, Rosacea, and Related Disorders. Clinical Dermatology: 162.
33. Held BL, Nader S, Rodriguez-Rigau LJ, et al. Acne and hyperandrogenism. *J Am Acad Dermatol* 1984; 10:223–226.
34. Goodfellow A, EA. Oral Spironolactone improves acne vulgaris and reduces sebum excretion. *Br J Dermatol* 1984; 111:209–214.
35. Colver GB, Dawber RPR. Cyproterone acetone and two doses of estrogen in female acne: a double blind comparison. *Br J Dermatol* 1988; 118:95–99.
36. Peck GL, Olsen TG, Yoder FW, et al. Prolonged remissions of cystic and conglobate acne with 13-cis-retinoic acid. *New Engl J Med* 1979; 300:329–333.
37. Strauss JS, RR, Shalita AR, Konecky E, Pochi PE, Comite H, Exner JH. Isotretinoin therapy for acne: results of a multicenter dose-response study. *J Am Acad Dermatol* 1984; 10(3):490–496.
38. Ward A, Brogden RN, Heel RC, et al. Isotretinoin: a review of its pharmacological properties and therapeutic efficacy in acne and other skin disorders. *Drugs* 1984; 28:6–37.
39. Falk ES, Stenvold SE. Long term effects of isotretinoin in the treatment of severe nodulocystic acne. Riv Eur Sci Med Farmacol 1992; 14:215–220.
40. Chivot M, Midoun H. Isotretinoin and Acne—a study of relapses. *Dermatologica* 1990; 180:240–243.
41. Peck GL, Olsen, TG, Butkus D, et al. Isotretinoin versus placebo in the treatment of cystic acne. *J Am Acad Dermatol* 1982; 6:735–745.

42. Dai WS, LaBraico JM, Stern RS. Epidemiology of isotretinoin exposure during pregnancy. *J Am Acad Dermatol* 1992; 26:599–606.
43. Farrell LN, Strauss JS, Stranieri AM. The treatment of severe cystic acne with 13-cisretinoic acid. Evaluation of sebum production and the clinical response in a multiple dose trial. *J Am Acad Dermatol* 1980; 3:602-611.
44. Levine R, Rasmussen JE. Intralesional corticosteroids in the treatment of nodulocystic acne. *Arch Dermatol* 1983; 119:480–481.
45. DeGroot L, PE. Thyroid carcinoma and radiation. A Chicago epidemic. *J Am Med Assoc* 1975; 225:487.
46. Van Scott E Yu RJ. Alpha hydroxy acids: procedures for use in clinical practice. *Cutis* 1989; 43:222–228.

16

Drug Therapy of Psoriasis

John Y. M. Koo and Jack Maloney
University of California at San Francisco Medical Center
San Francisco, California

I. INTRODUCTION

Before World War II, in the days of Dr. Goeckerman and Dr. Ingram, the mainstay of Western medicine for the treatment of psoriasis was limited to coal tar, anthralin, and ultraviolet B (UVB) phototherapy, supplemented by various adjunctive therapeutic measures such as salicylic acid and moisturizers. However, in the past half-century since the end of World War II, numerous therapeutic options have been devised to enrich the therapeutic armamentarium. These range from topical steroids in all different strengths, intralesional steroids, calcipotriene, tazarotene, and PUVA phototherapy to various systemic agents, such as methotrexate and the most recent FDA-approved addition, cyclosporine (Neoral). Despite this virtual explosion in therapeutic options, the management of psoriasis remains a challenge to clinicians. This is because of several peculiarities of psoriasis. First, although psoriatic plaques usually look similar from patient to patient, the way in which they respond to any particular treatment may be highly unpredictable. It is not unusual for one patient to respond beautifully to one medication, while the exact same medication has no efficacy for another patient with identical-looking psoriatic plaques. Moreover, even in patients who seem to have relatively responsive psoriatic lesions, one can frequently identify certain plaques that are much more resistant to treatment than the others. This is truly a mystery of psoriasis. For example, two psoriatic plaques with similar appearances might be treated with a systemic agent or phototherapy, and one plaque resolves completely while the other responds partially or not at all. These commonly observed phenomena defy currently popular genetic and immunological theories on the pathogenesis of psoriasis, since each individual is presumed to have the same genetic and immunological characteristics throughout his or her body. To improve resistant psoriasis, treatment modalities frequently need to be used creatively, with the sequential use of different combinations.

In addition to the challenges of trying to eradicate resistant psoriasis plaques, there is also the challenge of providing patients with an effective long-term maintenance strategy that is both safe and convenient. Some of the newer therapeutic modalities such as superpotent topical steroids or cyclosporine are ideally suited for use as ''quick fixes'' due to the rapidity of their onset of action. However, since psoriasis is a chronic disease, with many patients requiring ongoing, maintenance therapy to keep the condition under control, simply providing a ''quick fix'' may not be enough; one needs to devise a strategy for long-term control that has an optimal benefit-to-risk ratio. The clinician should carefully consider how to make the shift from the short-term solutions to a maintenance regimen, so as to minimize recurrence or rebound during the transitional period. Although phototherapy, especially UVB phototherapy, is generally thought to be safe for long-term use, it is not very convenient for busy, working individuals. On the other hand, the most reliable systemic agents, such as etretinate, cyclosporine, or methotrexate, are all associated with possible cumulative side effects. In view of this, the need for a safe and convenient agent for long-term use has yet to be fully met. As an interim measure, rotational therapy, in which the maintenance regimen is altered every year or two, or at some other periodic interval, is widely practiced in order to minimize the cumulative side effects to one organ system [1]. So, despite the enrichment in our therapeutic options over the past half-century, psoriasis continues to challenge us, and any new safe and effective addition to the therapeutic armamentarium is welcome.

The above discussion is meant to provide a general overview and the proper perspective for the current state of affairs with regard to drug therapy of psoriasis. In the next section, each individual agent will be discussed, one at a time, with an emphasis on clinically relevant information thought to be useful for the average practitioner. The order of presentation follows a ''1–2–3'' scheme, whereby topical therapies are discussed first, followed by drug therapy involved in phototherapy, and then systemic agents.

II. TOPICAL THERAPIES

A. Coal Tar

Coal tars have been used in the treatment of psoriasis since the nineteenth century, and although the therapeutic efficacy of crude coal tar in psoriasis is well known, we have only limited knowledge of its mode of action [2]. It may be used effectively as monotherapy or in combination with other treatment modalities [3]. The safety and efficacy of crude coal tar in conjunction with ultraviolet light B phototherapy was discovered and popularized by Dr. Goeckerman of the Mayo Clinic in the 1920s. Original Goeckerman therapy is conducted on an inpatient basis, in which black crude coal tar is applied liberally all over the patient's body; this tar is left on for 24 h per day. UVB phototherapy is administered before the tar is applied or after it is washed off. The Goeckerman regimen remains an intensive daily therapy that is usually conducted for a period of several weeks; however, nowadays it is often done on an outpatient basis. The black tar is usually available in a concentration of 2, 5, and 10%; salicylic acid or lactic acid, also in a concentration of 2, 5, or 10%, can be added to the tar to enhance the therapeutic effect in patients with thick, scaly lesions. Dr. Goeckerman also realized that, in addition to the topical treatments, UVB phototherapy needs to be optimized and, for many patients, this would mean a gradual increase in the millijoules of UVB used, until a dosage close to the minimal erythema dose is reached. Moreover, he recognized the need for intense, localized applications of light for more resistant lesions, such as psoriatic plaques on the shins. At the Mayo Clinic, where Goeckerman therapy was devised, truly recalcitrant lesions are often isolated by the use of zinc oxide paste to protect the normal skin, and a hot quartz lamp is used to deliver light at a level higher than the minimal erythema dose for added efficacy. In short, the use of black tar in an optimal concentration, combined with both aggressive and creative applications of UVB phototherapy, constitutes the Goeckerman regimen—a therapy that is probably still the fastest and safest treatment for psoriasis, with a reputation for long-term remissions [2].

Although the Goeckerman regimen has been practiced for more than half a century, patients receiving this treatment have experienced very few adverse systemic effects, other than salicylate toxicity, which may occur rarely when salicylic acid is applied topically in large amounts or at high concentrations [4]. Because of its proven track record of safety with regard to systemic side effects, Goeckerman therapy can be used to clear widespread, recalcitrant psoriasis among pregnant women, immunosuppressed patients, and children, or anyone for whom the use of other agents (e.g., methotrexate or PUVA phototherapy) may pose significantly more risk of toxicity.

Unfortunately, because of the cost-cutting measures taken by parties such as Medicare and insurance companies, access to Goeckerman therapy has been diminishing in recent years. Moreover, the use of brown tar (e.g., liquor carbonis detergens or "LCD") in place of black tar, combined with outpatient UVB therapy, has frequently been mislabeled as "modified Goeckerman." Brown tar is made from the extracts or refined products of crude coal tar, and is available in many different formulations for outpatient use; brown tar products, however, are markedly less effective than black tar. Thus, LCD, tar soaks, tar shampoos, etc., have some limited utility, but the gradual loss of the capacity to conduct true Goeckerman therapy is a significant therapeutic step backward, despite the advent of more convenient, systemic agents.

B. Anthralin

Anthralin was originally developed from an herbal medication called Goa powder in South America. It is moderately effective and quite safe in plaque psoriasis, both for short- and long-term use; the major side effect is occasional irritation. As for the mechanism of action, anthralin is known to have antimitotic activity and other effects at the cellular level; however, it is not clear which of these actions are therapeutic in psoriasis [5]. Anthralin has been extensively used in Europe, especially in England, as part of the Ingram regimen—a combination of anthralin and UVB phototherapy [6]. However, anthralin's potential to cause permanent staining on furniture, clothing, sinks, etc., has greatly limited its popularity in the United States. To rectify this situation, a new formulation of anthralin, called Micanol, was developed, in which anthralin is encased in a special lipid covering designed to break down and release anthralin only when Micanol is in contact with body temperature, thereby greatly diminishing the risk of staining [7,8]. In clinical trials, Micanol was found to be just as effective as traditional anthralin, but had a greatly reduced likelihood of staining the skin and other materials [9]. Therefore, the use of anthralin might see a resurgence with the availability of this new formulation.

Anthralin powder is commercially available. Therefore, anthralin can be compounded in various vehicles, such as a nonionic base cream, petrolatum, etc., to create a higher concentration for better efficacy. It is prepared in varying strengths, from 0.1% up to 10% or higher when specially compounded. If compounded, it is generally necessary to also add 3 to 10% salicylic acid, not only as a keratolytic, but, more importantly, as a preservative to retard the oxidation of anthralin. As mentioned, the main side effect of anthralin is irritation. Irritation is more likely to occur in the perilesional skin than on the psoriasis plaque itself. For this reason, the application of anthralin, especially at higher concentrations, needs to be limited to the lesional skin. Short contact treatment of 30 min or less will likely reduce irritation, and this short treatment period has been shown to be about as effective as conventional overnight treatment [10–12]. Anthralin is also available for scalp use, both in the traditional formulation (Drithoscalp) or as the new formulation, Micanol.

C. Topical Steroids

There are numerous topical steroids available, ranging from superpotent topical steroids to the very weak over-the-counter agents, such as 1% hydrocortisone.

As compared to eczema, psoriasis generally requires a stronger topical steroid to achieve an adequate response. The strongest topical steroids, clobetasol (Temovate) and halobetasol (Ultravate), are not only limited in the duration of their usage (generally 2 weeks' usage at a time), but also in the absolute amount of the medication that can be used per week (generally 50 g or less per week). The major side effects of topical steroids are skin atrophy and adrenal suppression, where the risk is greater as the strength of the topical steroid is increased.

The strongest of the topical steroids are ideal ''quick-fix'' agents in the treatment of psoriasis, because they have a rapid onset of action, and rarely cause any side effects such as irritation in the short term. However, for long-term use, topical steroids have serious shortcomings. Not only can topical steroids cause skin atrophy and adrenal suppression, but they may also show a diminished effectiveness with time, known as tachyphylaxis. Due to their potential for tachyphylaxis and a reputation for short remission periods, the long-term use of strong topical steroids as the mainstay of maintenance therapy may not be the optimal course of action.

D. Intralesional Steroids

Intralesional injections of triamcinolone in the usual concentration of 5 to 10 mg/cc is a very effective option for resolving small amounts of residual, truly recalcitrant, psoriatic lesions. Unlike topical steroids, intralesional steroids generally induce long remission periods. Intralesional steroids can also be effective in controlling localized pustular psoriasis. However, the usefulness of intralesional steroids is limited to only small areas of application, since excessive use can lead to a systemic steroid effect.

E. Systemic Steroids

Unlike the management of generalized eczema, the use of systemic steroids in the treatment of psoriasis is generally not recommended due to the well known risk of rebound and pustular conversion [13,14]. ''Rebound'' refers to the phenomenon whereby the psoriasis becomes more widespread and recalcitrant over time; this may occur as a consequence of treatment with systemic steroids. ''Pustular conversion'' refers to a situation in which plaque-type psoriasis converts to the more dangerous pustular lesions as the steroid effect wears off. Both of these phenomena are well documented. Because of the availability of other systemic agents such as methotrexate and cyclosporine, which can provide rapid improvement without the associated risk of rebound or pustular conversion, there is currently very little justification for the use of systemic steroids in the treatment of psoriasis [13].

F. Calcipotriene (Dovonex)

Calcipotriene (Dovonex), which is called calcipotriol in Europe, is a modified vitamin D molecule known to be efficacious in the treatment of psoriasis. It works by inhibiting the proliferation of keratinocytes and causing their terminal differentiation [15,16]. Calcipotriene is currently available in ointment, cream, or solution form. Calcipotriene ointment is slightly more efficacious than calcipotriene cream. When the ointment formulation was used twice per day in large clinical series, it was slightly more effective than fluocinonide (Lidex) ointment applied twice per day [17,18].

Calcipotriene is free of unwanted steroid effects such as skin atrophy, tachyphylaxis, and adrenal suppression, with the main side effect being lesional or perilesional irritation. Mild stinging, burning, or pruritus may occur in as many as one out of five patients when they initially use calcipotriene ointment, but in most cases, these sensations resolve over time. Only 2 to 3% of patients in the clinical studies had to terminate their participation due to persistent irritation [18]. In actual clinical usage, the irritation rate appears to be much lower, probably due to the flexibility the clinician has in modifying the regimen. For example, physicians can instruct patients to use calcipotriene ointment every other day, or in combination with topical steroids or phototherapy, which may decrease the likelihood of irritation from this agent. The use of more than 100 g per week of calcipotriene ointment can lead to symptomatic hypercalcemia [18,19]. In the pediatric age group, the administration of this agent should be conducted with regular assessments of serum or 24-h urine calcium levels, since the amount of calcipotriene ointment that is safe for each age group in the pediatric population has not been established.

Calcipotriene is more effective when applied twice per day versus once per day, especially during the first month of therapy. In fact, during this time period, the efficacy of calcipotriene ointment falls by approximately 50% when it is applied only once per day rather than twice per day [18]. Therefore, if the patient is not willing or able to use the ointment formulation twice per day due to its greasiness, the optimal regimen for that individual may involve the use of calcipotriene cream in the morning and ointment at night.

G. Tazarotene (Tazorac)

Tazarotene is a modified vitamin A molecule formulated as a topical agent for the treatment of psoriasis. It is FDA-approved for both the treatment of psoriasis and acne. Tazarotene appears to modulate three major pathogenic factors in psoriasis: keratinocyte hyperproliferation, abnormal keratinocyte differentiation, and the infiltration of inflammatory components [20]. The major advantage of this agent is that it works just as well applied once per day as twice per day, and it seems to induce a much longer remission of psoriasis than topical steroids [21]. It is recommended for use in patients with total body surface involvement of 20% or less; however, there are no known systemic side effects (apart from controversy regarding pregnancy risks) even when this agent is applied to a larger total body surface area.

Tazarotene is currently available as a 0.1% and 0.05% gel. In terms of clinical efficacy, tazarotene 0.1% gel applied once per day works about as well as fluocinonide (Lidex) cream applied twice per day [21]. The major side effect of tazarotene gel is its propensity to cause irritation. In clinical studies, approximately 10% of the subjects who used tazarotene 0.05% gel twice per day discontinued the study, and approximately 12% of those who used the 0.1% gel dropped out [22]. This is not surprising when one considers the fact that topical retinoids are known to be more irritating than most other topical agents. The total cumulative irritation rate, including complaints of "burning," "stinging," and other symptomatology, is approximately 20% of the clinical research subjects. However, in actual clinical usage, the irritation rate may again turn out to be significantly less because of the flexibility inherent in clinical practice; for example, tazarotene may be used every other day or in combination with a topical steroid to minimize the irritation.

In addition to first-line use just like any other topical agent, there is a theoretical possibility that tazarotene may find its niche as a therapeutic enhancer to other treatment modalities, including other topical therapies and phototherapy. With regard to the combination use of tazarotene gel and UVB phototherapy, a preliminary analysis of the clinical research data suggests there may be synergy between the two therapies. It takes approximately half the time for psoriatic plaques to show significant improvement when tazarotene 0.1% gel is used in combination with UVB phototherapy, versus UVB phototherapy used alone or in conjunction with the vehicle [23]. Moreover, topical retinoids are known to enhance penetration of other topical agents. Whether tazarotene gel actually enhances the efficacy of topical steroids or calcipotriene has yet to be shown, but there is every reason to believe that such a phenomenon may occur. The availability of tazarotene may prove critical in the clinician's capacity to effectively treat recalcitrant psoriasis plaques without having to resort to systemic agents or phototherapy, which may be more toxic or inconvenient.

III. MEDICATIONS USED IN PHOTOTHERAPY

Since UVB phototherapy does not require the concurrent use of topical or oral medications, psoralen, which is used for PUVA phototherapy, is the primary topic of this section. Psoralens are originally derived from plants and are known to be photosensitizing. They are activated by exposure to ultraviolet radiation, whereby the psoralen interacts with DNA pyrimidine base pairs and leads to an inhibition of DNA synthesis. The most widely used formulations of psoralen in the United States are 8-methoxypsoralen (8-MOP) and Oxsoralen-Ultra. Oxsoralen-Ultra is a newer formulation of 8-methoxypsoralen with more predictable and efficient bioavailability than 8-MOP. Consequently, since the introduction of Oxsoralen-Ultra, the old formulation of 8-MOP is rarely used. When Oxsoralen-Ultra is used, ultraviolet A (UVA) irradiation is conducted 1½ h after dosing, rather than 2 h later as with the 8-MOP formulation. The main advantage of the old formulation of 8-MOP over Oxsoralen-Ultra is that it is less likely to induce nausea, which is probably the most common side effect experienced by patients taking psoralen orally. Other common systemic side effects experienced by patients on psoralen include dizziness, headaches, and insomnia. The nausea from psoralen can be countered by several practical measures; these include: (1) splitting the dose so that the required dosage is taken 15 min apart; (2) ingesting psoralen with food; (3) scheduling treatments later in the day rather than first thing in the morning; and (4) use of ginger products, such as ginger snaps and commercially available ginger tablets, known to decrease nausea [24]. If these more conservative approaches fail, trimethobenzamide (Tigan) 250 mg or promethazine (Phenergan) 25 mg taken about 30 min before the ingestion of psoralen may be effective. If all of these measures fail, bath PUVA is a fool-proof way of avoiding nausea. A more recent development in this area includes the availability of 5-MOP in Europe. 5-MOP is a formulation of psoralen that is known to have a much lower propensity for causing nausea; unfortunately, it is not yet available in the United States.

The recommended dosage of Oxsoralen-Ultra, according to weight, is 0.4 mg/kg body weight [24]. A common misconception among clinicians is that one can use a dosage of psoralen that is lower than the recommended dose, as long as extra UVA exposure is given. Such an approach is not likely to work because psoralen is extensively metabolized during the first-pass effect through the liver. Thus, if patients are seriously underdosed with psoralen, it is questionable whether any of the psoralen compound would ever make it into the general circulation and to the skin. There are commercially available tests to check serum psoralen levels. Such laboratory evaluations are helpful in the management of patients who appear not to respond as expected, despite adequate dosages. An undetectable or grossly inadequate serum psoralen level would indicate that the patient is not receiving appropriate treatment. Since PUVA phototherapy is both expensive and time-consuming, any unorthodox regimen should include serum psoralen levels so as to avoid administering a "sham" treatment.

Topical PUVA phototherapy has one distinct advantage in that the topical application of psoralen circumvents systemic side effects such as nausea, headaches, and dizziness. Topical PUVA phototherapy includes bath, soak, and paint PUVA. Because topical psoralen is very photosensitizing, it is important to be extremely conservative and cautious in the application of UVA. For bath PUVA, the authors recommend that five capsules of 8-methoxypsoralen (50 mg) be dissolved in 8 ounces of boiling water, and then added to 100 L of warm bath water. For soak and paint PUVA, one uses the topical formulation of 8-methoxypsoralen; however, this is currently only available as a 1% lotion. According to the experience of most clinicians who practice topical PUVA therapy, there is uniform agreement that 1% lotion is more concentrated than can be safely used by most patients. Therefore, this medication is almost always diluted at least 10:1 (i.e., 0.1% concentration or less in alcohol) before applying to patients' skin for paint PUVA treatments. Since the topical psoralen used for paint PUVA is extremely photosensitizing, the dosimetry for UVA phototherapy generally starts at the lowest possible setting, usually 0.25 J/cm^2, and this exposure is increased only every two to three treatments and by minimal increments. This cautious application of UVA is recommended no matter what the patient's skin type. As for soak PUVA, the authors recommend diluting 1 cc of the 8-methoxypsoralen in 2 L water.

IV. SYSTEMIC MEDICATIONS FOR PSORIASIS

A. Methotrexate

Methotrexate has been successfully used for decades to treat severe cases of psoriasis. It is one of the most convenient ways to treat psoriasis, since methotrexate is taken orally just once per week. In the past, it was thought that dividing the dosage over a 24-h period might enhance its efficacy based on the theoretical model that methotrexate works by blocking cell replication. However, more recent thinking is that methotrexate may act by disabling a subset of T-lymphocytes rather than through blocking cell replication directly [25], and in terms of efficacy, there is no advantage to taking the medication in divided doses. Still, taking a once-per-week dosage of methotrexate in divided doses can be beneficial in decreasing the risk of nausea and vomiting in patients who are susceptible to these gastrointestinal side effects.

Because of the very small but finite risk of inducing acute hepatitis or bone marrow suppression, methotrexate is generally started with a minimal test dose to verify a patient's tolerance of this medication before a regular dose is given. This test dose usually consists of one or two tablets of methotrexate (2.5 mg each) given after a premethotrexate laboratory evaluation, which includes a CBC with platelets, BUN, creatinine, and liver function tests. For those cases in which there is a history of hepatitis or possible chronic carrier state, a hepatitis screen should be obtained. The CBC, platelet count, and liver function tests are repeated 1 week after the test dose. If there is no significant problem with the lab results, the patient is started on the regular starting dose, which usually ranges from four to six tablets (10–15 mg total) per week. One should be aware that several drugs, such as sulfonamides or salicylates, may interact with methotrexate, increasing its toxicity [26]. Nonsteroidal anti-inflammatory medications (NSAIDS) can decrease the renal elimination of methotrexate, thus changing its blood level; the three nonsteroidal anti-inflammatory medications recommended for use with methotrexate include ketoprofen (Orudis®), flurbiprofen (Ansaid®), and piroxicam (Feldene®) [27].

Methotrexate can have cumulative toxicity to the liver in terms of an increased risk of fibrosis or cirrhosis, especially when a cumulative lifetime dosage of 4 g is exceeded [28,29]. Liver biopsies are thus required at periodic intervals with long-term methotrexate use. According to the revised guidelines developed by the AAD Guideline Committee on Methotrexate, headed by Dr. Henry Roenigk, Jr., the first liver biopsy is recommended when a cumulative dose of 1.5 g is reached in patients who have no other risks of liver disease [30]. Due to the cumulative risk of inducing liver fibrosis or cirrhosis, methotrexate is not frequently viewed as the preferred agent to treat younger patients such as adolescents; phototherapy or another modality with less systemic toxicity is probably a healthier way to proceed in terms of long-term management. Short-term side effects of methotrexate include nausea, vomiting, anorexia, and fatigue; however, these symptoms are dose-related and reversible. Last, there have been nearly 50 reported cases of patients on long-term, low-dose methotrexate therapy for rheumatoid arthritis who have developed lymphoma. It was noted that many of these patients underwent spontaneous remission when the methotrexate therapy was discontinued [31]. Because of this new finding, the listing in the Physicians' Desk Reference was modified to reflect the possible risk of lymphoma with methotrexate use. Due to the hepatotoxicity and these other possible long-term side effects, methotrexate is best used sequentially with other treatment modalities such as PUVA phototherapy, Goeckerman therapy, oral retinoids, or cyclosporine to minimize the long-term, cumulative risks associated with methotrexate therapy.

B. Etretinate and Acitretin

Etretinate and acitretin are members of a class of therapeutic agents known as retinoids, which are vitamin A derivatives. Although their principal mechanism of action in psoriasis has not been clearly defined, they are known to have anti-inflammatory properties, as well as effects on cell proliferation and differentiation [32]. Etretinate has been available for the treatment of psoriasis for many years. However, the use of etretinate according to the FDA labeling [i.e., in high dose (at or close to 1 mg/kg/day) as a monotherapy] has been difficult to carry out, as a large proportion of patients experience multiple, annoying side effects at high doses. These side effects include mucocutaneous dryness, bone and muscle aches, diarrhea and other GI symptoms, hair loss, skin fragility, and others. Thus, etretinate is most often used in lower doses, either as a maintenance therapy or to enhance PUVA and UVB phototherapy. It is well established that etretinate, or other retinoids such as isotretinoin (Accutane), used at a lower dosage significantly enhances the efficacy of both PUVA and UVB phototherapy. This is referred to as Re-PUVA or Re-UVB phototherapy.

An active metabolite of etretinate known as acitretin (Soriatane) has recently become available in the United States. It has been used for many years in most other countries, including Canada. Acitretin has a much shorter half-life of 50 h, compared to the half-life of etretinate, which is approximately 80 to 100 days [32,33]. Consequently, acitretin is known to be safe in reproductive women, as long as there is an adequate length of time after the last dose of acitretin in which pregnancy is prohibited. In the United States, the required period of prohibition for conception is 3 years, due to findings that acitretin may be converted back to etretinate in the human body, a process that is enhanced by alcohol ingestion [34]. Therefore, it is important to instruct patients of reproductive age to not use alcohol during therapy with acitretin, and for several months after discontinuing acitretin therapy. Despite this requirement, dermatologists in the United States can finally use a psoriasis-indicated oral retinoid for reproductive women.

C. Cyclosporin

A new formulation of cyclosporine called Neoral was recently approved by the FDA in June 1997 for the treatment of psoriasis. The impressive efficacy of cyclosporine in the treatment of psoriasis has been known for more than a decade, and it has been widely used as a government-approved medication for psoriasis in practically all developed countries other than the United States for many years. Cyclosporine is believed to work by inhibiting the immune system-induced propagation of psoriasis, by preventing the activation of T cells [35]. The recommended upper limit of the dosage for dermatological use for the original formulation of cyclosporin, Sandimmune, is 5 mg/kg/day. The dose of Neoral required for successful treatment, however, is 15% lower than for Sandimmune [36]. The speed of improvement and the probability of successful treatment clearly correlates with the dosage used [37–39]. Consequently, there are two schools of thought with regard to how treatment with cyclosporine should be initiated. One is to start with a low or medium dose, such as 2.5 mg/kg/day, and to increase the dose only if an adequate response is not seen over a 1- to 3-month period. The other approach is to use cyclosporine at 5 mg/kg/day to rapidly control the psoriatic flare, and then decrease the dosage once the ''tables are turned'' on the psoriasis.* Outside the United States, dermatologists have had years of experi-

* The U.S. FDA recommends 4 mg/kg/day as the maximum dermatologic dose in the treatment of psoriasis.

ence using cyclosporine, and are therefore comfortable enough to use it even for moderate psoriasis. For these cases, a more conservative approach (i.e., initiating therapy with a moderate dosage) makes sense, since many of the moderate and routine cases will respond well without administering higher doses. On the other hand, in the United States, where dermatologists are less comfortable with this medication, cyclosporine is likely to be used only as a treatment of last resort for patients with severe, recalcitrant psoriasis. In that setting, short-term use with the maximum dosage might be more advantageous.

With respect to side effects, short-term use of cyclosporine (for 3 months duration or less) is arguably safer than the use of methotrexate. In healthy patients without contraindications such as preexisting hypertension, renal disease, active infection, etc., it is exceedingly unlikely that any acute, catastrophic adverse effects would occur with cyclosporine. Unlike methotrexate, in which a test dose is mandatory due to the possibility of acute, fulminant hepatitis or, in rare instances, myelosuppression, there is no test dose required before initiating therapy with the maximum dermatological dose of cyclosporine. For long-term use, the major concern centers on the risk of nephrotoxicity and hypertension. The accepted guideline for monitoring kidney function is to modify the dose of cyclosporin if the baseline creatinine increases by 30%.* The serum creatinine is checked 1 month after a dosage modification, and if the serum creatinine remains elevated by 30% or more, cyclosporine should be stopped until the creatinine returns to within 10% of the pretreatment value [37,40]. If one follows this guideline and there is no preexisting renal disease present, the chance of inducing clinically relevant, irreversible kidney damage is thought to be nil. Despite a fear that some American dermatologists have about the possibility of renal failure in psoriatic patients treated with cyclosporine, there has not been a single case documented world-wide of someone developing permanent kidney failure due to the use of cyclosporine for psoriasis within the established guidelines.

The continuous use of cyclosporine beyond 1 year is currently not recommended by the established guidelines. This is because the safety of cyclosporine beyond 1 year of continuous use, especially with regard to the risk of lymphoma or any systemic cancer, has not been adequately studied in large numbers of patients. However, the incidence of malignant lymphoma and skin cancer in psoriasis patients receiving cyclosporine is no greater than the incidence reported for PUVA and other systemic therapies, including methotrexate [41]. The current recommendation is to rotate patients onto some other therapy before or when the continuous use of cyclosporine has reached 1 year. After a period of "rest," treatment with cyclosporine can be restarted and continued for up to another year's duration. Since cyclosporine does not induce long-term remissions, it is

* The U.S. FDA recommends a change in dosage with a 25% increase in creatinine.

imperative that an alternative therapy, such as another systemic agent, phototherapy, or a combination thereof, be initiated in conjunction with the tapering of cyclosporine, so as to minimize the chance for recurrence of the psoriasis.

D. Hydroxyurea (Hydrea)

Hydroxyurea is considered to be a less toxic alternative to methotrexate, since it is not known to cause liver fibrosis or irreversible hepatic injury [42]. On the other hand, the therapeutic efficacy of hydroxyurea is somewhat unpredictable. Used as monotherapy, hydroxyurea in a dosage of 500 mg twice per day is thought to be effective in approximately half the cases [43,44]. It works as an antimitotic, blocking DNA synthesis [45,46]. The major possible side effect of hydroxyurea is myelosuppression leading to anemia, leukopenia, and thrombocytopenia. Some academicians believe that hydroxyurea shows therapeutic efficacy only when used at dosages high enough to affect blood counts; however, the authors' experience is that hydroxyurea may be effective without a change in blood counts, especially when it is combined with UVB or PUVA phototherapy. Hydroxyurea is known to induce megaloblastic erythrocyte changes in practically all patients who take this medication. However, macrocytosis by itself does not pose a risk to the patient, as long as a macrocytic anemia does not develop.

E. Sulfasalazine

Sulfasalazine, effective in inflammatory bowel disease and rheumatoid arthritis, is a medication that appears to work occasionally for patients with psoriasis. The effectiveness of sulfasalazine in psoriasis may be a result of anti-inflammatory effects, through its actions as a 5-lipoxygenase inhibitor and/or folate antagonist [47,48]. Due to its relative safety, sulfasalazine is often used when alternatives are limited in recalcitrant psoriasis. The starting dose is 500 mg three times daily. If there are no adverse reactions after 3 days, the dosage should be increased to 1 g three times per day. Adverse effects may include a hypersensitivity reaction, nausea, or abdominal pain [47,49].

F. 6-Thioguanine

6-Thioguanine is an antimetobolite that inhibits DNA synthesis through the inhibition of enzymes involved in purine metabolism [50,51]. 6-Thioguanine can be as effective as methotrexate in treating recalcitrant, generalized psoriatic cases [52]. However, the major concern with this agent is its propensity to induce sudden, catastrophic drops in blood counts. Because of this, the authors recommend that therapy with 6-thioguanine be started at a very low dose, such as half a tablet (i.e., 20 mg) twice per week, with weekly monitoring of blood counts (including platelets), as well as liver and kidney function tests. If the blood counts prove to be stable at this dose, a full dosage (40 mg) twice per week may be used. If necessary, the dose of 6-thioguanine can be increased to 40 mg every day; up to 80 mg per day may be administered with close monitoring of blood counts. 6-Thioguanine is not thought to be particularly toxic to either the liver or the kidneys [52]. For patients with limited therapeutic options, this agent can be a godsend.

V. CONCLUSION

In this chapter, drug therapies that are frequently used for the treatment of psoriasis were discussed one by one. It is important to remember that many of these medications are used in combination, and that it is recommended that therapeutic modalities be rotated periodically for those who require chronic, long-term maintenance therapy. However, a complete discussion regarding all possible combinations of these medications is beyond the scope of this chapter. Last, it should be mentioned that in non-Western countries such as China, there is a whole different pharmacopoeia used that specifically pertains to psoriasis and includes a variety of herbal medications [53]. However, there is limited availability of double-blind, placebo-controlled studies with regard to the safety and efficacy of these agents.

REFERENCES

1. Weinstein GD, White GD. An approach to the treatment of moderate to severe psoriasis with rotational therapy. J Am Acad Dermatol 1993;28:454–459.
2. Hjort N, Norgaard Mette. Tars. In: Roenigk HH and Maibach HI, eds. Psoriasis, 2nd ed. New York: Marcel Dekker, 1991:475–476.
3. Young E. The external treatment of psoriasis: a critical study. Br J Dermatol 1970; 82:510–515.
4. Maurer TA, Winter ME, Koo JYM, Berger TG. Refractory hypoglycemia: a complication of topical salicylate therapy. Arch Dermatol 1994;130:1455–1456.
5. Stern RS, Wu J. Psoriasis. In: Arndt K, Leboit P, Robinson J, Wintroub B, eds. Cutaneous Medicine and Surgery, An Integrated Program in Dermatology. Philadelphia: Saunders Co., 1996:295–321.
6. Ingram JT. Approaches to psoriasis. Br Med J 1953; 2:591–594.
7. Christensen OB, Brolund L. Clinical studies with a novel dithranol formulation (Miconol) in combination with UVB at day care centers. Acta Derm Venereol Suppl (Stockh) 1992;172:17–19.
8. Zanolli MD. Psoriasis and Reiter's syndrome. In: Sams WM Jr, Lynch PJ, eds. Principles and Practice of Dermatology, 2nd ed. New York: Churchill Livingstone, 1996: 352.
9. Van Der Vleuten CJM, Gerritsen MJP, De Jong EMGJ, Elbers M, De Jongh GJ, Van de Kerkhof PCM. A novel dithranol formulation (Micanol): The effects of monotherapy and UVB combination therapy on epidermal differentiation, proliferation,

and cutaneous inflammation in psoriasis vulgaris. Acta Derm Venereol (Stockh) 1996;76:387–391.

10. Schaefer H, Farber EM, Goldberg L, Schalla W. Limited application period for dithranol in psoriasis. Br J Dermatol 1980;102:571–573.
11. Scharz T, Gschnait F. Anthralin minute entire skin treatment. Arch Dermatol 1985; 121:1512–1515.
12. Lowe NJ, Ashton RE, Koudsi H, Verschoore M, Schaefer H. Anthralin for psoriasis: short-contact anthralin compared with topical steroids and conventional anthralin. J Am Acad Dermatol 1984;10:69–72.
13. Lahti A, Maibach HI. Systemic corticosteroids. In: Roenigk HH and Maibach HI, eds. Psoriasis, 2nd ed. New York: Marcel Dekker, 1991:559–562.
14. Champion RH. Treatment of psoriasis. Br Med J 1966;2:993–995.
15. Kragballe K, Wildfang IL. Calcipotriol (MC903), a novel vitamin D_3 analogue, stimulates terminal differentiation and inhibits proliferation of cultured human keratinocytes. Arch Dermatol Res 1990;282:164–167.
16. Binderup L, Bramm E. Effects of a novel vitamin D analogue (MC 903) on cell proliferation and differentiation in vitro and on calcium metabolism in vivo. Biochem Pharmacol 1998;37:889–895.
17. Bruce S, Epinette WW, Funicella T, Ison A, Jones EL, Loss R Jr, McPhee ME, Whitmore C. Comparative study of calcipotriene (MC903) ointment and fluocinonide ointment in the treatment of psoriasis. J Am Acad Dermatol 1994;31(5 pt 1): 755–759.
18. Koo JYM, Siebenlist J. Vitamin D analogues in the treatment of psoriasis. Submitted for publication.
19. Bourke JF, Berth-Jones J, Iqbal SJ, Hutchinson PE. High-dose topical calcipotriol in the treatment of extensive psoriasis vulgaris. Br J Dermatol 1993;129:74–76.
20. Esgleyes-Ribot T, Chandraratna RA, Lew-Kaya DA, et al. Response of psoriasis to a new topical retinoid, AGN 190168. J Am Acad Dermatol 1994;30:581–590.
21. Weinstein GD. Tazarotene gel: efficacy and safety in plaque psoriasis. J Am Acad Dermatol 1997;37(2 pt 3):S33–S38.
22. The Tazarotene Clinical Study Group. Tazarotene 0.1% and 0.05% gels compared with fluocinonide 0.05% cream in the treatment of plaque psoriasis: an investigator-masked study of safety, efficacy, and duration of therapeutic effect (poster). Presented at Clinical Dermatology 2000 International Congress, May 28–31, 1996;Vancouver, British Columbia, Canada.
23. Tazarotene 0.1% gel plus UVB phototherapy in the treatment of psoriasis. Presented at the World Conference of Dermatology; June 1997; Sydney, Australia.
24. Morison WL. PUVA therapy. In: Weinstein GD, Gottlieb A, eds. *Therapy of Moderate-to-Severe Psoriasis*. City: The National Psoriasis Foundation, Seattle, WA, 1993: 23–38.
25. Weinstein GD, Jeffes EWJ, McCullough JL. Cytotoxic and immunologic effects of methotrexate in psoriasis. J Invest Dermatol 1990;95(suppl):49S–51S.
26. Evans W, Christensen M. Drug interactions with methotrexate. J Rheumatol 1985; 12(suppl 12):15–20.
27. Tracy TS, Worster T, Bradley JD, Greene PK, Brater DC. Methotrexate disposition

following concomitant administration of ketoprofen, piroxicam and flurbiprofen in patients with rheumatoid arthritis. Br J Clin Pharm 1994;37(5):453–456.
28. Nyfors A. Liver biopsies from psoriatics related to methotrexate therapy. Acta Pathol Microbiol Scand 1977; 85(4):511–18.
29. Zachariae H, Schiodt T. Liver biopsy in methotrexate treatment. Acta Dermatol Venereol 1971; 51(3):215–20.
30. Roenigk HH, Auerbach R, Maibach HI, Weinstein GD. Methotrexate in psoriasis: revised guidelines. J Am Acad Dermatol 1988;19:145–156.
31. Georgescu L, Quinn GC, Schwartzman S, Paget SA. Lymphoma in patients with rheumatoid arthritis: association with the disease state or methotrexate treatment. Semin Arthritis Rheum 1997;26(6):794–804.
32. Gollnick HPM. Oral retinoids—efficacy and toxicity in psoriasis. Br J Dermatol 1996;135(suppl 49):6–17.
33. Phillips TJ, Dover JS. Recent advances in dermatology. New Engl J Med 1992;326: 167–178.
34. Larsen FG, Jakobson P, Knudsen J, Weismann K, Kragballe K, Nielsen-Kudsk F. Conversion of acitretin to etretinate in psoriatic patients is influenced by ethanol. J Invest Dermatol 1993;100(5):623–627.
35. Wong RL, Winslow CM, Cooper KD. The mechanisms of action of cyclosporin A in the treatment of psoriasis. Immunol Today 1993;14:69–74.
36. Gulliver WP, Murphy GF, Hannaford VA, Primmett DRN. Increased bioavailability and improved efficacy, in severe psoriasis, of a new microemulsion formulation of cyclosporin. Br J Dermatol 1996;135(suppl 48):35–39.
37. Koo JYM, Lee J. Cyclosporin: what clinicians need to know. Dermatol Clin 1995; 13(4):897–907.
38. Timonen P, Friend D, Abeywickrama K, Laburte C, von Graffenried B, Feutren G. Efficacy of low-dose cyclosporin A in psoriasis: results of dose-finding studies. Br J Dermatol 1990;122(suppl 36):33–39.
39. Ellis CN, Fradin MS, Messana JM, Brown MD, Siegel MT, et al. Cyclosporin for plaque-type psoriasis: results of a multidose, double-blind trial. New Engl J Med 1991;324(5):277–284.
40. Mihatsch MJ, Wolff K. Report of a meeting: consensus conference on cyclosporin A for psoriasis, February 1992. Br J Dermatol 1992;126:622.
41. Data on file, Novartis, Inc.
42. Baker H. Antimitotic drugs in psoriasis. In: Farber EM, Cox AJ eds. Psoriasis: Proceedings of the Third International Symposium. New York: Grune & Stratton, 1982: 119–126.
43. Moschella SL. Chemotherapy of psoriasis: ten years of experience. Int J Dermatol 1976;15:373–378.
44. Layton AM, Sheehan-Dare RA, Goodfield MJD, et al. Hydroxyurea in the management of therapy resistant psoriasis. Br J Dermatol 1989;121:647–653.
45. Boyd AS, Neldner KH. Hydroxyurea therapy. J Am Acad Dermatol 1991; 25(3): 518–524.
46. Bergsagel DE, Frenkel EP, Alfrey CP, et al. Megaloblastic erythropoiesis induced by hydroxyurea (NSC-32065). Cancer Chemother Rep 1964;40:15–17.
47. Gupta AK, Ellis CN, Siegel MT, Voorhees JJ. Sulfasalazine: a potential psoriasis therapy? J Am Acad Dermatol 1989;5(1):797–800.

48. Halasz CLG. Sulfasalazine as folic acid inhibitor in psoriasis. Arch Dermatol 1990; 126:1516.
49. Gupta AK, Ellis CN, Siegel MT, Duell EA, Griffiths CEM, et al. Sulfasalazine improves psoriasis. Arch Dermatol 1990;126:487.
50. Drug Evaluations Annual 1991, published by the American Medical Association 1990:1774.
51. Molin L, Thomsen K. Thioguanine treatment in psoriasis. Acta Derm Venereol (Stockh) 1987;67:85–88.
52. Zackheim HS, Glogau RG, Fisher DA, Maibach HI. 6-Thioguanine treatment of psoriasis: experience in 81 patients. J Am Acad Dermatol 1994;30(3):452–458.
53. Lin XR. Psoriasis in China. J Derm 1993;20(12):746–755.

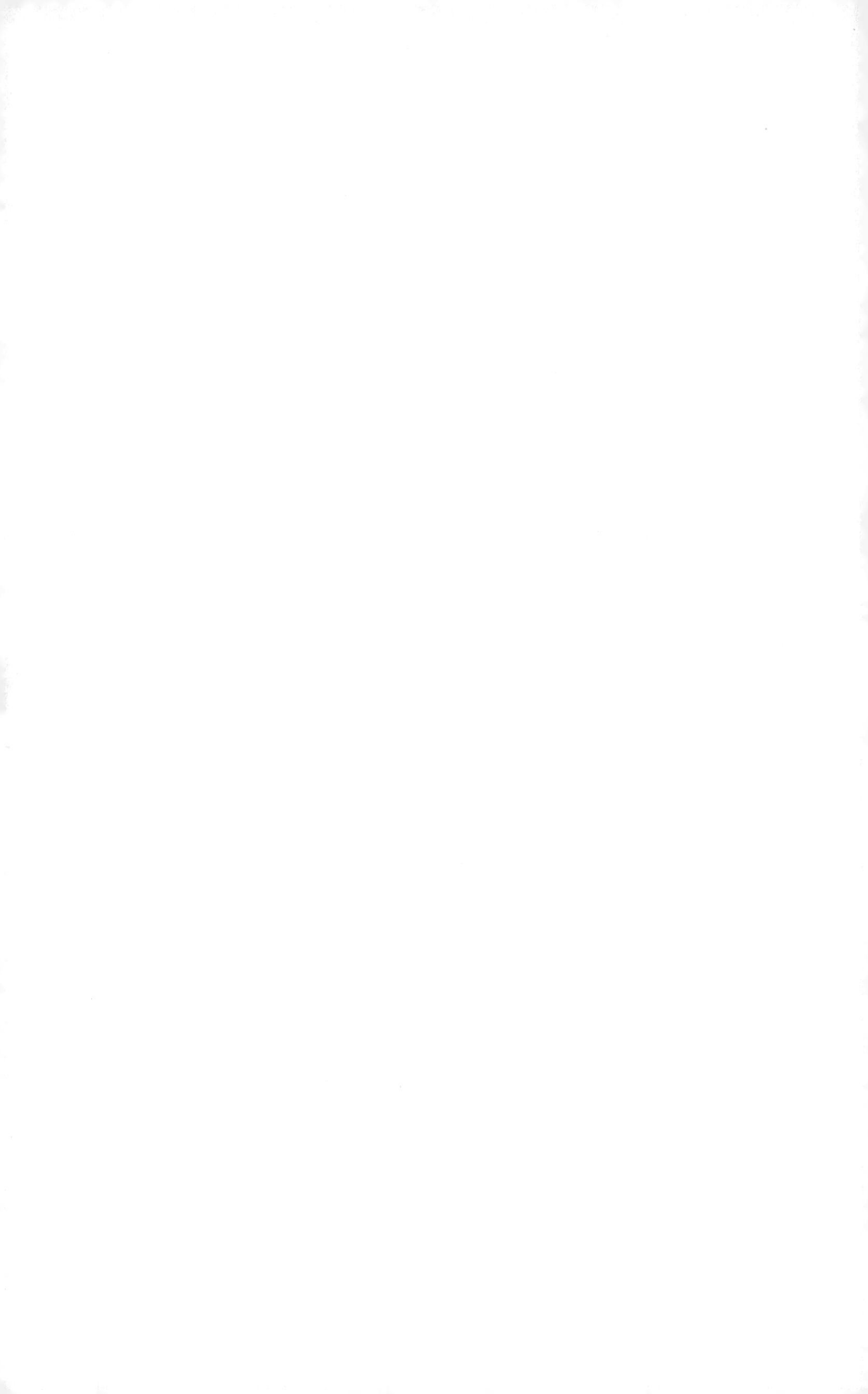

17

Drug Therapy of Urticaria

Malcolm W. Greaves
St. Thomas' Hospital
London, United Kingdom

Urticaria can be arbitrarily classified into acute (attacks of urticaria lasting less than 6 weeks), chronic (urticaria continuing on a daily or almost daily basis for 6 weeks or more), and intermittent (recurrent bouts of acute urticaria). Urticarial vasculitis will also be included in this chapter, as well as physical urticarias, urticaria pigmentosa (cutaneous mastocytosis), contact urticaria, and papular urticaria.

I. ACUTE URTICARIA AND ANGIOEDEMA

A. Etiology and Pathogenesis

An attack of widespread wheals with pruritus, with or without angioedema, lasting for days or a few weeks constitutes a typical attack of acute urticaria. Individual wheals, which usually manifest a central pale-colored or dull red swelling due to edema and a bright red surrounding flare, last less than 24 h and fade without leaving a mark in the skin. Angioedema may be subcutaneous or submucosal. In the latter instance, the oropharyngeal mucosa may be involved causing acute distress to the patient. Systemic symptoms are variable, but, unless the acute urticarial episode is part of an anaphylactic reaction to a drug (e.g., penicillin) or an insect sting, usually minimal.

Acute urticarial attacks if allergic in origin occur more commonly in atopic individuals and are usually due to a type 1 (Gell and Coombs) reaction involving IgE. However, identical acute urticarial reactions can occur due to nonimmunological causes (e.g., aspirin in an aspirin-sensitive individual or scombrotoxic fish poisoning). Common causes of acute allergic urticaria include drugs, especially penicillin, and foods, especially shell fish, and rarely infections [1]. No apparent cause can be found in at least half of acute urticaria attacks [1].

The pathological features of acute urticaria and angioedema are similar. Mast-cell degranulation is a pivotal event. Products of mast-cell activation, including histamine, eicosanoids (prostaglandins and leukotrienes), proteases (including tryptase), and cytokines all contribute to the clinical picture. Histamine is probably the main, if not the only, cause of itching. However, nonhistamine mediators contribute to the wheals and redness, thus accounting for the fact that histamine-evoked wheals last only a few minutes whereas the wheals of acute (and chronic "idiopathic") urticaria last individually up to 24 h. The acute urticarial wheal is also characterized histologically by scattered eosinophils, with release of eosinophilic granular material, perivascular neutrophil accumulation, and edema and vasodilation. The pathology of associated angioedema is essentially similar, except that the changes occur predominantly in the subcutis and submucosa, with more prominent edema.

B. Drug Treatment

Removal of any identifiable cause is the first consideration. However, even if a cause can be identified and withdrawn, it is often several days before the urticaria subsides and during this period symptoms need to be alleviated.

1. Antihistamines

The detailed pharmacology of the H_1- and H_2-antihistamines is described elsewhere in this volume and will not be considered here; this chapter will focus on their applications to the management of acute urticaria. Human skin blood vessels express both H_1 and H_2 histamine receptors [2]. Therefore, theoretically, both H_1- and H_2-antihistamines should have a role in the treatment of acute urticaria. In practice, although combination treatment by H_1- and H_2-antihistamines does produce greater relief than use of the same H_1-antihistamine alone, the outcome is statistically significant rather than clinically useful [3]. However, histamine-induced itching involves H_1- but not H_2-receptors [2]. Therefore, H_2 antagonists such as cimetidine and ranitidine are ineffective for relief of itching due to urticaria.

In the prescription of H_1-antihistamines for acute urticaria, a number of factors need to be considered. If the eruption is severe at nighttime, an oral sedative antihistamine is often preferred (e.g., 25 mg hydroxyzine). Daytime whealing and itching is often best controlled by a low-sedation antihistamine such as 10 mg loratidine or 180 mg fexofenadine. Cetirizine (10 mg) may also be useful for daytime management of acute urticaria, but does show mild sedative activity.

TABLE 1 Acute Urticaria/Angioedema—Drug Treatment

H_1-antihistamines
Daytime: Loratidine 10 mg, cetirizine 10 mg or fexofenadine 180 mg daily.
Nighttime: Hydroxyzine 25 mg.
Corticosteroids[a]: Tapering regime commencing with 30 mg prednisolone daily, with or without concurrent H_1-antihistamine administration.
Topical: 1% menthol cream or lotion ad lib.
Angioedema: As above, plus 0.5–1.0 mg epinephrine intramuscularly, repeated every 10–15 min until remission.

[a] Severely affected patients only.

2. *Corticosteroids*

A case can be made for a short, tapering course of oral corticosteroids in severe acute urticaria, especially when the cause has been identified and withdrawn. A reasonable regimen for an adult would be 30 mg prednisolone daily for 3 days, which can then be reduced by 5 mg daily every 3 days. H_1-antihistamines can also be prescribed concurrently.

3. *Angioedema*

Angioedema of the oropharynx is very frightening and should be treated vigorously by intramuscular injection of 0.5 to 1.0 mg epinephrine (adrenaline). This can be repeated every 10 to 15 min, depending on blood pressure and pulse rate, which should be monitored until clinically evident improvement occurs. The H_1-antihistamine chlorpheniramine, given intramuscularly in a 4-mg dosage, may also be useful. Diphenhydramine, either intravenously or intramuscularly, is also useful in acute attacks. Dose varies with body weight, ranging from 25 mg to 50 mg.

4. *Other Measures*

Acute urticaria is often intensely pruritic and patients often find the application ad lib of 1% menthol in aqueous cream to be very soothing. It can also be prescribed as a lotion (e.g., 1% menthol in calamine lotion).

Table 1 summarizes the drug treatment of acute urticaria.

II. CHRONIC URTICARIA AND ANGIOEDEMA

A. Etiology and Pathogenesis

The natural history of chronic urticaria is for spontaneous remission in an average of 2 to 5 years. Most textbooks on dermatology or allergy list food components, infections and infestations, and ''stress'' as causes of chronic urticaria. In practice, it is rarely possible to confirm the involvement of any specific factor from the previously mentioned categories [4]. The gold standard for implication of a food additive should be the placebo-controlled challenge trial with tests for reproducibility. On this basis, we [5] can identify a food additive as a culprit in only a handful of patients with chronic urticaria out of around 600 new patients attending our chronic urticaria service annually. Recent enthusiasm for the role of *Helicobacter pylori* is also misplaced according to our own and others' [6] experience.

Until recently, the culprit in the great majority of patients remained obscure. Recent evidence [7–10] indicates that up to 55% of patients with chronic ''idiopathic'' urticaria possess functional IgG antibodies directed against the high-affinity IgE receptor (FcεRI) or less commonly against IgE itself. These autoantibodies release histamine from human skin mast cells and blood basophils and appear to be the cause of the disease. Refinement of immunoassays and other laboratory diagnostic technologies may enable many of the apparently autoantibody negative chronic urticaria patients to be assigned to the autoimmune groups.

That histamine is a major mediator of the symptoms and signs of chronic urticaria has been demonstrated by measurement of tissue histamine levels directly in lesional skin [11]. However, like the wheals of acute urticaria, it is presumed that other mast-cell- or basophil-derived mediators also contribute to the redness and edema that may persist in an individual wheal for up to 24 h. Histological features include fibrin deposition, eosinophil, neutrophil, and lymphocyte accumulation. Immunoglobulin and complement components may be deposited perivascularly, and can be visualized by direct immunofluorescence examination [4]. In keeping with its autoimmune basis, autoantibody-positive chronic urticaria shows an increased frequency of certain HLA class 2 haplotypes [12].

B. Drug Treatment

Better understanding of the etiology has led to some advances in treatment.

1. *Antihistamines*

Whether or not an autoimmune etiology can be demonstrated in a patient with chronic urticaria, antihistamines still remain the mainstay of drug treatment. Unless the urticaria is exceptionally severe, the patient should be advised to take a combination of daytime low-sedation antihistamines and nighttime sedative antihistamines, depending upon the diurnal periodicity of the urticaria. Suggested combinations are the same as for acute urticaria. Patients with severe, unremitting chronic urticaria frequently experience depression and anxiety. Doxepin is a tricyclic antidepressant with potent antihistamine H_1- and H_2-receptor activity. It is useful in a single nighttime dose of 25 to 50 mg in depressed patients, but care should be taken to avoid combining it with other drugs that are metabolized by the cytochrome P-450 system of the liver, including terfenadine and astemizole. Cognitive function is also impaired during the morning after a nighttime dose of doxepin. Fifty percent of patients with chronic idiopathic urticaria also suffer from associated mucocutaneous angioedema. This may respond adequately to a combination of low-sedation and sedative H_1-antihistamines as previously described, but for severe oropharyngeal angioedema, parenteral adrenaline may be necessary as described for acute urticaria. Patients with chronic urticaria and mucosal angioedema also find an extemporaneous formulation of 2% ephedrine in water dispensed as a spray to be very useful and reassuring since it is portable. It is used as two to three puffs self-administered at the onset of the characteristic "tingling" sensation on the lips or tongue. Almost 40% of patients with chronic "idiopathic" urticaria also suffer from the physical delayed pressure urticaria and this may prove a major cause of disability. H_1-antihistamines are not generally effective against delayed-pressure urticaria, but anecdotally, cetirizine, a mildly sedative H_1-antihistamine, seems to have a better track record in this situation.

2. Corticosteroids

Long-term systemic corticosteroid therapy is not recommended for chronic urticaria. Increasingly high maintenance dosages will be required, with poor control, risk of rebound upon withdrawal, and inevitable side effects. Short, tapering courses are permitted, however, under exceptional circumstances and are usually effective. Prednisolone (30 mg) can be given daily for 3 days and reduced by 5 mg daily every 3 days. H_1-antihistamines can be prescribed concurrently. Oral steroids may also relieve delayed-pressure urticaria but high dosage is usually needed and, due to the chronicity of this physical urticaria, this treatment is not recommended.

3. Cyclosporine

The treatment of severe, persistent chronic urticaria is an unlicensed indication for this drug. However, recent studies attest to its effectiveness in severe antihistamine-resistant chronic urticaria [13,14]. It appears to be equally effective in both autoimmune and nonautoimmune chronic urticaria. It is ineffective in physical urticarias, including delayed-pressure urticaria. The normal dose range for chronic urticaria in 2.5 to 5 mg/kg/day. It is my practice to prescribe it for 2 to 3 months in the first instance. Control of the urticaria usually occurs within 1 week of commencing treatment. In a recent placebo-controlled double-blind study, two-thirds of patients receiving the active drug achieved control of their urticaria without serious side effects [15]. About one-third of responders remain in remission after cyclosporine withdrawal, one-third relapse but with less severe disease than prior to cyclosporine, and one-third experienced a full relapse. Only one patient of mine receiving cyclosporine experienced a urticaria rebound after withdrawal. Precautions, including close monitoring of renal function and blood pressure readings, need to be taken regularly in patients receiving cyclosporine.

4. Treatment of Autoimmune Chronic Urticaria

In patients with less severe disease that responds adequately to routine H_1-antihistamine treatment, no further measures should normally need to be attempted. In patients with severe recalcitrant autoimmune chronic urticaria, additional options are available. Unless there are contraindications, cyclosporine should be the first choice (see above). If the patient is unable to take cyclosporine or is poorly responsive, then intravenous immunoglobulin (IVIG) [16] or plasmapheresis [17] should be considered. Detailed descriptions of the use of these modalities in autoimmune chronic urticaria are beyond the scope of this chapter, but are covered in Refs. 16 and 17.

5. Other Drug Treatments

A number of other drug treatments have been reported to be effective in chronic urticaria, but the evidence is mainly anecdotal and lacks support from controlled clinical trials.

a. Ketotifen. Ketotifen is an H_1-antihistamine that is said to have additional mast-cell.stabilizing properties [18]. It is an effective antihistamine with significant sedative side effects and a tendency to cause weight gain. In the author's view it is neither worse nor better than its competitor sedative H_1-antihistamines. We [19] were unable to demonstrate evidence of mast-cell ''stabilization'' in patients with mastocytosis receiving this drug. It is normally prescribed in an oral dosage of 1 to 2 mg daily or at night.

b. Disodium Cromoglycate. Disodium cromoglycate is an effective mast-cell stabilizer in the lung; unfortunately, it has no effect on cutaneous mast cells [20] and, furthermore, it is not absorbed systemically to any significant degree after oral administration. Therefore, it is not surprising that we [19] were unable to demonstrate any reduction in urinary excretion of histamine and its metabolites in patients with urticaria pigmentosa. However, it may be useful in allaying any gastrointestinal symptoms in patients with mastocytosis (see below).

c. Beta Agonists. Secretion of histamine from human skin mast cells is regulated by levels of intracellular cyclic AMP [21], which in turn modulates evoked histamine secretion by these cells. Terbutaline, a beta-2 agonist with minimal cardiovascular action, has been used alone and in combination with ketotifen (see above) in patients with chronic urticaria with apparently encouraging results [22]. Terbutaline is administered orally in a dosage of 2.5 mg three times daily.

Table 2 Chronic Urticaria/Angioedema—Drug Treatment

H_1-antihistamines	Daytime: loratidine 10 mg, cetirizine 10 mg or fexofenadine 180 mg once daily. Nighttime: hydroxyzine 25 mg or doxepin 10 to 25 mg.
Corticosteroids	Not recommended. Occasionally a short, tapering regime commencing with prednisolone 30 mg daily with or without concurrent H_1-antihistamine administration.
Cyclosporin[a]	For severely incapacitated antihistamine-resistant patients only, in a dosage of 2.5–5.0 mg per kg body weight daily for up to 3 months.
Miscellaneous systemic drugs	
	Ketotifen 1 to 2 mg daily. Terbutaline 2.5 mg three times daily[a] with or without ketotifen.
Topical	1% menthol cream or lotion ad lib.
Angioedema	As above, plus epinephrine 0.5 to 1.0 mg intramuscularly, repeated every 10 to 15 min until remission. Regular use of an ephedrine, 2% aqueous spray (2–3 puffs as required), can also be used.
Autoimmune chronic urticaria	Any of above, plus intravenous immunoglobulin[a] (Ref. 16) or chronic plasmapheresis (Ref. 17).

[a] Unlicensed indication.

The options for drug treatment of chronic urticaria are summarized in Table 2.

III. INTERMITTENT URTICARIA

The range of drug treatments used is essentially identical with that for chronic urticaria.

IV. URTICARIAL VASCULITIS

Patients with urticarial vasculitis need to be distinguished from those with ''ordinary'' chronic urticaria (including those with autoimmune chronic urticaria) because the investigations and treatment of urticarial vasculitis differ in several important ways from that of chronic urticaria.

A. Etiology and Pathogenesis

Although certain distinguishing clinical features (duration of individual wheals greater than 24 h; residual pigmentation after wheals have subsided; induration;

poor response to H_1-antihistamines; associated systemic symptoms) may give a clue to the diagnosis, in most cases the clinical picture is indistinguishable from that of ''ordinary'' chronic urticaria. Angioedema occurs in about 40% of patients. In order to establish the diagnosis of urticarial vasculitis, a skin biopsy needs to be done to establish the major diagnostic histological criteria (endothelial cell swelling or damage; extravasation of red blood cells, leukocytoclasia). Other important diagnostic criteria include lowered serum complement $C^1 3$ and evidence of nephritis [4]. Although these are only present in a minority.

Urticarial vasculitis is due to immune complex deposition in the postcapillary venules of the skin and may be a cutaneous manifestation of an autoimmune connective tissue disease (especially systemic lupus erythematosus, rheumatoid arthritis, and Sjögrens syndrome). Other causes include hepatitis B or C infection, dysproteinemias, serum sickness, and drug hypersensitivity reactions. Urticarial vasculitis is a type III (immune complex-mediated) immunological reaction in the Gell and Coombs classification. Anti-FcεRI or anti-IgE antibodies are rarely associated with urticarial vasculitis.

B. Drug Treatment

No drug treatment has ever been demonstrated to be consistently effective in urticarial vasculitis. Antihistamines rarely bring about useful relief. Other proposed oral nonsteroid drugs include colchicine 0.5 to 1.5 mg daily, dapsone 50 to 100 mg daily, or hydroxychloroquine 200 to 400 mg daily. Oral corticosteroids may be effective in large doses (over 30 mg prednisone daily), but rapid relapse usually occurs if the dose is lower. Immunosuppressive drugs (azathioprine 1.5 mg per kg body weight, methotrexate 12.5 to 25 mg once weekly; cyclophosphamide 1.5 mg per kg daily) are rarely of value. The diagnosis and treatment of urticarial vasculitis has been comprehensively reviewed recently [23]; the range of drug treatments for urticarial vasculitis are summarized in Table 3.

TABLE 3 Urticarial Vasculitis—Drug Treatment

H_1-antihistamines:	Rarely effective; may relieve itch.
Corticosteroids:	May be effective in high dosage (greater than 30 mg prednisolone daily); side effects a problem.
Other suggested systemic treatments:	Colchicine 0.5 to 1.5 mg daily.
	Dapsone 50 to 100 mg daily.
	Hydroxychloroquine 400 mg daily.
	Cyclophosphamide 1.5 mg per kg daily.*
	Methotrexate 12.5 to 25 mg once weekly.*
Topical:	1% menthol cream or lotion may relieve itch.

* Severely affected, treatment-resistant patients only.

V. PHYSICAL URTICARIAS

Physical urticarias include symptomatic dermographism, cholinergic urticaria, delayed-pressure urticaria, cold contact urticaria, heat contact urticaria, solar urticaria, aquagenic urticaria, and vibratory angioedema. The etiology, pathogenesis, and drug treatment share many features in common. These common features will be discussed together. Important features specific to individual physical urticarias will be mentioned where appropriate under separate headings.

A. Etiology and Pathogenesis

The natural history of physical urticarias is for self-limiting chronicity. Most patients experience remission in an average time of 2 to 3 years [24]. Patients present with a history indicative of chronic urticaria; however, questioning reveals the importance of physical provocative factors in the generation of the wheals. These include rubbing or stroking (symptomatic dermographism); perpendicularly applied pressure (e.g., a tight belt, watch strap, or shoes) (delayed-pressure urticaria); exercise, a hot bath, or shower or emotions (cholinergic urticaria), contact with a cold or hot surface, cold or hot water or air (cold or hot contact urticaria, respectively); contact with water of any temperature (aquagenic urticaria); exposure to ultraviolet or visible light (solar urticaria); or application of a vibratory stimulus to the skin (e.g., gripping the handle of a lawn mower) (vibratory angioedema). With the exception of dermographism and aquagenic urticaria, physical urticarias may also present with angioedema. The underlying cause in most types of physical urticaria is unknown. Some (cold urticaria, symptomatic dermographism) can be passively transferred by serum [25,26] and are believed to involve IgE. More than one physical urticaria may occur concurrently in the same patient. Cold urticaria may also be due to circulating cold precipitating immunoreactants (cryoglobulins, cold agglutinins).

The importance of identifying patients with chronic urticaria in whom the sole or predominant problem is a physical urticaria is that it obviates the necessity for further laboratory or clinical investigation once the nature of the physical urticaria has been confirmed by appropriate challenge testing. With the exception of cryoglobulins and cold agglutinins in cold urticaria, no laboratory tests, skin-prick tests, exclusion diets, or other maneuvers are of any value in physical urticarias. The patient should be informed that the urticaria has to run its course and be treated symptomatically.

B. Drug Treatment

Most physical urticarias respond reasonable well to H_1-antihistamines. The combinations of low-sedative H_1-antihistamines by day and sedative antihistamines at night are essentially the same as for acute and chronic urticaria (Tables 1 and

2). Systemic corticosteroids and immunosuppressive drugs are not recommended for physical urticarias, with the possible exception of delayed pressure urticaria.

1. Symptomatic Dermographism

The response to H_1-antihistamines is usually good. Photochemotherapy with 8-methoxy psoralen and UVA irradiation (PUVA treatment) may be of value for the itching in some patients [27].

2. Cholinergic Urticaria

H_1-antihistamines are the mainstay of treatment. Anxiety-provoked attacks can be allayed by use of the beta-adrenergic blocking agent propranolol in a dosage of 20 to 40 mg twice daily; cholinergic urticaria is associated with lowered plasma levels of protease inhibitors [28]. Severely affected patients, especially those with associated severe pruritus and/or angioedema, have been successfully treated by the attenuated androgen danazol 200 mg three times daily. This treatment was of proven effectiveness in a double-blind placebo-controlled trial [29] in selected patients. The treatment is better tolerated by males than females, and regular evaluation of liver function needs to be carried out while receiving this treatment.

3. Delayed-Pressure Urticaria

This physical urticaria tends to be more persistent than other physical urticarias and is associated with chronic ''idiopathic'' urticaria in almost 40% of patients. Cetirizine is anecdotally believed to be the preferred H_1-antihistamine for delayed-pressure urticaria, but antihistamines are generally disappointing for this indication. Large doses of corticosteroids (e.g., prednisolone 30 mg or more daily) may be effective, but with inevitable troublesome side effects. Nonsteroidal anti-inflammatory drugs (e.g., colchicine, up to 1.5 mg daily) are recommended by some, but have been disappointing in the author's own experience [30]. The topical application of a nonsteroidal anti-inflammatory cream (benzydamine hydrochloride 3%) has anecdotally been found useful as a symptomatic treatment by delayed-pressure urticaria patients.

4. Cold Urticaria

The etiology is unknown in most patients. H_1-antihistamines are effective in most mildly to moderately affected patients. Cyproheptadine 4 mg has been the preferred antihistamine for this physical urticaria, but the author has been unimpressed. Cyproheptadine has marked sedative actions, causes troublesome weight gain, and is no more effective than modern, low-sedation antihistamines [31]. The author has used a combination of a beta-2 adrenergic blocking agent (salbutamol 2 to 4 mg two to four times a day) plus the phosphodiesterase inhibitor aminophylline (225 to 450 mg twice daily) with success in cold urticaria [32].

However, the use of aminophylline in this context is not recommended because of the narrow margin between effective and toxic plasma levels.

Severely affected patients with cold urticaria are extremely difficult to manage effectively. Cold tolerance (cold ''desensitization'') treatment is an option for the strongly motivated patient [33]. Systemic steroids and immunosuppressants are not recommended for cold urticaria.

5. Solar Urticaria

H_1-antihistamines are poorly effective in this distressing physical urticaria. Antimalarials (e.g., hydroxycloloroquine 400 mg daily) may be effective in some patients. Topical treatment with a sunscreen is a logical and often valuable treatment. The patient must first be phototested to determine the action spectrum of his or her photosensitivity. Once the active wavelength range has been determined, an appropriate sunscreen can be prescribed. Patients who are sensitive to long wavelength UV or visible light will require titanium-dioxide-based sunlight barrier creams. Tolerance treatment has also been reported to be useful in this physical urticaria [34] as has PUVA (8-methoxypsoralen UVA photochemotherapy) [35] with or without plasmapheresis. The drug treatment of physical urticarias is summarized in Table 4.

TABLE 4 Physical Urticarias—Drug Treatment

General:	H_1-antihistamines as outlined in Tables 1 and 2. Corticosteroids not recommended. Occasionally prednisolone can be prescribed for recalcitrant, disabling delayed-pressure urticaria. Immunosuppressives are ineffective and not recommended.
Symptomatic dermographism	PUVA (photochemotherapy with 8-methoxy psoralen and UVA) may relieve pruritus.
Cholinergic urticaria	Propranolol 20 to 40 mg twice daily, if anxiety is a provoking factor. Attenuated androgens in severely affected male patients (e.g., danazol 200 mg three times daily).
Delayed-pressure urticaria	Cetirizine is possibly the preferred H_1-antihistamine. Topical 3% benzydamine may give symptomatic relief.
Cold urticaria	Cold tolerance treatment (cold ''desensitization'') may be of value in strongly motivated patients.
Solar urticaria	After determining the action spectrum a suitable sunscreen should be prescribed. Tolerance treatment, PUVA, and plasmapheresis may be considered in severely disabled patients.

VI. URTICARIA PIGMENTOSA (CUTANEOUS MASTOCYTOSIS)

Mastocytosis frequently presents with cutaneous symptoms and signs. These are commonly due to direct skin involvement, but may be partly or entirely a consequence of systemic involvement, leading to release of histamine and probably other mediators that affect the skin.

A. Etiology and Pathogenesis

The cutaneous mast cell derives from a bone marrow progenitor stem cell termed CD-34. This cell reaches the skin via the blood stream. Mast cells in the skin express a protein-kinase-linked receptor termed c-KIT. Its natural ligand is stem cell factor also called c-KIT ligand. Its main sources in the skin are fiboblasts and keratinocytes. In cutaneous mastocytosis (urticaria pigmentosa), there is increased expression of soluble c-KIT. In these circumstances, mastocytosis is believed to be a reactive rather than a neoplastic process. A subset of mastocytosis seems to involve a different mechanism. In these patients there is a somatic point mutation of c-KIT mRNA. This mutation leads to the autoactivation of c-KIT. Some of these patients have an associated bone marrow hematological disorder. The pathogenesis of cutaneous mastocytosis has recently been reviewed [36]. The symptoms and signs of urticaria pigmentosa are due in part to the consequences of excessive histamine release from the abundant cutaneous mast cells in response to trivial mechanical stimuli, partly to associated melanin pigmentation, and also to systemic release of histamine, causing flushing and rarely rosacea.

B. Drug Treatment

Patients with any form of mastocytosis should avoid certain drugs known to activate mast cells. These include aspirin, iodine containing radiographic contrast media, codeine and morphine, muscle relaxants, and polymyxin. H_1-antihistamines are the standard treatment for patients with whealing and itching due to cutaneous mast-cell activation. The selection of H_1-antihistamines is essentially the same as for acute and chronic urticaria outlined in Tables 1 and 2. There may be a case for adding an H_2-antihistamine (cimetidine 400 mg twice daily with food) (care should be taken to avoid concurrent administration of cimetidine and doxepin) to combat gastric hyperacidity due to increased circulating histamine levels. Antihistamines also ameliorate flushing due to systemic histamine release. Results with oral disodium cromoglycate treatment (200 mg four times daily) have been conflicting. Two reports [37,38] seemed to show significant suppression of cutaneous gastrointestinal and neurological symptoms. However, in our hands [19], it was ineffective, and did not influence urinary excretion of histamine or its metabolites. Primarily effective in camouflaging the pigmentation, PUVA

Table 5 Urticaria Pigmentosa (Cutaneous Mastocytosis)—Drug Treatment

H_1-antihistamines:	As outlined in Tables 1 and 2. In addition, an H_2-antihistamine can be used to combat histamine-induced gastric hyperacidity.
Other treatments of possible value:	Oral sodium cromoglycate, 200 mg four times daily with food, may relieve any gastrointestinal symptoms.
	PUVA (oral 8-methoxypsoralen plus UVA photochemotherapy) brings about considerable cosmetic improvement.
	Potent topical steroid applications using clobetesol propionate 0.05%; clinical and biochemical improvement occurs but this treatment is inconvenient and there is the risk of systemic toxicity from percutaneous absorption.
	Human recombinant interferon-alpha, 3 million IU 3 times weekly for 12 to 24 weeks, suitable for severe systemically involved patients only.

(8-methoxy psoralen UVA photochemotherapy) has been used extensively to treat urticaria pigmentosa but may have little or no effect on mast-cell numbers or histamine content of irradiated skin [39]. More successful as a technique for reducing the excessive population of mast cells in the diseased skin, potent topical steroid therapy applied under occlusion each night has produced clear clinical as well as biochemical remission [40]. Our approach [41] has been to apply clobetesol propionate 0.05% under occlusion, using a plastic suit, for 6 weeks. This results in dramatic depletion of mast cells and histamine content of the treated skin. However, the treatment is inconvenient, the suit being hot in the summer with only reluctant patient compliance. Use of so-called ''soft'' topical steroids with reduced systemic side effects (e.g., fluticasone or mometasone) would be worth trying. Recently, there has been considerable interest in the treatment of more severe cutaneous mastocytosis with human recombinant interferon-alpha [42]. The treatment involves three times weekly injections of 3 million IU of interferon alpha for up to 12 months. The treatment is very expensive, of uncertain value, and regularly associated with side effects, especially influenza-like symptoms.

The therapeutic regimens available for urticaria pigmentosa are listed in Table 5.

VII. CONTACT URTICARIA

Contact urticaria may be immunological (e.g., latex allergy, foods) or nonallergic (nettle stings, ammonium persulphate in baking powder). Treatment is symptomatic using H_1-antihistamines as described in Tables 1 and 2. In addition, doxepin

5% cream is licensed in some countries for treatment of limited irritant or allergic reactions. It is applied twice or three times daily. Its main side effect is drowsiness due to percutaneous absorption. One percent menthol cream is a milder substitute (provided the offending allergen is unrelated to menthol). Obviously, the most important measure is to identify the culprit irritant or allergen and avoid it.

VIII. PAPULAR URTICARIA

Cutaneous reactions to insect bites may be either immunological or nonimmunological. A sting by a fire ant is most likely to be nonimmunological unless the patient had previously become sensitized. Reactions to mosquito bites are, in contrast, almost invariably due to an immunological response to the bite. Other common causes of papular urticaria include fleas, bed bug bites, tick bites, and lice infestation. Highly sensitized individuals show an immediate wheal and flare (typical urticarial) response to the bite, which is probably IgE- or possibly IgG4-mediated. More common is the delayed hypersensitivity response that presents as an itchy papule and may persist for days, weeks, or even months. Intractable pruritus is the main symptom.

Drug treatment can be divided into measures to lessen the likelihood of further bites (insect repellents such as dimethylphthalate insect repellent cream or lotion) and treatment of the bite itself. Secondary infection is common and needs to be treated by an antibacterial soak (1:10,000 potassium permanganate solution, or 0.5% silver nitrate lotion). Pruritus can often be allayed by a weak antipruritic such as menthol 1% aqueous cream. More intense pruritus can be treated by an oral H_1-antihistamine such as chlorpheniramine 4 mg. Doxepin 5% cream (see above) may also be useful. Topical corticosteroids are normally not indicated for papular urticaria. The problem has been recently reviewed [42].

REFERENCES

1. Zuberbier T, Ifflander J, Semmler C, Czarnetzki BM. Acute urticaria clinical aspects and therapeutic unresponsiveness. Acta Dermatol Venereol 1996; 76:295–297.
2. Greaves MW, Marks R, Robertson I. Receptors for histamine in human skin blood vessels: a review. Br J Dermatol 1977; 97:225–228.
3. Bleehen SS, Thomas SE, Greaves MW. Cimetidine and chlorpheniramine in the treatment of chronic idiopathic urticaria: a multicentre randomised double-blind study. Br J Dermatol 1987; 117:81–88.
4. Greaves MW. Chronic urticaria. New Engl J Med 1995; 332:1767–1772.
5. Black AK, Greaves MW, Champion RH, Pye RJ. The urticarias 1990. Br J Dermatol 1991; 124:100–108.
6. Valsecchi R, Pigatto P. Chronic urticaria and Helicobacter pylori. Acta Dermatol Venereol 1995; 78:440–442.
7. Hide M, Francis DM, Grattan CEH, Hakimi J, Kochan JP, Greaves MW. Autoanti-

bodies against the high affinity IgE receptor as a cause of histamine release in chronic urticaria. New Engl J Med 1993; 328:1599–1604.
8. Fiebiger E, Maurer D, Holub H, Reininger B, Hartmann G, Woisetschlager M. Serum IgG autoantibodies directed against the alpha chain of FCεRI: a selective marker and pathogenetic factor for a distinct subset of chronic urticaria patients. J Clin Invest 1995; 96:2606–2612.
9. Niimi N, Francis DM, O'Donnell BF, Hide M, Black AK, Winkelmann RK, Greaves MW, Barr RM. Dermal mast cell activation by autoantibodies against the high affinity IgE receptor in chronic urticaria. J Invest Dermatol 1996; 106:1001–1006.
10. Tong LJ, Balakrishnan G, Kochan JP, Kinet J-P, Kaplan AP. Assessment of autoimmunity in patients with chronic urticaria. J Allergy Clin Immunol 1997; 99:461–465.
11. Kaplan AP, HoraKova Z, Katz SI. Assessment of tissue fluid histamine levels in patients with urticaria. J Allergy Clin Immunol 1978; 61:350–354.
12. O'Donnell BF, O'Neill CM, Francis DM, Nimii N, Barr RM, Barlow A, Black AK, Welsh KI, Greaves MW. HLA class II associations in chronic idiopathic urticaria. Br J Dermatol 1999; 140:853–858.
13. Barlow RJ, Black AK, Greaves MW. Treatment of severe chronic urticaria with cyclosporin A. Eur J Dermatol 1993; 3:273–275.
14. Toubi E, Blant A, Kessel A, Golan TD. Low dose cyclosporin A in the treatment of severe chronic idiopathic urticaria. Allergy 1997; 52:312–316.
15. Grattan CEH, O'Donnell BF, Francis DM, Nimii N, Barlow RJ, Seed PT, Black AK, Greaves MW. Randomised double blind study of cyclosporin in chronic idiopathic urticaria. Br J Dermatol 2000 (in press).
16. O'Donnell BF, Barr RM, Black AK, Greaves MW. Intravenous immunoglobulin in autoimmune chronic urticaria. Br J Dermatol 1998; 138:101–106.
17. Grattan CEH, Francis DM, Slater NGP, Greaves MW. Plasmapheresis for severe unremitting chronic urticaria. Lancet 1992; 339:1078–1080.
18. Kuokanen K. A new antihistamine HD 20-511 compared with dimetinden (Fenestil retard) in the treatment of chronic urticaria. Acta Allergy 1977; 32:316–320.
19. Mallet AI, Norris P, Wong E, Greaves MW. The effect of disodium cromoglycate and ketotifen on the excretion of histamine and N-methylimidazole acetic acid in urine of patients with mastocytosis. Br J Clin Pharmacol 1989; 27:88–91.
20. Pearce CA, Greaves MW, Plummer VM, Yamamoto S. Effect of disodium cromoglycate on antigen-evoked histamine release from human skin. Clin Exp Immunol 1974; 17:437–440.
21. Yamamoto S, Greaves MW, Fairley VM. Cyclic AMP-induced inhibition of IgE-mediated hypersensitivity in human skin. Clin Exp Immunol 1973; 24:77–83.
22. Saihan EM. Ketotifen and terbutaline in urticaria. Br J Dermatol 1981; 104:205–206.
23. O'Donnell B, Black AK. Urticarial vasculitis. Int Angiol 1995; 14:166–174.
24. Warin AP, Champion RH. Urticaria, Vol 1. In: Rook A, ed. Major Problems in Dermatology. London: Saunders, 1974:12.
25. Murphy G, Zollman PE, Greaves MW, Winkelmann RK. Symptomatic dermographism (factitious urticaria)—passive transfer experiments from human to monkey. Br J Dermatol 1987; 116:801–804.

26. Misch K, Black AK, Greaves MW, Almosawi T, Stanworth DR. Passive transfer of idiopathic cold urticaria to monkeys. Acta Dermatovenereol 1982; 63:163–164.
27. Logan RA, O'Brien TJ, Greaves MW. The effect of psoralen photochemotherapy (PUVA) on symptomatic dermographism. Clin Exp Dermatol 1989; 14:25–28.
28. Eftekhari N, Ward AM, Allen R, Greaves MW. Protease inhibitor profiles in urticaria and angioedema. Br J Dermatol 1980; 103:33–39.
29. Wong E, Eftekhari N, Greaves MW, Milford Ward A. Beneficial effects of danazol on symptoms and laboratory changes in cholinergic urticaria. Br J Dermatol 1987; 116:553–556.
30. Lawlor F, Black AK, Milford Ward A, Morris R, Greaves MW. Delayed pressure urticaria objective evaluations of a variable disease using a dermographometer and assessment of treatment using colchicine. Br J Dermatol 1989; 120:403–408.
31. Wanderer AA, St Pierre JP, Ellis EF. Primary acquired cold urticaria double-blind comparative study of treatment with cyproheptadine, chlorpheniramine and placebo. Arch Dermatol 1977; 113:1375–1377.
32. Keahey TM, Greaves MW. Cold urticaria: dissociation of cold-evoked histamine release and urticaria following cold challenge. Arch Dermatol 1980; 116:174–177.
33. Bentley Phillips CB, Black AK, Greaves MW. Induced tolerance to cold urticaria caused by cold evoked histamine release. Lancet 1976; ii:63–66.
34. Ramsay CA. Solar urticaria treatment by inducing tolerance to artificial radiation and natural light. Arch Dermatol 1977; 113:1222–1225.
35. Hudson-Peacock MJ, Farr PM, Diffey BL, Goodship TLJ. Combined treatment of solar urticaria with plasmapheresis and PUVA. Br J Dermatol 1993; 128:440–442.
36. Greaves MW. Clinical and molecular correlations in mastocytosis. Malaysian Dermatol 1998; 11:11–14.
37. Soter NA, Austen KF, Wasserman SI. Oral disodium cromoglycate in the treatment of systemic mastocytosis. N Engl J Med 1979; 301:465–469.
38. Czarnetzki BM, Behrendt H. Urticaria pigmentosa clinical picture and response to oral disodium cromoglycate. Br J Dermatol 1981; 105:465–469.
39. Vella Briffa D, Eady RAJ, James P. Photochemotherapy (PUVA) in the treatment of urticaria pigmentosa. Br J Dermatol 1983; 109:67–75.
40. Barton J, Lavker RM, Schechter NM, Lazarus GS. Treatment of urticaria pigmentosa with corticosteroids. Arch Dermatol 1985; 121:1516–1523.
41. Lawlor F, Black AK, Murdoch RD, Greaves MW. Symptomatic dermographism: whealing mast cells and histamine are decreased in the skin following long-term application of a potent topical corticosteroid. Br J Dermatol 1989; 121:629–634.
42. Millikan LE. Papular urticaria. Semin Dermatol 1993; 12:53–56.

18

Therapies for Vitiligo

Pearl E. Grimes
Vitiligo and Pigmentation Institute of Southern California, and University of California at Los Angeles
Los Angeles, California

INTRODUCTION

Vitiligo is a common acquired disease that affects 1 to 2% of the population. It is characterized by one or multiple patches of depigmented skin (Fig. 1). Histologically there is an absence of cutaneous melanocytes. In addition, lymphocytic infiltrates have been described in the involved border and uninvolved skin of patients (1). The disorder may begin at any age but peak frequencies occur in the second and third decade. Females are affected more often than males. Studies show a familial incidence in 25 to 30% of patients with vitiligo. The disease can be precipitated by severe emotional stress, physical illness, bacterial and viral infections, sunburn, and physical trauma.

The precise cause of vitiligo is unknown. Proposed theories include genetic, neural, biochemical, self-destruction, viral, and autoimmune mechanisms (2–5). Vitiligo patients have an increased frequency of a variety of autoimmune diseases including hyperthyroidism (Graves' Disease), hypothyroidism (Hashimoto's Thyroiditis), Alopecia Areata, Rheumatoid Arthritis, Pernicious Anemia, and Addison's Disease. Detailed review studies addressing the causal origin of vitiligo, viewed in totality, suggest that vitiligo is probably a heterogeneous disease with multiple causes (2–5).

Vitiligo remains an emotional and cosmetically disfiguring condition. It impacts every racial and ethnic group. Despite the equal incidence in different racial and ethnic groups, the disease is cosmetically more disfiguring in darker-skinned individuals. Although significant therapeutic advances have occurred in the past 20 years, many dermatologists consider vitiligo an untreatable insignifi-

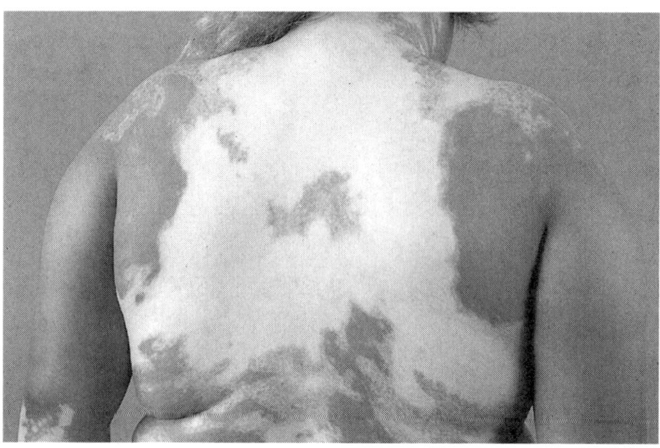

Figure 1 40-year-old male with generalized vitiligo.

cant cosmetic malady. A variety of medical and surgical therapies offer significant benefit for patients with this disease.

RATIONALE FOR CHOOSING THERAPEUTIC OPTIONS

Therapies for vitiligo include topical and systemic steroids, topical and systemic psoralen photochemotherapy, ultraviolet B (UVB) phototherapy, nutritional/vitamin supplementation, khellin, phenylalanine, immunomodulators, autologous melanocyte grafting, and a variety of other miscellaneous therapies. In severe cases, depigmentation may be indicated. Such therapies should be predicated on the age of the patient, extent of cutaneous surface involvement (severity), and activity or progression of the disease (Table 1). The disease can be divided into four stages based on severity of disease: limited (<10%) involvement, moderate (10–25%) involvement, moderately severe (26–50%) involvement, and severe disease (>50%) depigmentation.

MEDICAL THERAPIES

Corticosteroids

Topical, intralesional, intramuscular, and oral steroids have been used in patients with varying results (6–12). Low-, mid-, and high-potency topical steroids are used to repigment vitiliginous lesions. In general, low-potency steroids such as hydrocortisone 1% have minimal efficacy in patients. However, maximal results

Table 1 Therapeutic Approaches for Vitiligo

Stage I, II Disease*	Stage III, IV Disease†
Topical Steroids	Oral Photochemotherapy
Topical Photochemotherapy	Systemic Steroids (Oral, IM) (for stabilization)
PUVA-sol	Bath Photochemotherapy
In-Office PUVA	UVB Phototherapy
Bath Photochemotherapy	Narrow Band
Pseudocatalase/UVB	Broad Band
UVB Phototherapy	Oral Khellin/UVA
Narrow Band	L Phenylalanine/UV
Broad Band	Immunomodulators
L Phenylalanine/UV	Isoprinosine
Topical Khellin/UVA	Levamasole
Melagenena	Immunosuppressives
Calcipotriol/PUVA	Cyclosporine
Tar Emulsions	Cyclophosphamide
Vitamin Supplementation	Nitrogen Mustard
Autologous Melanocyte Grafting (stable lesions)	Depigmentation (severe, recalcitrant lesions)

* Stage I, <10% involvement; Stage II, 10–25% involvement. † Stage III, 26–50% involvement; Stage IV, >50% involvement.

are achieved with high-potency topical steroid preparations (6). Topical steroid–induced repigmentation has been reported in 9 to 92% of patients treated with this modality. Maximal repigmentation occurs on the face and neck (Fig. 2). Corticosteroid preparations probably alter aberrant immunological responses in patients with vitiligo.

Steroid side effects include atrophy, telangiectasias, hypertrichosis, and steroid acne. In light of side effects, particularly when using high-potency or Class I steroids, treatments should be used for 1 or 2 months, then interrupted for 1 month or tapered to a low-potency preparation.

Topical mid- to high-potency steroids are ideal initial treatments for patients with localized or limited disease involving less than 10% of the cutaneous surface. Low- to mid-potency preparations can also be safely used in very young children. High-potency or Class I steroids are recommended for older children and adults. If no clinical response is evident by 3 to 4 months, alternative topical therapies should be considered.

Several studies have documented the efficacy of intralesional steroids. However, this form of steroid administration is associated with a high frequency of steroid-induced atrophy.

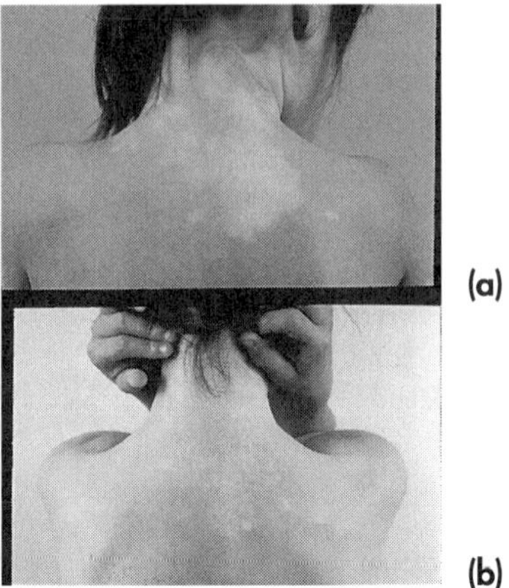

FIGURE 2 Repigmentation in a child treated with high-potency Class I topical steroids. (a) Before, (b) after.

Systemic steroids have been used as monotherapy or in combination with other therapies, such as oral psoralen photochemotherapy (PUVA) and levamisole, with mixed results (6,12). Short courses of systemic steroids are often indicated in patients with rapidly progressive moderate to severe vitiligo. An intramuscular injection of Kenolog 40 mg can be administered every 6 weeks for up to three injections to stabilize patients with progressive vitiligo (personal data, Vitiligo and Pigmentation Institute of Southern California, 1998). However, prolonged use of systemic steroids can be associated with weight gain, fluid retention, and other systemic steroid–induced side effects. Prolonged use of moderate- to high-dose steroid therapy is not indicated.

Psoralen Photochemotherapy (PUVA)

When compared with other medical therapies for vitiligo, topical and systemic PUVA therapies remain the mainstay for repigmenting vitiliginous lesions (Fig. 3). The use of psoralen preparations as repigmenting agents for vitiligo was described as early as 1400 B.C. (13). They were subsequently investigated by El Mofty in 1947 (14) when he documented the efficacy of oral and topical 8-methoxypsoralen (8-MOP) in combination with sunlight exposure. Fitzpatrick and others further expanded our experience with the psoralen drugs (15). The acronym PUVA was introduced in 1974 when Parrish, et al. used oral psoralens in combination with then newly developed high-intensity long wave (328–400 nm) ultraviolet phototherapy units (16). The psoralens are furocoumarin compounds, photodynamically active drugs that are capable of absorbing radiant energy (17).

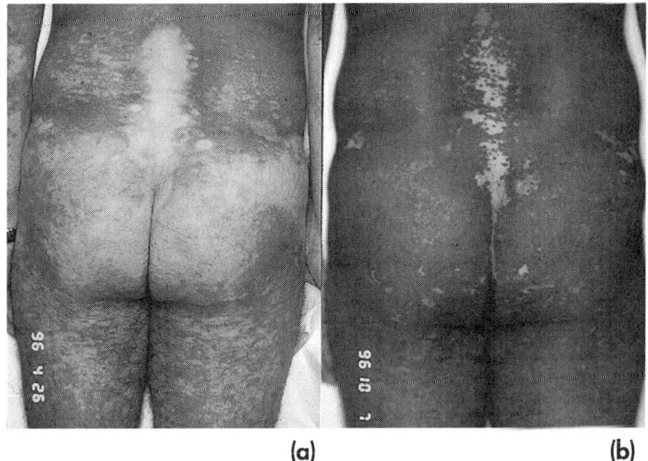

(a) (b)

FIGURE 3 Significant repigmentation in patient undergoing oral photochemotherapy. Approximately 100 treatments. (a) Before, (b) after.

The precise mechanism of action of psoralens and long-wave ultraviolet light in the treatment of vitiligo is unknown. Psoralens form monofunctional and bifunctional photoadducts that suppress DNA synthesis. In addition, studies have shown that PUVA stimulates proliferation and hypertrophy of melanocytes of the outer-root sheath of the hair follicle as well as melanocytes from the border of vitiliginous lesions (18,19). Repigmentation may indeed result from migration of these stimulated melanocytes into the area of depigmentation. In addition, in vitro studies suggest that PUVA therapy causes a depletion of epidermal growth factor receptors on melanocytes and also alters the expression of melanocyte surface antigens (20). PUVA may also alter type IV collagen secretion (21) and release circulating growth factors that stimulate cell proliferation (22). Evidence also suggests that PUVA alters cell-mediated immunological responses (23,24).

Topical Photochemotherapy

Topical photochemotherapy treatments can be administered in the office or in combination with sunlight. The choice of topical PUVA is predicated on the severity of vitiligo, distribution of lesions, and lifestyle of the patient. Topical in-office PUVA is appropriate for patients with less than 20 to 25% involvement (6,7). A thin coat of 0.01 or 0.1% methoxalen ointment (dilution of Oxsoralen Lotion 1%; ICN Pharmaceuticals, Costa Mesa, CA) is applied to the vitiliginous areas 30 minutes before UVA exposure. An initial UVA dose of 0.12 J is administered with increments of 0.12 J weekly according to the patient's skin type. After moderate asymptomatic erythema is achieved, the UVA dose is maintained at a dosage sufficient to retain erythema. The treated area is washed with soap and water immediately after UVA exposure. A broad-spectrum sunscreen is applied to sun-exposed treated areas before leaving the physician's office. The major advantages of this form of topical therapy are lower cumulative UVA exposures and lack of systemic or ocular toxicity. A mean repigmentation of 58% has been reported using this protocol (7). The major side effect of in-office topical photochemotherapy using 0.1% methoxalen ointment is severe phototoxic or blistering reactions and perilesional hyperpigmentation. Side effects can be minimized by making careful increments in UVA exposure as well as having the patient avoid additional sun exposure to the treated areas. Oxsoralen 0.1% should never be used in combination with sunlight exposure because of the known likelihood of developing severe phototoxic reactions.

In light of the inherent difficulties of in-office topical PUVA for many patients with vitiligo, particularly children, an alternative protocol can be followed using sunlight as a UVA light source. It is a therapeutic option for children and adults with less than 10% involvement. Patients apply a thin coat of methoxalen ointment 0.001% to the affected areas. Thirty minutes later, vitiliginous areas are exposed to sunlight for 15 to 30 minutes between 10:00 a.m. and 4:00 p.m. Affected areas can be treated daily or every other day. This approach minimizes the adverse reactions often associated with in-office topical PUVA using higher concentrations of Oxsoralen. Grimes reported a mean repigmentation of 71% in 125 patients treated with this therapeutic approach (7). Furthermore, costs are minimal and it provides increased availability of treatment to larger segments of the population. Side effects are minimal.

Oral Photochemotherapy

Previous studies have reported the efficacy of oral photochemotherapy (7,16,17). Oral photochemotherapy is usually reserved for patients with moderate to severe disease involving greater than 20 to 25% of the cutaneous surface. Oral psoralens generally are not used in children less than 9 years of age. The standard dose of 8-methoxypsoralen (8-MOP) is usually 0.3–0.4 mg/kg ingested 1.5 h before office UVA exposure. Ingestion with food minimizes side effects including headaches and gastrointestinal reactions. Initial UVA doses of 1 to 2 J are administered with increments of 0.5 to 1.0 J weekly until moderate asymptomatic erythema develops. As with topical PUVA, the UVA dose should be maintained at a level sufficient to retain erythema. Patients should always apply a broad spectrum sunscreen to exposed areas after treatment. In addition, in light of the ocular pharmacokinetics of 8-MOP, protective UVA sunglasses should be worn for 18 to 24 h indoors and outdoors after ingestion of 8-MOP.

5-Methoxypsoralen has been successfully used in combination with UVA for treating vitiligo and psoriasis (25,26). Clinical trials suggest that 5-MOP is comparable in efficacy to 8-MOP, but requires greater total UVA exposure. The frequency of cutaneous and gastrointestinal side effects is substantially less with 5-MOP.

Trimethylpsoralen (Trisoralen; ICN Pharmaceuticals, Costa Mesa, CA) is a viable alternative, but is less effective for patients that are unable to receive therapy at a PUVA treatment center. The appropriate Trisoralen dose is 0.6 to 0.8 mg/kg. After ingestion of Trisoralen, the initial sun exposure should be 5 min between 10:00 a.m. and 4:00 p.m. Subsequent sun exposure is increased by 5 minutes until lesional erythema appears. Treatments are given three times weekly.

Contraindications for oral PUVA treatment include cataracts, liver disease, and, in general, photosensitivity disorders. Side effects include headaches, nausea, vomiting, xerosis, pruritus, photoaging, diffuse hyperpigmentation, and hypertrichosis. The major advantages of oral PUVA include its effectiveness in controlling the progression of active disease and its lower frequency of blistering reactions.

Oral PUVA therapy has been associated with an increase in nonmelanoma and melanoma skin cancer in patients with psoriasis (27,28). However, similar documentation has not been reported in patients with vitiligo (29).

Factors that portend enhanced PUVA-induced repigmentation include young age (children), patient motivation, maintenance of adequate lesional phototoxicity, and location of lesions (7). Maximal repigmentation occurs on the face and neck.

Bath PUVA

Bath PUVA using a very dilute solution of methoxalen in water has been reported in patients with psoriasis and vitiligo (30,31). Although more photosensitizing than oral PUVA, compared with topical PUVA, it provides a uniform delivery of methoxalen to the skin and there is a substantial reduction in cumulative UVA exposure. Bath PUVA is also a therapeutic option in young children with moderate to severe disease when oral PUVA is contraindicated because of age restrictions.

L-Phenylalanine

Several studies have reported variable results of oral and topical L-phenylalanine in combination with UV light for repigmentation of vitiligo in both children and adults (32–34). Dosages have ranged from 50 to 200 mg/kg, 30 min to 1 h before UV exposure. The essential amino acid phenylalanine is a precursor of tyrosine, the substrate for melanin synthesis. The precise mechanism of action of phenylalanine is unknown; however, it may alter epidermal Langerhans cells (32) and inhibit antibody production. The major advantage of phenylalanine is its lack of side effects including phototoxicity. Therapeutic contraindications include phenylketonuria, skin cancer, pregnancy, lactation, prior radiation therapy, and arsenic exposure.

UVB Phototherapy

Recent studies have reported the benefits of UVB phototherapy (35). Westerhof (36) compared the efficacy and safety of narrow band (311 nm) UVB phototherapy with topical psoralen and UVA. Twenty-eight patients received topical PUVA twice weekly using a 0.005% concentration, whereas 78 patients received narrow band UVB twice weekly. Their results suggested that narrow band UVB treatment was as effective as topical PUVA with fewer side effects.

Khellin and UVA

Khellin is a furanochrome isolated from the seeds of ammi visnaji. It was used extensively in the 1940s and 1950s as a coronary vasodilator in the treatment of angina pectoris and asthma but subsequently abandoned for better treatments (6). It is not approved by the FDA for use in the United States; however, it has been administered orally and topically in combination with UVA or sunlight in other countries. Oral doses have ranged from 50 to 100 mg ingested 45 min to 2.5 h before UV exposure (37). A topical 2% preparation has also been used. Response rates vary (38–40). However, response rates of 70 to 77% have been reported (37), results comparable to PUVA-induced repigmentation. Unlike PUVA, khellin does not induce phototoxic erythema or hyperpigmentation of normal skin. It is also less mutagenic and carcinogenic in light of its induction of only monofunctional photoadducts. However, both oral and topical khellin have been associated with reversible elevations in liver transaminases (39,40).

Melagenina

Miyares-Cao (41) in 1976 first reported the efficacy of topical melagenina, a hydroalcoholic extract of human placenta in combination with infrared radiation. The initial product now called Melagenina I contains amino acids, free fatty acids, phospholipids, minerals, and other compounds. The most active component is an alpha lipoprotein that stimulates melanin synthesis and melanocyte proliferation. The alpha lipoprotein has been subsequently purified for production of Melagenina II, a compound with purported increased efficacy in clinical trials (42,43). Melagenina II has shown efficacy in the absence of infrared exposure.

Despite the initial favorable reports in 84% of 732 patients (41), subsequent repigmentation rates have varied (42,43). There have been no well-controlled trials evaluating the efficacy or safety of placental extract products for treatment of vitiligo.

Pseudocatalase Calcium with UVB Therapy

Schallreuter, et al. (44) reported the beneficial effects of pseudocatalase and calcium applied twice daily and twice weekly UVB exposure for patients with vitiligo. The rationale for this therapy was derived from previous studies that showed aberrant catalase and calcium homeostasis in patients. Of the 33 patients treated for a mean duration of 15 months, excellent repigmentation was reported in 90%. No controls were treated or patients with UVB alone. Hence, in light of the known beneficial effects of UVB therapy alone, further double-blind, well-controlled studies are necessary to document the efficacy of pseudocatalase and calcium.

Vitamin Supplementation

Montes (45) reported the efficacy of folic acid 1 mg, ascorbic acid 1000 mg, and biweekly vitamin B_{12} 1000 mg injections as repigmenting agents for vitiligo in eight patients. Juhlin and Olsson (46) treated 100 patients with Vitamin B_{12} 1 mg and folic acid 5 mg twice daily. Patients were encouraged to expose their skin to sun in the summer and UVB irradiation in the winter. Patients were monitored for 2 years. Some evidence of repigmentation occurred in 52%. Total repigmentation was observed in six patients. In addition, the disease stabilized in 64%.

I routinely start patients on high-dose multivitamins containing the B-complex vitamins, vitamin E, and ascorbic acid. Preliminary uncontrolled data suggest that vitamin supplementation is indeed beneficial in achieving stabilization of vitiligo. However, well-controlled blinded studies should be conducted to document the role of vitamins as repigmenting and/or stabilizing agents for vitiligo.

Immunomodulators

Abnormalities of both humoral and cell-mediated immune responses have been documented in patients with vitiligo (1–3). A rational therapeutic approach involves the use of immune modulatory drugs. The efficacy of several such agents has been reported for repigmentation of vitiliginous lesions. In a preliminary study, the efficacy and immunomodulatory effects of isoprinosine were assessed in 17 patients. Follicular and/or confluent areas of repigmentation were observed in six of the 12 patients completing the clinical trial (47). The drug had profound immunomodulatory effects at 14 weeks of therapy, ameliorating many of the observed baseline humoral and cell-mediated immunological abnormalities. Isoprinosine is not approved by the FDA for use in the United States. Levamisole has been used as a monotherapy and in combination with fluocinolone acetonide and topical clobetosol propionate 0.05% in 64 patients (48). Some degree of repigmentation was observed in 64% of patients treated with levamisole alone compared with 87% for levamisole and fluocinolone and 100% of the levamisole/clobetosol group. Nihei, et al. (49) reported the efficacy of suplatast fosilate in seven patients with vitiligo. Suplatast fosilate is an antiallergic agent that inhibits the transcription of T-cell IL-4m RNA. Of the patients treated, three showed improvement. In addition, it halted disease progression in three and reduced thyroid antibody titers in two patients.

The beneficial effects of cyclosporine and anapsos have been reported in patients with vitiligo (6,42). The immunosuppressive agents, cyclophosphamide, and nitrogen mustard have also been used as repigmenting agents (50,51).

Miscellaneous Therapies

A variety of additional therapies have been reported to offer some benefit in repigmenting vitiliginous lesions. They include Chinese herbal extracts, tar emulsions, tocopherol in combination with PUVA, minoxodil and PUVA, caleipotriol and PUVAsol, copper, dapsone, clofazamine, ACTH, melanocyte-stimulating hormone, and metharmon-F (sex steroid-thyroid hormone) (6,42,52,53).

Depigmentation

Monobenzylether of hydroquinone (MBEH, Benoquin; ICN Pharmaceuticals, Costa Mesa, CA) has been used as a depigmenting agent for patients with extensive vitiligo since the 1950s. In general, MBEH causes permanent irreversible destruction of melanocytes (6,54,55) and induces depigmentation locally and remote from the sites of application. Hence, the use of MBEH for other disorders of pigmentation is contraindicated.

Depigmentation is a viable therapeutic alternative in patients with greater than 50% cutaneous depigmentation who have shown recalcitrance to repigmentation or in individuals with extensive vitiligo who have no desire to undergo repigmentation therapies. Treatment should be initiated with a 10% concentration of MBEH applied twice daily because of irritancy induced by the full-strength preparation. The concentration should be gradually increased to 20% in 2 to 3 months if no irritation ensues. In an effort to limit absorption of this drug, the body should be depigmented regionally. I usually depigment the face and upper extremity areas first, then the lower extremity sites, and finally truncal areas. Depending on the percentage of residual pigmentation, this process may take 6 months to 2 years. During and on completion of this process, patients are permanently photosensitive; therefore, they must minimize inadvertent sun exposure and wear broad spectrum sunscreens.

The major side effects of MBEH therapy are dermatitis and pruritus, which usually respond to topical and/or systemic steroids (56). Other side effects include severe xerosis, alopecia, and premature graying (Grimes, unpublished data, 1998). In addition, conjunctival melanosis and corneal pigment deposition have been reported (6). These changes, however, do not interfere with visual acuity. Patients must be extremely careful to avoid inadvertent contact exposure of spouses or other intimate contacts to MBEH-treated skin for at least 2 to 3 hours after drug application.

SURGICAL THERAPIES

Surgical therapies for vitiligo are indicated for patients with stable, localized patches that have failed medical intervention. The major advantage of transplantation procedures is the transfer of a reservoir of healthy melanocytes to vitiliginous skin to undergo proliferation and migration into areas of depigmentation. These procedures are contraindicated in patients with a history of hypertrophic scars or keloids. Transplantation protocols differ by the methods used to collect and transplant tissue from the donor to the recipient site. Donor methods include shave biopsy, punch biopsy, cryoinduced blisters, suction blisters, and autologous cultured melanocytes. Recipient sites are prepared for grafting via punch biopsies, dermabrasion, suction blisters, cryoinduced blisters, or laser ablation. (57–68)

Autologous Suction Blister Grafts

Suction blister grafting for leukoderma was initially used by Falabella (57,58) to treat leukodermas in four patients in 1971. This technique involves the induction of epidermal vacuum pump–induced suction blisters or cryotherapy-induced blisters. The roof of the blisters are then transplanted to denuded achromic skin. The success of this method depends on blistering technique, location of the treated lesion, and type of vitiligo. Despite the cumbersome equipment often required for induction of suction blisters or the discomfort associated with liquid nitrogen blisters, the technique is associated with minimal scarring.

Autologous Punch Grafts

Punch grafts are an easy, efficient in-office method for repigmentation of small localized areas of vitiligo (Figs. 4,5). No special equipment is required. The technique involves collecting 1.5 to 2 mm punch grafts from donor sites such as the buttock area, outer thigh, or inner arm; the grafts are transplanted to recipient sites from which similar grafts have been removed (1,6,57). The major advantage of punch grafts include simplicity, ease of manipulation of the punch biopsy graft and lack of need for special equipment. Side effects include cobblestoning, koebnerization, and, in rare cases, infections. Cobblestoning improves and may completely disappear in 2 to 6 months (6).

Autologous Melanocyte Transplant

Lerner, et al. (59) first transplanted cultured autologous melanocytes to the depigmented skin of patients with piebaldism. Although initial melanocyte culture

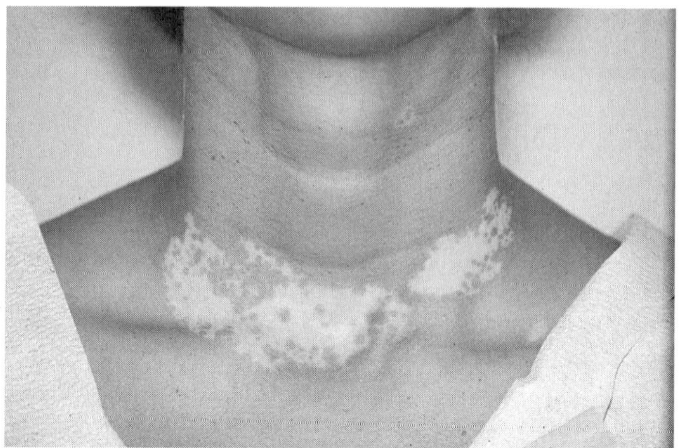

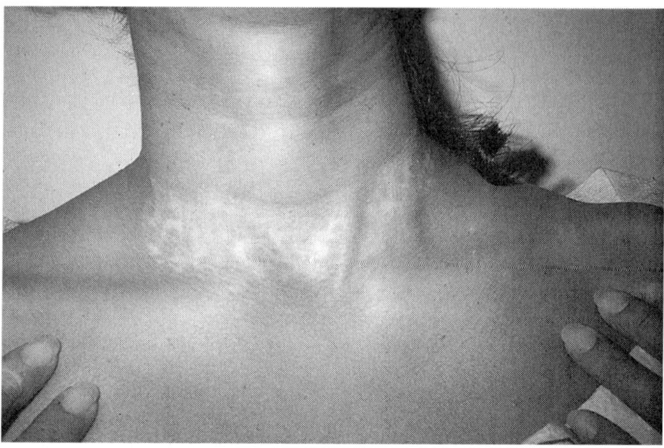

FIGURE 4 Repigmentation of neck/chest areas after autologous grafting.

technology involved the use of phorbol esters (tumor promotors), menlanocytes are now expanded in culture using physiological reagents (60,61) that contain natural melanocyte growth factors such as basic fibroblast growth factor. Mixed cocultures of melanocytes and keratinocytes have also been used. This technique involves culturing melanocytes and keratinocytes on collagen-coated membranes (62). Repigmentation results vary from 10 to 100% (58,60,61). Despite the success of cultured melanocyte transplantation, culture techniques remain tedious and expensive, requiring special technology and culture facilities.

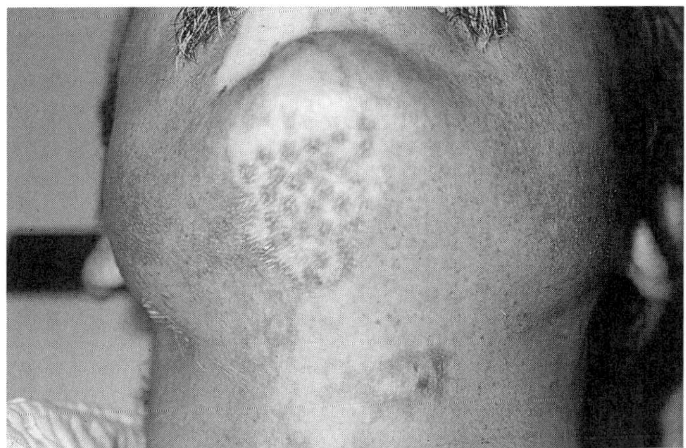

FIGURE 5 **Migration of pigment from 2 mm punch grafts.**

Olsson and Juhlin (63) reported a new technique that eliminates the need for cell culture. After removal of a 4 × 30 cm^2 skin sample, cells were mechanically separated in a trypsin/EDTA solution, centrifuged, and washed in a melanocyte medium. The melanocyte-enriched epidermal suspension devoid of stratum corneum and stratum granulosum was then transplanted to dermabraded vitiliginous skin. This technique has been successful in patients with vitiligo, piebaldism, and halo nevi.

Other Transplantation Techniques

Na, et al. (64) reported transplantation of single hairs collected from donor occipital scalp in 21 patients. Perifollicular pigment was observed in 71% in 2 to 8 weeks. Epidermal sheet grafts (65) involve the removal of ultrathin donor skin, which is then transpslanted to a dermabraded recipient site. In addition, the erbium-YAG laser and short pulse CO_2 laser are reported useful for skin ablation of the recipient graft site (66–68).

Micropigmentation (Tatooing)

This technique involves microsurgically implanting iron oxide pigment into the dermis of vitiliginous skin via a variety of commercially available micropigmentation units (6,69). Although dramatic results may be noted immediately after the procedure, the pigment often fades within 1 to 6 weeks of treatment. In addition, it is often extremely difficult to obtain an adequate pigment match with the patient's

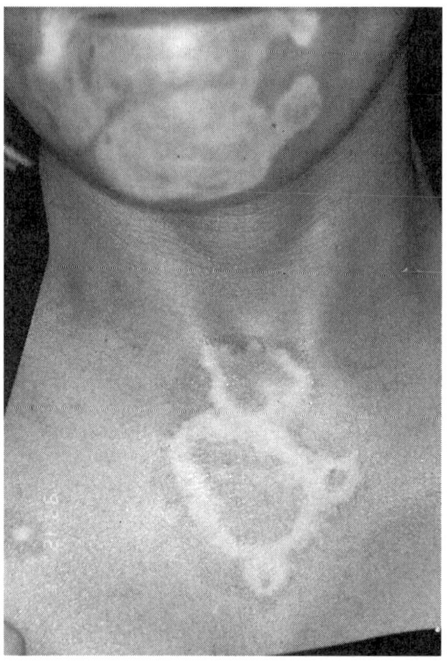

FIGURE 6 Koebnerization after micropigmentation of vitiliginous lesions.

normal skin tone. This becomes increasingly apparent as the pigment fades. Some patients develop koebnerization surrounding the treated site (Fig. 6). In light of these issues, micropigmentation is only recommended for treatment of lips, areas traditionally recalcitrant to other therapeutic modalities.

ADJUNCTIVE THERAPIES

Broad spectrum sunscreens are important adjunctive therapies for patients with vitiligo. Such agents minimize tanning, thereby limiting the contrast between vitiliginous and normal skin. In addition, sunscreens should be worn by all vitiligo patients to limit the susceptibility to sunburn and long-term photodamage. Broad spectrum photoprotective UVA/UVB sunscreens are recommended.

Cosmetic camouflage with stains, make-up, or self-tanning lotions is also practical and acceptable to some patients, particularly those with very limited involvement in exposed areas. In addition, many patients camouflage exposed lesions while undergoing therapies such as PUVA. These preparations should be removed before UVA exposure. Cosmetics and stains frequently used by vitiligo patients include Dermablend, Dermacolor, Vitadye, and Chromelin brands. Multiple self-tanning lotions containing dihydroxyacetone are also available. These lotions are most effective in skin types I to III.

Psychological counseling should be routinely considered in patients who are emotionally distressed by vitiligo. In addition, many patients report that communication with other vitiligo patients serves to enhance their coping mechanisms.

REFERENCES

1. Grimes PE. Diseases of hypopigmentation. In: Sams WM, Lynch PJ, eds. Principles and Practice of Dermatology. 2nd ed. New York: Churchill-Livingstone, 1996, pp. 873–885.
2. Boissy R, LePoole C. Vitiligo. Sem Cut Med Surg 16:3–14, 1997.
3. Kovacs SO. Vitiligo. J Am Acad Dermatol 38:647–666, 1998.
4. Schwartz RA, Janniger CK. Vitiligo. Cutis 60:239–244, 1997.
5. Grimes PE, Sevall JS, Wojdani A. Cytomegalovirus DNA identified in skin biopsy specimens of patients with vitiligo. J Am Acad Dermatol 35:21–26, 1996.
6. Grimes PE. Vitiligo: an overview of therapeutic approaches. Dermatol Clin 11:325–337, 1993.
7. Grimes PE. Psoralen photochemotherapy for vitiligo. Clin Dermatol 15:921–926, 1997.
8. Nordlund JJ, Halder RM, Grimes PE. Management of vitiligo. Dermatol Clin 11: 27–33, 1993.
9. Nordlund JJ, Grimes PE, Halder RM. Guidelines for treatment of vitiligo. J Am Acad Dermatol 15:921–926, 1997.
10. Kumari F. Vitiligo treated with topical clobetasol proponate. Arch Dermatol 120: 631–635, 1984.
11. Geraldez CB, Gutierrez G. A clinical trial of clobetasol propionate in Filipino vitiligo patients. Clin Therapeutics 9:474–482, 1987.
12. Farah FS, Kurban AK, Chaglassian HT. The treatment of vitiligo with psoralens and triamcinolone by mouth. Br J Dermatol 79:89–91, 1967.
13. El Mofty AM. Vitiligo and Psoralens. New York: Pergamon Press, 1968.
14. El Mofty AM. A preliminary clinical report on the treatment of leucoderma with *Ammi majus linn*. J Egypt Med Assoc 31:631–660, 1948.
15. Fitzpatrick TB. The psoralen story: photochemotherapy and photoprotection. Proceedings of the International Congrcss: Psoralens in 1988. 1989: pp. 5–10.
16. Parrish JA, Fitzpatrick TB, Shea G, et al. Photochemotherapy of vitiligo: use of orally administered psoralens and a high-intensity long-wave ultraviolet light system. Arch Dermatol 112:1531–1534, 1976.
17. Honig B, Morison WL. Photochemotherapy beyond psoriasis. J Am Acad Dermatol 31:775–790, 1994.
18. Ortonne JP, MacDonald DM, Micoud A, et al. PUVA-induced repigmentation of vitiligo: a histochemical (split DOPA) and ultrastructural study. Br J Dermatol 101: 1–7, 1979.

19. Cui J, Shen L, Wang G. Role of the hair follicles in repigmentation of vitiligo. J Invest Dermatol 97:410–416, 1991.
20. Kao CH, Hsen SY. Comparison of the effect of 8-methoxypsoralen (8-MOP) plus UVA (PUVA) on human melanocytes in vitiligo vulgaris and in vitro. J Invest Dermatol 98:734–740, 1992.
21. Morelli JG, Yohn JJ, Zekman T, et al. Melanocyte movement in vitro: role of matrix proteins and integrin receptors. J Invest Dermatol 101:605–608, 1993.
22. Abdel-Naser MB, Hann SK, Bystryn JC. Oral psoralen with UVA-A therapy releases circulating growth factor (A) that stimulates oil proliferation. Arch Dermatol 133: 1530–1533, 1997.
23. Morison WL. In vivo effects of psoralens plus longwave ultraviolet radiation on immunity. J Natl Cancer Inst 66:243–246, 1984.
24. Morison WT, Parrish JA, McAuliffe DJ, et al. Sensitivity of mononuclear cells to PUVA: effect on subsequent stimulation with mitogens and on exclusion of trypan blue dye. Clin Exp Dermatol 6:273–278, 1981.
25. McNeely W, Goa KL. 5-Methoxypsoralen: a review of its effects in psoriasis and vitiligo. Drugs 56:667–690, 1998.
26. Hann SK, Cho MY, Im S, et al. Treatment of vitiligo with oral 5-methyoxypsoralen. J Dermatol 18:324–329, 1991.
27. Stern RS, Lange R. Nonmelanoma skin cancer occuring in patients treated with PUVA 5 to 10 years after first treatment. J Invest Dermatol 91:120–124,1998.
28. Stern RS, Thibodeau LA, Kleinerman RA, et al. Risk of cutaneous carcinoma in patients treated with oral methoxsalen photochemotherapy for psoriasis. N Engl J Med 300:809–813, 1997.
29. Halder R, Battle EF, Smith EM. Cutaneous malignancies in patients treated with psoralen photochemotherapy (PUVA) for vitiligo. Arch Dermatol 131:734–735, 1995.
30. Lowe NJ, Ukingarten D, Bourget T, May LS. PUVA therapy for psoriasis: comparison of oral and bathwater delivery of 8-methoxypsoralen. J Am Acad Dermatol 14: 754–760, 1986.
31. Mai DW, Ossohuntro C, Dijksta J WE, Bailin P. Childhood vitiligo successfully treated with bath PUVA. Ped Dermatol 15:53–55, 1998.
32. Cormane RH, Siddiqui AH, Nangerman IM. Photochemotherapy of vitiligo with oral phenylalanine. J Invest Dermatol 80:367–370, 1983.
33. Antiniou C, Schulpis H, Michas T, et al. Vitiligo therapy with oral and topical phenylalanine and UVA exposure. Int J Dermatol 28:545–547, 1989.
34. Siddiqui AH, Stolk LML, Bhaggol R, et al. L-phenylalanine and UVA irradiation in the treatment of vitiligo. J Dermatol 188:215–218, 1994.
35. Koster W, Wisekmann A. Photherapie mit UV-B bei vitiligo. Z Hautkr 65:1022–1029, 1990.
36. Westerhof W, Nievweboer-Krobotova L. Treatment of vitiligo with UV-B radiation vs. topical psoralen plus UV-A. Arch Dermatol 133:1525–1528, 1997.
37. Abdel-Fattah A, Aboul-Enein MN, Wassel G, et al. An approach to the treatment of vitiligo by khellin. Dermatologica 165:136–140, 1982.
38. Ortel B, Tanew A, Honigsman H. Treatment of vitiligo with khellin and ultraviolet light. J Am Acad Dermatol 18:693–701, 1988.

39. Dushet P, Schwartz T, Pusch M, et al. Marked increase of liver transaminases after khellin and UVA therapy. J Am Acad Dermatol 21:592–593, 1989.
40. Orrecchia G, Perfetti L. Photochemotherapy with topical khellin and sunlight. J Dermatol 184:120–123, 1992.
41. Miyares-Cao C. Melagenina: a Cuban product. A new and effective drug for the treatment of vitiligo. Series of National Reports. Republic of Cuba, Havana, 1986.
42. Mandel AS, Haberman HP. Non-PUVA nonsurgical therapies for vitiligo. Clin Dermatol 15:907–919, 1997.
43. Suite M, Quamina DB. Treatment of vitiligo with topical melagenina—a human placental extract. J Am Acad Dermatol 24:1018–1019, 1991.
44. Schallreuter KU, Wood JM, Lemke KR, et al. Treatment of vitiligo with a topical application of pseudocatalase and calcium in combination with short-term UVB exposure: a case study on 33 patients. Dermatology 190:223–229,1995.
45. Montes LF, Diaz ML, Lajous J, Garcia NJ. Folic acid and vitamin B_{12} in vitiligo: a nutritional approach. Cutis 50:39–42, 1992.
46. Juhlin I, Olsson MJ. Improvement of vitiligo after oral treatment with vitamin B_{12} and folic acid and the importance of sun exposure. ACTA Derm Venereol 77:460–462, 1997.
47. Grimes PE, Wojdani A, Loeb LJ, et al. The effects of isoprinosine treatment on repigmentation and immunologic aberrations in vitiligo. J Invest Dermatol 98(abstr): 534, 1992.
48. Pasricha JS, Khera V. Effect of prolonged treatment with levamisole on vitiligo with limited and slow-spreading disease. Int J Dermatol 33:584–587, 1994.
49. Nihel Y, Nishibu A, Kaneko F. Suplatast fosilate (IPD), a new immunoregulator, is effective in vitiligo treatment. J Dermatol 25:250–255, 1998.
50. Gokdale BB. Cyclophosphamide and vitiligo. Int J Dermatol 18:92, 1979.
51. VanScott EJ, Yu RJ. Melanogenesis from topical mechlorethamine and analogues in skin of hairless mice and in vitiligo. J Invest Dermatol 65:476–478, 1975.
52. Parsud D, Saini R, Verma N. Combination of PUVAsol and topical calcipotriol in vitiligo. Dermatol 197:167–170, 1998.
53. Muto M, Furumoto H, Ohmura A, et al. Successful treatment of vitiligo with a sex steroid-thyroid hormone mixture. J Dermatol 22:770–772, 1995.
54. Oliver EA, Schwartz L, Warren LH. Occupational leukoderma. Arch Dermatol Syphylol 42:993–1014, 1940.
55. Mosher DB, Parrish JA, Fitzpatrick TB, et al. Monobenzylether of hydroquinone: a retrospective study of 18 severely affected patients. Br J Dermatol 97:669–679, 1977.
56. Nordlund JJ, Fazet B, Kirkwood J, Lerner AB. Dermatitis produced by applications of monobenzone in patients with active vitiligo. Arch Dermatol 121:1141–1144, 1985.
57. Falabella R. Epidermal grafting: an original technique and its application in achromic and granulating areas. Arch Dermatol 104:592–600, 1971.
58. Falabella R. Surgical therapies for vitiligo. Clin Dermatol 15(5):927–939, 1997.
59. Leiner AB, Halaban R, Klaus SN. Transplantation of human melanocytes. J Invest Dermatol 89:219–224, 1987.
60. Lontz W, Olsson MJ, Moellman G, et al. Pigment cell transplantation for treatment of vitiligo: a progress report. J Am Acad Dermatol 30:591–597, 1994.

61. Olsson MJ, Juhlin L. Transplantation of melanocytes in vitiligo. Br J Dermatol 132: 587–591, 1995.
62. Plott RT, Brysk MM, Newton R, et al. A surgical treatment for vitiligo: autologous cultured-epithelial grafts. J Dermatol Surg Oncol 15:1161–1166, 1989.
63. Olsson MJ, Juhlin I. Leucoderm treated by transplantation of basal cell layer enriched suspension. Br J Dermatol 138:644–648, 1998.
64. Na GY, Seo SK, Choi SK. Single hair grafting for the treatment of vitiligo. J Am Acad Dermatol 38:580–584, 1998.
65. Khan AM, Cohen MJ, Kaplan L, et al. Vitiligo: treatment by dermabrasian and epithelial sheet grafting. J Am Acad Dermatol 33:646–648, 1995.
66. Kahn AM, Ostad A, Moy RL. Grafting following short-pulse carbon dioxide laser deepithelialization. Dermatol Surf 22:965–968, 1996.
67. Kaufman R, Greiner D, Kypenberger S, Bernd A. Grafting in vitro cultured melanocytes onto laser-ablated lesions in vitiligo. Octa Derm Venereol 78:136–138, 1998.
68. Yang JS, Kye VC. Treatment of vitiligo with autologous epidermal grafting by means of pulsed erbium: YAG laser. J Am Acad Dermatol 38:280–282, 1998.
69. Halder RM, Pham H, Breadon JY, Johnson BA. Micropigmentation for the treatment of vitiligo. J Dermatol Surg Oncol 15:1092–1098, 1989.

19

Treatment of the Cutaneous Manifestations of Autoimmune Connective Tissue Diseases

Richard D. Sontheimer
University of Iowa College of Medicine
University of Iowa Health Care
Iowa City, Iowa

The cutaneous manifestations of the autoimmune connective tissue diseases (syn. rheumatic diseases) are extremely numerous and a comprehensive discussion of the management of all clinical entities in this category is not possible here. Therefore, this chapter will focus upon the management of the signature cutaneous changes of the three major autoimmune connective tissue diseases of greatest interest to the dermatologist—lupus erythematosus (LE), dermatomyositis (DM)/polymyositis (PM), and scleroderma/systemic sclerosis (SSC).

I. LUPUS ERYTHEMATOSUS

A hallmark feature of LE is heterogenous clinical expression and this is especially true with respect to skin disease. Isolated skin lesions that are never accompanied by systemic lupus erythematosus (SLE) disease activity are seen in some LE patients [e.g., isolated localized discoid lupus erythematosus (DLE)], while others have isolated skin lesions that occur as a forerunner of SLE [e.g., generalized DLE, subacute cutaneous LE (SCLE)], and still others have skin lesions occurring in conjunction with underlying SLE [e.g., acute cutaneous LE (ACLE)]. Anyone managing patients with cutaneous LE must always be cognizant of the status of underlying SLE disease activity.

The cutaneous manifestations of LE can be divided into those that are found upon skin biopsy to be histologically specific for LE (LE-specific skin disease) and those that are not histologically specific for LE (LE-nonspecific skin disease)

[1,2]. LE-specific skin disease is commonly referred to as cutaneous LE. LE-nonspecific skin lesions includes a diverse set of skin changes that are most commonly encountered in the setting of SLE but can be seen in unrelated disease settings as well (e.g., cutaneous small vessel leukocytoclastic vasculitis).

The three major categories of LE-specific skin disease are acute cutaneous lupus erythematosus (ACLE), subacute cutaneous lupus erythematosus (SCLE), and chronic cutaneous lupus erythematosus (CCLE). ACLE in its localized form is more commonly recognized as the photosensitive ''butterfly rash'' or ''malar rash'' of SLE, although more widespread forms do occur. Since most patients with ACLE have evidence of SLE, this form of cutaneous LE is most commonly managed within the context of systemic immunosuppressive therapy that is required to suppress the SLE disease activity (e.g., prednisone, azathioprine, and/or cyclophosphamide). The two forms of LE-specific skin disease most frequently managed by the dermatologist are SCLE and CCLE (the most common form being classic DLE). For the most part, these two categories of cutaneous LE respond to treatment in a parallel fashion to the local and systemic measures outlined in Table 1.

More comprehensive discussion of the cutaneous manifestations of LE, including color illustrations, can be found in Ref. 3.

A. Patient Education

Most cutaneous LE patients are photosensitive, with many reacting to both short-wavelength (UVB) and long-wavelength (UVA) ultraviolet light (UV). Such patients should avoid unnecessary exposure to natural sunlight (e.g., sunbathing) or artificial sources of UV (e.g., tanning booths, unshielded fluorescent lighting). In addition, exposure to mid-day sunlight (10 AM to 3 PM) should be avoided (a simple rule of thumb is if one's shadow is longer than one is tall it is relatively safe to be outside). Sunlight exposure at high altitudes and around highly reflective surfaces such as snow, sand, and water should be avoided. Broad-brimmed hats and tightly woven, long-sleeved shirts or blouses should be used. Special sun-protective clothing, although expensive, is available (e.g., Solumbra Ultra Sun Protective Clothing, Frogwear Sun Protective Clothing). Table 2 summarizes management issues relevant to photosensitivity in rheumatic skin disease patients.

Patients should also be advised to avoid photosensitizing drugs such as thiazides and diltiazem that can precipitate or exacerbate certain forms of cutaneous LE, such as SCLE. Patients should also be advised to discontinue cigarette smoking since it appears to be capable of antagonizing the beneficial effects of antimalarials (personal observation) and has been found to be a risk factor for cutaneous LE [4].

TABLE 1 A Therapeutic Ladder Approach to the Management of LE-Specific Skin Disease

- I. First Line
  - A. Sun avoidance/sun protection measures outlined in Table 2.
  - B. Local therapy
    - 1. Topical corticosteroids
      - a. Class I–III creams, ointments, gels, solutions
      - b. Impregnated tape (Cordran)
    - 2. Intralesional corticosteroids
      - a. Triamcinolone acetonide suspension 2.5–5.0 mg/mL
    - 3. Corrective camouflage cosmetics
      - a. Covermark
      - b. Dermablend
- II. Second Line
  - A. Systemic therapy: antimalarials
    - 1. Hydroxychloroquine (Plaquenil, Quineprox)
    - 2. Chloroquine (Aralen)
    - 3. Hydroxychloroquine + Quinacrine[a]
    - 4. Chloroquine + Quinacrine
- III. Third Line
  - A. Systemic therapy: other, nonimmunosuppressive anti-inflammatories
    - 1. Diaminodiphenylsulfone (Dapsone)
    - 2. Isotretinoin (Accutane)/Etretinate (Tegison)
    - 3. Gold (Auranofin, Myochrisine)
    - 4. Clofazamine (Lamprene)
    - 5. Thalidomide
- IV. Fourth Line
  - A. Systemic therapy: immunosuppressives
    - 1. Systemic corticosteroids (prednisone)
    - 2. Azathioprine (Imuran)
    - 3. Methotrexate
    - 4. Cyclophosphamide (Cytoxan)
- V. Investigational
    - 1. Phenytoin
    - 2. Sulfasalazine
    - 3. Anti-CD4 monoclonal antibody
    - 4. Photopheresis
    - 5. UVA-I phototherapy
- VI. Surgical
  - A. Dermabrasion
  - B. Laser

[a] Available in the U.S. through compounding pharmacies only.

TABLE 2 Sun Protection Measures for the Patient with Photosensitive Rheumatic Skin Disease

I. Sun Avoidance Measures
   A. Avoid excessive exposure to UV from natural sunlight that can occur during sunbathing, at high altitudes, around highly reflective surfaces such as snow, sand, and water.
   B. Avoid exposure to midday sunlight (10 AM–3 PM).
   C. Avoid artificial sources of UV (e.g., tanning booths, unshielded fluorescent lighting).
   D. Whenever possible, use umbrellas, broad-brimmed hats, and tightly woven, long-sleeved shirts or blouses. Specially designed (and expensive) sun-protective clothing is available from:
      1. Solumbra Ultra Sun Protective Clothing—Phone (800) 882-7860 for free catalog.
      2. Frogwear Sun Protective Clothing—Phone (800) 328-4440 for free catalog.

II. Broad-Spectrum Chemical Sunscreens of SPF 15 or Greater That Contain the Most Effective UVA Blockers
   A. Avobenzone (Parsol 1789)
      1. Shade UVA Guard (SPF 15)
      2. Antihelios-L (SPF 60) (not yet available in the U.S. at time of writing)
   B. Micronized titanium dioxide
      1. Bain de Soleil All Day Gentle Block (SPF 30)
      2. DuraScreen Lotion (SPF 30)
      3. Johnson's Baby Sunblock Lotion (SPF 15)
      4. Neutrogena Sunblock (SPF 15)
      5. Physician's Formula Chemical Free Sunscreen Lotion (SPF 25)
      6. Vaseline Intensive Care Blockout Moisturizing Sunblock Lotion (SPF 40)
      7. Solbar 50 (SPF 50)
      8. Antihelios-L (SPF 60) (not yet available in the U.S.)

III. Other Effective Broad Spectrum Chemical Sunscreens[a]
   A. Bullfrog Body Gel (SPF 36)
   B. Coppertone Sport Lotion (SPF 15)
   C. Solbar 30/Solbar 50

IV. Corrective Cosmetics for Disfiguring Skin Disease
   A. Covermark—Department store cosmetic counters or phone (800) 524-1120
   B. Dermablend Corrective Cosmetics—Department store cosmetic counters or phone (800) 631-2158

[a] Product choices represent author's personal opinion.

B. Local Medical Therapy

A ladder approach to the management of cutaneous LE similar to that recently employed by Fivenson [5] is presented in Table 1. Local therapy, including topical and intralesional corticosteroids, should always be maximized prior to initiating any systemic treatments.

1. Sunscreens

Regular use of adequate amounts of properly applied, water-resistant/waterproof broad-spectrum chemical sunscreens having a sun protection factor (SPF) of at least 15 should be encouraged. Since patients often apply considerably smaller amounts of sunscreen than are used to determine its SPF value [6]; some argue that products containing a SPF of at least 30 should be used to provide a ''real-life'' SPF of at least 15.

Avobenzone (Parsol 1789) and micronized titanium dioxide enhance a sunscreen's ability to provide broad-based UVA protection. Unfortunately, avobenzone has not previously been available in the United States in a product having a SPF of greater than 15. A listing of sunscreen products currently available in the United States that can be recommended for the patient with cutaneous LE can be found in Table 2.

Sunscreens should be applied at least 30 min prior to sun exposure and should be reapplied every 2 h while swimming or when in a hot, sweaty environment even if the product is advertised as water-resistant or waterproof. The use of wax-based sunscreen lipsticks around the eyes can prevent the stinging and burning sensations caused by many other sunscreen products used in this area. Concomitant use of sunscreens with other topical products such as insect repellant can reduce the effective SPF value of the sunscreen, perhaps due to vehicle incompatibility [7].

2. Topical Corticosteroids

Intermediate-strength preparations such as triamcinolone acetonide 0.025 to 0.1% for the face and superpotent topical class I agents such as clobetasol propionate 0.05% or betamethasone dipropionate 0.05% for other parts of the body produce the greatest benefit in cutaneous LE. Cyclical therapy consisting of daily application of a superpotent corticosteroid for 2 weeks followed by a 2-week rest period can minimize the risk of local complications such as steroid atrophy and telangiectasia. Occlusive therapy with corticosteroid-impregnated tape (e.g., flurandrenolide) can be of extra value, but also carries a higher risk of local side effects. The use of custom-fitted prostheses for compressive occlusion therapy with topical corticosteroids has also been advocated [8]. Ointments are preferred for more hyperkeratotic lesions such as hypertrophic DLE. Corticosteroid solutions, gels, and sprays are best when treating the scalp. Regrettably, even the most potent topical corticosteroids alone do not provide adequate improvement for the large majority of SCLE and DLE patients.

3. Other Topical Agents

Topical retinoids such as tretinoin (Retin-A) have been reported to be of occasional value in cutaneous LE [9]. A newer topical retinoid, tazarotene gel (Tazorac) has not yet been systematically studied in cutaneous LE. FK-506 has shown promise as a topical immunosuppressive in atopic dermatitis and theoretically might also be of value in cutaneous LE. Topically applied 5-fluorouracil [10] and nitrogen mustard [11] have also been recommended anecdotally.

4. Intralesional Corticosteroids

Because of the smaller numbers of lesions usually involved, intralesional corticosteroid therapy is generally more useful in DLE than SCLE. Triamcinolone acetonide suspension 2.5 to 5 mg/mL can be employed for the face, with higher concentrations being used in less sensitive sites. Intralesional corticosteroids can produce cutaneous and subcutaneous atrophy (deep injection into the subcutaneous tissue enhances this risk). A 30-gauge needle injected perpendicularly into the skin is preferred since it produces less discomfort. Active borders of lesions should be thoroughly infiltrated. Intralesional therapy can be of special value for particularly hyperkeratotic lesions that are unresponsive to topical corticosteroids. Unfortunately, most cutaneous LE patients have too many lesions to be managed exclusively by intralesional corticosteroid injections.

Preliminary reports of the successful use of intralesional antimalarials (e.g., chloroquine hydrochloride) [12] and antimalarials delivered percutaneously by iontophoresis [e.g., Plaquenil (hydroxychloroquine)] [13] have been presented.

5. Corrective Camouflage Cosmetics

Instruction in the proper use of a corrective camouflage cosmetic, such as Covermark for those with a light complexion and Dermablend for those having a dark complexion, can provide a temporary sanctuary from the often-staring eyes of the general public when confronted with chronic disfiguring skin disease such as cutaneous LE. Such products also serve as highly effective broad-spectrum sunscreens, since they contain physical sunscreens such as zinc oxide and are opaque [14].

B. Systemic Medical Therapy

1. Antimalarials

When local therapy proves inadequate, a trial of single-agent or combined aminoquinoline antimalarial therapy should be considered next. Such therapy is successful in producing skin disease remissions in approximately 70 to 90% of SCLE and classical DLE patients [15–18]. Therapy is initiated with hydroxychloroquine sulfate (Plaquenil, Quineprox), the usual dose being 400 mg per day by mouth for the average adult (6.5 mg/kg/day in adults and children). Six to eight weeks of treatment are usually required to reach equilibrium blood levels when full therapeutic benefit starts to occur. Once an adequate clinical response has been achieved, the daily dose should be decreased to a maintenance dose of 200 mg per day for at least a year to minimize chances of recurrence (some recommend even longer periods of inductive treatment). If no response is seen after 8 to 12 weeks of hydroxychloroquine therapy, quinacrine hydrochloride 100 mg per day can be added to the hydroxychloroquine without enhancing the risk of retinopathy [18,19]. Quinacrine is currently available in the United States only through compounding pharmacies. One such mail order pharmacy is the Panorama Pharmacy (Phone: 1-800-247-9767, email: PanoraP@aol.com). If, after 4 to 6 weeks, adequate clinical control has not been achieved, consideration should be given to replacing the hydroxychloroquine in the combination regimen with chloroquine diphosphate (Aralen) 250 mg per day [20,21]. Hydroxychloroquine and chloroquine should not be used together because of enhanced risk for retinal toxicity. In some patients chloroquine, might be more efficacious than hydroxychloroquine.

The risks of antimalarial retinal toxicity should be discussed with the patient and a pretreatment ophthalmological examination should be carried out. It is now recognized that the risk of antimalarial retinopathy is extremely rare if recommended daily dose maximums of these agents are not exceeded—hydroxychloroquine 6.5 mg/kg/day, chloroquine 4 mg/kg/day [22]. Patients should have follow-up ophthalmological evaluations every 6 to 12 months while on hydroxychloroquine or chloroquine therapy. Use of the self-administered Amsler Grid at home to detect the earliest evidence of visual field defects has become popular. There does not appear to be an upper limit on the ''safe'' total lifetime dose of these drugs if these daily maximum dosing recommendations are not exceeded.

Other antimalarial side effects include headache, gastrointestinal intolerance, pruritus, lichenoid drug eruptions, and mucosal or cutaneous pigmentary disturbance. Quinacrine can cause a yellow skin and scleral discoloration in fair-skinned individuals; however, this is completely reversible upon discontinuation of the drug. Genetic deficiency of glucose-6-phosphate dehydrogenase enzyme activity can potentiate the hemolytic effects of quinacrine and, less commonly, hydroxychloroquine and chloroquine.

Antimalarials must be used very cautiously in patients having overt or subclinical porphyria cutanea tarda for fear of producing acute hepatotoxicity when treated with therapeutic doses of antimalarials for cutaneous LE. Each of the aminoquinoline antimalarials can rarely produce bone marrow suppression. This potentially fatal complication has been reported more frequently with quinacrine, although this appears to be virtually nonexistent at doses not exceeding 100 mg/day [23]. The American College of Rheumatology considers the risk of hematological and hepatic toxicity from hydroxychloroquine in a daily dosage of 6.5 mg/kg/day or less for rheumatoid arthritis to be so low as not to require any form of baseline or follow-up blood test monitoring [24]. Although recent data indicate that the risk is relatively low, women should be cautioned that it would be best not to become pregnant while on antimalarials. High-dose antimalarial treatment used in the past was associated with toxic psychosis, grand mal seizures, neuromyopathy, and cardiac arrhythmias. These problems are only rarely encountered today using the lower daily dosing regimen.

Some use a brief tapering course of prednisone to more rapidly suppress acutely symptomatic skin disease while waiting for longer-acting agents such as antimalarials to work.

2. Nonimmunosuppressive Anti-Inflammatory Therapy

Nonimmunosuppressive anti-inflammatory drugs such as diaminodiphenylsulfone (Dapsone), isotretinoin (Accutane), etretinate (Tegison), gold (Auranofin, Myochrysine), clofazimine (Lamprene), and thalidomide have been conventionally used in the antimalarial-resistant cutaneous LE patient.

Dapsone (diaminodiphenylsulfone) 100 to 200 mg/day is of relatively greater value in treating ''bullous SLE'' [25,26]. The author has had relatively little positive experience in treating SCLE or DLE patients with this agent, although others have reported benefit in isolated cases within a few weeks after starting therapy [27–29]. Hematological, hepatic, and renal toxicity can occur with this drug which requires frequent monitoring.

Systemic retinoids such as isotretinoin (Accutane), etretinate (Tegison), and acitretin (Soriatane) at approximately 0.5 to 1.0 mg/kg/day have been shown to significantly improve SCLE and hypertrophic DLE lesions [26,30–33]. Mucocutaneous dryness and teratogenicity are considerable problems with these agents. Patients should use sunscreens judiciously while being treated with these agents to minimize their tendency to aggravate photosensitivity. Hair loss and peeling of the hands and feet are seen more often with etretinate. Other less commonly encountered side effects include drug-induced hepatitis, hypertriglyceridemia, and the diffuse idiopathic skeletal hyperostosis (DISH) syndrome.

In 1981 cofazimine (Lamprene) 100 mg/day was reported to be of value in annular SCLE [34]. Gastrointestinal intolerance can be a problem and, at higher doses, clofazimine has been reported to precipitate in mesenteric arteries resulted in splenic infarction [35]. A pink to brownish-black skin pigmentation, which can persist for months to years after discontinuing the drug, develops in most patients on long-term clofazimine therapy. These problems have limited its use in cutaneous LE.

Oral gold [auranofin (Ridaura)] or parenteral gold [aurothiomaleate (Myochrysine; aurothioglucose (Solganal)] can also be used in cutaneous LE patients with resistant disease [36,37]. Gold frequently has mucocutaneous toxicity and, less commonly, has hematological, renal, and pulmonary toxicity. Careful monitoring for toxicity is required when using any form of gold.

Thalidomide, 100 to 200 mg/day, can be very effective in managing antimalarial refractory SCLE and DLE in a relatively short time frame [38–42]. Because of its notorious teratogenicity, a new, compassionate-use investigational drug permit from the FDA has been required for use in the United States (thalidomide is expected to be approved very soon by the FDA for use in erythema nodosum leprosum). Other side effects of thalidomide include somnolence, constipation, and sensory neuropathies.

Less conventional nonimmunosuppressive drugs that have been reported to be of value in refractory cutaneous LE but whose value remains to be confirmed include: alpha-interferon [43–46], phenytoin [47], sulfasalazine [48–50], and danazol [51,52]. Vitamin E has also been suggested anecdotally to be of benefit in cutaneous LE; however, a more recent controlled trial failed to confirm this [53].

3. Phototherapy

Low fluence total body UVA-I exposure has recently been suggested to be of therapeutic benefit in SCLE patients [54]; however, this treatment modality remains to be confirmed in independent controlled clinical trials. Photopheresis has also been claimed in uncontrolled trials to be of value in cutaneous LE accompanied by SLE [55].

4. Immunosuppressive Therapy

On rare occasion, LE skin disease is severe enough to consider using immunosuppressive agents such as systemic corticosteroids (prednisone, pulse methylprednisolone) [56], azathioprine (Imuran) [57], methotrexate [17], or cyclophosphamide (Cytoxan). Hydroxychloroquine used in conjunction with methotrexate appears to ameliorate to some degree the hepatotoxic gastrointestinal side effects of methotrexate [58] and this combination might be of particular value in the management of refractory cases of cutaneous LE. Immunotherapy with agents such as anti-CD4 monoclonal antibody has recently been reported to be of value in difficult cases of cutaneous LE [59]. Each of the drugs mentioned in this paragraph can have severe and, at times, potentially fatal side effects and should be used with considerable caution.

C. Special Considerations Concerning Variant Clinical Forms of CCLE

Even with minimal trauma, LE panniculitis/profundus lesions tend to break down and ulcerate. Therefore, the trauma of intralesional corticosteroid therapy should be approached with considerable caution since even this form of trauma can at times cause complications. Most cases of LE panniculitis/profundus can be managed successfully with single agent or combined antimalarial therapy [60]; however, some will require more aggressive treatment with systemic corticosteroids. Thalidomide [61] and gold [62] have also been used in refractory LE panniculitis/ profundus patients.

Hypertrophic DLE lesions that do not respond to single-agent or combined antimalarial therapy have been reported to respond to treatment with systemic retinoids such as isotretinoin (Accutane) [33]. Azathioprine has been advocated for those patients having antimalarial-resistant palmar/plantar DLE [57]. The majority of LE tumidus and mucosal DLE lesions will respond to antimalarial therapy.

D. Surgical Therapy

Any form of surgical manipulation of cutaneous LE lesions or nonlesional skin of LE patients carries the risk of aggravating LE skin disease activity (i.e., isomorphic response or Köebner phenomenon). Thus, procedures such as dermabrasion for DLE scar revision should be approached very cautiously, preferably while the patient is on active treatment with antimalarials to prevent disease reactivation.

Cryotherapy was used to treat cutaneous LE prior to the availability of corticosteroids and antimalarials. More recently, pulsed-dye and argon lasers

Table 3 Management of LE-Nonspecific Skin Disease

LE-Nonspecific Skin Lesions	Treatment Options
Cutaneous vasculitis	Colchicine, dapsone, antimalarials, SIT[a]
Alopecia (nonscarring)	SIT
Raynaud's/Sclerodactyly	Nifedipine
Rheumatoid nodules	Treatment optional, SIT
Calcinosis cutis	Surgical debridement of symptomatic lesions, SIT
"Bullous SLE"	Dapsone, SIT
Urticaria	Antihistamines, SIT
Papulonodular mucinosis	SIT
Cutis laxa/anetoderma	SIT
Erythema multiforme	SIT
Leg ulcers	Anticoagulation, SIT
Livedo reticularis	Anticoagulation, SIT
Lichen planus	Topical corticosteroids, SIT

[a] SIT = systemic immunosuppressive therapy for underlying SLE.

have been used to treat cutaneous LE [63–65]. However, overzealous use of the argon laser on the nose has also been reported to precipitate cutaneous LE [66].

Comprehensive discussions of the management of cutaneous LE can be found elsewhere [1,5,67–69].

E. LE-Nonspecific Skin Disease

Space limitation here does not allow a comprehensive discussion of the management of LE-nonspecific skin disease, which is presented in outline form in Table 3. The reader is referred to other sources for a more thorough discussion of this subject [1].

II. DERMATOMYOSITIS

In juvenile and adult forms of classic DM, a highly characteristic pattern of skin lesions is accompanied by a histopathologically specific pattern of skeletal muscle inflammation that initially produces weakness in the shoulder and hip girdle musculature [70–72]. A highly similar, if not identical, pattern of muscle inflammation and weakness can occur in some patients who never develop skin lesions (i.e., polymyositis). Some patients can have weakness as a result of another, somewhat different, pattern of muscle inflammation that also is not associated with skin lesions (inclusion body myositis). The muscle inflammation seen in DM is associated with increased blood levels of skeletal muscle enzymes such as creatine kinase and aldolase, as well as characteristic electromyography (EMG) changes and diagnostic muscle biopsy findings. Muscle assessment with imaging techniques such as magnetic resonance imaging, ultrasound, and ^{31}P spectroscopy can also be of value in identifying myositis [70,71]. Patients having both the skin and muscle manifestations of DM require more aggressive forms of immunosuppressive therapy from the outset.

In approximately 60% of patients with classic DM, the skin and muscle changes appear concurrently, while in approximately 30% of classic DM patients, the skin manifestations precede the muscle symptoms by a period of up to 6 months. In approximately 10 to 20% of patients with DM, the hallmark skin changes of DM can occur as an isolated clinical finding for periods of 6 months or longer. Such patients have been referred to as amyopathic DM (syn. dermatomyositis siné myositis) [73,74]. In some patients, skin lesions of DM can persist without muscle weakness for as long as two decades (personal unpublished observation) while in others clinical evidence of muscle disease develops after several years [75]. It has been proposed that patients having only skin lesions of DM for 6 to 24 months be classified as having ''provisional amyopathic DM'' and those having such skin lesions for longer than 24 months be classified as having ''confirmed amyopathic DM'' [71,76].

Adult-onset classical DM [77] and perhaps amyopathic DM as well [78] can be a sign of evolving occult malignancy, especially ovarian carcinoma in women. Other organ systems that can occasionally be affected in DM patients include the heart, lungs, gastrointestinal tract, and eyes [70,72,79]. The myositis-specific autoantibody Jo-1 is seen more commonly in DM patients who develop interstitial lung disease. Other myositis-specific antibodies include Mi-2, which has been especially associated with the cutaneous manifestations of DM and SRP which have been associated with rapidly progressive, potentially fatal systemic disease. No serological marker has yet been identified for amyopathic DM.

The color and distribution of the skin changes are of considerable diagnostic importance [70]. The primary skin change is a highly pruritic confluent macular violaceous erythema (cutaneous LE is usually not pruritic). This violaceous skin coloration is often referred to as a heliotrope erythema or the ''heliotrope rash,'' especially when referring to periorbital involvement (the heliotrope is a purple-to-violet colored flower that tracks the course of the sun). Hyperkeratosis can be seen to develop overlying the violaceous erythema as the lesions evolve. The hallmark distribution of DM skin lesions includes the periorbital regions, malar aspects of the face, V-area of the neck, scalp, posterior neck and shoulders (shawl sign), and extensor aspects of the shoulders, arms, forearms, hands, and fingers. A hallmark cutaneous feature of DM is confluent macular violaceous erythema overlying the bony prominences including the elbows, knees, knuckles, and medial malleoli (Gottron's sign). Atrophic violaceous papules overlying the knuckles (Gottron's papules) combined with periungual telangicctasia and ragged cuticles represent a pathognomic cutaneous constellation of DM.

A. Patient Education

A laddered approach to the management of the cutaneous manifestations of DM is presented in Table 4. The same precautions concerning UV light avoidance and photoprotection described above for cutaneous LE patients should be followed by DM patients, since cutaneous involvement in DM is often exacerbated by UVB/UVA. All classic and amyopathic DM patients should have a sex- and age-appropriate evaluation for associated internal malignancy. Women should receive state-of-the-art screening for ovarian carcinoma, including transvaginal ultrasonography and blood CA-125 levels in addition to pap smear and bimanual pelvic examination. Reevaluation for internal malignancy should be carried out at 6 to 12-month intervals following diagnosis for at least the first 2 years of their illness. An amyopathic DM patient experiencing any evidence of muscle weakness or other symptoms of systemic DM involvement (e.g., pulmonary or cardiovascular symptoms) should bring this to the attention of their physician. Asymptomatic DM patients should be reevaluated for the development of muscle

TABLE 4 Therapeutic Ladder Approach to Management of the Cutaneous Manifestations of Dermatomyositis

I. First Line
   A. Sun avoidance/sun protection measures presented in Table 2
   B. Local therapy
      1. Class I to III topical corticosteroid creams, ointments, gels, solutions, tape
      2. Topical antipruritic agents
         a. Substantive emollients (e.g., Eucerin®, Aquaphor, Vaseline)
         b. Nonsensitizing topical antipruritics
            i. Menthol, camphor (Sarna)
            ii. Pramoxine (Prax)
            iii. Lubriderm with 1/4% menthol and 1/2% phenol
   C. Systemic therapy
      1. Antihistamines
         a. Doxepin (Sinequan) at bedtime as tolerated
         b. Hydroxyzine (Atarax, Vistaril) during day as tolerated
         c. Loratadine (Claritin) for those who must remain alert
         d. Cetirizine (Zyrtec) for those who must remain alert
II. Second Line
   A. Systemic anti-inflammatory agents
      1. Antimalarials
      2. Dapsone
III. Third Line
   A. Systemic immunosuppressives
      1. Prednisone
      2. Methotrexate
      3. Azathioprine (Imuran)
   B. Systemic immunomodulators
      1. High-dose i.v. gamma globulin
IV. Fourth Line
   A. Systemic immunosuppressives
      1. Chlorambucil (Leukeran)
      2. Cyclosporine (Neoral)
V. Surgical
   A. Surgical debridement of cutaneous calcium deposits

weakness on a regular basis (i.e., exams for muscle weakness, creatine kinase, and aldolase blood level determinations).

B. Local Medical Therapy

Local therapy should include the regular use substantive, broad-spectrum sunscreens as described above for LE patients. The skin manifestations of DM are characteristically extremely pruritic and at times patients can experience disability from intense itching alone. To combat pruritus, substantive bland emollients (e.g., Eucerine, Aquaphor, plain Vaseline) should be employed liberally, especially following bathing. Nonsensitizing topical antipruritics such as Sarna, Prax, and Lubriderm with 1/4% menthol and 1/2% phenol can also be helpful. The use of potent topical corticosteroids as described for LE patients above can provide some degree of relief from cutaneous inflammation and pruritus. Special attention should be directed to scalp burning and pruritus, which at times can be so severe as to be disabling. Class I corticosteroid scalp solutions used in conjunction with corticosteroid sprays can provide some degree of relief. Even after these local measures, systemic antipruritic therapy is usually required in all but the most mildly affected cases.

C. Systemic Medical Therapy

1. Nonimmunosuppressive Agents

Potent sedating antihistamines such as doxepin (Sinequan) 10 to 25 mg can be helpful especially at night. Nonsedating antihistamines such as loratadine (Claritin) 10 mg and cetirizine (Zyrtec) 5 to 10 every morning can provide some degree of relief. For those not requiring a nonsedating antihistamine during the day, hydroxyzine (Atarax, Vistaril) 25 to 50 mg po qid can provide a less costly alternative.

Single-agent or combination antimalarial therapy used as described above for cutaneous LE can sometimes provide relief for the cutaneous manifestations of DM [80–82]. Unfortunately, in the author's personal experience, antimalarials are much more effective in cutaneous LE than cutaneous DM. Dapsone has recently been suggested to be of value in cutaneous DM [83]. It is the author's experience that Dapsone can be helpful, most often in patients having the more limited forms of cutaneous DM.

2. Immunosuppressive Agents

Prednisone 60 to 80 mg/day has traditionally been the drug of choice for patients having both the cutaneous and muscle manifestations of DM. In acutely ill patients, intravenous pulse therapy with methylprednisolone can be used. This has become increasingly popular in the management of juvenile DM [84]. It has been suggested that early intervention with systemic corticosteroids in patients having classic DM has been associated with a better disease outcome [85]. It has also been suggested that early intervention with systemic corticosteroids in amyopathic DM might be associated with an improved prognosis [73], but this remains to be confirmed with systematic studies. The cost-benefit ratio of systemic corticosteroids in the management of patients having only the cutaneous manifestations of DM must be carefully weighed.

Approximately 25% of classic DM patients do not respond adequately to systemic corticosteroids [86]. A number of other immunosuppressive drugs can be used in this setting and for patients who cannot tolerate the numerous side effects of high-dose corticosteroids. Methotrexate (10–25 mg/week) [87] and azathioprine (Imuran) (1–2 mg/kg/day) [88] are often used for classic DM patients who have not responded to prednisone alone. These drugs can also be of benefit to the severely symptomatic amyopathic DM patient afflicted with only the cutaneous manifestations of DM who has not responded to local measures and antimalarials. High-dose iv gamma globulin [89–91], chlorambucil (2–6 mg/day) [92], cyclophosphamide (1–2 mg/kg/day) [88], and cyclosporine (5 mg/kg/day) [93] can be used for the most severely affected patients who have not responded to the previously discussed agents.

3. Cutaneous Calcium Deposits

Medical treatment of cutaneous calcium deposits that occur most commonly in the juvenile form of the disease has been virtually impossible [94]. Numerous approaches based on various rationales have been tried, including aluminum hydroxide suspension (15–20 mL four times per day) [95–97], probenecid (250 mg/day) [98,99], potassium para-amino benzoic acid (15–25 g/day) [100], warfarin (1 mg/day) [101,102], EDTA [103], and colchicine (1.2–1.8 mg/day) [104]. The most recent enthusiasm has centered around diltiazem [105], although data from a controlled clinical trial are not yet available.

D. Surgical Therapy

Surgical excision of symptomatic cutaneous calcium deposits can provide some degree of relief for this difficult complication [106].

More comprehensive reviews of the cutaneous aspects of classic and amyopathic DM, including discussion of treatment, can be found elsewhere [70–72,107].

III. SCLERODERMA

Scleroderma is a term commonly used to refer to two forms of autoimmune cutaneous sclerosis—localized scleroderma and systemic sclerosis (SSC). Thickened, hardened, leather-like skin is the defining clinical aspect of both localized scleroderma (morphea, linear scleroderma) [108] and SSC (limited-cutaneous SSC and diffuse-cutaneous SSC) [109].

The key clinical distinction between the localized and systemic forms of scleroderma is the presence or absence of vascular and cutaneous involvement of the fingers and/or hands (acral involvement) and systemic disease. Acral changes are hallmarks of SSC reflecting the systemic vasculopathy that is characteristic of this systemic disease process. Such acral changes are absent in patients with morphea and linear scleroderma.

Other organ systems that can be affected by SSC include the musculoskeletal system, kidneys, gastrointestinal tract, heart, and lungs. Renal involvement, in the context of malignant hypertension, is one of the most frequent causes of death in scleroderma patients. Patients can also succumb from lung and heart involvement. Although both localized scleroderma (morphea and linear scleroderma) and SSC are idiopathic forms of scleroderma that can be associated with qualitatively similar autoimmune abnormalities, it is extremely rare for a patient who presents with any form of localized scleroderma to subsequently make the transition to SSC.

Sclerodermatous skin changes can also occur as a result of a rather wide array of unrelated, nonautoimmune disorders and environmental stimuli (the pseudosclerodermas). Discussion of these clinical entities can be found elsewhere [109,110].

The cutaneous manifestations of localized scleroderma include: plaque-type morphea, linear scleroderma (including the en coup de sabre form of linear scleroderma and Perry-Romberg facial hemiatrophy), generalized morphea, morphea profunda (subcutaneous morphea), guttate morphea, and keloidal morphea. A full discussion of these entities can be found elsewhere [108].

The most common initial manifestation of SSC is Raynaud's phenomenon. Over time, the acral sclerodermatous skin changes appear following the onset of Raynaud's phenomenon. Raynaud's phenomenon can appear in young women as an isolated clinical phenomenon without progression to SSC (i.e., Raynaud's disease). The presence of periungual nailfold microvascular change and centromere autoantibodies can help distinguish Raynaud's phenomenon associated with SSC from isolated Raynaud's disease.

Two patterns of disease progression can be seen in SSC [109]. Patients with the limited cutaneous form of SSC (syn. CREST syndrome) usually present with Raynaud's phenomenon followed by the development of sclerodermatous involvement of the fingers (sclerodactyly), hands, forearms, face, and V-area of neck and upper chest. Matt-like telangiectasia are particularly common in affected areas of skin. Digital infarcts/ulcers are a frequent problem and become especially painful when complicated by secondary bacterial infection. These patients also frequently suffer from distal dysphagia due to sclerodermatous involvement of the musculature of the esophagus. Cutaneous calcium deposits can form in areas of chronically affected skin, especially over the hands and elbows. Patients with the CREST syndrome tend to have very slow progression of the disease in the lungs—fatal pulmonary fibrosis and/or pulmonary artery hypertension can occur after 10–20 years. Centromere autoantibody is a serological marker for the CREST syndrome.

Patients with the diffuse cutaneous form of SSC also usually present with Raynaud's phenomenon and go on to develop many of the other features described above for CREST syndrome patients. However, their disease differs from that of patients with the CREST syndrome by progressing more rapidly to involve large areas of skin on the proximal extremities and trunk. Affected areas of skin often display hyperpigmentation and hypopigmentation, frequently in a distinctive salt and pepper pattern (such pigmentary changes can also be seen in CREST syndrome patients). This more widespread distribution of cutaneous involvement correlates with an increased risk of developing more aggressive forms of systemic disease and a higher risk for early death. Renal and cardiopulmonary disease dictate prognosis to the greatest degree in this setting. Topoisomerase-I autoantibody (syn. Scleroderma-70) represents a serological marker for this more severe form of SSC.

The cutaneous changes of both localized scleroderma and SSC typically evolve through three stages. The early inflammatory, edematous stage is replaced by a fibrotic stage that eventually evolves into an atrophic stage. Most treatment modalities for this disorder have a better chance of working if they are begun during the initial inflammatory, edematous stage.

A. Patient Education

Patients having Raynaud's phenomenon should avoid cold exposure and use layered clothing and electrically warmed gloves and mittens whenever possible. Cigarette smoking should be discontinued as well as the use of vasoconstricting medications containing ergotamine, beta-blockers, and sympathomimetic amines, including pseudoephedrine in over-the-counter decongestant/allergy preparations and ephedrine in nutritional supplements. The use of vibrational tools should be curtailed and environmental stimuli such as silica or polyvinyl chloride exposure known to be capable of precipitating or exacerbating this illness should be avoided. Stress management techniques, including temperature biofeedback training, can mitigate an important trigger factor for Raynaud's attacks. Some patients can abort or shorten a Raynaud's attack by rapidly rotating their arms as if attempting to pitch a softball underhanded.

B. Local Medical Therapy

Table 5 summarizes the various local and systemic forms of treatment that have been suggested or shown to be of symptomatic value to patients with scleroderma [108,110–113]. Unfortunately, there is no definitive form of therapy for any form of localized scleroderma or systemic sclerosis. However, symptomatic improvement can be expected with treatment.

The benefit of local therapy should not be overlooked in scleroderma. Because sclerodermatous skin is often dry and pruritic, the same moisturization and

Table 5 Therapeutic Options for the Management of the Cutaneous Manifestations of Scleroderma

I. Local Therapy
   A. Topical moisturizers and antipruritics
   B. Topical antibiotics for ulcers
      1. Mupirocin (Bactroban)
   C. Semiocclusive dressings for ulcers
      1. DuoDerm
      2. Tegaderm
   D. Topical vasodilators
      1. Nitroglycerine ointment
   E. Topical and intralesional corticosteroids for early, inflammatory lesions
II. Systemic Therapy
   A. Systemic antibiotics for secondarily infected ulcers
   B. Vasodilators
      1. Calcium channel blockers
         a. Nifedipine, amlodopine, diltiazem, felodipine, isradipine, nicardipine
      2. Alpha-adrenergic receptor blockers
         a. Prazosin, terazosin, and doxazosin
   C. Anticoagulants/antiviscosity
      1. Aspirin and dipyridamole (Persantine)
      2. Pentoxifylline (Trental)
      3. Low-molecular-weight heparin
      4. Prostaglandins and prostaglandin analogues
         a. iloprost
         b. cicaprost
      5. Serotonin antagonist
         a. ketanserin
   D. Nonimmunosuppressive agents of questionable value: Antibiotics, aminoquinoline antimalarials, colchicine, phenytoin sodium (Dilantin), potassium aminobenzoate (POTABA), dimethyl sulfoxide (DMSO), sulfasalazine (Azulfidine), plasmapheresis
   E. Immunomodulatory/antifibrotic
      1. d-Penicillamine
   F. Immunosuppressive drugs
      1. prednisone
      2. azathioprine
      3. chlorambucil
      4. cyclosporine
      5. antithymocyte globulin

TABLE 5 Continued

G. Investigational
  1. Photopheresis
  2. Calcitonin gene-related peptide
  3. Relaxin
  4. Ultraviolet light therapy (PUVA, UVA-I)
  5. Interferon-gamma

III. Surgical Therapy
  A. Cervical or digital sympathectomy for severe Raynaud's phenomenon
  B. Surgical debridement of cutaneous calcium deposits

antipruritc measures described above for DM patients should be employed in scleroderma patients. Topical and intralesional corticosteroids can be of some benefit in early, edematous phase scleroderma lesions. The fingertip ulcerations that can complicate severe Raynaud's phenomenon can benefit from broad-spectrum topical antibiotics such as mupirocin (Bactroban). Semiocclusive dressings, such as DuoDerm or Tegaderm, used in conjunction with topical antibiotics can promote ulcer healing to some degree. Topical vasodilators such as nitroglycerine ointment, when applied to the intact skin surrounding digital ulcers, may promote healing in some patients.

C. Systemic Medical Therapy

1. Nonimmunosuppressive Agents

Painful digital ulcers secondary to Raynaud's phenomenon are often secondarily infected and can benefit from systemic antibiotics. Orally administered, long-acting calcium channel blockers such as nifedipine (30–90 mg/day) have become the mainstay for treating Raynaud's phenomenon. Other calcium channel blockers including amlodopine, diltiazem, felodipine, isradipine, and nicardipine have also been used in patients with Raynaud's phenomenon [112,113]. Peripheral alpha-adrenergic receptor blockers such as prazosin, terazosin, and doxazosin have also been used for Raynaud's symptoms. Anticoagulation and platelet-directed therapy such as subcutaneous low-molecular-weight heparin, aspirin 81-325 mg/day, and dipyridamole (Persantine) 50–100 mg tid qid, and pentoxifylline (Trental) 400 mg tid have also been used. Drugs that have been used for severe Raynaud's phenomenon that are not currently available in the United States include intravenous and oral prostaglandins and prostaglandin analogues including iloprost and cicaprost as well as the serotonin antagonist, ketanserin.

A number of miscellaneous, systemic nonimmunosuppressive agents have been anecdotally reported to be of benefit for the cutaneous manifestations of scleroderma. These include antibiotics, aminoquinoline antimalarials, colchicine, phentytoin sodium (Dilantin), potassium aminobenzoate (POTABA), dimethyl sulfoxide (DMSO), sulfasalazine (Azulfidine), and plasmapheresis. However, there is currently little evidence from controlled clinical trials to support the routine use of any of these agents. The author's personal experience suggests that systemic corticosteroids and antimalarial therapy can provide some degree of symptomatic relief during the early inflammatory/edematous phase of the disease. However, systemic corticosteroids should be used cautiously in SSC, since such drugs could exacerbate a major complication of this disease—malignant hypertension with ensuing renal failure.

There is now a wide clinical experience to suggest that long-term therapy with d-penicillamine can be of some value for the cutaneous and systemic manifestations of morphea/localized scleroderma and SSC [111–113]. The main limitations with this drug are its slow onset of action (up to 18 months) and the fact that therapeutic doses of d-penicillamine (750-1000 mg/day) are often associated with serious side effects, including bone marrow suppression and renal toxicity.

2. Phototherapy

PUVA and UVA-I phototherapy have recently been suggested to be of benefit for localized scleroderma in open trials [121–125]. Preliminary evidence indicates that some of these treatment regimens can enhance dermal collagenase expression. However, the overall clinical value of this treatment approach remains to be seen.

3. Immunosuppressive Agents

A number of immunosuppressive drugs in addition to prednisone, including azathioprine, chlorambucil, cyclosporine, and antithymocyte globulin, have also been used in scleroderma; however, there is little evidence from controlled clinical trials to suggest that any of these agents has a significant, long-term impact on either the cutaneous or systemic manifestations of scleroderma (data reviewed in Refs. 111–113).

4. Investigational Agents

Recent investigational approaches include photopheresis [114], intravenous calcitonin gene-related peptide [115], and relaxin [116]. There is considerable hope that biological response modifiers, such as gamma-interferon, might prove to be of value in the long-term management of this difficult disease [117,118].

Although usually unsuccessful, medical therapy for cutaneous calcinosis has been attempted with the same agents described above for DM.

D. Surgical Therapy

Both cervical sympathectomy or digital sympathectomy have been used for severe Raynaud's phenomenon. While these procedures can provide some degree of initial relief, symptoms often recur over time. Surgical excision of symptomatic cutaneous calcium deposits can also be of value in this setting.

Pulse dye laser therapy has been used to successfully treat scleroderma telangiectasia [119]. Autologous fat transfer has also been used for linear scleroderma/facial hemiatrophy.

More inclusive overviews of the diagnosis and management of localized scleroderma/SSC can be found elsewhere [108–112,120].

IV. OTHER RHEUMATIC SKIN DISEASES

Skin changes can be encountered in other rheumatic diseases such as Sjögren's syndrome, rheumatoid arthritis, Behçet's disease, primary systemic vasculitis, and Reiter's syndrome. Comprehensive discussion of the treatment of the cutaneous manifestations of these entities as well as other disorders that affect both the skin and musculoskeletal system can be found elsewhere [3].

REFERENCES

1. Sontheimer RD, Provost TT. Lupus Erythematosus. In: Sontheimer RD, Provost TT, eds. Cutaneous Manifestations of Rheumatic Diseases. Baltimore: Williams & Wilkins, 1996.
2. Sontheimer RD. The lexicon of cutaneous lupus erythematosus—a review and personal perspective on the nomenclature and classification of the cutaneous manifestations of lupus erythematosus. Lupus 1997; 6:84–95.
3. Sontheimer RD, Provost TT. Cutaneous Manifestations of Rheumatic Diseases. Baltimore: Williams & Wilkins, 1996.
4. Brown K, Petri M, Goldman D. Cutaneous manifestations of SLE: associations with other manifestations of SLE and with smoking. Arthritis Rheumat 1996; 39(suppl):S291 (abstr).
5. Fivenson DP. Nonsteroidal treatment of autoimmune skin diseases. Dermatol Clin 1997; 15:695–705.
6. Diffey BL. Sunscreens, suntans and skin cancer. People do not apply enough sunscreen for protection. Br Med J 1996; 313:942.
7. Montemarano AD, Gupta RK, Burge JR, Klein K. Insect repellents and the efficacy of sunscreens. Lancet 1997; 349:1670–1671.
8. Maggio KL, Singer MT, James WD. Clinical pearl—discoid lupus erythematosus—treatment with occlussive compression. J Am Acad Dermatol 1996; 35:627–628.
9. Seiger E, Roland S, Goldman S. Cutaneous lupus treated with topical tretinoin: a case report. Cutis 1991; 47:351–355.

10. Vena GA, Coviello C, Mastrolonardo M, Foti C, Angelini G. Topical 5-fluorouracil in the treatment of discoid lupus erythematosus—preliminary study over two years. J Dermatol Treat 1996; 7:167–169.
11. Wallace DJ. Cytotoxic drugs. In: Wallace DJ, Hahn BH, eds. Dubois' Lupus Erythematosus, 4th ed. Philadelphia: Lea & Febiger, 1993:588–595.
12. Everett MA, Coffey CM. Intradermal administration of chloroquine. Arch Dermatol 1961; 83:977–979.
13. Kutintschev M, Chlebarov S. Treatment of lupus erythematosus by iontophoresis with plaquenil. Z Haut Geschlechtskr 1967; 42:676–678.
14. Kaye ET, Levin JA, Blank IH, Arndt KA, Anderson RR. Efficiency of opaque photoprotective agents in the visible light range. Arch Dermatol 1991; 127:351–355.
15. Dubois EL. Antimalarials in the management of discoid and systemic lupus erythematosus. Sem Arthr Rheum 1978; 8:33–51.
16. Sontheimer RD. Subacute cutaneous lupus erythematosus: a decade's perspective. Med Clin North Am 1989; 73:1073–1090.
17. Furner BB. Treatment of subacute cutaneous lupus erythematosus. Int J Dermatol 1990; 29:542–547.
18. Costner M, Sontheimer RD. Antimalarial therapy in photosensitive dermatoses. Dermatol Ther 1997; 4:86–99.
19. Chung HS, Hann SK. Lupus panniculitis treated with a combination therapy of hydroxychloroquine and quinacrine. J Dermatol 1997; 24:569–572.
20. Feldman R. The association of the two antimalarials chloroquine and quinacrine for treatment-resistant chronic and subacute cutaneous lupus erythematosus. Dermatology 1994; 189:425–427.
21. Lipsker D, Piette J-C, Cacoub P, Godeau P, Frances C. Chloroquine-quinacrine association in resistant cutaneous lupus. Dermatology 1995; 190:257–258.
22. Lanham JG, Hughes GRV. Antimalarial therapy in SLE. Clin Rheum Dis 1982; 8:279–299.
23. Wallace DJ. The use of quinacrine (Atabrine) in rheumatic diseases: a re-examination. Sem Arthr Rheum 1989; 18:282–297.
24. Anonymous. Guidelines for monitoring drug therapy in rheumatoid arthritis. American College of Rheumatology Ad Hoc Committee on Clinical Guidelines. Arthr Rheum 1996; 39:723–731.
25. Hall RP, Lawley TJ, Smith HR, Katz SI. Bullous eruption of systemic lupus erythematosus. Ann Intern Med 1982; 97:165–170.
26. Ruzicka T, Meurer M, Braun-Falco O. Treatment of cutaneous lupus erythematosus with etretinate. Acta Dermatol Venereol (Stockh) 1985; 65:324–329.
27. McCormack LS, Elgart ML, Turner ML. Annular subacute cutaneous lupus erythematosus responsive to dapsone. J Am Acad Dermatol 1984; 11:397–401.
28. Fenton DA, Black MM. Low-dose dapsone in the treatment of subacute cutaneous lupus erythematosus. Clin Exper Dermatol 1986; 11:102–103.
29. Holtman JH, Neustadt DH, Klein J, Callen JP. Dapsone is an effective therapy for the skin lesions of subacute cutaneous lupus erythematosus and urticarial vasculitis in a patient with C2 deficiency. J Rheumatol 1990; 17:1222–1225.
30. Newton RC, Jorizzo JL, Solomon AR, Sanchez RL, Daniels JC, Bell JD, Cavallo

T. Mechanism-oriented assessment of isotretinoin in chronic or subacute lupus erythematosus. Arch Dermatol 1986; 122:170–176.

31. Ruzicka T, Meurer M, Bieber T. Efficacy of acitretin in the treatment of cutaneous lupus erythematosus. Arch Dermatol 1988; 124:897–902.
32. Furner BB. Subacute cutaneous lupus erythematosus response to isotretinoin. Int J Dermatol 1990; 29:587–590.
33. Green SG, Piette WW. Successful treatment of hypertrophic lupus erythematosus with isotretinoin. J Am Acad Dermatol 1987; 17:364–368.
34. Crovato F. Clofazimine in the treatment of annular lupus erythematosus. Arch Dermatol 1981; 117:249–250.
35. McDougall AC, Horsfall WR, Hede JE, Chaplin AJ. Splenic infarction and tissue accumulation of crystals associated with the use of clofazamine (Lamprene B663) in the treatment of pyoderma gangrenosus. Br J Dermatol 1980; 102:227–230.
36. Haxthausen H. Treatment of lupus erythematosus by intravenous injections of gold chloride. Arch Dermatol 1930; 22:77–90.
37. Dalziel K, Going G, Cartwright PH, Marks R, Beveridge GW, Rowell NR. Treatment of chronic discoid lupus erythematosus with an oral gold compound (Auranofin). Br J Dermatol 1986; 115:211–216.
38. Naafs B, Bakkers EJM, Flinterman J, Faber WR. Thalidomide treatment of subacute cutaneous lupus erythematosus. Br J Dermatol 1982; 107:83–86.
39. Knop J, Bonsmann G, Happle R, Lundolph A, Matz DR, Mifsud EJ, Macher E. Thalidomide in the treatment of sixty cases of chronic discoid lupus erythematosus. Br J Dermatol 1983; 108:461–466.
40. Volc-Platzer B, Wolff K. Treatment of subacute cutaneous lupus erythematosus with thalidomide. Der Hautarzt 1983; 34:175–178.
41. Holm AL, Bowers KE, McMeekin TO, Gaspari AA. Chronic cutaneous lupus erythematosus treated with thalidomide. Arch Dermatol 1993; 129:1548–1550.
42. Stevens RJ, Andujar C, Edwards CJ, Ames PRJ, Barwick AR, Khamashta MA, Hughes GRV. Thalidomide in the treatment of cutaneous manifestations of lupus erythematosus—experience in sixteen consecutive patients. Br J Rheumatol 1997; 36:353–359.
43. Charley MR, Sontheimer RD. Clearing of subacute cutaneous lupus erythematosus around molluscum contagiosum lesions. J Am Acad Dermatol 1982; 6:529–533.
44. Nicolas J-F, Thivolet J, Kanitakis J, Lyonnet S. Response of discoid and subacute cutaneous lupus erythematosus to recombinant interferon alpha 2a. J Invest Dermatol 1990; 95(suppl):142S–145S.
45. Thivolet J, Nicolas JF, Kanitakis J, Lyonnet S, Chouvet B. Recombinant interferon $\alpha 2a$ is effective in the treatment of discoid and subacute cutaneous lupus erythematosus. Br J Dermatol 1990; 122:405–409.
46. de Jong EM, van Erp PE, Ruiter DJ, Van de Kerkhof PCM. Immunohistochemical detection of proliferation and differentiation in discoid lupus erythematosus. J Am Acad Dermatol 1991; 25:1032–1038.
47. Rodriguez-Castellanos MA, Barba Rubio J, Barba Gomez JF, Gonzalez Mendosa A. Phenytoin in the treatment of discoid lupus erythematosus. Arch Dermatol 1995; 131:620–621.

48. Delaporte E, Piette F, Bourjot D, Duneton-Bitbol V, Bergoend H. Treatment of chronic lupus erythematosus with sulfasalazine. Presse Med 1994; 23:95–96.
49. Delaporte E, Catteau B, Sabbagh N, Gosselin P, Breuillard F, Doutre MS, Broly F, Piette F, Bergoend H. Treatment of discoid LE by sulfasalazine—11 observations. Ann Dermatol Venereol 1997; 124:151–156.
50. Artuz F, Lenk N, Deniz N, Alli N. Efficacy of sulfasalazine in discoid lupus erythematosus. Int J Dermatol 1996; 35:746–748.
51. Englert H, Hughes GVR. Danazol and discoid lupus. Br J Dermatol 1988; 119: 407–409.
52. Torrelo A, España A, Medina S, Ledo A. Danazol and discoid lupus erythematosus (letter). Dermatologica 1990; 181:239.
53. Yell JA, Burge S, Wojnarowska F. Vitamin E and discoid lupus erythematosus. Lupus 1992; 1:303–305.
54. McGrath H Jr. Prospects for UV-A1 therapy as a treatment modality in cutaneous lupus erythematosus and systemic LE. Lupus 1997; 6:209–217.
55. Knobler RM, Graninger W, Lindmaier A, Trautinger F. Photopheresis for the treatment of lupus erythematosus: preliminary observations. Ann NY Acad Sci 1991; 636:340–356.
56. Goldberg JW, Lidsky MD. Pulse methylprednisolone therapy for persistent subacute cutaneous lupus. Arthr Rheum 1984; 27:837–838.
57. Callen JP, Spencer LV, Bhatnagar Burruss J, Holtman J. Azathioprine: an effective, corticosteroid-sparing therapy for patients with recalcitrant cutaneous lupus erythematosus or with recalcitrant cutaneous leukocytoclastic vasculitis. Arch Dermatol 1991; 127:515–522.
58. Fries J, Singh G, Lenert L, Furst D. Aspirin, hydroxychloroquine, and hepatic enzyme abnormalities with methotrexate in rheumatoid arthritis. Arthr Rheumat 1990; 33:1611–1619.
59. Prinz JC, Meurer M, Reiter C, Rieber EP, Plewig G, Riethmuller G. Treatment of severe cutaneous lupus erythematosus with a chimeric CD4 monoclonal antibody, cM-T412. J Am Acad Dermatol 1996; 34:244–252.
60. Chung HS, Hann SK. Lupus panniculitis treated by a combination therapy of hydroxychloroquine and quinacrine. J Dermatol 1997; 24:569–572.
61. Sorg C. Macrophages in acute and chronic inflammation. Chest 1991; 100(suppl): 173S–175S.
62. Irgang S. Lupus erythematosus profundus. Report of an example with clinical resemblance to Darier-Roussy sarcoid. Arch Dermatol Syph 1940; 42:98–108.
63. Nurnberg W, Algermissen B, Hermes B, Czametzki B, Kolde G. Treatment of discoid lupus erythematosus with argon laser. J Invest Dermatol 1995; 104:689 (abstr.).
64. Núñez M, Boixeda P, Miralles ES, De Misa RF, Ledo A. Pulsed dye laser treatment in lupus erythematosus telangiectoides. Br J Dermatol 1995; 133:1010–1011.
65. Núñez M, Boixeda P, Miralles ES, De Misa RF, Ledo A. Pulsed dye laser treatment of telangiectatic chronic erythema of cutaneous lupus erythematosus. Arch Dermatol 1996; 132:354–355.
66. Wolfe JT, Weinberg JM, Elenitsas R, Ubertibenz M. Cutaneous lupus erythematosus following laser-induced thermal injury. Arch Dermatol 1997; 133:392–393.

67. Callen JP. Management of antimalarial-refractory cutaneous lupus erythematosus. Lupus 1997; 6:203–208.
68. Callen JP. Management of skin disease in lupus. Bull Rheum Dis 1997; 46:4–7.
69. Drake LA, Dinehart SM, Farmer ER, Goltz RW, Graham GF, Hordinsky MK, Lewis CW, Pariser DM, Skouge JW, Webster SB, Whitaker DC, Butler B, Lowery BJ, Sontheimer RD, Callen JP, Camisa C, Provost TT, Tuffanelli DL. Guidelines of care for cutaneous lupus erythematosus. J Am Acad Dermatol 1996; 34:830–836.
70. Euwer RL, Sontheimer RD. Dermatomyositis. In: Sontheimer RD, Provost TT, eds. Cutaneous Manifestations of Rheumatic Diseases. Baltimore: Williams & Wilkins, 1996.
71. Euwer RL, Sontheimer RD. Dermatologic aspects of myositis. Curr Opin Rheumatol 1994; 6:583–589.
72. Sontheimer RD. Dermatomyositis. Chapter 173. In: Freedberg IM, Eisen AZ, Wolff K, Austen KF, Goldsmith LA, Katz SI, et al. Fitzpatrick's Dermatology in General Medicine, 5th ed. New York: McGraw Hill, 1999.
73. Euwer RL, Sontheimer RD. Amyopathic dermatomyositis (dermatomyositis sine myositis). Presentation of six new cases and review of the literature. J Am Acad Dermatol 1991; 24:959–966.
74. Euwer R, Sontheimer RD. Amyopathic dermatomyositis—a review. J Invest Dermatol 1993; 100:124S–127S.
75. Krain L. Dermatomyositis in six patients without initial muscle involvement. Arch Dermatol 1975; 111:241–245.
76. Euwer RL, Sontheimer RD. Amyopathic dermatomyositis: a review. J Invest Dermatol 1993; 100:124S–127S.
77. Cherin P, Piette JC, Herson S, Bletry O, Wechsler B, Frances C, Godeau P. Dermatomyositis and ovarian cancer: a report of 7 cases and literature review. J Rheumatol 1993; 20:1897–1899.
78. Whitmore SE, Rosenshein NB, Provost TT. Ovarian cancer in patients with dermatomyositis. Medicine 1994; 73:153–160.
79. Targoff IN. Diagnosis and treatment of polymyositis and dermatomyositis. Comprehens Ther 1990; 16:16–24.
80. Woo TY, Callen JP, Voorhees JJ, Bickers DR, Hanno R, Hawkins C. Cutaneous lesions of dermatomyositis are improved by hydroxychloroquine. J Am Acad Dermatol 1984; 10:592–600.
81. Olson NY, Lindsley CB. Adjunctive use of hydroxychloroquine in childhood dermatomyositis. J Rheumatol 1989; 16:1545–1547.
82. Cosnes A, Amaudric F, Gherardi R, Verroust J, Wechsler J, Revuz J, Roujeau JC. Dermatomyositis without muscle weakness: long-term followup of 12 patients without systemic corticosteroids. Arch Dermatol 1995; 131:1381–1385.
83. Konohana A, Kawashima J. Successful treatment of dermatomyositis with dapsone. Clin Exp Dermatol 1994; 19:367.
84. Malleson PN. Controversies in juvenile dermatomyositis. J Rheumatol Suppl 1990; 23:1–2.
85. Ramirez G, Asherson RA, Khamashta MA, Cervera R, D'Cruz D, Hughes GR.

Adult-onset polymyositis-dermatomyositis: description of 25 patients with emphasis on treatment. Semin Arthr Rheum 1990; 20:114–120.
86. Oddis CV, Medsger TA Jr. Current management of polymyositis and dermatomyositis. Drugs 1989; 37:382–390.
87. Zieglschmid-Adams ME, Pandya AG, Cohen SB, Sontheimer RD. Treatment of dermatomyositis with methotrexate: presentation of ten cases and review of the literature. J Am Acad Dermatol 1995; 32:754–757.
88. Bohan A, Peter JB, Bowman RL, Pearson CM. Computer-assisted analysis of 153 patients with polymyositis and dermatomyositis. Medicine 1977; 56:255–286.
89. Dalakas MC, Illa I, Dambrosia JM, Soueidan SA, Stein DP, Otero C, Dinsmore ST, McCrosky S. A controlled trial of high-dose intravenous immune globulin infusions as treatment for dermatomyositis [see comments]. N Engl J Med 1993; 329: 1993–2000.
90. Esteve E, Cambie MP, Serpier H, Vanderbroere-Bouquet A, Bellaiche P, Kalis B. Paraneoplastic dermatomyositis: efficacy of intravenous gammaglobulin. Br J Dermatol 1994; 131:917–918.
91. Collet E, Dalac S, Maerens B, Courtois JM, Izac M, Lambert D. Juvenile dermatomyositis: treatment with intravenous gammaglobulin. Br J Dermatol 1994; 130: 231–234.
92. Sinoway PA, Callen JP. Chlorambucil. An effective corticosteroid-sparing agent for patients with recalcitrant dermatomyositis [see comments]. Arthr Rheum 1993; 36:319–324.
93. Grau JM, Herrero C, Casademont J, Fernandez-Sola J, Urbano-Marquez A. Cyclosporine A as first choice therapy for dermatomyositis. J Rheumatol 1994; 21: 381–382.
94. Ansell B. Is there a treatment for the calcinosis of juvenile dermatomyositis? Br J Rheumatol 1990; 29:263.
95. Nassim JR, Connolly CK. Treatment of calcinosis universalis with aluminium hydroxide. Arch Dis Child 1970; 45:118–121.
96. Wang WJ, Lo WL, Wong CK. Calcinosis cutis in juvenile dermatomyositis: remarkable response to aluminum hydroxide therapy. Arch Dermatol 1988; 124: 1721–1722.
97. Nakagawa T, Takaiwa T. Calcinosis cutis in juvenile dermatomyositis responsive to aluminum hydroxide treatment. J Dermatol 1993; 20:558–560.
98. Dent CE, Stamp TCB. Treatment of calcinosis circumscripta with probenecid. Br Med J 1972; i:216.
99. Skuterud E, Sydnes OA, Haavik TK. Calcinosis in dermatomyositis treated with probenecid. Scand J Rheumatol 1981; 10:92–94.
100. Rowell NR, Goodfield MJD. The connective tissue diseases. In: Champion RH, Burton JL, Ebling FJG, eds. Textbook of Dermatology, 5th ed. London: Blackwell Scientific Publications, 1992:2163–2294.
101. Berger RG, Featherston GL, Raason RH. Treatment of calcinosis universalis with low dose warfarin. Am J Med 1987; 83:72–76.
102. Martinez-Cordero E, Lopez-Zepeda J, Choza-Romero F. Calcinosis in childhood dermatomyositis [letter]. Clin Exp Rheumatol 1990; 8:198–200.

103. Herd JK, Vaughan JH. Calcinosis universalis complicating dermatomyositis. Arthr Rheum 1964; 7:259–271.
104. Taborn J, Bole GG, Thompson GR. Colchicine suppression of local and systemic inflammation due to calcinosis universalis in chronic dermatomyositis. Ann Intern Med 1978; 89:648–649.
105. Oliveri MB, Palermo R, Mautalen C, Hubscher O. Regression of calcinosis during diltiazem treatment in juvenile dermatomyositis. J Rheumatol 1996; 23:2152–2155.
106. Shearin JC, Pickrell K. Surgical treatment of subcutaneous calcifications of polymyositis or dermatomyositis. Ann Plast Surg 1980; 5:381–385.
107. Drake LA, Dinehart SM, Farmer ER, Goltz RW, Graham GF, Hordinsky MK, Lewis CW, Pariser DM, Skouge JW, Webster SB, Whitaker DC, Butler B, Lowery BJ, Sontheimer RD, Callen JP, Camisa C, Provost TT, Tuffanelli DL. Guidelines of care for dermatomyositis. J Am Acad Dermatol 1996; 34:824–829.
108. Greenberg AS, Falanga V. Localized cutaneous sclerosis. In: Sontheimer RD, Provost TT, eds. Cutaneous Manifestations of the Rheumatic Diseases. Baltimore: Williams and Wilkins, 1996:141–155.
109. Tuffanelli DL. Systemic sclerosis. In: Sontheimer RD, Provost TT, eds. Cutaneous Manifestations of the Rheumatic Diseases. Baltimore: Williams and Wilkins, 1996: 115–139.
110. Drake LA, Dinehart SM, Farmer ER, Goltz RW, Graham GF, Hordinsky MK, Lewis CW, Pariser DM, Skouge JW, Webster SB, Whitaker DC, Butler B, Lowery BJ, Sontheimer RD, Callen JP, Camisa C, Provost TT, Tuffanelli DL. Guidelines of care for scleroderma and sclerodermoid disorders. J Am Acad Dermatol 1996; 35:609–614.
111. Pope JE. Treatment of systemic sclerosis. Rheumat Dis Clin N Am 1996; 22:893–907.
112. Legerton CW, Smith EA. Case management study: Raynaud's phenomenon. Bull Rheum Dis 1997; 45:6–8.
113. Wigley FM, Flavahan NA. Raynaud's phenomenon. Rheum Dis Clin N Am 1996; 22:765 ff.
114. Rook AH, Freundlich B, Jegasothy BV, Perez MI, Barr WG, Jimenez SA, Rietschel RL, Wintroub B, Kahalch MB, Varga J. Treatment of systemic sclerosis with extracorporeal photochemotherapy. Results of a multicenter trial. Arch Dermatol 1992; 128:337–346.
115. Wigley FM. Raynaud's phenomenon and other features of scleroderma, including pulmonary hypertension. Curr Opin Rheumatol 1996; 8:561–568.
116. Unemori EN, Bauer EA, Amento EP. Relaxin alone and in conjunction with interferon-gamma decreases collagen synthesis by cultured human scleroderma fibroblasts. J Invest Dermatol 1992; 99:337–342.
117. Hein R, Behr J, Hündgen M, Hunzelmann N, Meurer M, Braun-Falco O, Urbanski A, Krieg T. Treatment of systemic sclerosis with gamma-interferon. Br J Dermatol 1992; 126:496–501.
118. Hunzelmann N, Anders S, Fierlbeck G, Hein R, Herrmann K, Albrecht M, Bell S, Muche R, Wehnercaroli J, Gaus W, Krieg T. Double blind, placebo-controlled study of intralesional interferon gamma for the treatment of localized scleroderma. J Am Acad Dermatol 1997; 36:433–435.

119. Nunez M, Miralles ES, Boixeda P, Arrazola JM, Ledo A. Pulsed dye laser treatment of cutaneous vascular lesions in CREST syndrome. J Dermatol Treat 1994; 5:219–221.
120. Mitchell H, Bolster MB, LeRoy EC. Scleroderma and related conditions. Med Clin N Am 1997; 81:129–149.
121. Gruss C, Stucker M, Vonkobyletzki G, Schreiber D, Altmeyer P, Kerscher M. Low dose UVA1 phototherapy in disabling pansclerotic morphea of childhood. Br J Dermatol 1997; 136:293–294.
122. Kerscher M, Meurer M, Sander C, Volkenandt M, Lehmann P, Plewig G, Rocken M. PUVA bath photochemotherapy for localized scleroderma—evaluation of 17 consecutive patients. Arch Dermatol 1996; 132:1280–1282.
123. Kerscher M, Dirschka T, Volkenandt M. Treatment of localised scleroderma by UVA_1 phototherapy. Lancet 1995; 346:1166.
124. Morita A, Sakakibara S, Sakakibara N, Yamauchi R, Tsuji T. Successful treatment of systemic sclerosis with topical PUVA. J Rheumatol 1995; 22:2361–2365.
125. Scharffetter-Kochanek K, Goldermann R, Lehmann P, Hölzle E, Goerz G. PUVA therapy in disabling pansclerotic morphoea of children. Br J Dermatol 1995; 132:830–831.

20

Pruritus

Larry E. Millikan
Tulane University Medical Center
New Orleans, Louisiana

Andreas D. Katsambas
University of Athens
A. Syngros Hospital
Athens, Greece

I. PRURITUS

The challenge of pruritus is a continuing one, since no underlying cause is found in many patients. It is a significant medical problem, with some surveys showing it as the cause for two million office visits a year. Of these patients, 48% considered pruritus as a problem interfering with their social activities during the day, 46% interfering with their social activities at night. Sixty percent noted problems sleeping, and 12% had problems at work and school. Therefore, this is a medical challenge that has been seen by practitioners on a fairly frequent basis. Mild symptoms respond to moisturizers and OTC remedies, but most severe cases result in a visit to the dermatologist.

The subject of pruritus always brings forth concern for underlying etiology. Serious, sometimes potentially fatal, diseases can present with the symptoms of pruritus. The history from the patient is as important as the care in the patient with urticaria. One should question in depth previous medical history, including medications and any recent changes in them. Allergies and the history of atopy is also important. Lifestyle review should include occupation and possible exposure to contactants and irritants, bathing oils, pets, and possible ectoparasites. Recent history should cover hobbies, travel history, as well as social/sexual activities. The cause of the pruritus may become obvious after a careful history or will at least allow a more focused workup.

A. Generalized Pruritus

The physiology of pruritus is becoming better understood. The interactions of neurotransmitters and the A and C fibers are better understood. A fibers seem to be protective and relieve itch, while the C fibers are the excitatory circuits and usually the culprits in the symptomatology. In general, the mediating agents most likely to cause itching are histamine and substance P, and less likely are certain injectable proteins, 5-hydroxy tryptamine, and calcitonin. The latter three more likely will cause pain upon release in the tissue. Opiates have long been known to potentiate pruritus, and their primary role often is to potentiate histamine-initiated pruritus. This evolving understanding of various agents is gradually allowing us to focus on better methods of treatment to provide specific therapy for such mechanisms [1]. The use of doxepin as a very potent blocker of the H1-receptor (775 times greater than diphenhydramine, and 56 times greater than hydroxyzine) is a good example of information evolving from the understanding of the basic pathophysiology. Similarly, the use of capsaicin as a specific inhibitor of substance P has allowed an alternative approach to therapy, albeit with some significant side effects. The approach to diagnosis and therapy relates to the pattern in regard to generalized or localized, and diurnal, seasonal, or perennial. These all are important factors in the initial evaluation and history. The list of causes for generalized pruritus is long, in contrast to the more obvious, but not necessarily more treatable, localized pruritus.

Three areas of system disorders most likely play a significant role in acquired acute pruritus: renal disease, hepatic disease, and abnormalities of the hematopoietic system. In regard to liver disease, several mechanisms are operative, but the most common relates to associated cholestasis with liver problems. The hepatic cholestasis secondary to drugs is very common, and the patient's history should be reviewed for the use of anabolic steroids, cephalosporins, diethylpropamide, cimetidine, erythromycin, nonsteroidal anti-inflammatory agents, nicotinic acid, oral contraceptives, as well as occasionally penicillin, phenothiazine, Dilantin and tolbutamide. Other drugs are continually being added to the list, so this is an area that must be continually revised and reviewed. Hepatitis can also be a major factor, and the pruritus associated with hepatitis may occur through cholestatic changes; other mechanisms still remain to be elucidated. This can occur with both hepatitis B and with hepatitis C [2], although the more usual cutaneous symptomatology relates to erythema multiforme, urticaria, or urticarial vasculitis [3]. With renal disease, often the itching precedes frank biochemical changes of advanced renal failure. The etiology here is not entirely clear, but parathyroid hormones, calcium levels, phosphate, magnesium, and middle molecular weight substances are deemed the most productive areas. Itching can often be controlled by regulation of the dialysis, which suggests some insight into the underlying mediators. Such patients are seen with less frequency by dermatologists at the present time, as dialysis centers have become much more adept at controlling pruritic symptoms. We have found UVB as perhaps the best supplemental therapy for some of these very symptomatic patients.

Hematopoietic disease is the third area of significant systemic disease to be evaluated. Classically, polycythemia vera was associated with bath pruritus; leukemias and lymphomas may also present similarly, as well as monoclonal gammopathies that can directly induce pruritus or lead to renal failure, which can induce a pruritus of renal origin. Cutaneous T-cell lymphoma or mycosis fungoides has long been associated with pruritus, but this usually evolves over a very long-term history of pruritus and rarely is associated with acute evolution of pruritic symptoms.

Infections and infestations, real or imagined, also play a role in this group of patients. Infections include varicella and rubella in young patients, and the presence of HIV infection in older patients. The patient with HIV infection who is pruritic may have a variety of causes for this symptomatology. The papular and pruritic eruptions seen in AIDS patients at the time of uremia and seroconversion have long been one of the major, early signs of the disease. With more advanced disease and significant repression of the CD4 population, one can see infections or ectoparasites as contributing to the symptomatology. The so-called ''crusted scabies'' are very common in these patients, folliculitis can contribute to the pruritic symptoms, as well as a rather unique condition—eosinophilic pustular folliculitis. In many of these patients, the possibility of a drug etiology must also be carefully sought, as well as evaluation of the liver and renal status as possible contributors to the symptomatology.

Sea bathers eruption is an infestation that is usually easily diagnosed because of the patient's recent history of exposure, but sometimes can be a confusing call. Imagined infestations (neurotic excoriations), as well as real ones such as scabies and other ectoparasites, also need to be considered when there is appropriate distribution of the pruritus.

B. Localized Pruritis

Localized pruritus may give important clues as to the etiology, and is less likely to be associated with widespread cutaneous or systemic disease. Localized pruritus can be further dissected in regard to patterning (i.e., linear, and regional). The linear aspects on any part of the body suggest the possibility of a contact dermatitis, especially when the linear pattern follows clothing or potential exposure to contactants such as Rhus. Perhaps the most difficult treatment challenges are localized pruritus of the inguinal anal region and the scalp. In the scalp, often this is related to psoriasis or an ongoing folliculitis, and the psoriasis is often extremely recalcitrant to virtually all forms of therapy. Pruritus ani, pruritus vulvi, and pruritus scroti often are chronic, sometimes flared by maceration and infection, but are classical examples of a potentiated itch scratch cycle, and this becomes extremely difficult to treat [4]. Optimally anogenital pruritus also should be evaluated when it is acute for an association with venereal disease, ectoparasites, and other parasites such as pin worms. It should be borne in mind that the scabies mite and crab lice are often seen on the skin and nits are hallmark; body lice may retreat to the seams of the underclothing and not be obvious on the initial examination. Pruritus of the hands and feet often is related to chronic diseases of the hands and feet, psoriasis, pompholyx, and contact dermatitis. In older patients, the distal lower extremities are a frequent site of pruritus, and sometimes difficult to treat. Often the pruritus-associated excoriations become secondarily infected and this is compounded by cardiovascular compromise and chronic lymphedema. Here the treatment has to be multifocal, persistent, anti-infective, as well as symptomatic. Some neurological disorders should be considered, including the midback pruritus associated with notalgia paresthetica, and sometimes associated with macular amaroid. Other patterned dermatomal pruritic symptoms can be seen with disorders of the peripheral nervous system. But in these cases, the symptoms are often more likely to be pain rather than pruritus.

For the dermatologist, several skin diseases may present with significant pruritus. Psoriasis was traditionally considered a pruritic disorder, but in reality it is not always such.

Lichen planus is more uniformly pruritic, as is eczema, atopic disease, and dermatitis herpetiformis.

As noted in Table 1, many dermatological conditions can present with pruritus which in some cases may be seasonal. Patients with atopic dermatitis tend to be more affected during the winter, with secondary xerosis of the skin; some patients with atopy have severe problems with miliaria and sweat disorders in the summer. In the elderly, one can note pruritus, asteatosis, and dermatitis heimalis from the dry air in the winter, and in the southern parts of the country this can be almost perennial because of the presence of air-conditioning, which also tends to lower significantly the relative humidity. The key in many of the dermatological conditions is the history and the cutaneous examination.

The workplace is of importance to the practitioner, as symptomology may be related to contact dermatitis, for this represents 40% of occupational illnesses [5]. Key causes here include oleoresins, rubber, wool, nickel, and the various caine anesthetics. The workup is of great importance because an obvious etiology will prompt specific therapy instead of the usual nonspecific symptomatic treatment. Therefore, the appropriate workup, as indicated briefly in Table 2, should be undertaken in most patients who do not respond to initial steps in diagnosis therapy. When the initial workup has determined no other significant medical

Table 1 Dermatologic Causes of Pruritis

Urticaria
Psoriasis, pityrias rubra pilaris
LP
Atopic dermatitis
Dermatitis herpetiformis
Occupational
Contact-
Allergies
Irritant (Fiberglas)
Arthropods
Insect Bites-
Grain mites, etc.
Mosquitoes, etc.
Ectoparasite
Pediculosis
Phthirius
Sarcoptes
Pityriasis rosea
CTCL
Stasis dermatitis

Table 2 Workup

CBC
Differential + smear + sedimentation rate
Chemistries
Include
liver function
renal; bun CR clearance
Thyroid Evaluation
Biopsy and immunofluoresence
As indicated
Patch testing
Photopatch testing
Immunoglobulins IGE, IGA, IGG, IGM,
SPEP (suspect monoclonalgammopathy)

reasons for pruritus, then treatment often will be successful, beginning with topical therapy and concomitant use of oral/systemic therapy. In mild cases, this is largely limited to the use of antihistamines, most of which are problematic because of sedating side effects. However, with the use of the new agents—the so-called ''nonsedating'' antihistamine medications—treatment has become easier. This group is covered in depth in Chapter 12.

C. Therapy

The patient seeing the physician for complaints of pruritus is primarily interested in relief from same. There are reasons to aggressively pursue systemic workup; this should be done at the same time as therapy is undertaken. It has often been this author's experience that essential pruritus, or pruritus due to trivial causes, responds to symptomatic therapy. However, there are exceptions to every rule.

1. Nonpharmacological Approaches

There are nonpharmacological approaches to the treatment of pruritus, and these are easily started at the time of the first patient–physician encounter. Such therapy includes the use of ultraviolet light, which can provide very significant relief from pruritus. The problem for the patient is that sometimes symptoms are at first worsened by treatment with ultraviolet light. Ultraviolet light provides some hardening of the skin, relieving, perhaps, dermatitis, and furthermore may have some effect on mast cells and other potential sources of pruriogens within the skin.

Ultraviolet B is our preferred nonpharmacological treatment regimen [1,6]. This must be carefully monitored to avoid potential severe reactions such as sunburn. Initial exposure time relates to skin type, potency of light box, and past history of photo exposure. UVA is usually slower to give relief, but avoids the problem of sunburn and is easier to regulate in any given patient—this is the obvious reason that UVA is the usual modality in the tanning centers. UVA penetrates more deeply into the dermis, and this is the likely reason UVA therapy is so effective in mastcell disease, being able to affect many of the several sources of histamine and other pruriogenic amine release.

In initiating therapy, the clinician must be aware of the status of the light source(s). Age of the bulbs may significantly alter the output and, hence, the duration of exposure. Usual UV sources can provide enough diffuse light in less than 1 min. The minimal erythema is the desirable goal. This often results in diminished pruritus and ''hardening'' of the skin, making it more resistant to future pruritic stimuli.

UVA is usually simpler to administer, usually beginning with 1/2 to 1 J exposure on the first visit. Several treatments usually result in symptom relief. This is the most effective approach to treating pruritus resulting from mast-cell disorders. Severe pruritus may also require the addition of psoralens in a PUVA protocol; this has recently been found to be very effective, especially in the pruritus from skin diseases such as atopic dermatitis and psoriasis which are most severe in description.

Soaks are also very effective, and tub soaks with emollients and moisturizers are certainly a key part of the treatment of the elderly patient, with significant asteatosis accompanying or causing the pruritus. Soaks can be done several times a day and could include colloidal oatmeal, other bath oils and surface acting agents (Aveeno®, Alpha Keri®, and others) that contain Triton X45 or other surfactants, and, most importantly, the use of tars (such as Balnetar®). Tars with their multiple effects on the epidermis, when incorporated in a bath oil, seem to provide significant relief for many patients. However, a major caution is the fact that most of these tar preparations have the potential of staining surfaces other than porcelain. One should check the facilities available and, even more importantly, warn the patient. Patients should be cautioned to avoid slipping in the tub when bath oils are used, especially elderly patients. In addition, since many older patients with significant arthritis have difficulty getting in and out of the tub and rely on showers for general cleanliness, soaks to relieve their symptoms are not easily accomplished. If showers are the only option, use of new moisturizing cleansers (Calgon, Eucerin Shower Therapy®, and others is an option). In cases of severe pruritus, the patient can also utilize the hospital physical therapy system, hubbard tank soaks, or whirlpool treatments. Home health care may also provide another avenue for the patient to get the appropriate soaks. Additional modalities include the use of emollients for pruritus occurring during the dry winter months, when these patients often present with classical findings of asteatosis, asteatotic eczema, and the initial itch–scratch cycle that tends to put the patient in a recurring cycle of itching–scratching–itching.

2. Topical Pharmacological Therapy

Chronic pruritus will lead to significant secondary changes in the skin, with thickening and scaling of the epidermis, many secondary excoriations, and an epidermal response of thickening (lichenification); in some biopsies, an apparent increase in the appearance and size of cutaneous innervation with prominence of cutaneous neuroreceptors is apparent. Blocking the receptors and the resulting pruritus can be done with both topical and systemic agents. Topical steroids, especially those in emollient bases or with soothing gels, can decrease the pruritic symptoms and give the patient significant relief. Chronic use of steroids has a downside—cutaneous atrophy—that can be a serious concern in the elderly patient who already has some preexisting dermatological changes or cutaneous atrophy from chronic sun damage. Alternatively, there are numerous over-the-counter preparations available containing menthol, camphor, and other soothing agents and emollients. Several of these include lotions, such as Sarna® and Sarna® with incorporation of hydrocortisone, may be quite effective for mild-to-moderate pruritic symptoms. The appearance of underlying inflammation accompanying the pruritus may predicate the use of steroids as a cutaneous anti-inflammatory agent. Often by the time they appear in a dermatologist's office, patients have already availed themselves of most topical agents containing the above-mentioned additives, and therefore more extensive prescription therapy is indicated. Traditional agents available by prescription include topical agents containing pramoxine (Prax®) and its formulations. The most effective single topical agent is doxepin, which provides effective relief through its effect on histamine. Patients will often try topical substances containing Benadryl, but in a certain percentage of patients this can result in sensitization that can be a significant complication of OTC topical therapy. The use of topical doxepin (Zonalon®) has become a standard for treatment because the incidence of sensitization is less than 1% and side effects of drowsiness are essentially no greater than the use of topical Benadryl and other topical antihistamines. Other topical agents that may be useful may contain topical analgesics, such as lidocaine, and here, again, precautions must be taken so as not to induce a contact sensitivity that will complicate effective therapy.

Steroids may be the treatment of choice (with or without tars added) for some dermatological diseases presenting with pruritus, such as psoriasis, lichen planus, and pityriasis rubra pilaris. Similarly, topical agents with ultraviolet may be the treatment of choice for patients with eczema. Contact eczema, when it creates symptoms of pruritus, will require very strong class I or II steroids, often in a gel formulation. Gel formulations are very soothing, but are potentially very drying in the winter months, and may not be a useful option in the elderly who already have significant asteatosis. When large areas of the skin are involved, it is usually appropriate to use low-cost bulk steroids (Class III Triamcinolone), with Class I steroids used aggressively in any trigger points.

The Class I steroids (Ultravate®, Temovate®, Diprolene®, Psorcon®, and others) are often the first round of therapy to be used for a short period of time to aggressively decrease cutaneous inflammation and sensitivity. (Topical steroids are dealt with in greater detail in Chap. 1.)

Once initial relief of the severe symptoms has been accomplished, the patient can then be downgraded to a class II, III, or IV steroid, with the most cost-effective agents being the various formulations, generic and otherwise, of triamcinolone, which can be obtained in bulk quantities. The usual algorithm for the treatment of pruritus topically and systemically is included in Table 3.

3. Systemic Therapy

Minor and localized pruritus may respond to topical therapy. Patients with significant and generalized pruritus need systemic therapy. For acute onset, systemic

Table 3 Therapy of Pruritus

	1. Remove cause: drug, contactant
	2. Nonspecific treatment
Mild symptoms	emollients—correct asteatosis
	menthol
	camphor
	pramoxine
	3. Topical treatment—prescription
	Steroids–class I–III
	Antihistamines—Zonalon (doxepin)
	4. Systemic antipruritics
	Antihistamines
	Nonsedating
Mild/moderate symptoms	Loratadine (Claritin) 10 qd.
	Fexofenidine (Allegra) 50 qd.
	Low sedation
	Cetirizine (Zyrtec)10 mg qd.
	Sedating
	Hydroxyzine Atarax—25 mg HS 10 b.i.d.
	Cyproheptidine (Peri Actin 4 mg ii HS i b.i.d.
	Anti-H_2-Doxepin .025 HS
Severe symptoms	Steroids
	Prednisone 1 mg/kg taper ↓ 25% q. 4–6 D.
	Depot—Kenalog 40 1 cc
	Celestone 1 cc
When all else fails	
	1. Hemoperfusion
	2. Oral charcoal
	3. Cholestyramine
	4. Capsaicin
	5. Lidocaine
	6. Intralesional steroids (for localized pruritus and trigger points)

steroids are often used to nonspecifically diminish the patient's symptoms. This is the major treatment for acute contact dermatitis, and, in circumstances with a self-limited disorder, may be all that is necessary. Dosage under these circumstances ranges from 1.0 to 1.5 mg/kg, and the dosage is key. Insufficient dosage is the main reason for failure, and is increasingly the case in the modern overweight population. A taper is begun as soon as relief of symptoms is achieved, and tapers should be gradual, over the course of 14 to 21 days. The use of steroid-sparing agents, such as dapsone, gold, the tetracyclines, niacinamide, and others may be a very useful adjunct to shorten the course of steroids and control the pruritus. These are dealt with elsewhere in this book.

The mainstay for treatment of pruritus is the use of antihistamines blocking the H_1- and H_2-receptor sites [1,6]. Modern classification of the anti-H_1s includes the traditional sedating, the newer mildly sedating, and the newest nonsedating groups of antihistamines. Of the traditional antihistamines, Benadryl® and Chlor-Trimeton®, which are available over the counter in the United States, are perhaps the most widely used by the patients prior to seeking medical attention. The two most important drugs in this group are hydroxyzine and cyproheptadine, which are the mainstay for most patients, and will also very effectively treat pruritus associated with urticaria and urticarial vasculitis. The newest group of anti-H_1s include loratadine and fexofenadine, which have supplanted the initial drugs in this category, astemizole and terfenadine [7]. These drugs see little usage nowadays, and indeed have been withdrawn in some countries because of the significant side effects related to the cytochrome P-450 3A interactions, and cardiac toxicity with use of certain combinations of drugs. The problem with drug interactions has become an increasing concern, and much of these interactions center around certain dermatological drugs, including the systemic. Significant drugs in these interactions are noted in Chapter 4: antifungal therapy. The usual approach is to initiate therapy with loratadine or fexofenadine daily, adding one of the sedating or mildly sedating antihistamines at bedtime. Hydroxyzine 25 mg HS is often very useful, but here again the dosage should relate to the weight of the patient. Dosage in milligrams per kilogram is key here: 25 mg HS is our usual therapy for 70-kg patients, but is adjusted downward and upward according to the weight of patient. Doses of Claritin® (loratadine) and Allegra® (fexofenadine) can similarly be adjusted upward. Additional benefits can sometimes be obtained by the use of cetirizine (Zyrtec®), a metabolite of hydroxyzine, which still has some mild sedating effects, but achieves the benefits of hydroxyzine without as great a concern over its effect on alertness and fine motor function. In the United States, dosage is 10 mg. Allegra's U.S. dosage is 50 mg, but is available at different dosages around the world. The use of H_2-blockers has become significant, especially in difficult and challenging patients. H_2-blockers include cimetidine and its derivatives. Doxepin is an ataractic but has significant anti-H_1 and anti-H_2 activity. Therefore, it is the next line in therapy when control is not achieved with the standard usage and adjustment of anti-H_1 agents.

The challenge of pruritus is a very significant one for the dermatologist who is best equipped to evaluate all the potential causes, and has the training to coordinate nonspecific topical therapy with effective prescription agents, both in topical and systemic forms. The appropriate evaluation of such patients also largely can be done most efficiently in the dermatologist's office. There are few patients that are as grateful as those whose symptoms have been minimized or eliminated. The statement that pruritus is a minor problem to the physician—unless he or she is the patient—was never more true. Today, with the tradition of compounding old remedies and the newer pharmacopeia available, effective therapy can be instituted with great benefit to the patient.

REFERENCES

1. Millikan LE. Treating pruritus: what's new in safe relief of symptoms? Postgrad Med 1996; 99(1):173–184.
2. Dega H, Frances C, Dupin N, Lebre C, Simantov A, Callot C, Laporte JL, Blot C, Opolon P, Poynard T, Chosidow O. Pruritus and the hepatitis C virus. The MULTIVIRC unit. Annu Dermatol Venereol J 1998; 125(1):9–12.
3. Monroe EW. Therapy of acute and chronic urticaria. J Eur Acad Dermatol 1997; 8: 511–17.
4. McKay M. Vulvodynia, scrotodynia, and other chronic dysesthesias of the anogenital region (including pruritus ani). In: Bernhard JD, ed. Itch—Mechanisms and Management of Pruritus. New York: McGraw-Hill, 1994:161–84.
5. Sampson HA. Atopic dermatitis. Ann Allergy 1992; 69:469–79.
6. Bernhard JD. General principles, overview, and miscellaneous treatments of itching. In: Bernhard JD, ed. Itch—Mechanisms and Management of Pruritus. New York: McGraw-Hill, 1994:367–84.
7. Monroe EW. Chronic urticaria: Review of non-sedating H_1 antihistamines in treatment. J Am Acad Dermatol 1998; 19:842–849.

21

Treatment of Hair and Nail Disorders

Anne M. Farrell and Rodney P.R. Dawber
Churchill Hospital
Oxford, United Kingdom

I. INTRODUCTION

Hair and nails are two ectodermal structures whose appearance carries important social signals. Disorders involving the hair and nails often cause great psychological distress and can significantly impair the patient's self-esteem and social functioning. Severe nail pathology can also impair the functional ability of that digit. Dermatologists, in being able to diagnose and offer treatment for hair and nail disorders, can play a vital role in improving patients' quality of life. Recent years have seen advances in our understanding of the pathophysiology of a number of hair and scalp disorders and their treatment. We will consider the most frequently encountered hair and nail disorders where pharmacological treatments can prove beneficial.

II. HAIR DISORDERS

A. Androgenetic Alopecia

Although common baldness is a genetically determined physiological event occurring during the lifespan of most men and women, since ancient times there has been a tendency by physician and laymen alike to regard it as an abnormality. Other terms used to describe it include androgenetic alopecia, pattern baldness, and male pattern baldness, although the latter term is misleading when applied to the common baldness seen in women. In men, the typical appearance of temporal recession, frontal recession, and thinning over the vertex has been well described

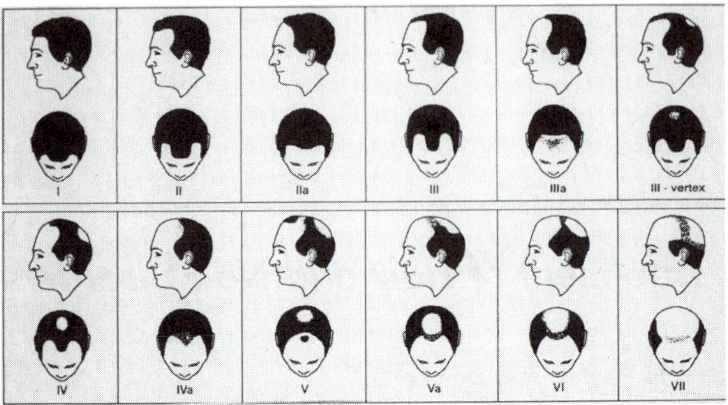

Figure 1 **Typical pattern of androgenetic alopecia seen in men (after Norwood, 1975).**

by Hamilton and later by Norwood and is easily recognized (Fig. 1). In women, although some do develop a similar pattern to men, the majority demonstrate a diffuse pattern of loss with sparing of the frontal hairline as described by Ludwig (Fig. 2) [1].

The physiological change involves shortening of the anagen phase of the hair cycle and consequent increase in the proportion of telogen hairs. Linear growth, however, is only minimally reduced. Structurally, there is progressive transformation of terminal hair follicles into ''vellus'' (miniaturized) follicles, but these differ from true primary vellus follicles by still retaining some remnants

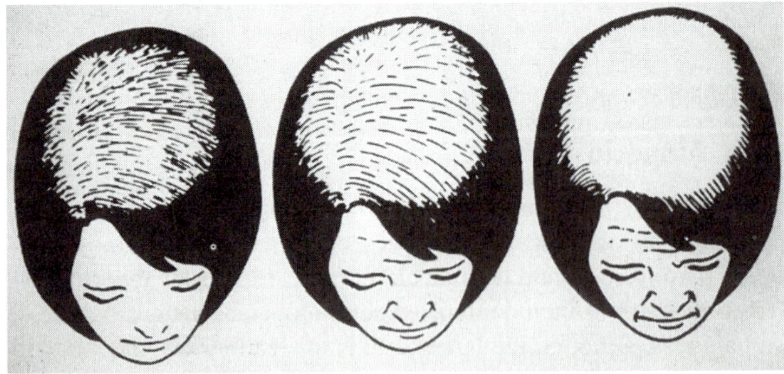

Figure 2 **Typical pattern of androgenetic alopecia seen in women (Ludwig pattern).**

of the erector pili muscles. Histologically, the earliest change is a focal perivascular basophilic degeneration in the lower third of the connective tissue sheath of anagen hair follicles [2]. This is followed by a perifollicular lymphocytic infiltrate at the level of the sebaceous duct and destruction of the connective tissue sheath, the remains of which can be seen early in the process as ''streamers.'' The result is that in the balding scalp most of the follicles are short and small with some quiescent terminal follicles and a wide range of hair shaft diameters compared with nonbald scalp. Reduced blood flow to the involved scalp has also been demonstrated, but whether this precedes or follows the baldness is unknown.

There appears to be a genetic predisposition and a number of studies have attempted to determine the mode of inheritance. One such study was that of Smith and Wells [3], who reported that among the first-degree relatives of 56 women with common pattern baldness, 54% of males and 23% of females over the age of 30 years were similarly affected. They proposed that the mode of inheritance was either dominant, with increased penetrance in the male, or multifactorial. Others have also supported the concept of a multifactorial inheritance. However, it is as yet unclear as to whether early (before the age of 30 years) and late-onset baldness have different patterns of inheritance. It is anticipated that gene linkage studies will identify genes involved in the inheritance of androgenetic alopecia in the future.

Early theories that a disturbance of sebaceous activity is a causative agent in common baldness have not been substantiated. Maibach [4] found no difference in the rate of production of sebum in bald and fully haired men and, in another study, no qualitative differences were found in the skin surface lipids [5].

The role of androgens and their interaction with genetic factors was demonstrated by Hamilton [6], who reported that baldness did not occur in 10 eunuchoids, 10 men castrated at puberty and 34 men castrated during adolescence, but that administration of testosterone led to baldness in those who were genetically predisposed. On discontinuing testosterone, the baldness did not progress, but it did not reverse either. Furthermore, males suffering from syndromes of androgen insensitivity such as 5α-reductase deficiency fail to develop temporal recession after puberty [7]. However, a number of studies have failed to show a correlation between testosterone levels and baldness in men [8,9], although these studies did show a correlation of baldness with urinary dehydroepiandrosterone [8] and elevated serum dehydroepiandrosterone sulfate [9]. In women, however, the degree of baldness may be associated with reduced concentrations of sex hormone binding globulin and therefore elevated levels of ''free'' circulating testosterone [10]. A significant number of women presenting with diffuse hair loss have evidence of polycystic ovary syndrome [11]. The maximum change in hair pattern occurs after menopause, when estrogen levels decline and a more ''androgenetic'' environment occurs. In premenopausal women with androgens within the normal female range, baldness only occurs in those with a strong genetic predisposition. In those women with a less strong genetic predisposition, baldness only occurs when androgen production is increased or drugs with androgen-like activity are taken. There are some women, however, who do not develop baldness despite having significantly abnormal levels of androgens, although they do typically have hirsutism. It appears that the essential inherited factor responsible for androgenetic alopecia is the manner in which the follicles of the frontal and vertex regions of the scalp react to androgens, in particular dihydrotestosterone. It is well established that the pilosebaceous unit can metabolize a wide range of androgens. Although the androgen metabolism of sebaceous glands has been extensively studied, the androgen metabolism of hair follicles has proved more difficult to study, principally because the plucked anagen hair follicles leave behind some of the germinative matrix and all of the dermal papilla. However, improving ability to culture dermal papillary cells has enabled the demonstration of androgen receptors on dermal papillary cells and their ability to metabolize a range of androgens [12,13]. The weak androgen dehydroepiandrosterone can be converted to androstenedione which, in turn, can be converted to testosterone and then to the more potent 5α-dihydrotestosterone (DHT) (Fig. 3). The enzyme involved in the latter conversion is 5α-reductase. Work in young balding men has shown a substantial increase in the production of DHT in frontal anagen hair follicles compared to frontal hair follicles in nonbalding men [14]. Bingham and Shaw demonstrated in 1973 that some individuals had increased 5α-reductase activity in the balding scalp compared to the nonbalding scalp [15]. Furthermore, men with 5α-reductase deficiency do not develop androgenetic alopecia. Two isoforms of this enzyme exist. The type 1 isoenzyme is found predominantly in the skin, located in sebaceous glands, epidermal and follicular keratinocytes, dermal papilla cells, sweat glands, and fibroblasts. The type 2 isoenzyme is found in the liver, prostate, epididymis, seminal vesicles, and inner root sheath of the hair follicle [16–18]. Sawaya and Price [18] reported that both forms of 5α-reductase isoenzyme were present in frontal hair follicles of women and men with andro-

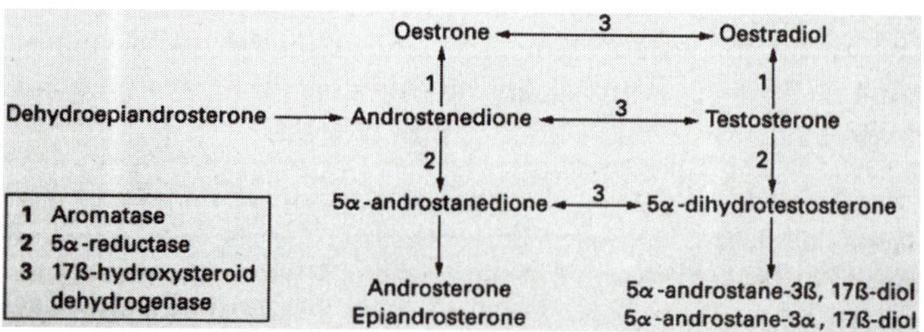

FIGURE 3 Pathways of androgen metabolism.

genetic alopecia and lower levels were also present in the occipital (more androgen-resistant) hair follicles. In women, frontal hair follicles had 40% more of both isoenzyme forms than occipital follicles while in men the figure was 60%. In addition, men had approximately 3.5 times more of each isoenzyme in frontal hair follicles than women. In both sexes, the 5α-reductase isoenzymes were located predominately in the outer root sheath.

Androgen receptors have been demonstrated in the dermal papillae of both anagen and telogen hairs and the outer root sheath [18,19]. Higher levels of the androgen receptor have been reported in cultured papillae from androgen-responsive sites such as the beard and moustache compared with the nonbalding scalp [20]. Using scalp biopsies, Sawaya and Price [18] demonstrated that both male and female subjects with androgenetic alopecia had 30% more androgen receptors in frontal hair follicles than occipital hair follicles, and that the androgen receptor content in females was 40% less than the amount found in men for both frontal and occipital regions. In the same subjects they also studied levels of cytochrome P-450-aromatase (AROM), a microsomal enzyme that converts testosterone and 4-androstenedione to estradiol and estrone, respectively, and found that frontal hair follicles in the women had approximately six times more AROM than frontal follicles in the men and that occipital follicles in the women had approximately four times more AROM than occipital follicles in the men. In the women, the frontal hair follicles had approximately half the AROM of occipital follicles, suggesting that AROM may be an important enzyme limiting the level of androgens in hair follicles of women by converting androgens to estrogens [18].

1. Treatment of Androgenetic Alopecia

A number of drugs when given systemically have been reported to lead to an improvement in androgenetic alopecia as part of a general hypertrichosis. These include diazoxide, minoxidil, viprostol, benoxaprofen, and cyclosporin A [21]. However, only minoxidil has shown some effectiveness when used topically.

Minoxidil is a piperidinopyrimidine derivative and a potent vasodilator which is effective in treating severe hypertension. When applied topically as a 2% solution twice daily it has been demonstrated to result in the conversion of some vellus to terminal hairs, and moderate to dense regrowth of hair in 24% to 59% of individuals [21,22]. However, a uniform covering of the bald areas was seen in less than 10% of subjects studied, and those male patients who respond best are younger, have a smaller area of hair loss, and are at the early stages of balding [24]. The recently available 5% solution gives slightly enhanced results. In women with androgenetic alopecia a double-blind application of 2% topical minoxidil solution resulted in significantly more new hair growth than application of placebo [25]. However, the benefits only last for as long as the topical minoxidil is applied and on discontinuing the applications 3 months later the hair loss returns to what it would have been had the minoxidil not been used. Its mode of action is uncertain—it does not have antiandrogenic properties. Wester et al. [26] demonstrated an increase in scalp cutaneous blood flow, but this was only statistically significant for the 5% solution and in this study vehicle alone also affected blood flow and a positive control was not included. When Bunker and Dowd [27] studied the effect of minoxidil on cutaneous blood flow and included a positive control with established vasoactivity they found no difference. A recent study demonstrated that minoxidil increases the expression by dermal papillary cells of vascular endothelial growth factor (VEGF), an endothelial cell-specific mitogen [28]. The hair cycle is characterized by increased vascularization of the dermal papilla during the anagen phase associated with increased VEGF production by the dermal papillary cells, while in telogen there is loss of the capillary network in the dermal papilla associated with decreased VEGF expression. It may be, therefore, that minoxidil increases production of VEGF and maintains vascularization at the level of the dermal papillae.

Topical minoxidil appears to be safe, the main side effect being occasional local irritation and a low incidence of contact dermatitis. Although an average of less than 1.4% is absorbed through the skin surface the following theoretical side effects may occur: sodium and water retention, tachycardia, and aggravation of angina pectoris. Therefore, the recommended dose should not be exceeded and topical minoxidil should be avoided in those with ischemic heart disease and used with caution in those with hypertension. Some patients treated with minoxidil develop hirsutism particularly over the forehead and temples that usually resolves as the minoxidil continues to be used. Topical tretinoin may also have some effectiveness since Bazzano et al. [29] demonstrated that topical 0.025% tretinoin also stimulated hair growth in 58% of subjects studied and the combination of 0.025% topical tretinoin with 0.5% minoxidil was more effective than 0.5% minoxidil alone.

Other therapeutic measures that have been reported to lead to some improvement in individual cases are drugs with anti-androgenic properties including cyproterone acetate, spironolactone, cimetidine, ketoconazole, and flutamide, but such reports of their efficacy are ''uncontrolled'' [30]. Because of their antiandrogenic properties, these have been predominantly used in females, although when cyproterone acetate was used to treat persistent male sex offenders, androgenetic alopecia in these men was said to improve. Of these drugs only cyproterone acetate has been studied extensively, although even these studies concentrated on its effect on hirsutism with its effects on the scalp hair being reported as an incidental finding. It acts by blocking the androgen receptor binding site thus preventing steroid/receptor interaction with DNA. Regimes that have been used include cyproterone acetate 100 mg daily from day 5 to 14 of the menstrual cycle plus ethinyl estradiol 50 μg from day 5 to 25, although this regime was associated with side effects [31]. Attempts to reduce the dose of cyproterone acetate to 2 mg daily plus ethinyl estradiol 50 μg did not reliably maintain the improvement gained on the higher dose regime [32]. Another study reported that three women treated cyclically for a year with cyproterone acetate 50 mg daily for 10 days plus ethinyl estradiol 40 μg daily for 21 days following the withdrawal bleed experienced some improvement [33]. However, there are no long-term prospective trials of its use and, although it is sometimes prescribed on a named patient basis, there are no product licenses anywhere in the world for its use in androgenetic alopecia. Side effects include lassitude, weight gain, breast tenderness, loss of libido, and nausea and because it has the potential to feminize a male fetus it should be used in conjunction with an oral contraceptive. Both the cyproterone acetate and ethinyl estradiol increase the risk of thromboembolic disease in those with a personal or family history of thromboembolic disease. Therefore, disturbances of the coagulation system must be ruled out before these medications are prescribed and patients should be advised to discontinue the medication and seek medical advice if they develop thrombophlebitis, leg swelling, shortness of breath, chest pains, or severe headaches. It should also be avoided in those with severe diabetes with vascular changes and sickle-cell anemia. There has also been concern about the hepatic effects of cypoterone acetate: fulminant hepatitis has occasionally been reported in patients receiving it for prostate cancer (although at high doses of 200–300 mg). If hepatotoxicity occurs, it is usually after several months of treatment and therefore liver function tests should be performed in any patient who develops symptoms of hepatotoxicity. Although there have been reports of hepatocellular cancer associated with its use, including women treated for hyperandrogenic conditions [34], this is extremely rare and it is possible that other factors played a role in such cases [35].

Burke and Cunliffe [36] reported a subjective improvement with oral spironolactone (200 mg od), which is mildly antiandrogenic and which has been more extensively studied in acne and hirsutism [30]. Side effects included mood swings, irregular menses, and breast tenderness. Another small study claimed success with high-dose cimetidine (300 mg 5 times daily) believed to be mediated through androgen receptor blockade [37]. Flutamide is a pure antiandrogen that has also been effective in hirsutism but there are only anectdotal reports of its effectiveness in androgenetic alopecia [30]. It has also been reported to be potentially hepatotoxic and regular monitoring of liver function tests is recommended.

Topical antiandrogens have also been tried, including topical progesterone, which proved ineffective. However, small studies with topical 11α-hydroxyprogesterone and 17α-estradiol showed some benefit [38,39].

A recent promising development for future treatment of androgenetic alopecia is finasteride. This is a selective type II 5α-reductase inhibitor. The observations that patients who are deficient in 5α-reductase do not develop androgenetic alopecia and that elevated levels of DHT are present in scalps with androgenetic alopecia, led to finasteride being tried as a potential therapeutic agent in men with common baldness [40,41]. In phase III studies, finasteride 1 mg/day orally resulted in decreases in the level of DHT in the scalp and serum compared with placebo, and increased scalp hair in all parameters including scalp hair counts, patient self-assessment, investigator assessment, and global photography. The safety and tolerability is excellent and at a dose of 1 mg/day there are no significant adverse effects including no clinically important changes in LH, FSH, or testosterone or significant impairment in fertility compared with placebo. However, because of its potential feminizing effect on the male fetus, it is contraindicated in women who are or may be pregnant.

B. Alopecia Areata

The characteristic presentation of alopecia areata is the appearance of a well-circumscribed, totally bald smooth patch often with the presence of exclamation-mark hairs at the border (Figs. 4–6). In the majority of cases, the lesion is asymptomatic and may be noticed by the patient only by chance, although some patients do complain of local irritation or paresthesia preceding the hair loss. It has been claimed that the scalp is the first site to be affected in 60% of cases but any site of the body may be involved. The subsequent progress is varied; the initial patch of hair loss may regrow within a few months or new areas of hair loss may develop, in some cases resulting in diffuse hair loss. Several studies have shown varying incidences of recovery or progression to complete bladness. In Chicago, the duration of the initial attack was less than 6 months in 33%, and less than 1

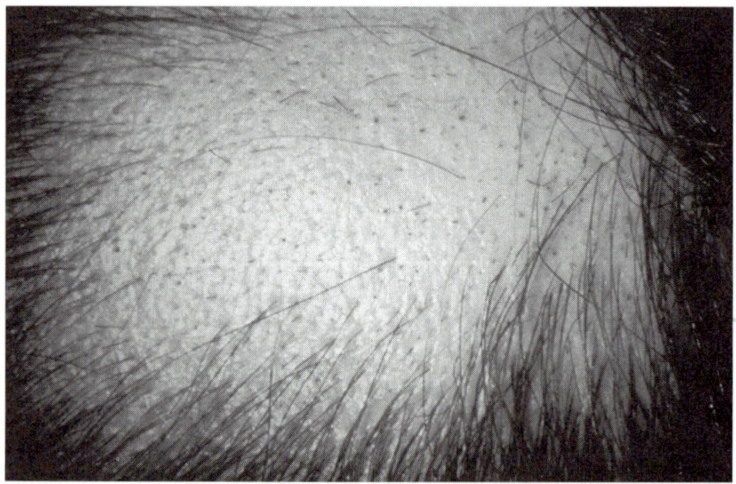

FIGURE 4 Well-circumscribed patch of hair loss in alopecia areata.

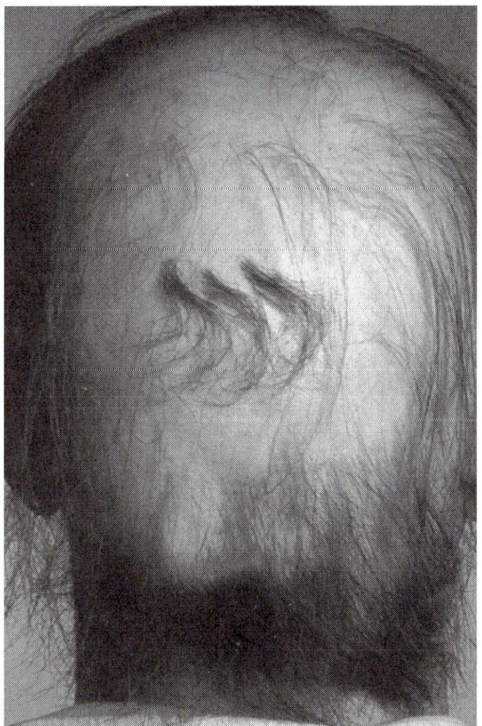

FIGURE 5 Widespread alopecia areata.

year in 50% [42]. However, 33% never recovered from the initial attack and in those patients followed up for 20 years the incidence of relapse was 100%. Muller and Winkelmann [43] reported that only 1% of children and 10% of adults with alopecia totalis showed complete regrowth. The prognosis seems to differ pre- and postpuberty. In the Chicago series of those patients developing alopecia areata prepuberty, 50% became totally bald and none recovered, while of those developing it after puberty only 25% became totally bald and 5.3% recovered. It also appears that alopecia areata occurring in atopics has a worse outcome.

The precise etiology is uncertain but a genetic predisposition appears to be important with a high incidence of family history in reports from a number of countries, and several reports of its occurrence in twins. The condition also shows an increased incidence in atopic individuals and those with Down's syndrome. Reports that alopecia areata is associated with an increased frequency of autoimmune diseases, including thyroid disease, vitiligo, Addison's disease, pernicious anemia, systemic lupus erythematosus, and rheumatoid arthritis have been inter-

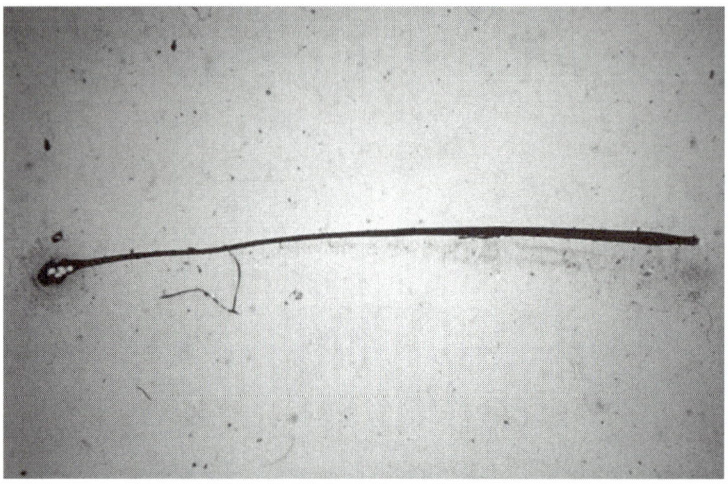

FIGURE 6 Alopecia areata: Exclamation-mark hair.

preted as evidence for an autoimmune origin. Further evidence for an autoimmune role in the pathogenesis of alopecia areata is the presence of a lymphocytic infiltrate in and around hair follicles. Immunohistochemistry has demonstrated that this infiltrate is largely T cells with increased numbers of Langerhans cells [44]. However, several studies using direct immunofluorescence have failed to demonstrate the presence of antifollicle antibodies in affected scalps and, although deposition of complement at the hair follicle basement membrane has been reported in alopecia areata, it has also been reported in normal scalp and male pattern baldness. Alopecia areata differs from other recognized autoimmune diseases in that it does not result in complete loss of function of the target organ but rather in a temporary switching off of hair follicle activity that can return to normal, suggesting that the target in alopecia areata may be a controlling growth factor or its receptor.

1. Treatment of Alopecia Areata

One of the principal problems in assessing the efficacy of any treatment in alopecia areata is the potential for natural recovery. To date, there is no completely specific or reliable treatment and the majority of reports of therapeutic effectiveness are anecdotal.

The earliest treatments were nonspecific irritants and anecdotal claims for improvement were made for phenol, benzylbenzoate, UVB in erythematous doses, and dithranol. However, the scientific evidence for the efficacy of these treatments is poor.

Systemic corticosteroids result in regrowth of hair in many cases, but on discontinuing the treatment most of these patients relapse so that the majority of authors have felt that there was insufficient evidence of prolonged benefit to justify the potential systemic adverse reactions [45]. Pulsed intravenous methylprednisolone (250 mg b.d. for 3 days) was reported to prevent progression of recent-onset alopecia areata [46], but another study reported it to be ineffective in alopecia totalis [47]. Some benefit was suggested in studies combining systemic steroids with topical or intralesional steroids, or topical minoxidil, or cyclosporine, but the numbers of patients in these studies were small. There have also been occasional reports of the effectiveness of topical corticosteroids such as fluocinolone [48]. However, regrowth of hair tends to occur in those cases in which it was most likely to have occurred spontaneously anyway, and folliculitis may be a significant side effect. Intralesional steroids have been shown to be beneficial in some cases, administered either by needle injection [49] or jet injection [50]. Porter and Burton reported that response appeared to be in an ''all or nothing'' fashion [49]. However, skin atrophy is an important side effect that can occur not only at the site of injection but also in a linear fashion following the direction of lymph flow [51]. Because of this, the use of intralesional steroids should be principally for accelerating regowth in well-circumscribed and cosmetically disfiguring areas of hair loss.

Another approach has been the use of potent sensitizers to produce a contact dermatitis that may sometimes be associated with regrowth of the hair. Dinitrochlorobenzene (DNCB) was among the chemicals used for this purpose: after sensitization was achieved using concentrations of up to 2%, once-weekly applications were applied at a concentration sufficient to achieve a mild inflammatory response (from concentrations as low as 0.0001%). A variety of success rates were reported, ranging from 10 to 78%, the worst response being seen in patients with alopecia totalis and patients with a family history of alopecia areata and a personal or family history of atopy [52]. The mechanism by which contact sensitivity leads to hair regrowth is uncertain, but hypotheses include attraction of effector T cells to the area or localized antigen competition. However, following reports of the potential carcinogenicity of DNCB, other sensitizing chemicals were studied, including squaric acid dibutyl ester (SADBE) [53]. When used as a 2% solution, some authors have reported a success rate of up to 70%, although others [54] found it no more effective than placebo. Other sensitizers that have been reported to be beneficial include *Primula obconica* and diphencyprone [55]. The latter is the sensitizer now most frequently used. It is capable of inducing significant regrowth in a minority of cases but well over 50% of those regaining hair will subsequently lose it. However, the side effects of the induced dermatitis and the risk of sensitizing the medical staff administering the chemicals has diminished the routine practical use of contact sensitization in alopecia areata.

Some groups have reported that treatment with PUVA, using oral 8-methoxypsoralen, is beneficial in up to 60% of cases [56,57]. Lassus et al. reported that oral 8-methoxypsoralen was as effective as topical 8-methoxypsoralen with approximately 70% responding, but between 20 to 40 treatments were required [57]. Other reports in the literature vary from poor response to approximately 45% of cases responding, and with the same degree of relapse occurring in up to 90% up on discontinuation of treatment [58]. Again, patients with alopecia totalis or atopy responded poorly. The exact mechanism of action is uncertain but may be due to the irritant effect of the PUVA, or the immunological changes that occur in the skin after PUVA treatment. Although some patients appear to respond well to PUVA, the overall poor response rate and the high doses of UVA often required have led many dermatologists to avoid using it for alopecia areata.

Topical minoxidil was initially reported to be beneficial [59], although subsequent double-blind and dose-responsive studies were less encouraging [55]. However, another study using 3% minoxidil reported that 9 of 20 patients with 25 to 99% hair loss at the start of the study developed cosmetically acceptable hair regrowth at 64 weeks follow-up [60]. The highest response was reported using 5% topical minoxidil [61], with regrowth in 85% of severe cases, although in the majority of cases this was not cosmetically acceptable. Oral minoxidil, 5 mg twice daily, gave a faster response rate than the 5% minoxidil solution but cosmetically acceptable improvement was still only 18% [62]. The use of oral minoxidil was also restricted by its tendency to cause generalized hypertrichosis.

Oral cyclosporin A has been shown to produce hair regrowth in some cases, but also induces general hypertrichosis, renal, and immunological side effects [63]. There have also been reports of its effectiveness when used in low doses with prednisolone [64], although other authors were unable to confirm this and have been reluctant to use it because of its toxicity.

Topical cyclosporin A has been tried in concentrations of 5 to 10% and, although it produces hair regrowth better than placebo, this regrowth was patchy and sporadic [65]. Recent studies have demonstrated that topical applications of the immunomodulatory drug FK506 can induce hair regrowth in the Dundee experimental bald rat (DEBR), which has been developed as an animal model for alopecia areata, and this might prove to be a treatment applicable to human alopecia areata in the future [66].

Oral administration of the immunomodulatory agent inosine pranobex (inosiplex, Isoprinosine, or Imunovir) has also been reported to be beneficial in some patients, but this effect was often lost within two to three weeks of stopping treatment [67]. However, other studies were unable to confirm this [68].

C. Cicatricial Alopecia

Cicatricial or scarring alopecia refers to alopecia that is associated with loss of hair follicles. Several independent processes can result in this endpoint, including trauma, infiltration by benign or malignant tumors, infection (e.g., tuberculosis, syphilis, fungal infections, leishmaniasis, and herpes zoster), and inflammatory processes (e.g., lichen planus, cicatricial pemphigoid). When all the clinically and histologically recognized causes have been excluded, the two remaining syndromes are folliculitis decalvans and pseudopelade.

In the early stages, scarring is not always easily identified clinically and it may be necessary to re-examine the patient on a number of occasions. Additional clinical features that are helpful in deciding the cause include the presence of folliculitis, follicular plugging, telangiectasia, or broken hairs. Hairs should be obtained from the edge of the bald area for microscopy and culture and, if biopsies are felt to be indicated, the most useful are several punch biopsies taken from early lesions. The most common of the conditions causing scarring alopecia will be discussed individually.

D. Pseudopelade

In 1885, Brocq described a scarring alopecia that he termed ''pseudopelade,'' but for many years there was confusion about the nomenclature. Pseudopelade is now regarded as a syndrome in which destruction of the follicles leads to permanent patchy baldness but in which there is no clinical evidence of folliculitis or inflammation. However, lichen planus can produce a very similar picture and some authors have reported that on the basis of associated skin findings and pathology some cases of pseudopelade are caused by lichen planus. Lupus erythematosus can also result in similar changes and therefore many authors believe that pseudopelade is the end result of one of a number of different pathological processes. Biopsies taken from clinically normal scalp at the edge of a plaque of pseudopelade show numerous lymphocytes in the upper two thirds of the follicles; later, as the follicles and sebaceous glands are destroyed, the epidermis may remain relatively normal or atrophic, and the dermis densely sclerotic adjacent to the affected follicles. Follicular plugging is not a characteristic feature.

The condition most commonly affects middle-aged women, although men and children may also be affected. The typical presentation is that the patient discovers a small bald patch by chance and this is often located on the apex. Occasionally there is slight preceding irritation. The involved patch is smooth and slightly depressed and in the early stages there may be some diffuse or perifollicular erythema and the clinically involved hairs at the margin of the patch are very easily extracted (Fig. 7). In most cases, the progress of the disease is

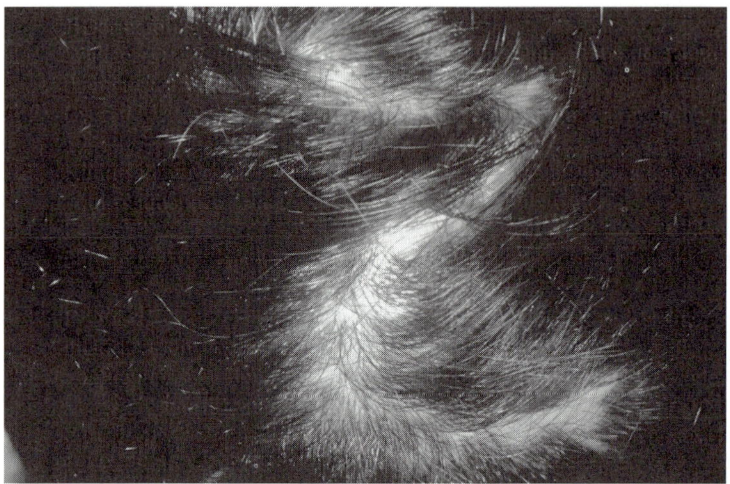

FIGURE 7 Early stage of pseudopelade showing erythema.

very slow, resulting in small round patches that can still be easily concealed by the patient. But in some cases a more rapid course can result as individual patches become confluent, resulting in almost complete baldness after 2 years. The current treatment is unsatisfactory and, in those cases where the condition does not appear to be secondary to lichen planus or lupus erythematosus, there is no recognizable treatment. Intralesional steroids do not appear to alter the progress of the disease. At present, the only option is autografting from unaffected to scarred scalp in cases where there is no longer active inflammatory change.

E. Folliculitis Decalvans and Tufted Folliculitis

In 1888, Quinquaud described a form of scarring alopecia of the scalp in which chronic pustular folliculitis at the advancing margin was a notable clinical feature. As successive crops of pustules develop, at the margins of the round or oval patches of alopecia, the area of the scarring alopecia slowly extends (Fig. 8). A similar process can involve other body sites, particularly the beard and pubic areas, axillae, and thighs. Both scalp and body involvement can coexist. Scalp involvement occurs in men from adolescence upward and women aged 30 to 60 years, but it may also rarely occur in infancy. Involvement of sites other than the scalp is predominantly seen in men. *Staphylococcus aureus* is grown from the pustules in most cases. A defect in the patient's immune response to the organisms has been postulated, although investigations of patients presenting with this condition usually reveal no evidence of an immunological defect. Histo-

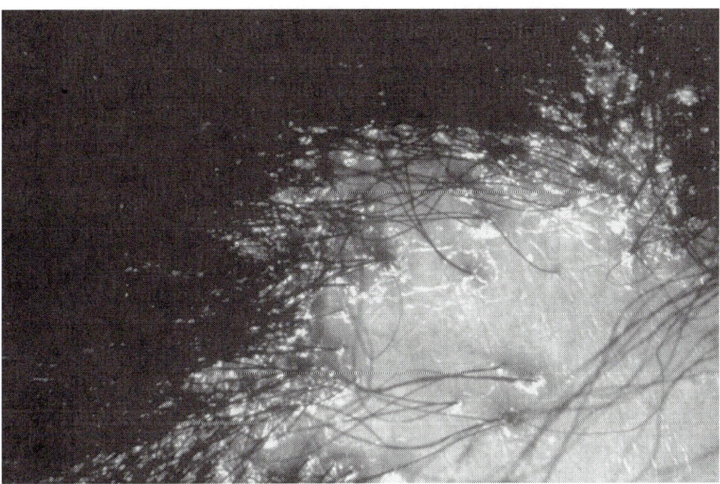

FIGURE 8 Folliculitis decalvans showing crops of pustules that result in patches of scarring alopecia.

logical examination shows inflammation in which lymphocytes predominiate with relatively few polymorphs, some plasma cells, and the occasional giant cell [69]. It is thought that scarring may be the result of damage to the stem cells in the ''bulge'' area.

Tufted folliculitis may be a secondary phenomenon observed in this and other inflammatory scalp disorders due to inflammation and scarring around the superficial parts of the adjacent follicles, resulting in close grouping or ''tufting'' of hairs (Fig. 9) [70].

Systemic antibiotics have been used and may prevent extension of the disease but usually for only as long as they are administered. There are anecdotes of topical fusidic acid and oral zinc sulfate being beneficial. Brozena et al. reported a single case which, after only minimal improvement with several courses of antibiotics, resolved after a 10-week course of rifampicin [71]. More recently, Powell et al., in a larger series of patients, have confirmed the effectiveness of rifampicin (300 mg b.i.d.) in combination with clindamycin [69].

F. Lichen Planus

Lichen planus affecting the trunk and limbs may commence at any age and is a relatively common condition seen in general dermatology clinics. However, significant involvement of the scalp is relatively rare. In one study of 307 cases of lichen planus [72], significant scalp involvement was only seen in 10 patients.

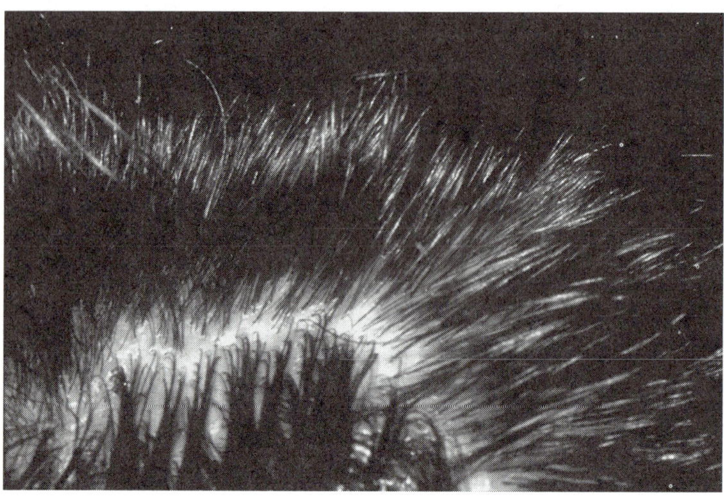

Figure 9 Tufted folliculitis.

However, the incidence of scalp lichen planus is problably higher than this as such reports tend to exclude patients in whom alopecia, classified as pseudopelade, is the only site of involvement. The typical clinical presentation is of a middle-aged female with recent onset of violaceous papules, erythema, and scaling that progresses to follicular plugging and scarring (Fig. 10). The follicular plugs are eventually shed from the scarred areas, which remain white and smooth, although plugs are often seen at the margins of the scarred area if the disease is progressing. However, often by the time the patient attends for consultation all that is clinically apparent is irregular white scarring and the condition is labeled as ''pseudopelade.'' It is the finding of typical lesions of lichen planus elsewhere including the oral mucosa which points towards the diagnosis. Biopsies usually need to be obtained from early lesions if they are to be informative. Two variants of lichen planus—bullous lichen planus and lichen plano-pilaris—have a higher incidence of scalp involvement and may have a rapid progression with fast onset of extensive scarring alopecia. A number of drugs including gold, mepacrine, para-aminosalicylic acid, aminophenazole, and phenothiazine derivatives can also produce lichen planus-like eruptions that, if involving the scalp, can result in a scarring alopecia, and a careful drug history should be taken to exclude this.

Potent topical steroids, intralesional steroids, or even a short course of systemic steroids may be helpful in some cases where active inflammatory changes are evident. In severe cases, azathioprine or cyclosporin may also be considered. However, once the scarring has occurred, it is irreversible and the only interven-

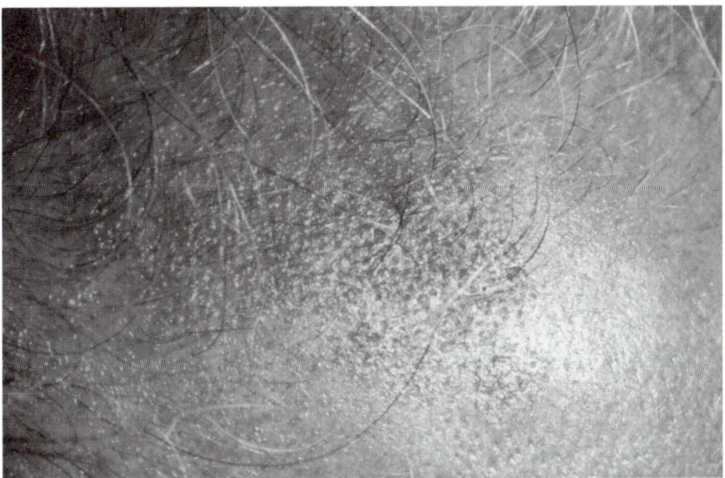

FIGURE 10 Lichen planus demonstrating erythema, scarring, and follicular accentuation.

tion that might lead to a cosmetic improvement is surgical once the condition has ''burned itself out.''

G. Graham-Little (Lassueur-Graham-Little, Piccardi-Lassueur-Little) Syndrome

This condition is characterized by the development of progressive scarring alopecia of the scalp (in some reported cases associated with follicular plugging) with loss of pubic and axillary hair and the rapid onset of kertatosis pilaris. It is believed by some to be a variant of lichen planus. No recognized treatment is known other than surgical treatment for areas of scarring.

H. Frontal Fibrosing Alopecia

This condition, seen in middle-aged or elderly women in particular, is probably a variant of follicular scarring lichen planus. As the name implies, it is a scarring alopecia that commences anteriorly and spreads posteriorly toward the vertex of the scalp. There is no effective pharmacological treatment once the scarring has occurred, but potent topical steroid applied to the margin may help slow its progression.

I. Scarring Follicular Keratosis

A number of syndromes have been described characterized by keratosis pilaris, associated with inflammatory change and eventual destruction of affected hair follicles. Among them are atrophoderma vermiculata, keratosis pilaris atrophicans faciei, and keratosis pilaris decalvans. No reliable treatments are recognized, although there have been a few anecdotal reports of topical and oral retinoids being helpful.

J. Lupus Erythematosus

Scalp changes can occur in both the systemic and chronic forms of lupus erythematosus. At least 50% of cases of acute systemic lupus erythematosus have diffuse shedding of the hair, erythema of the scalp, and dry fragile broken hairs, so-called ''lupus hair,'' particularly at the frontal margin. However, scarring alopecia is seen less frequently in the acute systemic form than in the discoid lupus erythematosus form where scalp lesions occur in approximately 20% of men and 50% of women. The typical clinical appearance of discoid lupus eythematosus involving the scalp is an itchy, erythematous, scaly area that extends irregularly and leaves scarring (Fig. 11). Histology at the early stage will show follicular plugging and basal liquefaction and a positive lupus band on immunofluorescence, but in more advanced cases histology may only show scarring.

Treatment with potent topical steroids may reduce the erythema and inflammation and halt the progression of the disease, but this may need to be supplemented with systemic corticosteroids and/or antimalarials. For cases that fail to respond to these measures, other therapeutic measures that have been used include dapsone, retinoids, and oral gold [73,74]. However, no pharmacological

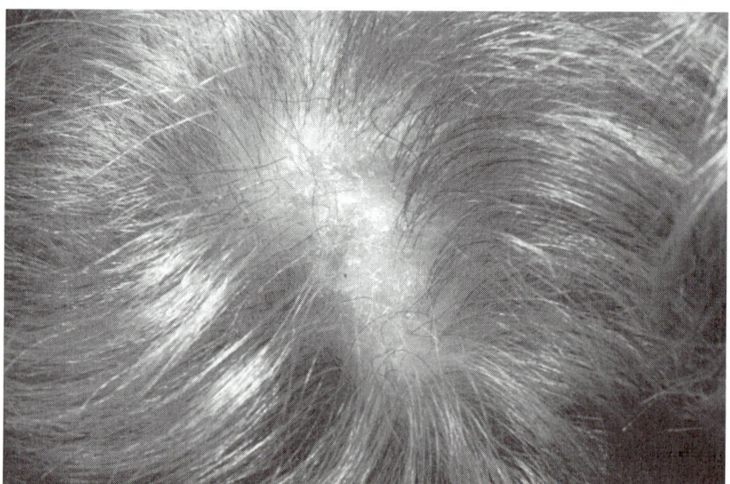

FIGURE 11 Discoid lupus erythematosus showing erythema and scarring.

measures can reverse scarring once it has occurred, although in cases where the disease has ''burned out,'' surgical excision of the scarred areas is an option.

K. Cicatricial Pemphigoid (Benign Mucosal Pemphigoid)

This subepidermal blistering disorder predominantly involves the eyes and mucous membrane. It can involve skin elsewhere and the scalp is one site that is more frequently involved (Fig. 12). Involvement of mucosal sites and direct immunofluorescence demonstrating linear deposits of IgG, IgA, and complement at the dermo–epidermal junction aid the diagnosis. Potent topical steroid may partly inhibit the process in some cases. For unresponsive lesions, there is controversy as to whether introducing systemic corticosteroids for nonmucosal lesions is justified as they are not always beneficial.

L. Erosive Pustular Dermatosis of the Scalp

This condition occurs in the elderly. Clinically it presents as erythema and crusting of the scalp and pustulation is evident below and at the margins of the crusting (Fig. 13). Swabs of these pustules show no significant bacterial growth. As the process progresses, scarring alopecia ensues and squamous cell carcinoma has been reported within the scars [75]. Potent topical steroids such as 0.05% clobeta-

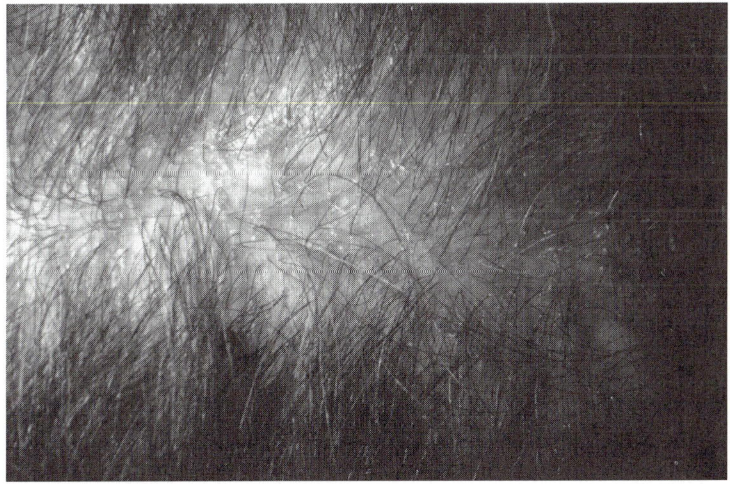

FIGURE 12 Cicatricial pemphigoid.

sol propionate twice daily suppress it and there have also been anecdotal reports of it responding to oral zinc sulfate.

M. Scalp Ringworm (Tinea Capitis)

Of the dermatophytes the genera *Microsporum* and *Trichophyton* are capable of invading hair. Table 1 summarizes the organisms recognized as invading human hair and, in the case of the zoophilic fungi, the animals from which the human

Table 1 Fungi That Cause Scalp Ringworm

Type	Distribution and host
Anthropophilic	
Microsporum audouini	Worldwide
M. ferrugineum	China, Japan, parts of Russia, Central and E. Africa*
Trichophyton rubrum (rarely affects the scalp)	Widespread endemic: extension from Asia
T. schoenleini	Widespread, but uncommon in most areas: common in the Middle East, N. Africa
T. tonsurans	Widespread: common in parts of Latin America
T. violaceum	Dominant in many parts of Africa*, Central and S. Europe, Middle East†
T. gourvilii	W. Africa
T. megninii	S. Europe, Africa
T. soudanense	Central Africa
T. yaoundi	Africa
Zoophilic	
Microsporum canis	Worldwide (Cats and dogs)
M. equinum	(Horses)
M. nanum	(Pigs)
M. persicolor	W. Europe (Field-vole)
Trichophyton mentagrophytes	Worldwide (Many species: reservoirs in rodents)
T. verrucosum	Widespread (Cattle)
T. equinum	Widespread (Horses)
T. erinacei	Europe, New Zealand (Hedgehogs)
T. quinckeanum	Widespread, but generally rare (Mice: may be transmitted to man by cats and dogs)
T. simii	India (Monkeys)
Geophilic	
Microsporum gypseum	Widespread (Soil: man infected by contact with soil or from infected animals)

*Verhagen (1976).
†Asgari & Sutevl (1973).

usually acquires the fungus. At least one species, *Microsporum gypseum*, is geophilic in that it normally resides in the soil. The worldwide distribution of dermatophytes outlined in Table 1 is constantly being updated, with increasing movements of populations around the world, and as more is learned about fungal species in parts of the world where mycology has been poorly studied in the past [76]. In the past, scalp ringworm in the United States, was predominantly caused by the *Microsporum* species *M. canis* and *M. audouini*, but in the last 40 years *Trichophyton tonsurans* has become the most common causative organism. In Europe, *M. canis* remains a frequent cause.

The pattern of pathology depends on the mode of growth of the fungus within the hair shaft and the host's immune response to it. In some dermatophytes in certain patients the infection can be acutely inflammatory and self-limiting, while with other dermatophytes, or the same dermatophyte in different patients, the infection manifests as chronic scaling and broken hairs that eventually resolve without scarring (Fig. 14). Other dermatophyte infections typically run a prolonged course resulting in permanent scarring, but scarring can also be seen in some patients infected with dermatophytes that generally tend not to scar other patients.

Work into the pathogenesis of scalp ringworm was largely performed by Kligman in the 1950s with *M. audouini*. After inoculation of the fungus into the scalp (usually as a result of minor trauma), the fungal hyphae grow centrifugally in the stratum corneum and grow down the keratin shafts of hairs that are in the active growing phase. By the seventh day, fungus is detectable 1 mm above

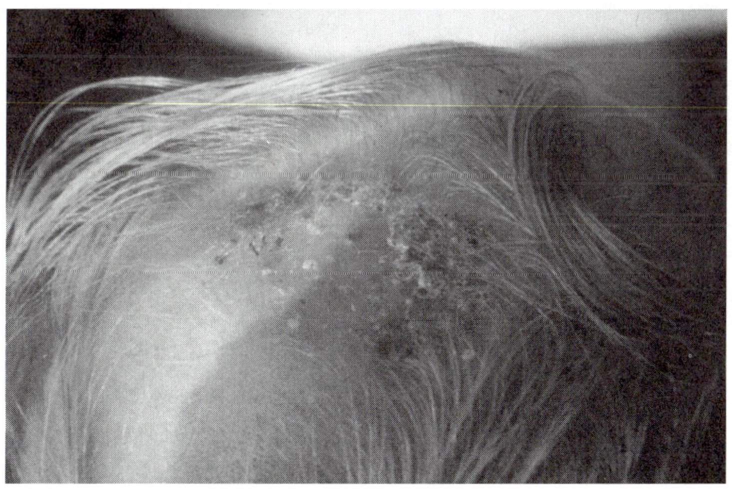

FIGURE 13 Erosive pustular dermatosis of the scalp.

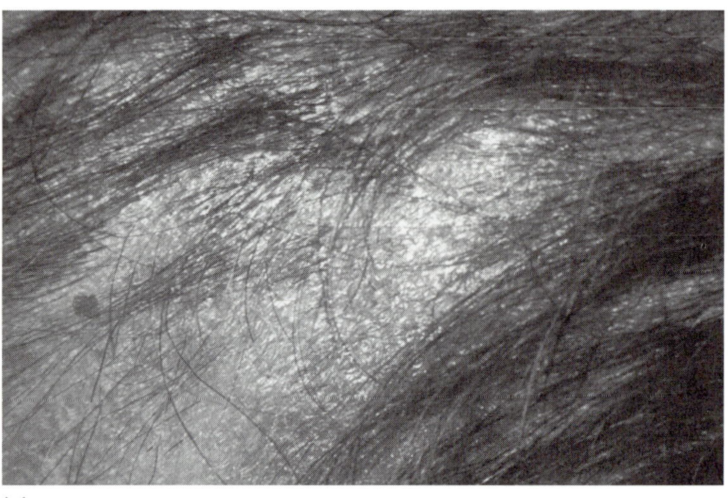

(a)

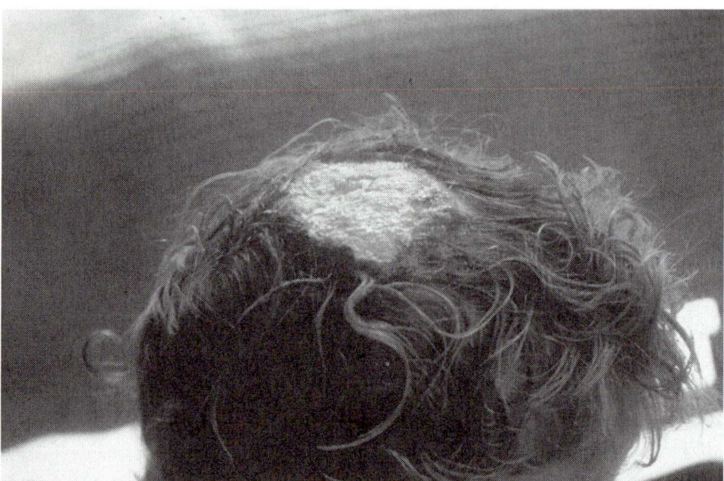

(a)

FIGURE 14 (a) Ringworm infection of the scalp causing scaling of the scalp and broken hairs. (b) Ringworm infection of the scalp causing an acute inflammatory reaction (kerion).

the hair bulb and as the hair grows the fungus moves up with the hair within the keratin and is visible above the surface by the 14th day. The infected hair is brittle and breaks easily. The fungus continues to grow in the stratum corneum so that other hairs are also involved and this continues until a stage of host–parasite equilibrium is reached in which fungus is present within the infected follicles but no longer present in the stratum corneum. The infection tends to resolve spontaneously after 7 months, but the precise mechanism of this spontaneous resolution is not fully understood. *M. canis* is another species that has also been studied in this way and demonstrates a similar sequence, although invasion of the hairs occurs more rapidly and resolution, often accompanied by inflammatory changes, usually occurs within 3 months.

Although there are no such extensive, detailed studies for other species, the pattern of infection is probably similar for most dermatophytes differing principally in rate of growth, duration of infection, and extent of host immune response. However, the dermatophytes can be divided on the basis of their pattern of hair invasion. Two patterns are recognized: ectothrix pattern (e.g., *Trichophyton mentagrophytes*, *T. verrucosum*, and *Microsporum sp.*), where the hyphae grow within the hair shaft but emerge through the hair surface to release their spores, and endothrix pattern (e.g., *T. tonsurans, T. violaceum*, and *T. soudanense*) where the hyphae within the hairs form spores that fill the cortex of the hair and remain within the hair shaft. Because of the greater degree of hair damage in the endothrix pattern, the hairs break off closer to the surface of the scalp than in the ectothrix pattern.

Diagnosis is made by identification of fungus on hair microscopy and culture. This can be aided by the use of Wood's light as some species demonstrate fluorescence.

If access to antifungals is economically available, then they are the treatment of choice in scalp ringworm. Although many of the noninflammatory infections or kerions caused by zoophilic species may well resolve spontaneously, coexisting lesions elsewhere on the scalp may persist for some time. Griseofulvin was for many years the main treatment for scalp ringworm and in many countries is still the only antifungal drug licensed for use in children. It is derived from *Penicillium griseofulvum* and is active against dermatophytes but not bacteria, *Nocardia* sp., *Candida albicans*, aspergillus, or *Malassezia furfur* (pityriasis versicolor). It is thought to act by disrupting fungal mitotic spindle structure, thereby preventing fungal cell mitosis. Therefore, it is fungistatic rather than fungicidal and accumulates in the keratin of the stratum corneum, hair, and nails, rendering them resistant to invasion by fungus. However, because griseofulvin has a relatively low affinity for keratin, its concentration in keratin declines in parallel with those in plasma, and treatment must be continued for as long as it takes infected keratin to be replaced by resistant keratin. Although this is usually 6 to 8 weeks, the treatment may need to be given for longer until there is good regrowth of uninfected hair and mycological cure has been achieved. Resistance to griseofulvin among dermatophytes is rare.

The usual dose of griseofulvin microsize is 500 to 1000 mg for adults, or 10 mg/kg body weight for children, and it can be administered in single or divided doses. Following oral administration, griseofulvin is absorbed principally from the duodenum and peak concentrations of the drug occur approximately 4 h after dosing. Absorption is enhanced by fatty food or by administering in reduced particle size (micronization). It is primarily bound to serum albumin and it is the free plasma concentration that determines the tissue distribution. Plasma levels remain at 1 to 2 μg/mL while in the skin concentrations measure 12 to 25 μg/g.

Griseofulvin has a half-life of 9 to 24 h and is metabolized in the liver, the main metabolite being 6-methylgriseofulvin which is microbiologically inactive and is excreted in the urine. Unmetabolized griseofulvin is excreted in feces.

The effectiveness of the griseofulvin is also improved with local hygiene measures and in very severe cases by cutting the hair in and around the infected area and applying tolnaftate cream or Whitfield's ointment daily. Antifungal shampoos containing ketoconazole, selenium sulfide, or povidone-iodine are useful adjunct therapies for the patient and close contacts. In kerions, griseofulvin treatment does not necessarily prevent the formation of scarring and additional treatment with corticosteroids may be beneficial [77]. Single doses of griseofulvin are sometimes effective. Friedman et al. [78] reported that of 22 children infected with *M. audouini* and treated with a single 3-g dose, 21 were cured; Van Breuseghem et al. [79] reported 93% cure rates in 72 children in the Congo treated with a single 1.5-g dose. Such single-dose regimes may be particularly useful in countries where access to griseofulvin is limited.

Griseofulvin is a relatively nontoxic drug and has been available since 1958 with a good safety profile, but occasional side effects include gastrointestinal upset, headaches, fatigue, and transient rashes including photosensitivity. The headache can sometimes be overcome by reducing the dose and then slowly increasing it again. Other, less frequently reported side effects include dizziness, granulocytopenia, leukopenia, confusion, toxic epidermal necrolysis, and peripheral neuropathy. Griseofulvin may also interact with other drugs including phenobarbitone, warfarin, and contraceptives. It may also be responsible for precipitating porphyria cutanea tarda in predisposed individuals and should not be administered to patients with established porphyria, hepatocellular failure, or lupus erythematosus. There have been some case reports suggesting that griseofulvin may produce human fetal abnormalities and therefore women should not become pregnant during or within 1 month of griseofulvin treatment. It may also damage sperm cells and therefore males should avoid fathering children within 6 months of treatment.

A significant advance has been the development of the azole compounds and allylamines, synthetic antifungals that are fungicidal compared to griseofulvin, which is fungistatic. Ketoconazole (an imidazole) was the first of these to be developed as an oral agent, but its use is limited by expense and side effects, particularly hepatotoxicity. Its action is blockade of the cytochrome P-450–dependent demethylation stage in the conversion of lanosterol into ergosterol which is involved in the formation of the fungal cell membranes. It is active against *Candida* as well as dermatophytes and is usually given at a dose of 200 mg daily with food, although the dose can be increased to 400. Peak absorption occurs 2 h after oral administration and absorption is reduced when gastric acidity is reduced by antacids or class 2 histamine antagonists.

It is contraindicated in patients with preexisting liver disease. In courses longer than 2 weeks, liver function tests should be measured after the first 2 weeks, at 4 weeks, and then at monthly intervals, since although elevations in serum transaminases may be insignificant and transient they may be early evidence of hepatotoxicity. If they are significantly elevated, then liver function tests must be performed at weekly intervals until transaminases return to normal, but if they remain significantly elevated or if the patient develops jaundice, fever, dark urine, or pale stools, treatment with ketoconazole should be discontinued and liver function tests monitored until they return to normal. Liver damage is usually reversible on discontinuing the drug but occasional fatalities have been reported usually where the drug was continued despite development of symptoms of hepatitis. Other side effects include gastrointestinal disturbance, headaches, transient rashes, thrombocytopenia, paresthesia, dizziness, alopecia, oligospermia, and occasionally a disulfiram-like reaction to alcohol. Its blocking of other cytochrome P-450–dependent pathways can result in other side effects (e.g., impairment of adrenal androgen metabolism can cause gynecomastia in men). Among the drugs with which it interacts are cyclosporin A, warfarin, chlordiazepoxide, tacrolimus, corticosteroids, alfentanil, taxanes, and possibly busulphan. It should not be given with astemizole, cisapride, or terfenadine. Its efficacy is reduced by rifampicin, isoniazid, and phenytoin. When administered in high doses to rats (>80 mg/kg), ketoconazole causes fetal abnormalities and is therefore contraindicated in pregnancy. Studies comparing the efficacy of griseofulvin with ketoconazole have given inconsistent results [80,81].

Because of its potential hepatotoxicity and its cost, ketoconazole has been largely superseded by itraconazole, a triazole whose mode of action is similar to that of ketoconazole but which has fewer side effects [82]. Peak plasma concentrations are reached 1.5 to 3 h after administration, but absorption is reduced when gastric acidity is reduced and in patients with achlorhydria, such as some AIDS patients and patients receiving H_2-antagonists; taking itraconazole with a cola beverage helps absorption. Its elimination half-life from the plasma is 20 h. It is metabolized by the liver to a large number of metabolites. Itraconazole can be detected on the skin surface within hours of administration, this initial phase of drug delivery to the skin occurring predominantly via the eccrine sweat. Some days later, larger amounts of itraconazole reach the stratum corneum by excretion in the sebum and by binding to the basal cells. It accumulates in keratin and persists in skin for 1 to 4 weeks after stopping treatment and in nails for up to 9 months, since elimination from keratinized structures is related to epidermal elimination rather than redistribution to the systemic circulation. The most frequent side effect is gastrointestinal, but others include headache, dizziness, transient rashes, and very occasionally peripheral neuropathy. Although the incidence of hepatic problems is less than with ketoconazole, rare cases of hepatitis and cholestatic jaundice have been reported, mainly in patients treated for more than 1 month, so it is advisable to monitor liver function in patients receiving treatment for more than 1 month. Liver function tests should also be performed in any patients who develop symptoms suggestive of hepatitis such as nausea, vomiting, or jaundice, and patients who have a history of liver disease treatment should only receive itraconazole if the expected benefit outweighs the risk of hepatic damage. Because itraconazole can inhibit metabolism of drugs by the cytochrome 3A family, it can cause elevated plasma levels of such drugs. In particular, terfenadine, astemizole, cisapride, and HMG-CoA reductase inhibitors such as midazolam, triazolam, and simvastatin should not be used with itraconazole. Other drugs whose concentration is increased by itraconazole include warfarin, phenytoin, digoxin, cyclosporin A, methylprednisolone, and possibly tacrolimus. When administered at high concentrations in rats (40 mg/kg/day), it causes fetal malformation and is therefore contraindicated in pregnancy; women of childbearing age are advised to use adequate contraception during therapy and for up to 1 month after discontinuing therapy. Itraconazole has been reported to have been used successfully in children without hepatotoxic effects [82–84]. In an open study, children with tinea capitis receiving itraconazole 100 mg/day continuous treatment for a median of 6 weeks exhibited clinical response and mycological cure rates of 94% and 89%, respectively, 2 weeks after completion of therapy [82]. However, in many countries, including the United Kingdom and the United States, it is not yet licensed for use in children. Because itraconazole is highly lipophilic and keratinophilic there has been interest in administering it as pulse therapy. Gupta et al. recently reported the use of itraconazole pulse therapy in children consisting of 5 mg/kg per day for 1 week and then, if clinically necessary, a second or third pulse each of 1 week duration 2 weeks after completion of the previous pulse [83]. Of 10 children studied with this regime, one, two and three pulses resulted in complete clinical and mycological cure in one, six, and three patients, respectively, and no clinical adverse effects or laboratory abnormalities were observed.

Fluconazole is a related drug that is also effective against a variety of dermatophytes and *Candida* but is used less frequently than itraconazole. In a open-label study in 27 children, Solomon et al. reported that fluconazole at a dose of

6 mg/kg per day for 20 days resulted in 89% of patients showing clinical and mycological cure at 4 months, compared to 60% of patients when a dose of 3 mg/kg per day was used and only 25% of patients when a dose of 1.5 mg/kg per day [85] was used. No clinical or laboratory adverse effects were noted. However, in many countries including the United Kingdom and the United States, it has not yet received license for treating children.

Another of the newer oral antifungal drugs is terbinafine, a member of the allylamine family. It acts by inhibiting the epoxidation of squalene, a step that is necessary in the formation of fungal cell membrane and has a wide spectrum of antifungal activity [86]. A single oral dose of 250 mg results in peak plasma concentration within 2 h. Terbinafine binds strongly to plasma protein and rapidly diffuses through the dermis to concentrate in the lipophilic stratum corneum. It is also secreted in the sebum so that high concentrations are achieved in hair follicles, hair, and sebum-rich skin, and is detectable in the nail plate within the first few weeks of commencing therapy. The principal side effects are gastrointestinal, occurring in 5% of patients, skin rashes in 3%, headaches, joint pains, dizziness, and paresthesia. Severe skin reactions (e.g., toxic epidermal necrolysis, Stevens–Johnson syndrome) can occur occasionally [86], and loss of taste has been reported in 0.6%, but usually resolves on discontinuing the drug. Rarely, neutropenia, thrombocytopenia, and agranulocytosis have been reported. Cases of hepatotoxicity have been reported on occasion, so treatment must be discontinued if the patient shows signs of developing hepatic failure. Patients with a past history of liver disease or preexisting stable chronic liver dysfunction should be carefully monitored. If there is a history of chronically abnormal but stable liver function tests or a creatinine clearance of less than 50 mL/min, these patients should receive half the adult dose. Otherwise, it is a safe drug. It does not interfere with drugs that are metabolized by the cytochrome P-450 pathway and animal studies did not suggest any fetal toxicity. However, since there is no clinical experience of its use in pregnant women, it should be avoided in pregnancy. An open study of terbinafine given to 82 patients (predominantly children) for 1, 2, or 4 weeks at a dose of 62.5 to 250 mg according to the patient's weight, gave overall cure rates of 44.4%, 57.1%, and 77.8%, respectively [87]. *T. tonsurans* infection responded excellently to terbinafine although *Microsporum* species responded less well. There were no significant side effects in any of the patients and no detectable abnormalities in liver function tests or lipid profile in patients randomly selected for blood examination. The dosage for children with dermatophytosis is 3 to 6 mg/kg per day as follows: children weighing less than 20 kg should receive a dose of 62.5 mg daily; children weighing 20 to 40 kg, a dose of 125 mg daily; and children weighing more than 40 kg, a dose of 250 mg daily [88]. However, in many countries, including the United Kingdom and the United States, terbinafine is not yet licensed for treatment of children.

N. Psoriasis

In psoriasis, scalp involvement is common and may be the initial site; sometimes the scalp remains involved continually for many years while lesions elsewhere on the body come and go. The clinical patterns may range from pink plaques covered in a silvery scale resembling those seen in other parts of the body, to patchy scaling or at the other end of the clinical spectrum layers of asbestos-like scale (pityriasis amiantacea) (Fig. 15a and 15b). Hair loss may occur but is usually reversible. Very severe disease can result in scarring alopecia, but this is rare.

In mild cases, treatment with a tar-based or keratolytic shampoo is sufficient. More severe cases often respond well to topical tar or dithranol preparations rubbed onto the areas for a few hours, then washed out and/or a topical steroid preparation applied [89]. Topical calcipitriol may also prove effective [90].

O. Folliculitis Keloidalis Nuchae (Acne Cheloidalis, Acne Keloidalis)

This chronic inflammatory folliculitis of the nape of the neck occurs exclusively in men and seems to be more common in Negroids. Many, but not all, of the patients will have had acne vulgaris. Clinically there are follicular papules and pustules that progress to keloidal papules. The precise cause is uncertain but genetic factors may also play a role and histologically there is a chronic folliculitis and foreign body granulomatous reaction around the hair. Treatment with topical antibacterial agents or systemic antibiotics may help but rarely effects a complete cure. The keloids may be successfully excised by plastic surgery.

P. Dissecting Cellulitis of the Scalp (Perifolliculitis Capitis Abscedens et Suffodiens)

This condition was first described in 1905 by Nobl of Vienna and occurs predominantly in male patients between the ages of 18 and 40, and more frequently in Negroids than Caucasoids. Clinically firm skin-colored nodules develop on the vertex and later become soft and fluctuant. These become confluent with other nodules forming interconnecting tubular ridges and sinuses from which blood-stained pus can exude. These ridges form against a background of scalp redness and edema and patchy hair loss. Histologically the follicles are destroyed by a florid folliculitis followed by a chronic granulomatous infiltrate containing foreign-body giant cells. The etiology is uncertain ana no specific organism can be cultured from the isolated lesions, although some authors have suggested that it is a form of hidradenitis suppurativa of the scalp.

Treatment is difficult. At the early stage, oral oxytetracycline or erythromycin can help reduce the inflammatory reaction and some practitioners have found

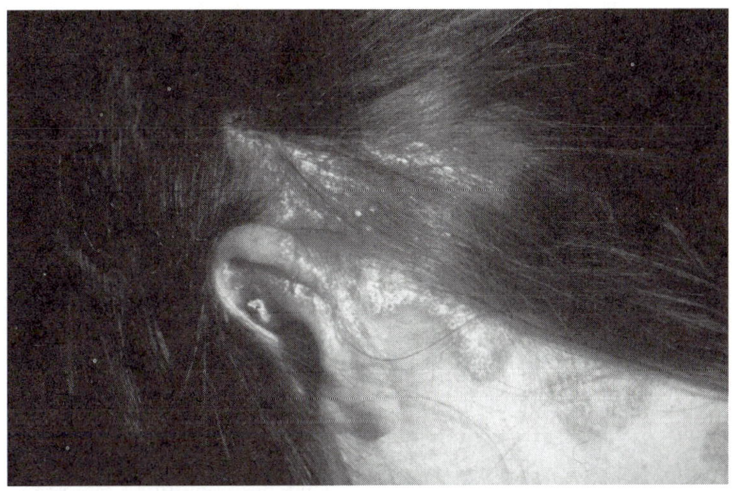

(a)

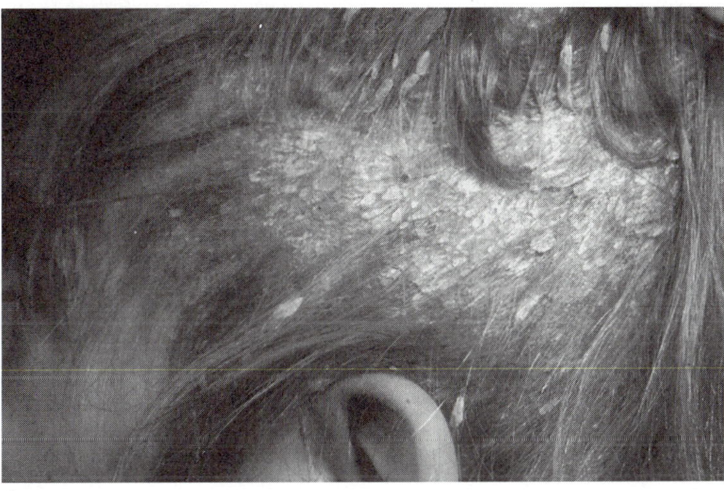

(b)

FIGURE 15 (a) Red plaques of psoriasis involving the hairline. (b) Pityriasis amianatacea.

benefit from combining these with systemic corticosteroids. Recent studies have shown benefit from isotretinoin [91].

Q. Pityriasis Capitis (Pityriasis Simplex, Dandruff)

This near-physiological scaling of the scalp is most common at about the age 20 when it is estimated that about half the Caucasian population develop it. The etiology is uncertain, but the peak incidence at this age suggests an androgenic influence. The role of *Pityrosporum ovale* has been debated for many years. Application of yeast inhibitors to one-half of the scalp produced a greater reduction in pityriasis than application of antibacterial agents to the other side of the scalp [92]. However, others attribute the increased numbers of *P. ovale* in pityriasis capitis to be secondary to the increased scaling [93].

Treatment with selenium sulfide (which has been shown to reduce epidermal turnover time), zinc pyrithione, or zinc omadine (which are said to reduce yeast populations) is usually effective in most patients, although there are some patients in whom these are ineffective. Those who have proposed a role for yeasts have suggested treatment with imidazole compounds [e.g., Nizoral shampoo (ketoconazole)]. In patients with more severe pityriasis, particularly if associated with seborrhea, a tar preparation rubbed into involved areas on the scalp and washed out after a few hours with a tar shampoo may be effective.

R. Seborrheic Dermatitis

Pityriasis capitis is regarded by many as the mildest form of seborrheic dermatitis that is characterized by erythematous flaky areas often associated with greasy yellowish scales. The hairline and postauricular areas are most frequently involved and involvement of the eyebrows, nasolabial folds and sternum can also be seen. It often responds to the same treatments outlined for pityriasis capitis, but if it is extensive then daily applications of a corticosteroid lotion may be helpful. Azole shampoos (e.g., ketoconazole) or 2% fluconazole shampoo is often effective; for more severe cases, a preparation containing tar and sulfur or Oil of Cade ointment rubbed into the scalp at least 2 h before shampooing can be helpful. Topical lithium succinate has also been suggested to be safe and effective [94].

III. NAILS

The most common nail problem encountered by the dermatologist is infection by dermatophyte fungi (onychomycosis) or chronic paronychia. Other frequently encountered nail disorders are psoriasis, and rarer nail problems include the inflammatory dermatoses such as lichen planus and spongiotic trachyonychia. Treatment of these will be dealt with in turn.

A. Onychomycosis

Onychomycosis is frequently preceded by tinea pedis and also appears more commonly in nails that are abnormal beforehand (e.g., from psoriasis or trauma). Fungal nail infections have been divided by the pattern of fungal growth: (1) superficial; (2) distal; and (3) proximal, and all of these can result in whole nail dystrophy (total dystrophic onychomycosis) (Fig. 16).

1. Superficial White Onychomycosis

This pattern is fairly rare and is usually confined to the toenails (Fig. 17). White, superficial patches appear on the nail plate and the principal organisms causing this pattern are summarized in Table 2. A rare variant is superficial black onychomycosis caused by *Scytalidium dimidiatum*.

2. Distal and Lateral Subungal Onychomycosis

This is the more common pattern of onychomycosis where the fungal infection commences in the onychodermal band and reaches the underside of the nail via the hyponychium, or alternatively from the lateral nail folds if the stratum corneum has already been colonized by dermatophytes (Fig. 18). The most common organism causing this pattern of onychomycosis is *Trichophyton rubrum*, but other organisms are listed in Table 2. The typical clinical pattern is that early infection is evident as white or yellow streaks at the free edge of the nail, at

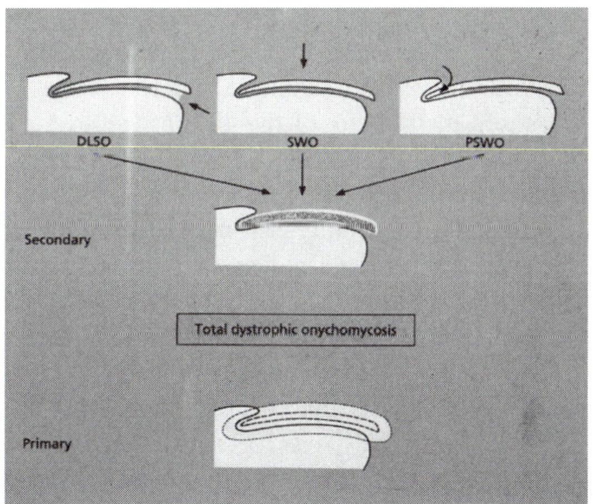

FIGURE 16 Diagram to show the site of invasion and types of onychomycosis. DLSO, distal and lateral subungal onychomycosis; SWO, superficial white onychomycosis; PSWO, proximal subungal white onychomycosis.

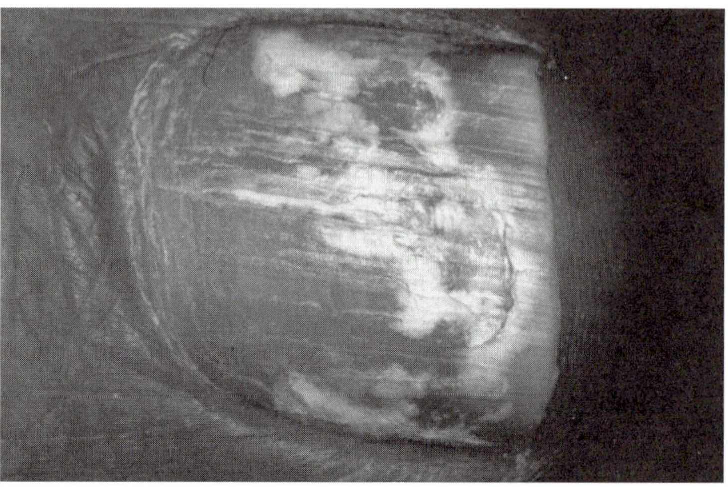

FIGURE 17 Superficial white onychomycosis.

the lateral nail fold, and progresses to thickening and onycholysis of the nail. Occasionally, these organisms, particularly the moulds, produce brown pigmentation of the affected nail.

3. Proximal Onychomycosis

This is caused by the organism invading via the cuticle and the ventral aspect of the proximal nail fold usually from a preexisting infection of the adjacent stratum corneum (Fig. 19). The infection may remain within the superficial layers of the nail plate or may invade the more distal parts of the nail matrix so that the deeper layers of the nail plate are also involved. The most common cause for the pattern is *T. rubrum*, but other causes are listed in Table 2. A rapidly progressing form of proximal white subungual onychomycosis has been described in patients with AIDS. Paronychia is an important predisposing cause of proximal superficial onychomycosis, particularly by *Candida*. The paronychia usually involves the hands and is seen three times more frequently in women than men. Predisposing factors are repeated hand washing and immersion in water, occlusion, handling carbohydrate-rich food, hyperhidrosis, diabetes mellitus, hormonal disturbance, corticosteroids, and systemic antibiotics. The nail fold changes tend to be worst over the lateral margins and, as the nail matrix becomes involved with the infection and inflammation, the nail plate deformity develops with irregular grooves, ridges, and pits. Ideally, the presence of fungi should be demonstrated on microscopy and culture before commencing treatment as the clinical signs of onychomycosis can sometimes be mimicked by other nail conditions.

Table 2 Organisms Causing Nail Infections

Organisms Causing Distal and Lateral Subungual Onychomycosis (DLSO)	
Dermatophytes	*Trichophyton rubrum, T. interdigitale, E. floccosum, T. schoenleinii, T. tonsurans, T. soudanense, T. erinacei, T. verrucosum, T. concentricum, T. violaceum, T. canis*
Yeasts	*Candida albicans, C. parapsilosis* (also *C. tropicalis* in cases with preexisting onycholysis)
Moulds	*Scopulariopsis brevicaulis, Hendersonula toruloidea* (also known as *Scytalidium dimidiatum*), *Scytalidium hyalinum* (In cases with preexisting onycholysis, various species of moulds have been isolated including *Aspergillus* and *Penicillium*)
Organisms Causing Superficial White Onychomycosis	
Dermatophytes	*Trichophyton interdigitale* (*M. persicolor, T. rubrum*[a], *T. equinum*)
Yeasts	*C. albicans* (only in infants)
Moulds	*Acremonium* and *Fusarium* spp., *Aspergillus terreus*
Organisms Causing Proximal White Onychomycosis	
Dermatophytes	*T. rubrum, T. megnini, T. schoenleinii, E. floccosum*
Yeasts	*Candida*
Moulds	*S. dimidiatum, S. hyalinum, Fusarium spp.*

[a] In this case, fungal elements are found deep in the nail plate.

Topical treatment is often disappointing: a tioconazole paint applied twice daily yields reported cure rates of no more than 20 to 22%, but it may be beneficial if used in addition to griseofulvin [95]. Contact sensitivity to the imidazoles has been reported. Amorolfine nail lacquer 5% applied twice daily has been reported to produce recovery in up to 70% of cases where there is no lunula involvement [96]. Ciclopirox 8% nail lacquer has also been reported to be beneficial [96].

For many years, griseofulvin given in daily doses of 500 to 1000 mg for adults was the principal systemic treatment. However, because of the slow rate at which toenails grow, it usually needs to be given for 12 to 24 months and, even then, meta-analysis shows a mycological cure rate of 24.5%, with a relapse rate of 40%, 3 to 12 months after end of therapy [97]. Factors that may influence whether the fungal infection responds to griseofulvin include the penetration of the drug into the nail keratin, leakage of the drug from the nail, the rate of nail growth, and resistance of the fungus to the drug. It has been suggested that addition of cimetidine enhances the effect of griseofulvin but this needs further assessment [98]. However, griseofulvin is not effective against *Candida*.

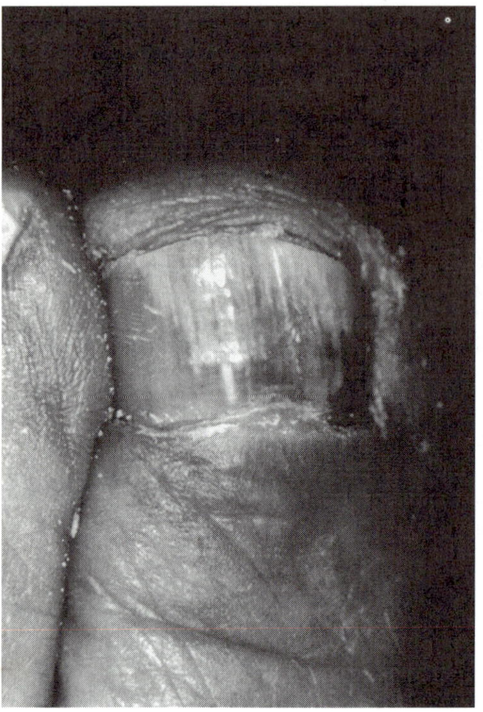

FIGURE 18 Distal and lateral subungal onychomycosis.

Because of this, griseofulvin has largely been superceded by terbinafine, although in many countries, including the United Kingdom and the United States, it has not yet received license for use in children. When terbinafine is given to adults at a dose of 250 mg daily for 6 weeks for fingernail infections and 12 weeks for toenail infections, it produces a clinical and mycological cure in approximately 80% of cases. The rate of clinical improvement in the appearance of the nails depends on the rate of growth of the nail; therefore, the clinical signs of improvement may be slow to appear, particularly in the toenails. One double-blind study compared treatment of onychomycosis of toenails with terbinafine 250 mg daily given for either 6 or 12 weeks and found that the mycological cure rate at 48 weeks after commencing therapy in the 6-week group was 56% compared with 82% for the 12-week group [99]. An alternative regime of terbinafine 500 mg for 1 week every month produced mycological cure in 16 out of 18 cases [100]. Itraconazole has also been shown to be effective against a variety of dermatophytes involving the nails, including *Candida*, but is not effective against *Scytalidium*. It is lipid-soluble and rapidly penetrates the nail and can be

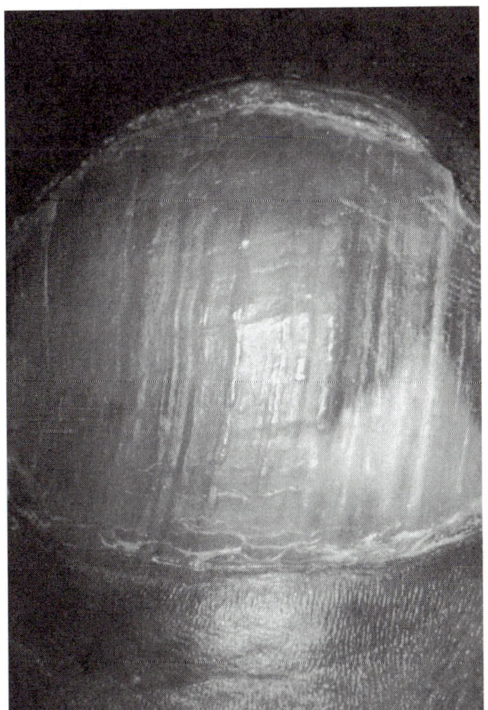

FIGURE 19 Proximal onychomycosis.

detected within the nail within 2 weeks of commencing therapy. When given as 200 mg daily for 3 months, the cure rate is over 90% for fingernails and over 70% for toenails, and the recurrence rate is only 11% [101]. Itraconazole persists in the nail plate for about 9 to 12 months from the start of therapy even though it is present in low to negligible concentrations in the plasma within 7 to 14 days of stopping therapy. For this reason, there has been interest in itraconazole pulse therapy using regimes such as 200 to 400 mg itraconazole daily for 1 week every month for 3 months [102,103]. Once the treatment period is completed, or if there is still evidence of persisting fungal infection, this can be treated by continuing the systemic therapy or changing to topical amorolfine. In one study undertaken to compare itraconazole continuous therapy (given as 200 mg daily for 3 months) with itraconazole pulse therapy given as 400 mg daily for 1 week a month for 3 months), at 12 months after commencing treatment mycological cure rates were 66% for continuous therapy and 69% for pulse therapy [102]. The authors observed that, although there was no significant difference between the two groups in outcome, the pulse therapy group needed half the dose of the continuous therapy group. Ketoconazole is generally not used because of its potential hepatotoxicity and its cost.

Pharmacoeconomic analysis of the treatment of onychomycosis of the toenail with griseofulvin, terbinafine, or itraconazole (continuous or pulse) suggest that terbinafine or pulse therapy with itraconazole are the two most cost-effective treatments, with no significant difference between them [97].

Cutting or filing the nail plate or total or partial nail ablation surgically can help the effectiveness of topical or systemic antifungals. An alternative method to reduce the nail plate bulk is by using urea ointment (40% urea, 5% white beeswax or paraffin, 20% anhydrous lanolin, 25% white petrolatum, 10% silica gel type H) applied to the nail plate, after masking the surrounding skin with tape, and occluding it under cellophane for 1 week. Alternative preparations to urea ointment are 20% urea (Onychomal) and 10% salicylic acid ointment under occlusion for 2 weeks, or the incorporation of 1% bifonazole into the urea paste or 50% potassium iodide ointment in anhydrous lanolin plus 0.5% iodochlorohydroxyquinine. It should also be remembered that fungal infections are more likely to occur in nails subject to repeated trauma and good podiatry is important in preventing recurrences. Podiatry alone may be all that is necessary in mild fungal onycholysis in the elderly.

4. Candida Onychomycosis

As mentioned above, itraconazole and terbinafine can also be effective against *Candida*. Other antifungals such as amphotericin B, intravenous miconazoles, and oral clotrimazole have also been used in the past with limited success. An important part of successfully treating candidal infection of the nail is prevention of excessive immersion of the fingers in water and drying the hands well after hand washing. Onycholysis can be treated by trimming back the onycholytic nail and some authors have achieved suppression of growth of *Candida* by daily applications to the exposed nail bed of miconazole, clotrimazole, 4% thymol in chloroform, or 15% sulfacetamide in 70% ethyl alcohol [96]. Chronic *Candida paronychia* can also be treated by at least twice-daily applications of topical antifungals (ideally in lotion form) to the groove between the nail plate and the proximal nail fold. This twice-daily application is usually required for 3 months and works as effectively as systemic therapy with ketoconazole. When treating chronic mucocutaneous candidiasis (Fig. 20), the dose of ketoconazole may need to be increased to 400 or 600 mg daily and, once remission has been obtained, the dose of ketoconazole should be stopped as resistance has been reported to develop when low-dose (200 mg daily) ketoconazole is continued.

Fluconazole, another azole drug of the triazole group, is also very effective against *Candida*. It has proved particularly valuable in the treatment of superficial *Candida* infection in patients with AIDS and because of its high degree of water

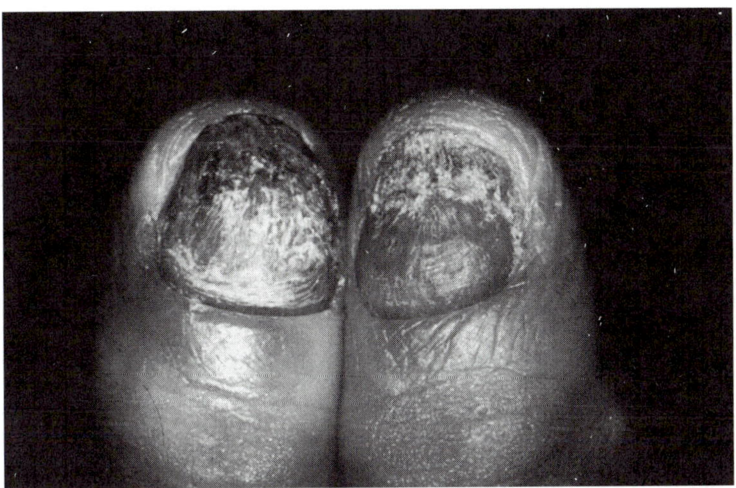

FIGURE 20 Nail changes in chronic mucocutaneous candidiasis showing bulbous appearance of the digits with erythema and swelling of the proximal and lateral nail folds and hyperkeratosis of the nail bed.

solubility it rapidly penetrates the nails and has proved to be very useful in treating both candidal and dermatophyte infections of the nail [104]. It is also thought to be less hepatotoxic than ketoconazole.

5. Infection by Nondermatophyte Moulds

This is often difficult to eradicate. For those moulds that tend to produce the superficial white onychomycosis pattern (e.g., *Acremonium, Aspergillus*, or *Fusaruim*), abrasion of the nail followed by topical therapy with econazole, clotrimazole, 28% tioconazole, amorolfine, ciclopiroxolamine, 8% ciclopirox, or 10% glutaraldehyde can be effective. However, mould infections involving deeper layers (e.g., *S. brevicaulis, Pyrenochaeta unguium-hominis, S. dimidiatum*, or *S. hyalinum*) are notoriously unresponsive to topical and systemic antifungal treatments. In such cases, the best chance of eradication is by repeated chemical removal of the nail followed by local applications of keratolytics and antifungal agents.

B. Psoriasis

Involvement of the nails in psoriasis is common and has been reported in up to 50% of cases but in the lifetime of any one patient the incidence probably approaches nearer 80 to 90%. The clinical features are, in order of decreasing frequency: pitting, discoloration, onycholysis, subungal hyperkeratosis, nail plate abnormalities, and splinter haemorrhages (Fig. 21a and 21b). Treatment of nail psoriasis is often difficult, but excessive manicuring should be avoided as it can lead to deterioration due to provoking the Koebner phenomenon. Fungal infection may also be a complicating factor and a high index of suspicion should be maintained and nail clippings sent for microscopy and culture if fungus is suspected.

Several topical treatments have been tried, including 1% fluorouracil solution dissolved in propylene glycol applied twice daily for 6 months and gently massaged around the margin of the nail [105]. Although success rates with this are not high, it can prove helpful in nails where pitting and hypertrophy are predominant defects, but should be avoided where there is onycholysis as it can lead to deterioration. Twenty percent urea plus 1% fluorouracil has also been reported to be helpful. High potency topical corticosteroids (i.e., flucinolone acetonide, triamcinolone acetonide, beta-methasone) applied under occlusive dressings such as nonporous tape or plastic gloves can be occasionally helpful and can be used for short and repeated periods, although care must be taken to avoid steroid atrophy. Mixing the topical steroid with 5 to 10% benzoyl peroxide or 0.1% retinoic acid cream may increase efficacy. Intralesional injection of long-acting steroids can also be helpful when administered to involved nail matrix and/or nail bed, and a suspension of triamcinolone acetonide mixed with equal parts sterile saline has been reported to be beneficial when injected at volumes of 0.2 to 0.4 mL per nail [106]. De Berker and Lawrence reported results of injecting triamcinolone acetonide (0.4 mL, 10 mg/mL) into the nail bed and matrix, 0.1 mL being injected at each of four periungal sites following ring block [107]. This was repeated at 3-month intervals. During injection, the 25-gauge needle was held in place either manually or by reusable sterile glass syringe with a Luer lock in order to prevent separation of the needle and syringe due to the pressure of the injection. The authors reported that subungual hyperkeratosis, thickening, and ridging showed a good response in almost all the 19 patients studied, while onycholysis and pitting improved in approximately 50% of cases. However, possible side effects are hemorrhage, pain, and reversible atrophy, and there have been rare reports of epidermoid implantation cysts.

There have also been reports of benefit from twice-daily applications of calcipitriol to the nail bed. Topical cyclosporin has also been reported to be very effective in an anecdotal report [108].

Systemic treatment with methotrexate and cylcosporin has proved beneficial in nail psoriasis when commenced for psoriasis elsewhere, but, because of their side-effect profile, they are rarely used for psoriasis affecting only the nails unless it is causing significant functional impairment. Although retinoids have proved helpful for many patients with widespread body psoriasis and some authors have reported very good results in nail psoriasis, others have reported disap-

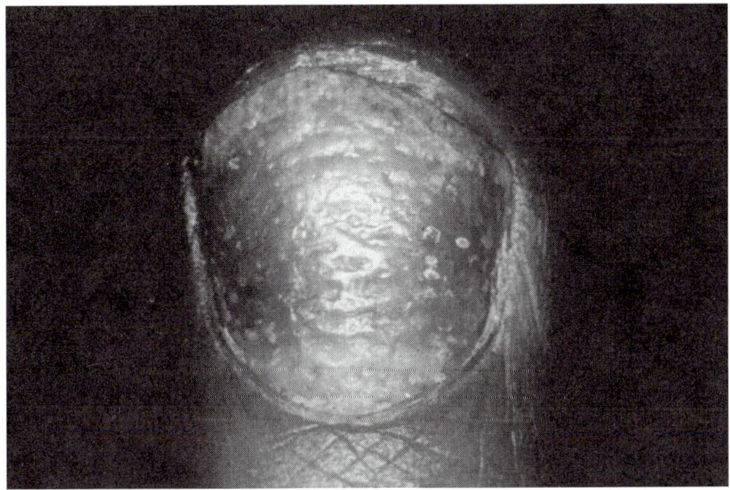

(a)

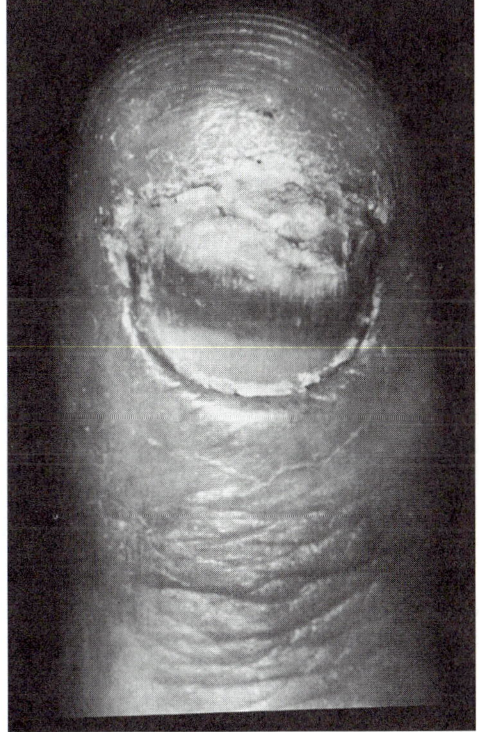

(b)

FIGURE 21 (a) Multiple nail pits due to psoriasis. (b) Distal subungual hyperkeratosis in psoriasis; note inflammatory brown margin.

pointing results with exacerbation of pitting and onycholysis and increased sensitivity to external pressure.

Photochemotherapy with either systemic or topical psoralen can be beneficial and complete clearance has been reported. However, overall response of psoriatic nails to photochemotherapy is not impressive and pitting in particular does not respond [109]. In addition photochemotherapy can be complicated by photo-onycholysis, subungal hemorrhage, and pigmentation of the nail bed.

Pustular psoriasis involving the nails and acrodermatitis continua of Hallopeau can show improvement with localized PUVA, and retinoids can also be beneficial although there is a high risk of recurrence 1 to 3 months after treatment is discontinued [110]. Combined retinoid and PUVA has been reported to reduce the rate of relapse. Other treatments that have been reported to show some improvement include topical mechloretamine, 5% fluorouracil cream, intramuscular triamcinolone, and nimesulid [106].

The nail involvement of Reiter's syndrome is often clinically and histologically indistinguishable from that of psoriasis. Antibiotics, steroids, and nonsteroidal anti-inflammatory drugs do not result in any improvement in the nails but PUVA or retinoids may be helpful. In resistant cases, combined therapy with methotrexate, aromatic retinoid, and prednisolone has been reported to be beneficial [106].

C. Lichen Planus

Involvement of one or more nails is seen in 10% of patients with lichen planus. One of the earliest clinical signs that may be seen is bluish or red discoloration of the dorsal nail fold with or without swelling, which indicates that the proximal nail matrix is involved and that nail plate changes are likely to follow. The clinical appearance depends on the extent of matrix involvement—if only a small portion of the matrix is involved, then only a small depression in the nail plate may result. If more extensive areas of the nail matrix are involved, then longitudinal grooves, fissuring, and distal splitting occur as the disease progresses, producing progressive thinning of the nail plate (Fig. 22a and 22b). Pterygium is the final hallmark of severe nail matrix involvement and is irreversible. If the lichen planus process is involving the nail bed it can result in marked subungual hyperkeratosis. Clinically similar changes may also be seen in graft-versus-host disease and drug-associated lichen-planus-like reactions.

Lichen planus of the nail is usually accompanied by lichen planus elsewhere, which aids the diagnosis. However, in those cases where no skin pathology can be seen elsewhere, nail biopsy is necessary to establish the diagnosis from other acquired and congenital causes of nail dystrophy. Often the disease is mild and resolves spontaneously and no treatment is necessary, but in those severe cases with rapid progression potent topical or systemic steroids are indi-

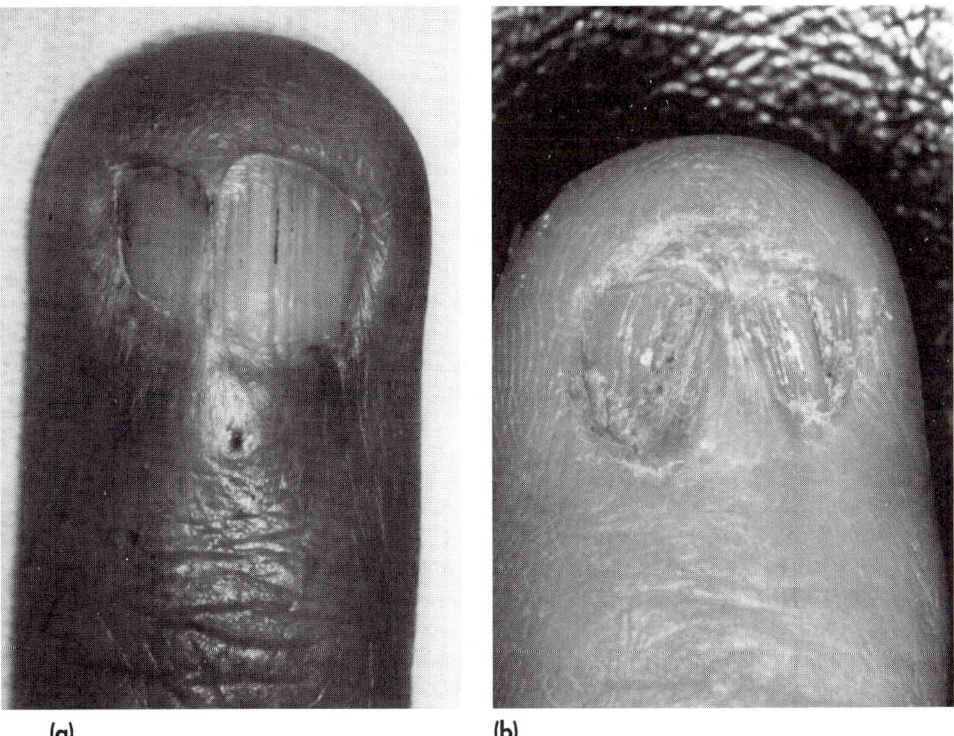

(a) (b)

FIGURE 22 (a) Early lichen planus of the nail. (b) More advanced lichen planus of the nail.

cated. The scarring and atrophic varieties may require up to 60 mg of prednisolone to arrest disease progression, but of course such high doses should only be used in those cases with very aggressive disease and no contraindications. Some benefit has also been obtained from the use of oral retinoids.

D. Discoid Lupus Erythematosus

Like lichen planus, the diagnosis is often suspected because of typical skin involvement elsewhere. Clinically, although the signs are not pathognomic, the diagnosis can be suspected because of the combination of typical red–blue coloring of the nail bed and alterations of the nail plates that lead to crumbling. The skin around the nails can be normal or reddish with brown–grey adherent scale. Some clinical improvement can be obtained with potent topical steroids.

E. Alopecia Areata

In addition to the hair changes noted above, nail changes in alopecia areata are relatively common, although quoted frequencies in the literature range from 7% to 66% of cases. Onychodystrophy can occur before the onset of hair loss, but its presence does not imply a poor prognosis. Clinical features include pitting, ridging, with surface onychorrhexis, cross fissures, Beau's lines, or transverse lines of intermittent pits, and, as the disease progresses, koilonychia, thinning of the nail plate, thickening of the nail plate (more rarely), and, in most severe cases, shedding of the nails. Hair regrowth is usually accompanied by an improvement in the nail dystrophy over several months. In some cases, injection of corticosteroid into the matrix results in improvement. Oral corticosteroids may be helpful, but should not be recommended for routine use.

F. Spongiotic Trachyonychia

Tosti et al. described 13 patients with trachyonychia (rough nails) in whom biopsy showed spongiotic inflammation of the nail apparatus [111]. Immunologically it appears to be a T-cell-mediated process and it has been suggested that it is a variant of alopecia areata. Some patients show a good response to low-dose systemic steroids.

G. Darier's Disease

Nail signs in Darier's disease are very common and classically appear as longitudinal, subungal red or white streaks, or both, associated with distal wedge-shaped subungal keratoses. The red or white streaks often end with a V-shaped notch at the free edge of the nails. In addition, the nails tend to become fragile with ridges appearing that often crack, and some patients develop keratotic papules on the proximal nail folds. Although treatment with aromatic retinoids can improve the generalized skin problems, they tend not to improve the nail changes [112].

H. Hailey–Hailey Disease

In one study more than half of 44 patients examined had longitudinal white bands but, in contrast to Darier's disease, nail fragility is not a feature and the nail changes are asymptomatic.

REFERENCES

1. Venning VA, Dawber RPR. Patterned androgenic alopecia. J Am Acad Dermatol 1988; 18:1073–1077.
2. Kligman AM. The comparative histopathology of male-pattern baldness and senescent baldness. Clin Dermatol 1988; 6(4):108–118.

3. Smith MA, Wells RS. Male-type alopecia, alopecia areata and normal hair in women. Arch Dermatol 1964; 89:95–98.
4. Maibach HI, Feldman R, Payne B, Hutshell T. Scalp and forehead sebum production in male pattern alopecia. In: Baccareda-Boy A, Moretti G, Fray JR, eds. Biopathology of Pattern Alopecias. Base: Karger, 1968:171–190.
5. Bloom RE, Wood S, Nicolaides N. Hair fat composition in early male pattern alopecia. J Invest Dermatol 1955; 24:97–101.
6. Hamilton JB. Male hormone stimulation is a prerequisite and an incitent in common baldness. Am J Anat 1942; 711:451–480.
7. Peterson RE, Imperato-McGinely J, Gautier T, Sturla E. Male pseudohermaphroditism due to steroid 5α-reductase deficiency. Am J Med 1977; 62:170–191.
8. Phillipou G, Kirk J. Significance of steroid measurements in male pattern alopecia. Clin Exp Dermatol 1981; 6:53–56.
9. Pitts RL. Serum elevation of dehydroepiandrosterone sulfate associated with male pattern baldness in young men. J Am Acad Dermatol 1987; 16:571–573.
10. Miller JA, Darley CR, Karkavitsas K, Kirby JD, Munro DD. Low sex-hormone binding globulin levels in young women with diffuse hair loss. Br J Dermatol 1982; 106:331–336.
11. Futterweit W, Dunif A, Yeh HC, Kingsley P. The prevalence of hyperandrogenism in 109 consecutive female patients with diffuse alopecia. J Am Acad Dermatol 1988; 19:831.
12. Messenger AG, Thornton MJ, Elliott K, Randall VA. Androgen responses in cultured human hair papilla cells. J Invest Dermatol 1988; 91:382 (abstr).
13. Murad S, Hodgins MB, Oliver RF, Jahoda CA. Comparative studies of androgen receptors and metabolism in dermal papilla cells cultured from human and rat hair follicles. J Invest Dermatol 1986; 87:158 (abstr).
14. Schweikert H, Milewich L, Wilson JD. Aromatization of androstenedione by isolated human hairs. J Clin Endocrinol Metab 1975; 40:413–419.
15. Bingham KD, Shaw DA. The metabolism of testosterone by human male scalp skin. J Endocrinol 1973; 57:111–121.
16. Chen W, Zouboulis CC, Orfanos CE. The 5 alpha-reductase system and its inhibitors. Recent developments and its perspective in treating androgen-dependent skin disorders. Dermatology 1996; 193(3):177–184.
17. Eicheler W, Aumuller G, Happle R, Hoffmann R. Differential distribution of steroid 5α-reductase isoenzymes in human skin. J Invest Dermatol 1994; 103:403.
18. Sawaya ME, Price VH. Different levels of 5α-reductase type I and II, aromatase, and androgen receptor in hair follicles of women and men with androgenetic alopecia. J Invest Dermatol 1997; 109:296–300.
19. Choudhury R, Hodgins MB, Van der Kwast TH, Brinkman AO, Boersma WJA. Localisation of androgen receptors in human skin by immunohistochemistry: implications for the hormonal regulation of hair growth, sebaceous glands, and sweat glands. J Endocrinol 1991; 133:467.
20. Randall VA, Thornton MJ, Messenger AG. Cultured dermal papilla cells from androgen-dependent human hair follicles (e.g. beard) contain more androgen receptors than those from non-balding areas of scalp. J Endocrinol 1992; 133:141.
21. Simpson NB, Barth JH. Hair patterns: hirsutism and androgenetic alopecia. In: Dawber R, eds. Diseases of the Hair and Scalp. Oxford: Blackwell, 1997:67–123.

22. Savin RC. Use of topical minoxidil in the treatment of male pattern baldness. J Am Acad Dermatol 1987; 16:696–704.
23. Olsen EA, Weiner MS, Delong ER, Pinnell SR. Topical minoxidil in early male pattern baldness. J Am Acad Dermatol 1985; 13:185–192.
24. De Villez RL. Topical minoxidil therapy in hereditary androgenetic alopecia. Arch Dermatol 1985; 121:197–202.
25. Jacobs JP, Szpunar CA, Warner ML. Use of topical minoxidil therapy for androgenetic alopecia in women. Int J Dermatol 1993; 32:758–762.
26. Wester RC, Maibach HI, Guy RH, Novak E. Minoxidil stimulates cutaneous blood flow in human balding scalps: pharmacodynamics measured by laser doppler velocimetry and photopulse plethysmography. J Invest Dermatol 1984; 82:515–517.
27. Bunker CB, Dowd PM. Alterations in scalp blood flow after the epicutaneous application of 3% minoxidil and 0.1% hexylnicotinate in alopecia. Br J Dermatol 1988; 117:668–669.
28. Lachgar S, Charveron M, Gall Y, Bonafe JL. Minoxidil upregulates the expression of vascular endothelial growth factor in human hair dermal papilla cells. Br J Dermatol 1998; 138:407–411.
29. Bazzano GS, Terezakis N, Galen W. Topical tretinoin for hair growth promotion. J Am Acad Dermatol 1986; 15:880–883.
30. Shaw JC. Antiandrogen therapy in dermatology. Int J Dermatol 1996; 35(11):770–778.
31. Hammerstein J, Meckies J, Leo-Rossberg I, Moltz L, Zielske F. The use of cyproterone acetate (CPA) in the treatment of acne, hirsuitism and virilism. J Steroid Biochem 1975; 6:827–836.
32. Dawber RPR, Sonnex T, Ralfs I. Oral antiandrogen treatment of common baldness in women. Br J Dermatol 1982; 107(suppl 22):20 (abstr).
33. Mortimer CH, Rushton H, James KC. Effective medical treatment for common baldness in women. Clin Exp Dermatol 1984; 9:342–350.
34. Watanabe S, Yamasaki S, Tanae A, Hibi I. Three cases of hepatocellular carcinoma among cyproterone users. Lancet 1994; 344:1567–1568.
35. Rabe T, Feldmann K, Grunwald K, Runnebaum B. Liver tumours in women on oral contraceptives. Lancet 1994; 344:1568–1569.
36. Burke BM, Cunliffe WJ. Oral spironolactone therapy for female patients with acne, hirsutism or androgenic alopecia. Br J Dermatol 1985; 112:124–125.
37. Aram H. Treatment of female androgenetic alopecia with cimetidine. Int J Dermatol 1987; 26:128–130.
38. Van Der Willigen AH, Peereboom-Wynia JDR, Van Joost T, Stolz E. A preliminary study of the effect of 11α-hydroxyprogesterone on the hair growth in men suffering from androgenetic alopecia. Acta Dermato-Venereol 1987; 67:82–85.
39. Orfanos CE, Vogels L. Lokaltherapie der alopecia androgenetica mit 17α-astradiol. Dermatologica 1980; 161:124.
40. Dallob AL, Sadick NS, Unger O et al. The effect of finasteride, a 5α-reductase inhibitor on scalp skin testosterone and dihydrotestosterone concentration in patients with male pattern baldness. J Clin Endocrinol Metab 1994; 79:703–706.
41. Walsh DS, Dunn CL, James WD. Improvement in androgenetic alopecia (stage V)

using topical minoxidil in a retinoid vehicle and oral finasteride. Arch Dermatol 1995; 131:1373–1385.

42. Walker SA, Rothman S. Alopecia areata. A statistical study and consideration of endocrine influences. J Invest Dermatol 1950; 14:403.
43. Muller SA, Winkelamm RK. Alopecia areata. Arch Dermatol 1963; 88:290–297.
44. Weisner-Menzel L, Happle R. Intrabulbar and peribulbar accumulation of dendritic OKT-6 positive cells in alopecia areata. Arch Dermatol Res 1984; 276:333–334.
45. Dillaha CJ, Rothman S. Treatment of alopecia areata totalis and universalis with cortisone acetate. J Invest Dermatol 1952; 18:5–6.
46. Perriard-Wolfensberger J, Pasche-Koo F, Mainetti C, Labarthe MP, Salomon D, Saurat JH. Pulse of methylprednisolone in alopecia areata. Dermatology 1993; 187: 282–285.
47. Burton JL, Shuster S. Large doses of glucocorticoid in the treatment of alopecia areata. Acta Dermato-Venereol 1975; 55:493–496.
48. Pascher F, Kurtin S, Andrade E. Assay of 0.2% fluocinolone acetonide cream for alopecia areata and totalis. Dermatologica 1970; 141:193–202.
49. Porter D, Burton JL. A comparison of intralesional triamcinolone hexacetonide and triamcinolone acetonide in alopecia areata. Br J Dermatol 1971; 85:272–273.
50. Abell E, Munro DD. Intralesional treatment of alopecia areata with triamcinolone acetonide by jet injection. Br J Dermatol 1973; 88:55–59.
51. Kikuchi I, Horikawa S. Perilymphatic atrophy of the skin. Arch Dermatol 1975; 111:795 (letter).
52. Daman LA, Rosenberg EW, Drake L. Treatment of alopecia areata with dinitrochlorobenzene. Arch Dermatol 1978; 114:1036–1038.
53. Happle R, Kalvaran KJ, Buchner U, Echternacht-Happle K, Goggelmann W, Summer JH. Contact allergy as a therapeutic tool for androgenetic alopecia: application of squaric acid dibutylester. Dermatologica 1980; 161:289.
54. Tosti A, De Padova MP, Minghetti G, Veronesi S. Therapies versus placebo in the treatment of patchy alopecia areata. J Am Acad Dermatol 1986; 15:209–210.
55. Happle R, Hausen BM, Wiesner-Menzel L. Diphencyprone in the treatment of alopecia areata. Acta Dermato-Venereologica 1983; 63:49–52.
56. Claudy AL, Gagnaire D. PUVA treatment of alopecia areata. Arch Dermatol 1983; 119:975–978.
57. Lassus A, Kianto W, Johansson E, Juvakoski T. PUVA treatment for alopecia areata. Dermatologica 1980; 161:298–304.
58. Mitchell AJ, Douglass MC. Topical photochemotherapy for alopecia areata. J Am J Dermatol 1985; 12:644–649.
59. Fenton DA and Wilkinson JD. Alopecia areata treated with topical minoxidil. J R Soc Med 1982; 75:963–965.
60. Price VH. Topical minoxidil (3%) in extensive alopecia areata, including long term efficacy. J Am Acad Dermatol 1987; 16:737–744.
61. Fiedler-Weiss VC, West DP, Buys CM, Rumsfield JA. Topical minoxidil dose-response effect in alopecia areata. Arch Dermatol 1986; 122:180–182.
62. Fiedler-Weiss VC, Rumsfield JA, Buys CM, West DP, Wendrow A. Evaluation of oral minoxidil in the treatment of alopecia areata. Arch Dermatol 1987; 123:1488–1490

63. Gupta AK, Ellis CN, Cooper KD, Nickoloff BJ, Ho VC, Chan LS, Hamilton TA, Tellner DC, Griffiths CEM, Voorhees JJ. Oral cyclosporin for the treatment of alopecia areata. J Am Acad Dermatol 1990; 22:242–250.
64. Teshima H, Urabe A, Irie M, Nakagawa T, Nakayama J, Hori Y. Alopecia universalis treated with oral cyclosporin A and prednisolone: immunologic studies. Int J Dermatol 1992; 31:513–516.
65. Thomson AW, Aldridge RD, Sewell HF. Topical cyclosporin in alopecia areata and nickel contact dermatitis. Lancet 1986; ii:971–972.
66. McElwee KJ, Rushton DH, Trachy R, Oliver RF. Topical FK506: a potent immunotherapy for alopecia areata? Studies using the Dundee experimental bald rat model. Br J Dermatol 1997; 137:491–497.
67. Galbraith GMP, Thiers BH, Jensen J, Hoehler F. A randomised double-blind study of inosiplex (isoprinosine) therapy in patients with alopecia totalis. J Am Acad Dermatol 1987; 16:977–983.
68. Berth-Jones J, Hutchinson PE. Treatment of alopecia totalis with a combination of inosine pranobex and diphencyprone compared to each treatment alone. Clin Exp Dermatol 1991; 16:172–175.
69. Powell J, Dawber RPR, Gatter K. Follicultis decalvans: The range of histological findings. (Communication) Br Soc Dermatopathol Jan 1998.
70. Pujol RM, Garcia-Patos V, Mateu-Ravella A, Casanova JM, Moragas JM de. Tufted hair folliculitis: a specific disease? Br J Dermatol 1994; 130:259–260.
71. Brozena SJ, Cohen LE, Fenske NA. Folliculitis decalvans—response to rifampicin. Cutis 1988; 42:512–515.
72. Altman J, Perry HO. The variations and course of lichen planus. Arch Dermatol 1961; 84:179–191.
73. Dalziel K, Going G, Cartwright PH, Marks R, Beveridge GW, Rowell NR. Treatment of chronic discoid lupus erythematosus with an oral gold compound (auranofin). Br J Dermatol 1986; 115:211–216.
74. Lo JS, Berg RE, Tomecki KJ. Treatment of discoid lupus erythematosus. Int J Dermatol 1989; 28:497–507.
75. Caputo R, Veraldi S. Erosive pustular dermatosis of the scalp. J Am Acad Dermatol 1993; 28:96–98.
76. Schwartz RA, Janniger CK. Tinea capitis. Cutis 1995; 55:29.
77. Rasmussen JE, Ahmed AR. Trichophytin reactions in children with tinea capitis. Arch Dermatol 1978; 114:371–372.
78. Friedman L, Derbes VJ, Tromovitch TA. Simple dose therapy of tinea capitis. Arch Dermatol 1960; 82:415–418.
79. Van Breuseghem R, Gatti F, Ceballos JA. Mass treatment of scalp ringworm by a single dose of griseofulvin. Int J Dermatol 1970; 9:59.
80. Gan VN, Petruska M, Ginsburg CM. Epidemiology and treatment of tinea capitis: ketoconazole vs. griseofulvin. Pediatr Infect Dis J 1987; 6:46–9.
81. Tanz RR, Herbert AA, Burton Esterly N. Treating tinea capitis. Should ketoconazole replace griseofulvin. J Pediatr 1988; 112:987–91.
82. Degreef H. Itraconazole in the treatment of tinea capitis. Cutis 1996; 58:90–93.
83. Gupta AK, Alexis ME, Raboobee N, Hofstader SLR, Lynde CW, Adam P, Summerbell RC, Doncker PDE. Itraconazole pulse therapy is effective in the treatment

of tinea capitis in children: an open multicentre study. Br J Dermatol 1997; 137: 251–254.

84. Greer DL. Treatment of tinea capitis with itraconazole. J Am Acad Dermatol 1996; 35(4):637–640.
85. Solomon BA, Collins R, Sharma R, Silverberg N, Jain AR, Sedgh J, Laude TA. Fluconazole for the treatment of tinea capitis in children. J Am Acad Dermatol 1997; 37:274–275.
86. Gupta AK, Lynde CW, Lauzon GJ, Mehlmauer MA, Braddock SW, Miller CA, Del Rosso JQ, Shear NH. Cutaneous adverse effects associated with terbinafine therapy: 10 case reports and a review fo the literature. Br J Dermatol 1998; 138: 529–532.
87. Kullavanijaya P, Reangchainam S, Ungpakorn R. Randomized single-blind study of efficacy and tolerability of terbinafine in the treatment of tinea capitis. J Am Acad Dermatol 1997; 37:272–273.
88. Elewski E. Cutaneous mycoses in children. Br J Dermatol 1996; 134(suppl 46) 7–11.
89. Dawber RPR. Aspects of treatment of scalp psoriasis. J Dermatol Treat 1989; 1(2): 103–105.
90. Klaber MR, Hutchinson PE, Pedvis-Leftick A, Kragballe K, Reunala TL, Van de Kerkhof PCM, Johnsson MK, Molin L, Corbett MS, Downess N. Comparative effects of calcipotriol solution (50μg/mL) and betamethazone 17-valerate solution (1mg/ml) in the treatment of scalp psoriasis. Arch Dermatol 1994; 131:678–683.
91. Scerri L, Williams HC, Allen BR. Dissecting cellulitis of the scalp: response to isotretinoin. Br J Dermatol 1996; 134:1105–1108.
92. Schuster S. The aetiology of dandruff and the mode of action of therapeutic agents. Br J Dermatol 1984; 111:235–242.
93. Leyden JJ, McGinlay KJ, Kligman AM. Role of microorganisms in dandruff. Arch Dermatol 1976; 112:333.
94. Gould DJ, Davies MG, Kersey PJW, Kenicer K, Green C, Strong A, Hammill E, Moss MY, Smith Y. Topical lithium succinate—a safe and effective treatment for seborrhoeic dermatitis. Br J Dermatol 1988; 119(suppl 33):27–28 (abstr).
95. Hay RJ, Clayton YM, Moore MK. A comparison of tioconazole 28% nail solution versus base as an adjunct to oral griseofulvin in patients with onychomycosis. Clin Exp Dermatol 1987; 12:175–177.
96. Hay RJ, Baran R, Haneke. Fungal (onychomycosis) and other infections involving the nail apparatus. In: Baran R, Dawber RPR eds. Diseases of the Nails and Their Management, 2nd ed. Oxford: Blackwell, 1994:97–134.
97. Gupta AK. Pharmacoeconomic analysis of oral antifungal therapies used to treat dermatophyte onychomycosis of the toenails. Pharmacoeconomics 1998; 113: 1–15.
98. Presser SE, Blank H. Cimetidine: adjunct in treatment of tinea capitis. Lancet 1981; 1:108–109.
99. Tausch I, Brautigam M, Weidinger G, Jones TC. The Lagos V Study Group. Evaluation of 6 weeks treatment of terbinafine in tinea unguium in a double blind trial comparing 6 and 12 weeks therapy. Br J Dermatol 1997; 136:737–742.
100. Tosti A, Piraccini BM, Stinchi C, Venturo N, Bardazzi F, Colombo MD. Treatment

of dermatophyte nail infections: an open randomized study comparing intermittent terbinafine therapy with continuous terbinafine treatment and intermittent itraconazole therapy. J Am Acad Dermatol 1996; 34:595–600.

101. Willemsen M, de Doncker P, Willems J, Woestenborghs R, Ven de Velde V, Heykrants J, Cutsem JV, Cauwenbergh G, Roseeuw D. Post treatment itraconazole levels in the nail. J Am Acad Dermatol 1992; 26:731–735.

102. Havu V, Brandt H, Heikkila H, Hollmen A, Oksman R, Rantanen T, Saari S, Stubb S, Turjanmaa K, Piepponen T. A double-blind, randomized study comparing itraconazole pulse therapy with continuous dosing for the treatment of toe-nail onychomycosis. Br J Dermatol 1997; 136:230–234.

103. De Doncker P, Gupta AK, Marynissen G, Stoffels P, Heremans A. Itraconazole pulse therapy for onychomycosis and dermatomycoses: An overview. J Am Acad Dermatol 1997; 37:969–974.

104. Grant SM, Clissold SP. Fluconazole. A review of its pharmacodynamic and pharmacokinetic properties and therapeutic potential in superficial and systemic mycoses. Drugs 1990; 39:877–916.

105. Frederiksson T. Topically applied fluorouracil in the treatment of psoriatic nails. Arch Dermatol 1974; 110:735.

106. Baran R, Dawber RPR. The nail in dermatological diseases. In: Baran R, Dawber RPR eds. Diseases of the Nails and Their Management, 2nd ed. Oxford: Blackwell, 1994:97–134.

107. De Berker DAR, Lawrence CM. A simplified protocol of steroid injection for psoriatic nail dystrophy. Br J Dematol 1998; 138:90–95.

108. Tosti A, Guerra L, Bardazzi F, Lanzarini. Topical cyclosporin in nail psoriasis. Dermatologica 1990; 180:110.

109. Marx L, Scher RK. Response of psoriatic nails to oral photochemotherapy. Arch Dermatol 1980; 116:1023–1024.

110. Baran R. Retinoids and the nails. J Dermatol Treat 1990; 1:151–154.

111. Tosti A, Fanti PA, Morelli R, Bardazzi F. Spongiotic trachyonychia. Arch Dermatol 1991; 127:584–585.

112. Burge SM, Wilkinson JD, Miller AJ, Ryan TJ. The efficacy of an aromatic retinoid, Tigason (etretinate), in the treatment of Darier's Disease. Br J Dermatol 1981; 104: 675–680.

22

Dapsone

David P. Jacobus
Jacobus Pharmaceutical Company, Inc.
Princeton, New Jersey

INTRODUCTION

This chapter on dapsone and dermatology is divided in several parts to mirror the breadth of dermatology, interest in both infectious and noninfectious disease, important questions of immunology, the safe handling of dapsone, and new uses for the future. Dapsone is best understood by dermatologists and infectious disease specialists.

As with many modern medications, Dapsone has at least two very diverse functions. The well-recognized activities include the control of dermatitis herpetiformis, a noninfectious disease, and of infectious diseases such as leprosy, *Pneumocystis carinii* pneumonia, and falciparum malaria as a para-aminobenzoic acid (PABA) antagonist.

Dapsone has been well established as effective in rheumatoid arthritis, a disease in which polymorphs are considered to play only a limited role. If dapsone were to be managed in rheumatoid arthritis in the same way as in dermatitis herpetiformis, this activity would not be recognized. In fact, no disease-modifying–activity drug would be found if any were handled as salicylates or prednisone are handled in rheumatoid arthritis or as dapsone is managed in dermatitis herpetiformis.

The mechanism of action in rheumatoid arthritis is not understood. It is likely that as knowledge develops, there will be diseases treated primarily by dermatologists that have comparable mechanisms. Rheumatoid arthritis is a common disease, so timing and response rates are well established and can serve as a pattern to read the myriad and perceptive case reports in infrequent dermatological diseases where dapsone usage is important. Because the clinical and laboratory parameters of rheumatoid arthritis are different, the emphasis in this report is on timing and duration of treatment and the timeline of responses.

Complicating the study of all disease-modifying agents in rheumatoid arthritis is the fact that for none of them is a recruitment of a responder close to 100%; the usual range is 40–60%. A further complication is that all patients with rheumatoid arthritis escape after a decade; the original disease-modifying agent and all subsequent ones fail to work, yet these agents have been established as essential for the management of rheumatoid arthritis other than sulfapyridine. Other disease-modifying antirheumatic drugs (DMARD) do not work in dermatitis herpetiformis or other dermatological conditions. However, if a similar recruitment rate and escape exists for an unusual dermatological disease, then the development of controlled data will not be easy.

Three Patterns of Usage

There are at least three different clinical patterns of usage:

1. The full response occurs within 1 or 2 days and an equally fast relapse occurs on withdrawal. These patients can be titrated on introduction, especially if higher doses are needed. The prompt relapse, often obtained by history, can be used to evaluate the titration and adjust the dosage in long-term patients. Almost but not all patients respond. The response is generally never lost so patients can require dapsone for decades.

Dermatitis herpetiformis is an example of this timeline. In dermatitis herpetiformis, the response is prompt, lost within 24–48 hours when discontinued in a properly titrated patient, and considered to be achieved by preventing polymorph-leukocytes from attacking self. Multiple mechanisms have been proposed for this activity. Erythema elevatum diutinum is in this class.

2. No response is seen for about a month followed by a steady gain in the next few weeks achieving almost all the improvement to be achieved although some gain does not occur until the ninth month. Withdrawal is followed by the reciprocal time line with no change for several weeks, then the beginning of relapse, and so on. Perhaps because of the time line the dosage is usually fixed. Generally not more than two thirds of the patients respond. The response is usually lost at the end of a decade with the patient ''escaping'' disease control.

The effect of dapsone in rheumatoid arthritis is an example of the aforementioned timeline. In rheumatoid arthritis, in five prospective well-controlled trials, dapsone is a DMARD comparable to d-penicillamine, injectable gold, sulfasalazine, or sulfapyridine. These drugs take 4 to 6 weeks to start to set up housekeeping and improve laboratory parameters, which are also improved in cases of spontaneous recovery. The dosage is usually not titrated. The effects last 4 to 6 weeks after the drugs are stopped. Generally, no more than two thirds of patients respond. In patients with continuing disease activity, ''escape'' before the end of a decade is customary with alternate members of the class not effective on introduction.

There is no agreement as to how dapsone or other DMARDS work, although the mechanism must be different from anti-inflammatory steroids such as prednisone or immunosuppressive drugs such as methotrexate. These timelines may be important when considering dapsone for dermatological conditions other than dermatitis herpetiformis. Cicatricial pemphigoid may be in this class.

3. In leprosy and other infectious diseases, dapsone has anti–PABA activity, which results from the inhibition of dihydropteroic acid synthase. The effect can be potentiated by concurrent administration of appropriate dihydrofolate reductase (DHFR) inhibitors. Other diseases include *Pneumocystosis carinii*, sometimes with trimethoprim potentiation for treatment, toxoplasmosis usually with pyrimethamine potentiation, and malaria such as *Plasmodium falciparum*, also usually with pyrimethamine; there is no effect on *P. vivax* and also no effect on bacterial pathogens such as *E. coli, staphylococci*, etc.

HISTORY

Dapsone, first synthesized in 1908 [1], was found effective in the treatment of tuberculosis in the guinea pig but not tolerated when given at a clinical dosage of a gram per day. The extraordinary sensitivity of *M. leprae* led to its clinical usage in leprosy as the first modern anti-leprosy drug. In the 1950s, there were approximately 15 million patients with leprosy. The World Health Organization (WHO) hoped that 5 million were on dapsone at any one time. There are now about 2 million with leprosy. Generally, the dosage was 50 mg per day for life which was increased to 100 mg per day in the 1960s. A multidrug 2-year program still includes dapsone for the remaining patients.

Stephen Katz [2] has reviewed the initial history of sulfapyridine by Costello [3] in 1947, the now-unavailable water-soluble bis methanesulfonate derivative of dapsone by Cornbleet [4] in 1951, and the parent compound dapsone by Kruizinga and Hamminga [5] in 1953. Dermatitis herpetiformis patients who do not adhere to a gluten-free diet generally take these drugs forever after the initial diagnosis. In the United States and Great Britain, numerous patients have had more than 20 years of continuous administration at a level of 100 mg per day under good follow-up with no disease other than dermatitis herpetiformis.

The third major use is in immunosuppressed patients (HIV, cancer, or transplant) as an alternative to sulfamethoxazole with trimethoprim for prophylaxis against *Pneumocystis carinii* pneumonia. Because of adverse reactions to sulfamethoxazole, half the HIV patients in the United States needing prophylaxis are on dapsone.

For leprosy, dermatitis herpetiformis, and immunosuppressed patients the medication is generally continued through pregnancy, other intervening diseases, and medications.

NONINFECTIOUS DISEASES

Dermatitis Herpetiformis

Dapsone and sulfapyridine are the mainstays of treatment of dermatitis herpetiformis [2,6]. Both medications produce a prompt improvement in the signs and symptoms of the disease.

Titrations

Although the modern practice often includes a gradual upward titration of the initial dosage of dapsone, naive patients started on 150 mg per day respond promptly from a few hours to within 48 hours. When a patient has been properly titrated, missing a single day or 2 days at the most of administration can lead to a flare in disease. It has been my practice to recommend that if a patient can miss more than 2 days without detecting a flare, then the daily dosage can and should be reduced. Lesions on the face are generally the most resistant. Properly titrated patients may continue to have facial lesions as well as an occasional vesicle elsewhere in the classical extensor distribution pattern.

Dosage adjustment in each patient is an important part of dapsone management. Because of excellent disease control, patients commonly state that a ''gluten-free diet'' was not effective so they continue to use dapsone or sulfapyridine to control the cutaneous lesions without instituting a gluten-free diet.

There are relatively few reports of the dosage range to control dermatitis herpetiformis. Of the 30 dapsone patients reported by Katz [6], nine were on 25–75 mg/day, 17 on 100–200 mg/day, three were on 250–300 mg/day, and one on 400 or more mg/day. This dosage range is compatible with the labeling ''if full control is not achieved within the range of 50–300 mg/daily, higher doses may be tried.'' However, I agree with Katz that the majority of patients are controlled on 100 mg per day. Neither dapsone nor sulfapyridine have an effect on the gastrointestinal component of the disease.

Gluten-Free Diet

A gluten-free diet is the only way to correct the intestinal lesion. Symptoms of celiac disease are usually not present in patients with dermatitis herpetiformis, presumably because of the fact that the small gut lesion covers only one third of the jejunum. Fry [7] has reported on the long-term follow-up of dermatitis herpetiformis with dapsone and with and without a gluten withdrawal: if the initial dosage is more than 50 mg/day, the average time to achieve a dosage reduction is 9 months with a range of 4–30 months. The average time to stop all dapsone is 33 months with a range of 10–86 months. Thus, there is an asynchronous effect with a reduction in the dapsone dosage generally occurring within the first year whereas the cessation of dapsone administration takes 3 years. The reduction in dosage generally coincides with the healing of the gut, which occurs with the initiation of a strict gluten-free diet, whereas the prolonged probably reflects the insoluble nature of immunoglobulin deposits in the dermal papilla.

A strict gluten-free diet is difficult. Fry [7] has graded the diet as Grade 1, strict no gluten intake; Grade 2, very occasional gluten intake and usually unintentional; and Grade 3, small quantities taken intentionally, but no more than once a week. Fry considers that patients with a Grade 3 compliance were deemed not to be adhering to the diet and, therefore, were told to take a normal diet. Fry had two patients in Grade 3; neither had a reduction in dosage.

Fry [7] reported that only 23 of his original 78 patients were able to maintain a strict gluten-free diet for up to 14 years. He reported that for some patients who had been able to stop dapsone, small and occasional gluten intake did not precipitate the rash. However, in those patients still taking dapsone, gluten intake often produced a flare-up of the skin lesions. Fry's report includes a follow-up on eight patients whose disease was controlled only by a gluten-free diet. Three of the eight had no immunoglobin A (IgA) deposits in the uninvolved skin after having been on the diet for 10, 14, and 14 years respectively, although 4 years previously these three patients had had IgA deposits still in the skin. In the remaining five patients not needing dapsone, IgA was still present in the skin. The deposits take a long time to clear.

Potential Complications of an Open Gut

The excellent dermatological control achieved by dapsone and sulfapyridine without substantial effect on the gastrointestinal track leads to the patient having a long-term open gut. If the drugs were less effective, then there would perhaps be a greater willingness to adhere to a strict gluten-free diet. Because dapsone facilitates the patient not going on a strict gluten-free diet, it is worth discussing the management of a long-term patient in relationship to the open gut.

Reduced B_{12} absorption is not confined to dermatitis herpetiformis patients. Lindenbaum et al. [125] reports that among the 548 surviving members of the Framingham cohort, that B_{12} deficiency was prevalent in 12%.

Peripheral Motor Neuropathy

We consider that an important part of the management of dapsone is the differential diagnosis between a peripheral motor neuropathy attributable to the drug versus a peripheral motor and sensory neuropathy attributable to the open gut. Perhaps as expected, peripheral motor neuropathy literature indicates that a higher dosage is needed, but 20 or 30 years of dapsone at 100 mg a day may well also produce a motor neuropathy. A long-term open gut may well also produce a subclinical (subhematologic) B_{12} deficiency, which is inherently correctable. Because dapsone facilitates the patient staying on a normal diet, we think this problem deserves attention in those patients who do not reduce their dapsone dosage or improve their B_{12} intake. Dapsone can produce a motor neuropathy that is generally considered to be a pure motor neuropathy without a sensory component, but there is only one literature report of a daily dosage as low as 100 mg.

B_{12} deficiency is common even without an open gut. Pennypacker et al. [9] reported in a Veterans Hospital session that in male patients over 65 with no known disease that there was a 14.5% prevalence of vitamin B_{12} deficiency as shown by an elevation in methylmalonic acid and homocysteine, both of which responded to parenteral vitamin B_{12}. The serum vitamin B_{12} level was insensitive for screening. The Pennypacker study involved the screen of 152 consecutive outpatients to find 29 patients with a serum level less than 300 pg/mL. Although it is generally agreed that 200 pg/mL probably indicates a deficiency state, 17 of 29 (59%) had abnormal methylmalonic acid and homocysteine levels. Beck [8,10] has reported that B_{12} is the only valid therapy, and that despite long contention, a convincing case has yet to be made for neuropathy or myelopathy attributable to a pure folate deficiency. Additional folic acid will stimulate B_{12} metabolism and deplete B_{12} stores in the central nervous system. Folic acid alone will accelerate both neuropsychiatric complications and posterior chord lesions. Lifelong B_{12} therapy is required as long as the gut remains open.

The classic symptoms of B_{12} deficiency are those of primary pernicious anemia with macrocytic erythrocytes and hypermature polymorphonuclear leukocytes. However, in pernicious anemia, absorption of B_{12} can be sufficient to keep erythrocyte indices abnormal even though insufficient B_{12} is absorbed to maintain the central nervous system. As a result, there can be long-term psychic and cognitive abnormalities [8] in the central nervous system, as well as loss of posterior cord function with peripheral signs of tingling along with reduced vibratory and position sense usually beginning in the feet.

Because an elderly dermatitis herpetiformis patient on a long-term normal diet must have more than 10% chance of a correctable folate deficiency, we consider that patients who have tingling in the feet or reduced position of vibratory sense need to have careful evaluation of the differential diagnosis between dapsone motor toxicity and B_{12} deficiency. Rather than advise a patient to consume oral B_{12}, we recommend that the diagnosis be established authoritatively. For B_{12} deficiency, our objective is to make certain that the patient receives sufficient B_{12} to correct the neurological lesions rather than just the hematological abnormalities.

Administration of parenteral B_{12} to a patient with primary pernicious anemia will result in an immediate and stunning sense of improved well being, but the cord lesions are generally considered to be irreversible. Both male and female patients with the full open gut of celiac disease have reduced fertility.

Erythema Elevatum Diutinum

Erythema elevatum diutinum (EED) is a rare disease characterized by red, purple, and yellowish papules and nodules usually distributed symmetrically over extensor surfaces. The disease is interesting in that the lesions show a leukocytoclastic vasculitis with a dense infiltrate primarily of neutrophils and occasional monocytes. Katz [11] has described five cases, four of whom were treated with dapsone. When the proper dosage is obtained, the response occurs within 12–48 hours. When equilibrium was established, two of the four cases were managed with 100 mg per day, but the other two were between 200 and 250 mg daily, thus showing that half the time higher-than-usual dosages are needed. Not all patients have been tried on these dosages. For example, Cream et al. [12] report two patients: one responded to 100 mg per day, the other failed to respond on 150 mg/day. Wilkinson et al. [13] report a series of 13 patients, nine of whom had a trial of dapsone with a maximum dosage of 150 mg/day. Four of the nine had a good response on 100 per day, four had a partial response on 100 a day, and the one patient on 150 mg failed to respond. The results are compatible with the Katz report in which half the patients needed 200–250 mg/day to control the disease.

In the Katz report, two of the five EED patients had abnormal neutrophil chemotaxis at baseline that was normalized on Dapsone. Four also had an arthus-like reaction to the streptokinase/streptodornase skin test (SKSD) with a marked improvement on dapsone. The improvement in clinical symptoms is accompanied by an improvement in these laboratory measurements.

Cicatricial Pemphigoid

Cicatricial pemphigoid has a low frequency of spontaneous remission. The disease may be intermittent, but patients can have extensive disease with severe scarring of mucosal surfaces. The oral mucosa is usually involved. Ahmed et al. [14] report that 65% of CP patients have ocular lesions, which usually begin unilaterally, but within 2 years are often bilateral. As all mucosal surfaces are involved, patients may be first diagnosed in ophthalmology or ear, nose, and throat (ENT) clinics. Progression of the conjunctival lesions can lead to blindness. Rogers et al. [15] reported that 20 of 24 patients responded with partial or complete control to dapsone to a graduated program beginning with 25 mg daily for 3 days then increasing 25 mg per day every 3 days, achieving 150 mg daily by the 17th day. Patients responded between 2 and 12 weeks with the median response time at 4 weeks. The highest dosage used was 200 in two of 24 patients. Rogers et al. [15] reported that the oral lesions responded before the ophthamalogical lesions.

Tauber et al. [16] have reported that cicatricial pemphigoid can lead to progressive corneal scarring and neovascularization which, if untreated, is eventually progressive, leading to profound visual loss. The progression is slow with periods of remission, but explosive exacerbation can occur. Surgical trauma often triggers rapid deterioration. But Foster's group [17,18] has shown that cataract surgery can be performed in ocular cicatricial pemphigoid under cover of dapsone and other agents. Topical therapeutic strategies are not considered effective in this systemic disorder. Of the 20 patients, 14 were on dapsone (11 dapsone only), six were on azothioprim (five azothioprim alone), and eight were on cyclophosphamide (four cyclophosphamide alone). No patient was on prednisone alone, but it was coadministered to four of the 20 patients.

We have been told that dapsone is considered essential for patients with cicatricial pemphigoid who need ophthalmic surgery [17,18] and that there are sufficient data to support the development of an official indication describing how to use dapsone for cicatricial pemphigoid.

Bullous Pemphigoid

Korman [19] in his review of bullous pemphigoid states that the treatment of bullous pemphigoid is aimed at controlling the resulting pathological process rather than the primary cause. Little is known about why patients form antibodies directly against the bullous pemphigoid antigen. The usual treatment has been corticosteroids, locally or systemically with systemic dosages often between 40 and 80 mg prednisone per day. Dapsone and sulfapyridine play a minor role. However, Pearson and Rogers [20] reported in 1977 that three of 41 (7%) patients on prednisone responded to the addition of dapsone or sulfapyridine with three additional patients having a partial response, approximately half of the successful rate Rook and Waddington [126] reported for sulfapyridine where four of 17 patients were controlled, seven had a partial response, and six had no effect. Pearson and Rogers provide the details on the response time of five of their six patients to sulfapyridine. The daily dosage ranged from 2 to 4 g per day with the time of response between 10 and 21 days. One patient who stopped sulfapyridine went 6 weeks before relapse. Of the two patients with long-term follow-up, one after 2 years required 500 mg daily and one after 15 months was able to discontinue sulfapyridine. Because spontaneous remission is expected, those few patients who respond should be retitrated regularly through a drug-withdrawal or dosage-reduction program.

Brown Recluse Spider

A brown recluse spider can inject a few microliters of venom that can produce a localized necrotic lesion in man, guinea pigs, and rabbits. An initial erythema in patients with a severe bite is followed by a lesion that increases steadily over the next 3 days to culminate in a central necrotic lesion 2 or 3 cm across with a surrounding erythema 15 cm in diameter. The center can slough out, leading to an ulcer that can progress across fascial layers and that often leaves a scar when healed by secondary intention.

The tissue damage in a severe bite is not attributable to the direct toxicity of the venom or its active ingredient, phospholipase [21]. Dapsone has no effect on the phospholipase. Polymorphonuclear leukocytes (PMN) appear early and are essential for the progression of the lesion, because in rabbits, depletion of PMN by nitrogen mustard inhibited leukocyte infiltration and hemorrhage [22]. In addition, depletion of circulating complement in guinea pigs by the parenteral administration of zymosan also resulted in a marked reduction of edema. The results support the conclusions that both PMN infiltration and complement are essential for the progression of the lesion.

Martin and Kachel [23] showed that depsone protected endothelium cells from neutrophil injury by inhibiting the respiratory burst of neutrophils. Patel et al. [24] report that in a similar system, an in vitro cell culture system containing Loxosceles venom PMNs were attracted to the endothelium cells after 3 hours. By 6 hours, 40% of the PMNs were adherent to the endothelium tissue. In this system the venom, when exposed directly on the PMNs, also had no effect on PMNs. Patel considered that the endothelium cells, when stimulated by the venom, led to a disregulated PMN response with an inappropriate accumulation and activation of the patients' own PMNs.

Based on the histological accumulation of PMNs in brown recluse spider bite lesions, King and Rees [25] administered dapsone to an acutely bitten patient. They reported that, although the lesion was advanced, dapsone appeared to stop the progression to a slough. Their work has not been fully accepted; some physicians remain supportive of early excision whereas others opt for high-dose steroid treatment. At the clinical level there is a technical difficulty in establishing data on the efficacy of any treatment. The amount of venom injected by the spider is not controlled. The patient arrives at a variable time. The bite is retrospectively deemed to be a brown recluse spider bite when the characteristic sequence has appeared, often with extensive tissue damage. Lastly, in the presence of a high morbidity, there has been an unwillingness to do a proper randomized trial of patients with severe bites.

Because the venom can be collected from spiders, pooled, and characterized, laboratory experiments to show activity before or after envenomation are possible. These experiments have a specific dose response and need to be carefully controlled themselves. All views, including a negative animal experiment [26] and references to well-conducted positive experiments [27], are summarized in Reference 28.

My own reading is that there is no doubt that the lesions are associated with extensive polymorph infiltration, that prednisone does not produce a significant inhibition of polymorph accumulation or polymorph activation, and that a study of early surgery versus dapsone was in favor of dapsone [29]. In the absence of obtaining a G6PD determination, I recommend the immediate administration of 50 mg dapsone, keeping the lesion cool with a dry ice pack and, if possible, keeping the bite elevated. The patient should be watched for the next several hours, after which time the dosage can be topped up to 100 mg. One hundred milligram per day may be enough, but many bites, especially severe bites, have been treated with a total of 200 mg per day. The dosage should be divided for better tolerance, especially because patients with serious envenomation appear to have a greater frequency of nausea or other adverse effects than is generally seen. I am not certain if administration of the drug after the lesion has sloughed out has any effect. I think the dapsone should be stopped at the end of the second week. Because the bite progresses in a matter of hours, my recommendation is that emergency rooms should be prepared to administer dapsone promptly after making a diagnosis.

Rheumatoid Arthritis

Rheumatoid arthritis is generally not managed by dermatologists, but the timing of the response of the disease parameters is instructive and might be relevant to rare conditions such as relapsing polychondritis.

After the initial observation of McConkey et al. [30] in 71 patients, there are now four prospective placebo-controlled trials [31–34] showing that dapsone is effective in rheumatoid arthritis. It is classified as a DMARD as is injectable gold, d-penicillamine, and sulfapyridine. Not all patients with active rheumatoid arthritis respond to a disease-modifying medication. The magnitude of the response is generally considered not to be affected by the dosage, although the response rates, which range between 40–70%, are modestly dose dependant. Why one patient responds and another does not is not understood. In nonresponders, usually one disease-modifying agent after another is tried. These agents have no analgesic activity. In addition to clinical improvement, there is improvement in the laboratory parameters, which usually are resistant to steroids. If present, the responsive laboratory parameters are an elevated rheumatoid factor (either IgM or IgG directed against the FC portion of the immunoglobulin) and an elevated sedimentation rate. These parameters also improve in spontaneous remission; hence, these drugs are called ''disease-modifying drugs'' although the effect on protection against joint damage is less well established.

All of the DMARD medications have a very comparable course. Characteristically nothing happens until the end of the first month when the patient says she can first sleep through the night. On immediate examination there is generally no change in the joint score, firmness of grip, or laboratory parameters such as sedimentation rate and rheumatoid factor. However, over the next several weeks to 2 months, there is a dramatic improvement in the joint score, clinical performance, and in the laboratory. These improvements are generally complete by the end of the third month with one exception: improvement in the anemia associated with active rheumatoid arthritis does not commence until the ninth month. Dapsone patients can also have an initial loss of an additional 1–2 g of hemoglobin during the initial 2 months. In the Grindulis and McConkey study of 84 patients [35] the average hemoglobin decreased from 12 to 11 g in the first 6 weeks, but the loss exceeded 2 g in only 10%. Anemia led to the discontinuation of dapsone treatment in 6% of patients. The average hemoglobin rose after 6 weeks, reflecting the compensation to dapsone therapy. However, even after 36 weeks the average hemoglobin was 11.5 in comparison to 12.3 at baseline.

When the DMARDS are stopped, the patient goes through the reciprocal time line. In patients with active disease it is generally believed that all patients who have had a favorable response will eventually "escape."

Methotrexate and to some extent other immunosuppressive agents such as cytoxan and azathioprine are essential for the management of rheumatoid arthritis. Generally, immunosuppressive drugs are easier to manage in that the magnitude of immunosuppression can be increased by raising the dosage. For the disease-modifying drugs, it is generally considered that the magnitude of the response cannot be enhanced through an increase in dosage. At most, such increases in dosage increase the number of patients responding.

In summary, dapsone, as well as the other disease-modifying agents such as injectable gold and d-penicillamine and sulfapyridine, on the basis of well-controlled placebo trials is a clearcut clinical benefit along with an improvement in laboratory parameters such as rheumatoid factor and sedimentation rate. However, for all of these disease-modifying agents in rheumatoid arthritis, 4–6 week administration is needed before the signs of clinical response begin. When these drugs are stopped, there is a similar delay before the disease begins to relapse. The response times and the relapsed times are, therefore, in marked contrast to the responsive of a few hours to several days seen in properly titrated dermatitis herpetiformis or EED patients. The reasons for these long response times with disease-modifying agents are not understood. By analogy, in some chronic diseases it is not unreasonable to consider a 6 week course of dapsone or sulfapyridine in the management of a difficult problem.

INFECTIOUS DISEASES

Leprosy

Dapsone was first tried in tuberculosis of guinea pigs in 1938 and 1939. It was effective, but the projected dose of 1 g per day was not tolerated in the clinic. In 1941, dapsone was shown to be safe and effective against mycobacterium leprae at the U.S. Public Health Facility at Carville, Louisiana. Initially, it was the only drug and was administered for life in patients with lepromatous leprosy and 10 years in patients with tuberculoid leprosy. Additional agents, such as Rifampin with enhanced bactericidal activity, were soon found. Our current recommendation for lepromatous leprosy is daily dapsone for 2 years with a daily administration of 600 mg of Rifampin. Under the WHO, the daily Rifampin is replaced with monthly Rifampin. Usually a third drug is coadministered such as clofazimine or ethionamide. The purpose of coadministration is to achieve a rapid decrease in the bacterial count, so that the chances of the development of resistance are reduced.

Worldwide resistance of dapsone has changed the sensitivity, so now the drug is just bacteriostatic. When dapsone was first studied Shephard [36] found a bacteriocidal response.

In 1981, the WHO recommended for multibacillary leprosy that multidrug therapy continue for 2 years and consist of daily dapsone, monthly rifampicin, and clofazimine, although in the United States we recommended that rifampicin be administered daily. For tuberculoid leprosy, the WHO recommends dapsone and rifampicin for 6 months. Because the logistics of treatment of leprosy patients is still cumbersome and the results continue to be good, the WHO recommended in 1997 that consideration be given to further shortening the treatment period for multibacillary disease to 12 months. The objective is to eliminate leprosy as a public health problem by reducing the prevalence below one patient per 10,000.

Pneumocystis carinii Pneumonia

In 1987, Metroka et al. [37] first showed activity of dapsone in the clinic would provide prophylaxis against the development of *Pneumocystis carinii* pneumonia (PCP). Laboratory evidence and additional clinical studies have followed. There are now 200 publications on the use of dapsone for the treatment of prophylaxis of PCP and sometimes the associated toxoplasmosis infections. Dapsone is now recommended by the Centers for Disease Control and Prevention (CDC) [38] as an alternative to sulfamethoxazole-trimethoprim. A recent review summarizing these clinical studies, the mechanisms of action, and clinical trials has been published by W. Hughes [39].

As previously discussed, because sulfamethoxazole-trimethoprim has a high frequency of adverse reactions, patients switch to a daily dosage of 100 mg of dapsone as recommended in the CDC Guideline. Generally, cross-reactions do not occur. Beaumont et al. [40] report that among 75 such switched patients only 6% had an adverse reaction comparable to the sulfamethoxazole-trimethoprim reaction. Before highly active antiretroviral therapy became available, patients were maintained on dapsone prophylaxis for the remainder of their life. It is worth noting that these patients were on a large number of therapeutic agents.

Malaria

The most common use of dapsone has been a tablet containing 100 mg of dapsone and 12.5 mg of pyrimethamine, known as Maloprim and used as a once-a-week prophylaxis for travelers in areas of modest chloroquine resistance. The medication has been mainly supplanted by the use of pyrimethamine with a long-acting sulfonamide. There are more cases of agranulocytosis associated with this combination than there are with dapsone alone, even though the dapsone dosage is only 100 mg per week. I feel that caution should be exercised when dapsone is coadministered with folic acid antagonists.

DAPSONE PHARMACOKINETICS

Absorption and Distribution

Dapsone is well absorbed in both animals and man [41]. In clinical studies, serum levels appear within 15 min after oral ingestion, so that absorption from the stomach is prompt. In some individual patients, serum levels reach a peak within the first hour, suggesting that in those patients absorption is complete before the material leaves the stomach. Three independent studies [42–44] have shown that absorption is not influenced by gastric pH, although a letter [45] was published that discussed the failure to achieve Pneumocystis prophylaxis in long-term dapsone patients and speculated that the absorption would be retarded if the gastric contents were neutralized. These reports have since shown that the absorption is not influenced by a change in gastric pH. The quick absorption of dapsone in humans [46–49] has been confirmed in animal studies for the mouse [50], rat [59], rabbit [51], and dog [52–54]. Rifampin shortens the half-life and lowers serum dapsone levels [55–56]; the effect is important in PCP where rifampin or ansamycin can induce a failure of prophylaxis [37]. The pharmacokinetics in HIV-infected children indicate that for those under 2 years of age the dosage should be 2 mg/kg [57,58] in contrast to the calculated 1 1.5 mg/kg achieved by the fixed PCP prophylaxis of 100 mg daily.

From both a clinical and laboratory viewpoint, the volume of distribution of dapsone is large. Leprosy is a disease of poorly vascularized tissues such as peripheral nerves, the pinna, and the anterior chamber of the eye, yet dapsone is known to be effective in treating these lesions. Concentrations in peripheral nerves are comparable to those in the serum. The measured volume of distribution in humans is comparable to the distribution of water. Central nervous system concentrations, spinal fluid concentrations, and plural fluids extrusions are all within 50% of the serum concentration [127].

The half-life of dapsone ranges between 24 and 48 h [59] but with a range of up to 4 days. The absolute bioavailability of dapsone is between 84 and 104%

in adult volunteers [52] with a peak concentration between 2 and 8 h [46]. The absorption half-life is 1.1 h with linear pharmacokinetics. Dapsone is about 70% bound to serum albumin. The acetyl metabolite is almost completely bound.

In a study of eight pediatric patients aged 1 to 11 years on either tablets or a liquid preparation available through an investigational new drug application (IND), the median peak serum level was 1 h with a C_{max} between 0.7 and 2.4 μ/mL [58]. In a prospective trial for the prevention of PCP in pediatric patients, the daily dosage had to be increased to from 1 mg/kg to 2 mg/kg [60].

Excretion

Dapsone is excreted through the kidney [61], the bile, and the gut. Alexander et al. [62] reported that after the administration of a single dose of 100 mg radiolabeled dapsone to nine normal volunteers and nine dermatitis herpetiformis patients, the concentration in the urine peaks at 12 h. About 30% of the total dosage is excreted in the first 24 h and 70% in the first 5 days. Israili et al. [59] administered 20 mg radio dapsone to three normal volunteers. Two volunteers with a serum half-life of 23 h excreted 93 and 62% respectively; a third volunteer with a half-life of 17 hours excreted 77% in the first 2 days, 90% in 9 days, with 11% in the feces.

The acetylated metabolites of dapsone will have a greater degree of plasma binding than free dapsone so acetylation (along with the enterohepatic cycle) will contribute to the long half-life. The dog does not acetylate dapsone. Dapsone clearance has been found in the dog to be proportional to glomerular blood flow [54] with no evidence of tubular secretion.

Probenecid, which blocks tubular secretion, does not have a significant effect on dapsone serum levels. Neither dapsone nor its metabolites have structural features such as a carboxyl group that are associated with tubular secretion. Without tubular secretion, probenecid will have no activity. There is one mistitled literature report [63] that has often been included in surveys that probenecid blocks excretion; the renal excretion of some dapsone metabolites are reduced but serum dapsone levels are not changed significantly. The report is not carried in the labeling.

Biliary excretion and an enterohepatic cycle does occur in both man and animals [54,55,59,64]. In patients with normal renal function, biliary secretion amounted to 1–6% of the amount in the urine. However, in cases of overdosage, biliary excretion is a significant route of elimination. The administration of activated charcoal can produce a 50% change in the slope of the projected half-life. Neuvonen et al. [65] reported in two patients who had ingested 1 g of dapsone that the half-life was reduced from 36 or 50 h to 12.5. Charcoal has been successfully used in pediatric and adult dapsone overdosage [66–68]. The results suggest that biliary secretion increases in overload. By extrapolation and because very little dapsone is excreted intact in the urine, biliary excretion should become more important in cases of renal insufficiency.

Dapsone Diffusion

Because of excellent diffusion, dapsone will diffuse through the bowel wall so that such direct diffusion should be included when considering the multiple paths of excretion, and the bowel contents are considered to be in equilibrium with the serum levels.

Metabolism

N-acetylation and n-hydroxylation are two metabolic cycles that occur in all patients and most animal species. Dapsone was used to measure acetylation status and still remains a component of the five-drug ''cocktail'' (see the Branch paper [128]) used to characterize the P450 profile of patients. Early work emphasized that some patients were fast acetylators and others slow acetylators, but there is now agreement that the acetylator status does not influence the dosage required for the management of leprosy or dermatitis herpetiformis. In contrast to sulfonamides or p-aminobenzoic acid [129], dapsone is deacetylated so that there remains an equilibrium. The deacetylation rate is approximately one third of the acetylation rate. Both are considerably faster than the excretion rate, so the ratio does not change as a function of serum level. The phenomenon of deacetylation represents one of the specific differences between dapsone and p-aminobenzoic acid or other PABA analogs, such as the sulfonamides or p-aminosalicylic acid [129]. Acetylation of sulfonamides usually eliminates (permanently) antibacterial activity. Deacetylation of dapsone undoubtedly contributes to the relatively long duration of effect after episodic administration. If the excretion of dapsone should be prolonged in renal disease deacetylation will maintain activity, in contrast to sulfonamides which will accumulate the inactive acetyl metabolite.

Hydroxylation of the amine of dapsone to the end hydroxyl analog has been widely shown in patients and in animals [69–71]. This n-hydroxylamine metabolite is the source of red cell toxicity. As with acetylation, there is an active cycle in which dapsone is oxidized to the hydroxylamine. The hydroxylamine in turn can be reduced back to dapsone, although some is further oxidized to products that are conjugated and excreted.

When dapsone is absorbed, the first pass through the liver results in an undetermined amount of microsomal hydroxylation to produce the hydroxylamine of dapsone, the known toxin. Much of the hydroxylamine is reduced back to dapsone by the hemoglobin in erythrocytes [69,72,73]. Every reduction has its corresponding oxidation, so the hemoglobin doing the reduction is in turn oxidized to methemoglobin. The methemoglobin is reduced back to hemoglobin by gluco-6-phosphate-dehydrogenase and methemoglobin reductase, which keeps the cycle going. The reaction of the hydroxylamine with hemoglobin is relatively slow [74], so the peak amount of hydroxylamine formation is related to the magnitude of the original dosage. Recognition of the role of hemoglobin leads to a logical schedule to improve tolerance; dividing the dosage results in a lower peak of the hydroxylamine and presents a smaller load to the recovery system.

The hydroxylamine is clearly established as the metabolite responsible for the toxicity of dapsone [75–77]. The methemoglobin cycle described above is relatively innocuous unless there is sufficient methemoglobin formed as to interfere with the need to transport oxygen. Methemoglobin by itself will not cause hemolysis. In the AIDS clinical trials group (ACTG) programs evaluating dapsone for PCP prophylaxis, 20% methemoglobin was the level usually selected in most study protocols that would trigger a modification in dosage.

Some hydroxylamine interacts with the stoma of erythrocytes with the resulting reduction of flexibility. The stiffening is comparable to the stiffening seen as erythrocytes age, so the net result is that the life span of erythrocytes are shortened. These erythrocytes are removed by the spleen. Typical figures are 100 mg a day or an initial reduction of 1–2 g of hemoglobin and the shortening of the life span to 110 days. There is a compensatory rise in the reticulocyte count with a return of the hemoglobin to near-normal levels but with the persistence of a shortened erythrocyte life span.

Reduction of hydroxylamine concentration will improve the tolerance of dapsone. Dividing the dosage seems the simplest. The in vitro kinetics suggest that the hemoglobin interaction with the hydroxylamine to produce methemoglobin will take 2–3 h. Metroka [45] reported that hemoglobin tolerance was improved in transfusion-dependent HIV patients if a dosage was converted from daily to twice daily and further improved when the dosage was converted to four times a day. Those results were expected because the peak hydroxylamine concentration should only be one quarter of the concentration if the drug is given all at once and the annealing of the hydroxylamine by the erythrocytes is slower.

Pharmacological attempts to improve tolerance have centered around the use of cimetidine to block the cytochrome P450 [70] leading to a lower production of the original hydroxylamine, but the improved tolerance is not important enough to merit the coadministration of a second medication.

There has been a controversy in the literature about which the isozyme of cytochrome P450 system is responsible for the oxidation of dapsone to its hydroxylamine. Mitra et al. [79] report that CYP2E1 is a high infinity enzyme that is relevant in vivo. They have shown that the administration of disulfiram 18 h before 100 mg of dapsone reduced the area under the hydroxylamine plasma curve by 65%; in contrast the acetyl dapsone concentration increased. The investigators also confirmed that the CYP3A4 was a low infinity isozyme and certainly relevant at in vitro concentrations of at least 24 μg/mL, about 10 times the upper concentration found in peripheral blood, but perhaps relevant for short periods in the portal system.

SPECIAL CONDITIONS

Cirrhosis

Branch reported that in patients with cirrhosis the dosage of dapsone does not need to be adjusted [80]. Microsomal hydroxylation was reduced and the percentage of acetylation appeared to be in the normal range. Patients with cirrhosis presumably have a reduced enterohepatic cycle.

Renal Disease

The management of dapsone in patients with end-stage renal disease has not been reported. There are data that indicate that either peritoneal or extracorporeal dialysis will remove dapsone. Until the data from an ongoing IND are available to determine if the enterohepatic cycle is sufficient, serum levels should be followed in end-stage renal disease.

One advantage dapsone has in end-stage renal disease, in addition to the enterohepatic cycle, is that dapsone is deacetylated as well as acetylated. In contrast, PABA, sulfonamides, and para-aminosalicylic acid are not deacetylated, so for these compounds in renal disease there is an increase in the inactive acetylated metabolites as well as a dependence on renal excretion. In contrast, dapsone will not be converted to an inactive metabolite.

Overdosage

The prominent event in overdosage is the development of methemoglobinemia. Nausea, vomiting, and hyperexcitability can appear in a few minutes after an overdosage. Methemoglobin-induced cyanosis, depression, and convulsions require prompt treatment. Methylene blue given slowly intravenously at a dosage of 1–2 mg/kg will reverse the cyanosis immediately, even during the injection. The effect is complete within 30 min but will have to be repeated if the methemoglobin reaccumulates as is usual with dapsone overdosage. Finch [81] has provided an excellent review of reports describing the use of methylene blue to control symptoms from sulfonamides used at high dosage in the late 1930s. Ascorbic acid is not clinically effective.

Interruption of the enterohepatic cycle with activated charcoal is important to the management of dapsone overdosage [65]. Oral charcoal should be continued for at least 3–4 days while symptoms of overdosage persist. Although dialysis will remove dapsone it has not been found useful, perhaps because of the large volume of distribution.

Cross-Sensitivity

Cross-sensitivity between dapsone and sulfonamides has always been assumed to exist, but a series of major trials and wide experience have called this assumption into question. In a prospective well-controlled trial, Bozzette et al. [82] evaluated 843 patients with HIV disease for prophylaxis against PCP before highly active antiretroviral therapy became available. Patients were randomized between dapsone 50 mg twice a day, sulfamethoxazole-trimethoprim 1 double strength (ds) twice a day, or aerosolized pentamidine. Patients who failed to tolerate one systemic drug were switched at full dosage to the other systemic drug. If they failed both systemic drugs, they were then switched to aerosolized pentamidine. These patients all had AIDS and are known to have a higher incidence of intolerance to both sulfamethoxazole-trimethoprim and dapsone than is seen in normal patients.

Toxicity was predefined and comparable for all three groups. Forty-seven percent of the sulfamethoxazole-trimethoprim, 47% of the dapsone, and 43% of the pentamidine patients all had grade 3 hematological adverse effects. For granulocytes, Grade 3 effects were seen in 40% sulfamethoxazole-trimethoprim, 34% dapsone, and 28% pentamidine patients. Rash was 16% in the sulfamethoxazole-trimethoprim, 9% in the dapsone, and 5% in the pentamidine group.

At the end of the study, 49% of the sulfamethoxazole patients and 58% of the dapsone patients were still assigned to their original medication (some at half dosage) in comparison with 88% of the aerosolized pentamidine group. However, the patients who were switched between the two systemic therapies because of adverse reactions were switched without desensitization. Not all patients tolerated the new systemic medication, but 31% of the sulfamethoxazole-trimethoprim patients tolerated dapsone and 24% of the dapsone-sensitive patients tolerated sulfamethoxazole-trimethoprim. Because the time of tolerance after switch was approximately the same as the initial time to intolerance we consider that in this patient population the response to the new medication represents the development of a new intolerance to a new medication rather than a hypersensitivity response to the prior treatment.

The data from this trial appear to be replicated at the national level. Almost all Pneumocystis patients needing prophylaxis against *Pneumocystis carinii* pneumonia are started on sulfamethoxazole-trimethoprim. Studies that enroll patients with advanced disease find that half the patients are on dapsone [83]. My conclusion is that cross-hypersensitivity between dapsone and sulfamethoxazole-trimethoprim is not a common event.

ADVERSE EFFECTS

Agranulocytosis

There were two major forms of toxicity that are not dose related. The first is agranulocytosis, which when severe can include all neutrophils, platelets, and be accompanied by elevated transaminases and skin rash [84–87]. The agranulocytosis can appear suddenly but generally the effect is gradual in onset. For example, Duhra [88] reports biweekly counts for a patient on 150 mg/day who had a gradual fall in white blood cell count (WBC) starting after the third week until the drug was stopped on the eighth week with a WBC of 1000; the fall continued for a week to a nadir of 450 before recovery the next week. Although this patient had neutropenia, elevated transaminases and thrombocytopenia occurred and were serious findings.

Cockburn for the Medicines Control Agency [89] reported that the earliest neutropenia was 3 weeks, the median was 8 weeks, and the longest were 10, 12, and 14 weeks, so continued diligence is appropriate. Hornsten et al. [90] in a survey of 17 years of dapsone usage reported that among the seven cases of agranulocytosis, one patient had been on 100 mg dapsone for 19 months before surviving a total bone marrow wipeout. The current recommendation is for a complete blood count (CBC) and liver functions to be performed weekly for the first month, monthly for the next 6 months, and semiannually thereafter. As stated by Hornsten, ''Patients should be instructed to seek medical care immediately in case of fever.''

Rash

Cutaneous reactions, especially bullous, include exfoliative dermatitis and are probably one of the most serious although rare complications of sulfone therapy. They are directly attributable to drug sensitization. Such reactions include toxic erythema, erythema multiforme, toxic epidermal necrolysis, morbilliform and scarlatiniform reactions, urticaria, and erytheme nodosum. If new or toxic dermatological reactions occur, dapsone therapy must be promptly discontinued and appropriate therapy instituted.

Immunosuppressed patients with AIDS have a higher frequency of adverse reactions than other population groups. Cutaneous adverse reactions in children were 17% [59].

Neuropathy

Peripheral motor neuropathy is a dose-related adverse effect of dapsone regularly seen in cases in subacute dapsone overdosage. The time of onset varies in relationship to the magnitude of the overdosage. For example, a patient on 700 mg for 1 month is more liable to have a motor neuropathy develop at the end of the month than a patient on 300 mg at the end of 6 months.

As can be seen from Table 1, with the exception of the leprosy patient reported by Jacob, motor neuropathy occurred on dosages in excess of 100 mg per day. A pure motor neuropathy would be unusual if it were attributable to leprosy, so this may well be a proper report about whether the lesion preceded dapsone therapy. Careful follow-up is appropriate.

Table 1 Neuropathy

Reference	Diagnosis	Dosage (mg/day)	Duration	% Recoverable	Pure Motor	Comment
99	DH	200	4 years	Partial over 3 months	Motor plus diminished vibration sense	
113	DH	300	24 months	"normal" after 2 years	Yes	
114	Subcorneal pustular dermatosis	≈600 (Plus 1–2 weeks 800)	4 months	Almost complete at 4 months for upper limbs, lower limbs almost complete at 12 months	Yes	
115	DH	300–400	21 months	Yes over 4 years	Yes	Rate of recovery is well documented
116	DH	300	10 months	Improved on 100 mg od in 6 months	Yes (No sensory component reported)	
117	Original diagnosis—neuritis secondary to leprosy	100 (Lowest dosage reported)	3 months	6 months	Yes	Thought not to have had leprosy, No discussion of original diagnosis
118	Cystic acne	200	2.5 months	1 week improvement; by 2 months almost full recovery.	Motor with loss of vibration sense	Slow acetylator
119	Alopecia mucinosa	500 (Off dapsone 500)	2.5 months 1 month 4 months	75 month recovery, almost full at 10 months with minimal proximal weakness.	Yes	

120	?	≈ 500	8 years	2 years upper limbs complete, lower limbs 4 years, lower limbs no further recovery	Paresthesia in the hand but not in the feet, mostly motor	
121	Case 1—Pyoderma gangrenosum	400	2.75 months	Complete in 1 year	Yes	
	Case 2—Acne conglobata	350	4 months	Partial at 3 months compete later	Yes	
122	DH	100 (occasional 200–400)	16 years	None at 4 months although later improved while on SP	Yes—but for mild loss of pinprick in one hand	Slow acetylator normal B_{12}
123	Herpes gestationis	200	2–6 months	Yes at 16 months	Minor sensory component	B_{12} is normal
124	DH	200–300	18 years	None at 4 months on 3 g SP	Tingling in both hands and feet, reduced sense of pinprick, light touch and vibration, motor weakness	Differential diagnosis included neuropathy secondary to gluten sensitivity; B_{12} and Schilling normal. This patient was considered by Guttman to be different from the usual motor neuropathy of dapsone.

Abbreviations: DH, dermatitis herpetiformis.

The differential diagnosis is between the relatively pure motor neuropathy of dapsone and the mixed neuropathy of HIV disease with pain and weakness, as well as the sensory neuropathy with posterior cord atrophy of Vitamin B_{12} deficiency. Dermatitis herpetiformis patients may have poor B_{12} absorption as a result of continued small bowel lesions. Both central and peripheral neurological lesions attributable to B_{12} deficiency can occur without abnormal hematological values. A sensory component in a patient on dapsone should be a signal to search for other causes of the neuropathy.

Recovery, especially if the disease is discovered early, is generally complete. The recovery is considered to be attributable to remyelination at about the rate of 1 inch a month, so severe cases may take at least 3 years for a reasonable recovery. The biochemical basis for the pathogenesis of the lesion has not been described in the literature.

The Nephrotic Syndrome

The nephrotic syndrome and massive edema without protein in the urine has been described in five cases, two of whom died [91–94]. The causal origin of this effect is not understood, but Kingman et al. [91] describe an increase in albumin catabolism in one patient that returned to normal off dapsone. Cowan and Wright [92] reported their patient slowly recovered on sulfapyridine, providing indirect support for the concept that the catabolism is attributable to a drug-albumin interaction. In all cases, dapsone had been started more than a year earlier, with one starting 11 years earlier. Hypoalbuminemia with or without proteinuria should lead to an immediate drug withdrawal and be intensively investigated. Belmont reported a classical nephrotic syndrome 3 weeks after the initiation of dapsone for dermatitis herpetiformis that resolved off the drug [95].

Fertility

There are reports of reduced fertility among dermatitis herpetiformis patients on either dapsone or sulfapyridine, but there are no reports in the literature on reduced fertility among patients with leprosy. The difference could reflect the difference in care generally given to patients with these two different diseases. Patients with leprosy are generally poor people in a poor country. However, patients with celiac disease who do not take dapsone have an open gut on a normal diet and a marked reduction in sperm count or amenorrhea. With the institution of a gluten-free diet, celiac patients gain normal bowel function in 1 month with a recovery of sperm count or normal cycling within 9 months. It is our recommendation that dermatitis herpetiformis patients with a concern about fertility be informed about the celiac patients and advised to follow a strict gluten-free diet.

In general, a patient will recover normal fertility within 1 year whereas dapsone will still be needed for up to 5 years.

Acute Psychiatric Reaction

Dapsone can cause an acute psychiatric reaction [96]. The symptoms abated promptly after withdrawal, reoccurred on rechallenge, and reoccurred on sulfapyridine. There are about 25 additional literature reports.

Dapsone Syndrome

The sulfone syndrome is a combination of fever, rash, hemolytic anemia, fulminating hepatitis, and often disseminated intravascular coagulation, which is usually considered to be attributable to a hypersensitive reaction. Generally, this combination is fatal. The adverse reaction usually starts during the first month with elevated liver functions, thrombocytopenia, neutropenia, fever, and rash. The first HIV patient to be reported with the sulfone syndrome [97] had an elevated bilirubin, lactic acid dehydrogenase (LDH), and serum glutamic oxaloacetic transaminase (SGOT) 20 times the upper level of normal within 1 week of starting dapsone prophylaxis. The medication was continued for 1 month and the patient was finally admitted with a fulminant hepatic failure. We feel that laboratory measurements, weekly for the first week, biweekly for the next 2 months, and semiannually thereafter provide protection to the patient. Because adverse reactions to dapsone are rare, there is a tendency not to follow this laboratory schedule. The patients not being closely followed in the laboratory should be carefully advised to report any new symptoms.

MECHANISM OF ACTION

A mechanism of action is not established. Our general statement is that dapsone prevents the attack of neutrophils on self, ie, the IgA antibodies deposited in the dermal papilla in dermatitis herpetiformis. If that is the correct description, it is still not a discussion of mechanism. My favorite mechanism is based on the data of Shigeura, et al. [98], which suggests that dapsone influences the incorporation of choline into lecithin of cells surfaces. It could follow that some receptors are changed with secondary effects such as an inhibition of neutrophil chemotaxis [99,100], of lysomal enzymes [101] or their release [102], an inhibition of leukocytes cytotoxicity [103], and/or effect on myeloperoxidase [104–106], an effect on the pillimer pathway [107], a change response to complement [108], suppression of the arthus reaction [109], and anti-inflammatory activity in rats [110]. Any mechanism has to explain the great specificity in dermatitis herpetiformis without an inhibition of the antibacterial component of neutrophil function or a general immunosuppression.

NEW USES

The usefulness of dapsone in a wide variety of dermatological conditions has led to suggested new uses based on comparable mechanisms and efficacy.

Chronic renal scarring secondary to pyelonephritis is the new usage that I find most intriguing because of a very credible series of experiments in rats. No patients have been treated.

Meylan et al. [111] in Switzerland have developed a rat model with acute pyelonephritis secondary to an ascending *E. coli* infection. These rats were then treated with dapsone for 3 days. There was no antibacterial effect, and no effect on superoxide production or lysosomal enzyme release. However, the dosage used produced an inhibition in the myeloperoxidase-mediated oxidation. The dapsone-treated animals sacrificed 2 months later had a 65% reduction of renal scars in comparison with controls. Because there was no antibacterial effect, no effect on acute inflammation, and no effect on the magnitude of PMN infiltration, the effect was considered by the investigators to be attributable to the prevention of oxidant-mediated tissue injury through the myeloperoxidase system. A clinical study should be initiated.

Steroid-Dependent Asthma

Martin and Kachel [23] showed that dapsone protected endothelial cells in tissue culture from neutrophil injury by inhibiting the respiratory burst. The mechanism is comparable to the experiment by Meylan et al. [111]. Berlow et al. [112] conducted an open study in 10 patients with stable steroid-dependent asthma. Patients were given 100 mg twice a day after a 1 month baseline. One patient showed no response, five were off steroid by 6 months, two additional patients by month 13, and the last two patients had a 74% reduction in steroid. The study must be replicated in a prospective placebo-controlled manner with the blind maintained in the clinic. The tissue culture experiment provides important support. We have had two INDs in place for which patients were not recruited on the argument that Berlow's work indicated that it was unethical to withhold dapsone.

Steroid-Dependent Pemphigus Vulgaris

To her credit, and with the support of seven participating dermatology centers, V. Werth at the University of Pennsylvania has launched a prospective placebo-controlled study to determine if dapsone will have a steroid-sparing effect in patients with steroid-dependent pemphigus vulgaris. Her study maintains the structure of the double-blind.

Potentiation of DHFR Antagonists

Dapsone has been coadministered with dihydrofolate reductase inhibitors for potentiation in malaria, tuberculosis, toxoplasma, and Pneumocystis. New uses in the field of malaria primarily involve coadministration with different DHFR inhibitors than have been available to date. These coadministration programs are the only ''new'' uses that would involve significant numbers of patients. They are not new with respect to the concept or expected activity. An example is Watkins' combination of dapsone with chlorproguanil for the treatment of acute falciparum malaria in Kenya [130].

REFERENCES

1. Fromm E, Wittmann J. Derivate des p-Nitro-thiophenols. Berichte d D Chem Gesellschaft 1908; 41: 145–147.
2. Katz SI. Sulfone (diasone) sodium for dermatitis herpetiformis. Arch Dermatol 1982; 118(10): 809–812.
3. Costello MJ. Sulfapyridine in the treatment of dermatitis herpetiformis treated and untreated. Arch Dermatol Syphilol 1947; 56: 614–628.
4. Cornbleet T. Sulfoxone (diasone) sodium for dermatitis herpetiformis. Arch Dermatol Syphilology 1951; 64: 681–687.
5. Kruizinga EE, Hamminga H. Treatment of dermatitis herpetiformis with diaminodiphenysulphone (DDS). Dermatologia 1953; 106: 386–394.
6. Katz SI. Dermatitis herpetiformis. Clinical, histologic, therapeutic and laboratory clues. Internat J Dermatol 1978; 17(7): 529–535.
7. Fry L, Leonard JN, Swain F, Tucker WFG, Haffenden G, Ring N, McMinn RMH. Long term follow-up of dermatitis herpetiformis with and without dietary gluten withdrawal. Br J Dermatol 1982; 197: 631–640.
8. Beck WS. Neuropsychiatric consequences of cobalamin deficiency. Stollerman GH, ed. Advances in Internal Medicine. St. Louis: Mosby Year Book, 1991: 33–56. 1991; 36: 33–56.
9. Pennypacker LC, Allen RH, Kelly JP, Matthews LM, Grigsby J, Kaye K, Lindenbaum J, Stabler SP. High prevalence of cobalamin deficiency in elderly outpatients. J Am Geriatr Soc 1991; 40: 1197–1204.
10. Beck WS. Erythrocyte disorders—anemias related to disturbance of DNA synthesis (megaloblastic anemias). Williams WJ, Beutler E, Erslev AJ, Lichtman MA, eds. Hematology. 3rd ed. New York: McGraw-Hill Book Co., 1983: 434–465.
11. Katz SI, Gallin JI, Hertz KC, Fauci AS, Lawley TJ. Erythema elevatum diutinum: skin and systemic manifestations, immunologic studies, and successful treatment with dapsone. Medicine (Baltimore) 1977; 56(5): 443–455.
12. Cream JJ, Levene GM, Calnan CD. Erythema elevatum diutinum: an unusual reaction to streptococcal antigen and response to dapsone. Br J Dermatol 1971; 84(5): 393–399.
13. Wilkinson SM, English JS, Smith NP, Wilson-Jones E, Winkelmann RK. Erythema

elevatum diutinum: a clinicopathological study. Clin Exper Dermatol 1992; 17(2): 87–93.
14. Ahmed AR, Kurgis BS, Rogers RS. Cicatricial pemphigoid. J Am Acad Dermatol 1991; 24(6): 987–1001.
15. Rogers RS, Seehafer JR, Perry HO. Treatment of cicatricial (benign mucous membrane) pemphigoid with dapsone. J Am Acad Dermatol 1982; 6(2): 215–223.
16. Tauber J, De La Maza MS, Foster CS. Systemic chemotherapy for ocular cicatricial pemphigoid. Cornea 1991; 10(3): 185–195.
17. De La Maza MS, Tauber J, Foster CS. Cataract surgery in ocular cicatricial pemphigoid. Ophthalmology 1988; 95(4): 481–486.
18. Neumann R, Tauber J, Foster CS. Remission and recurrence after withdrawal of therapy for ocular cicatricial pemphigoid. Ophthalmology 1991; 98(6): 858–862.
19. Korman NJ. Bullous pemphigoid. Dermatol Clin 1993; 11(3): 483–498.
20. Person JR, Rogers RS. Bullous pemphigoid responding to sulfapyridine and the sulfones. Arch Dermatol 1977; 113: 610–615.
21. Bernheimer AW, Campbell BJ, Forrester LJ. Comparative toxicology of *Loxosceles reclusa* and *Corynebacterium pseudotuberculosis*. Science 1985; 228: 590–591.
22. Smith CW, Micks DW. The role of polymorphonuclear leukocytes in the lesion caused by the venom of the brown spider, *Loxosceles reclusa*. Lab Invest 1970; 22(1): 90–93.
23. Martin WJ, Kachel DL. Reduction of neutrophil-mediated injury to pulmonary endothelial cells by dapsone. Am Rev Resp Dis 1985; 131: 544–547.
24. Patel KD, Modur V, Zimmerman GA, Prescott SM, McIntyre TM. The necrotic venom of the brown recluse spider induces dysregulated endothelial cell-dependent neutrophil activation. J Clin Invest 1994; 94: 631–642.
25. King LE, Rees RS. Dapsone treatment of brown recluse bite. JAMA 1983; 250(5): 648.
26. Phillips S, Kohn M, Baker D, Vander Leest R, Gomez H, McKinney P, McGoldrick J, Brent J. Therapy of brown spider envenomation: a controlled trial of hyperbaric oxygen, dapsone and cyproheptadine. Ann Emerg Med 1995; 25(3): 363–368.
27. Cole HP, Wesley RE, King LE. Brown recluse spider envenomation of the eyelid: an animal model. Opthalm Plast Reconstr Surg 1995; 11(3): 153–164.
28. Masters EJ. Images in clinical medicine. N Engl J Med 1998; 339: 379, 1944–1946.
29. Rees RS, Altenbern DP, Lynch JB, King LE. Brown recluse spider bites. A comparison of early surgical excision versus dapsone and delayed surgical excision. Ann Surg 1985; 202(5): 659–663.
30. McConkey B, Davis P, Crockson RA, Crockson AP, Butler M, Constable TJ. Dapsone in rheumatoid arthritis. Rheumatol Rehab 1976; 15: 230–234.
31. Swinson DR, Zlosnick J, Jackson L. Double-blind trial of dapsone against placebo in the treatment of rheumatoid arthritis. Ann Rheumat Dis 1981; 40: 235–239.
32. Fowler PD, Shadforth MF, Crook PR, Lawton A. Report on chloroquine and dapsone in the treatment of rheumatoid arthritis: 1 6-month comparative study. Ann Rheum Dis 1984; 43: 200–204.
33. Job-Deslandre C, Menkes CJ. Traitement de la polyarthrite rhumatoide par la dap-

sone. Revue du Rhumatisme et des Maladies Osteo-Articulaires 1989; 56(4): 313–316.

34. Haar D, Solvkjaer M, Unger B, Rasmussen KJE, Christensen L, Hansen TM. A double-blind comparative study of hydroxychloroquine and dapsone, alone and in combination, in rheumatoid arthritis. Scand J Rheumatol 1993; 22(3): 113–118.
35. Grindulis KA, McConkey B. Rheumatoid arthritis: the effects of treatment with dapsone on hemoglobin. J Rheumatol 1984; 11(6): 776–778.
36. Shepard CC. Chemotherapy of leprosy. Ann Rev Pharmacol 1969; 9: 37–50.
37. Metroka C, Lange M, Braun N, O'Sullivan M, Josefberg E, Jacobus D. Successful chemoprophylaxis for *Pneumocystis carinii* pneumonia with dapsone in patients with AIDS and ARC. Third International Conference on Acquired Immunodeficiency Syndrome, June 1–5. Abstract THP231 1987: 202.
38. 1999 USPHS-IDSA Guidelines for the Prevention of Opportunistic infections in persons infected with human immunodeficiency virus. MMWR 1999; 48: 1–59.
39. Hughes WT. Use of dapsone in the prevention and treatment of *Pneumocystis carinii* pneumonia: a review. Clin Infect Dis 1998; 27(1): 191–204.
40. Beumont MG, Graziani A, MacGregor RR. Safety of dapsone as PCP prophylaxis in HIV-infected patients with TMP/SMX intolerance. Program and Abstracts of the 34th Interscience Conference on Antimicrobial Agents and Chemotherapy (Orlando). American Society of Microbiology. Washington, DC, 1994: 168.
41. Ellard GA. Absorption, metabolism and excretion of di (p-aminophenyl) sulphone (dapsone) and di (p-aminophenyl) sulphoxide in man. Br J Pharmacol 1966; 26(1): 212–217.
42. Sahai J, Garber G, Gallicano K, Oliveras L, Cameron DW. Effects of the antacids in didanosine tablets on dapsone pharmacokinetics. Ann Intern Med 1995; 123(8): 584–587.
43. Slattery JT, Unadkat JD. Adverse reactions to co-trimoxazole in HIV infection. [Letter]. Lancet 1991; 338(8776): 1216.
44. Breen GA, Brocavich JM, Etzel JV, Shah V, Schaefer P, Forlenza S. Evaluation of effects of altered gastric pH on absorption of dapsone in healthy volunteers. Antimicrob Agents Chemother 1994; 38: 2227–2229.
45. Metroka CE, McMechan MF, Andrada R, Laubenstein LJ. Failure of prophylaxis with dapsone in patients taking dideoxyinosine. [Letter]. N Engl J Med 1991; 325(10): 747.
46. Zuidema J, Hilbers-Modderman ES, Markus FW. Clinical pharmacokinetics of dapsone. Clin Pharmacokinetics 1986; 11(4): 299–315.
47. Swain AF, Ahmad RA, Rogers HJ, Leonard JN, Fry L. Pharmacokinetic observations on dapsone in dermatitis herpetiformis. Br J Dermatol 1983; 108(1): 91–98.
48. Lammintausta K, Kangas L, Lammintausta R. The pharmacokinetics of dapsone and acetylated dapsone in serum and saliva. Internat J Clin Pharmacol Biopharm 1979; 17(4): 159–163.
49. Venkatesan K. Clinical pharmacokinetic considerations in the treatment of patients with leprosy. Clin Pharmacokinetics 1989; 16(6): 365–386.
50. Levy L, Biggs JT, Gordon GR, Peters JH. Disposition of the antileprosy drug, dapsone in the mouse. Proc Soc Exp Biol Med 1972; 140(3): 937–940.

51. Gordon GR, Shafizadeh AG, Peters JH. Polymorphic acetylation of drugs in rabbits. Xenobiotica 1973; 3(3): 133–150.
52. Pieters FA, Zuidema J. The absolute oral bioavailability of dapsone in dogs and humans. Int J Clin Pharmacol Ther Toxicol 1987; 25(7): 396–400.
53. Peters JH, Gordon R, Biggs JT, Levy L. The disposition of dapsone and monoacetyldapsone in the dogs (38516). Proc Soc Exp Biol Med 1975; 148(1): 251–255.
54. Biggs JT, Uhr AK, Levy L, Gordon RD, Peters JH. Renal and biliary disposition of dapsone in the dog. Antimicrob Agents Chemother 1975; 7(6): 816–824.
55. Gelber RH, Gool HC, Rees RJ. The effect of rifampin on dapsone metabolism. Proc West Pharmacol Soc 1975; 18: 330–334.
56. Zilly W, Breimer DD, Richter R. Pharmacokinetic interactions with rifampicin. Clin Pharmacokinetics 1977; 2(1): 61–70.
57. Gatti G, Loy A, Casazza R, Miletich F, Cruciani M, Bassetti D. Pharmacokinetics of dapsone in human immunodeficiency virus-infected children. Antimicrob Agents Chemother 1995; 39(5): 1101–1106.
58. Mirochnick M, Michaels M, Clarke D, Brena A, Regan AM, Pelton S. Pharmacokinetics of dapsone in children. J Pediat. 1993; 122(5): 806–809.
59. Israili ZH, Cucinell SA, Vaught J, Davis E, Lesser JM, Dayton PG. Studies of the metabolism of dapsone in man and experimental animals: formation of n-hydroxy metabolites. J Pharmacol Exper Ther 1973; 187(1): 138–151.
60. McIntosh K, Cooper E, Xu J, Mirochnick M, Lindsey J, Jacobus DP, Mofenson L, Yogev R, Spector SA, Sullivan JL, Sacks H, Kovacs A, Nachman S, Sleasman J, Bongura V, McNamara J. Toxicity and efficacy of daily vs. weekly dapsone for prevention of *Pneumocystis carinii* pneumonia in children infected with human immunodeficiency virus. ACTG 179 Study Team. AIDS Clinical Trials Group. Pediat Infect Dis J 1999; 18(5): 432–439.
61. Glazko AJ, Dill WA, Montalbo RG, Holmes EL. A new analytical procedure for dapsone. Application to blood-level and urinary excretion studies in normal men. Am J Trop Med Hyg 1968; 17(3): 465–473.
62. Alexander JO, Young E, McFadyen T, Fraser NG, Duguid WP, Meredith EM. Absorption and excretion of 35S dapsone in dermatitis herpetiformis. Br J Dermatol. 1970; 83(6): 620–631.
63. Goodwin CS, Sparell G. Inhibition of dapsone excretion by probenecid. Lancet 1969; 2(626): 884–885.
64. Andoh BY, Renwick AG, Williams RT. The excretion of 35S dapsone and its metabolites in the urine, feces and bile of the rat. Xenobiotica 1974; 4(9): 571–583.
65. Neuvonen PJ, Elonen E, Haapanen EJ. Acute dapsone intoxication: clinical findings and effect of oral charcoal and haemodialysis on dapsone elimination. Acta Med Scan 1983; 214(3): 215–220.
66. MacDonald RD, McGuigan MA. Acute dapsone intoxication: a pediatric case report. Pediat Emerg Care 1997; 13(2): 127–129.
67. Erstad BL. Dapsone-induced methemoglobinemia and hemolytic anemia. [Clinical conference]. Clin Pharm. 1992; 11(9): 800–805.
68. Hansen DG, Challoner KR, Smith DE. Dapsone intoxication: two case reports. J Emerg Med 1994; 12(3): 347–351.
69. Cucinell SA, Israili ZH, Dayton PG. Microsomal N-oxidation of dapsone as a cause

of methemoglobin formation in human red cells. Am J Trop Med Hyg 1972; 21(3): 322–331.

70. Uehleke H, Tabarelli S. N-hydroxylation of 4,4′-diaminodiphenylsuphone dapsone by liver microsomes, and in dogs and humans. Naunyn Schmiedebergs Arch Pharmacol 1973; 278(1): 55–68.
71. May DG, Porter JA, Uetrecht JP, Wilkinson GR, Branch RA. The contribution of n-hydroxylation and acetylation to dapsone pharmacokinetics in normal subjects. Clin Pharmacol Therapeutics 1990; 48(6): 619–627.
72. Coleman MD, Simpson J, Jacobus DP. Reduction of dapsone hydroxylamine to dapsone during methaemoglobin formation in human erythrocytes in vitro. IV. Implications for the development of agranulocytosis. Biochem Pharmacol 1994; 48(7): 1349–1354.
73. Reilly TP, Woster PM, Svensson CK. Methemoglobin formation by hydroxylamine metabolites of sulfamethoxazole and dapsone: implications for differences in adverse drug. J Pharmacol Exper Therap 1999; 288(3): 951–959.
74. Coleman MD, Jacobus DP. Reduction of dapsone hydroxylamine to dapsone during methaemoglobin formation in human erythrocytes in vitro II. Movement of dapsone across a semipermeable membrane into erythrocytes and plasma. Biochem Pharmacol 1993; 46(8): 1363–1368.
75. Glader BE, Conrad ME. Hemolysis by diphenylsulfones: comparative effects of DDS and hydroxylamine-DDS. J Lab Clin Med 1973; 81(2): 267–272.
76. Uetrecht J, Zahid N, Shear NH, Biggar WD. Metabolism of dapsone to a hydroxylamine by human neutrophils and mononuclear cells. J Pharmacol Exper Therapeutics 1988; 245(1): 274–279.
77. Jollow DJ, Bradshaw TP, McMillan DC. Dapsone-induced hemolytic anemia. Drug Metabol Rev 1995; 27(1–2): 107–124.
78. Coleman MD, Rhodes LE, Scott AK, Verbov JL, Friedman PS, Breckenridge AM, Park BK. The use of cimetidine to reduce dapsone-dependent methaemoglobinaemia in dermatitis herpetiformis patients. Br J Clin Pharmacol 1992; 34(3): 244–249.
79. Mitra AK, Thummel KE, Kalhorn TF, Kharasch ED, Unadkat JD, Slattery JT. Metabolism of dapsone to its hydroxylamine by CYP2E1 in vitro and in vivo. Clin Pharmacol Therap 1995; 58(5): 556–566.
80. May DG, Arns PA, Richards WO, Porter J, Ryder D, Fleming CM, Wilkinson GR, Branch RA. The disposition of dapsone in cirrhosis. Clin Pharmacol Therapeutics 1992; 51(6): 689–700.
81. Finch CA. Methemoglobinemia and sulfhemoglobinemia. N Engl J Med 1948; 239: 470–477.
82. Bozzette SA, Finkelstein DM, Spector SA, Frame P, Powderly WG, He W, Phillips L, Craven D, van der Horst C, Feinberg J. A randomized trial of three antipneumocystis agents in patients with advanced human immunodeficiency virus infection. NIAID AIDS Clinical Trials Group. N Engl J Med 1995; 332(11): 693–699.
83. El Sadr W, Murphy RL, Yurik TM, Luskin-Hawk R, Cheung TW, Balfour HH, Eng R, Hooton TM, Kerkering TM, Schultz M, van der Horst C, Hafner R. Atovaquone compared with dapsone for the prevention of *Pneumocystis carinii* pneumonia in patients with HIV infection who cannot tolerate trimethoprim sulfonamides or both. N Engl J Med 1999; 339(26): 1889–1895.

84. Smithurst BA, Robertson I, Naughton MA. Dapsone-induced agranulocytosis complicated by gram-negative septicaemia. Med J Austr 1971; 1: 537–539.
85. Levine PH, Weintraub LR. Pseudoleukemia during recovery from dapsone-induced agranulocytosis. Ann Internat Med 1968; 68: 1060–1065.
86. McKenna WB, Chalmers AC. Agranulocytosis following dapsone therapy. Br Med J 1958; 1: 324–325.
87. Ognibene AJ. Agranulocytosis due to dapsone. Ann Intern Med 1970; 72: 521–524.
88. Duhra P, Charles-Holmes R. Linear IgA disease with haemorrhagic pompholyx and dapsone-induced neutropenia. Br J Dermatol. 1991; 125(2): 172–174.
89. Cockburn EM, Wood SM, Waller PC, Bleehen SS. Dapsone-induced agranulocytosis: spontaneous reporting data. [Letter]. Br J Dermatol 1993; 128(6): 702–703.
90. Hornsten P, Keisu M, Wilholm BE. The incidence of agranulocytosis during treatment of dermatitis herpetiformis with dapsone as reported in Sweden, 1972 through 1988. Arch Dermatol 1990; 126: 919–922.
91. Kingham JGC, Swain P, Swarbrick ET, Walter JG, Dawson AM. Dapsone and severe hypoalbuminemia: a report of two cases. Lancet 1979; 2(8144): 662–664.
92. Cowan RE, Wright JT. Dapsone and severe hypoalbuminaemia in dermatitis herpetiformis. Br J Dermatol 1981; 104: 201.
93. Young S, Marks JM. Dapsone and severe hypoalbuminemia. Lancet 1979; 2(8148): 908–909.
94. Foster PN, Swan CHI. Dapsone and fatal hypoalbuminaemia. Lancet 1981; 2(8250): 806–807.
95. Belmont A. Dapsone-induced nephrotic syndrome. JAMA 1967; 200(3): 174–175.
96. Fine JD, Katz SI, Donahue MJ, Hendricks AA. Psychiatric reaction to dapsone and sulfapyridine. [Letter]. J Am Acad Dermatol 1983; 9(2): 274–275.
97. Chalasani P, Baffoe-Bonnie H, Jurado RL. Dapsone therapy causing sulfone syndrome and lethal hepatic failure in and HIV-infected patients. Southern Med J 1995; 87(11): 1145–1146.
98. Shigeura HT, He AC, Burg RW, Skelly BJ, Hoogstein K. Metabolic studies on diphenylsulfone derivatives in chick macrophages. Biochem Pharmacol 1975; 24: 687–691.
99. Abrens EM, Meckler RJ, Callen JP. Dapsone-induced peripheral neuropathy. Int J Dermatol 1986; 25(5): 314–316.
100. Harvath L, Yancey KB, Katz SI. Selective inhibition of human neutrophil chemotaxis to n-formyl-methionyl-leucyl-phenylalanine by sulfones. J Immunol 1986; 137: 1305–1311.
101. Mier PD, Van Den Hurk JJMA. Inhibition of lysosomal enzymes by dapsone. Br J Derm 1975; 93: 471–472.
102. Barranco VP. Inhibition of lysosomal enzymes. Arch Dermatol 1974; 110: 563–566.
103. Stendahl O, Molin L, Dahlgren C. The inhibition of polymorphonuclear leukocyte cytotoxicity by dapsone. J Clin Invest 1978; 62(1): 214–220.
104. Kazmierowski JA, Ros JE, Peizner DS, Wueppr KD. Dermatitis herpetiformis: effects of sulfons and sulfonamides on neutrophil myeloperoxidase-mediated iodination and cytotoxicity. J Clin Immunol 1984; 4(1): 55–64.

105. Uetrecht JP, Shear NH, Zahid N. N-chlorination of sulfamethoxazole and dapsone by myeloperoxidase system. Drug Metabol Disposition 1993; 21(5): 830–834.
106. Liu ZC, McClelland RA, Uetrecht JP. Oxidation of 5-aminosalicylic acid by hypochlorous acid to a reactive iminoquinone. Possible role in the treatment of inflammatory bowel diseases. Drug Metabol Disposition 1995; 23(2): 246–250.
107. Millikan LE, Conway FR. Effect of drugs on the pillemer pathway—dapsone. J Invest Dermatol. 1974; 62(abstr): 541.
108. Provost TT, Tomasi TB. Evidence for the activation of complement via the alternate pathway in skin diseases. II. Dermatitis herpetiformis. Clin Immunol Immunopathol 1974; 3: 178–186.
109. Thompson DM, Souhami R. Suppression of the arthus reaction in the guinea pig by dapsone. Proc R Soc Med 1975; 68(Abstr): 273.
110. Williams K, Capstick RB, Lewis DA, Best R. Anti-inflammatory actions of dapsone and its related biochemistry. J Pharm Pharmacol 1976; 28: 555–556.
111. Meylan PR, Markert M, Bille J, Glauser MP. Relationship between neutrophil-medicated oxidative injury during acute experimental pyelonephritis and chronic renal scarring. Infect Immun 1989; 57(7): 2196–2202.
112. Berlow BA, Liebhaber MI, Dyer Z, Spiegel TM. The effect of dapsone in steroid-dependent asthma. J Allergy Clin Immunol. 1991; 87(3): 710–715.
113. Epstein FW, Bohm M. Dapsone-induced peripheral neuropathy. Arch Dermatol 1976; 112(2): 1761–1762.
114. Fredericks EJ, Kugelman TP, Kirsch N. Dapsone induced motor polyneuropathy. A complication of prolonged treatment of subcorneal pustular dermatosis. Arch Dermatol 1976; 112(8): 1158–1160.
115. Gutmann L, Martin JD, Welton W. Dapsone motor neuropathy—an axonal disease. Neurology 1976; 26(6): 514–516.
116. Hubler WH, Solomon H. Neurotoxicity of sulfones: report of a case. Arch Dermatol. 1972; 106: 598–599.
117. Jacob AJ, Rajendran A, Menezes J, Vaz M. Dapsone induced motor polyneuropathy. Southeast-Asian J Trop Med Public Health 1992; 23(2): 341–343.
118. Koller WC, Gehlmann LK, Malkinson FD, Davis FA. Dapsone-induced peripheral neuropathy. Arch Neurol 1977; 34(10): 644–646.
119. Rapoport Am, Guss SB. Dapsone-induced peripheral neuropathy. Arch Neurol 1972; 27(2): 184–185.
120. Rosen I, Sornas R. Peripheral motor neuropathy caused by excessive intake of dapsone (avlosulfon). Archiv fur Psychiatrie Und Nervenkrankheiten. 1982; 232(1): 63–69.
121. Saqueton AC, Lorincz AL, Vick NA, Hamer RD. Dapsone and peripheral motor neuropathy. Arch Dermatol 1969; 100(2): 214–217.
122. Waldinger TP, Siegle RJ, Weber W, Voorhees JJ. Dapsone-induced peripheral neuropathy. Case report and review. Arch Dermatol 1984; 120(3): 356–359.
123. Wyatt EH, Stevens JC. Dapsone induced peripheral neuropathy. Br J Dermatol 1972; 86(5): 521–523.
124. Vivier AD, Fowler T. Possible dapsone-induced peripheral neuropathy in dermatitis herpetiformis. Proc R Soc Med 1974; 67(6): 439–440.
125. Lindenbam J, Rosenberg IH, Wilson PW, Stabler SP, Allen RH. Prevalence of

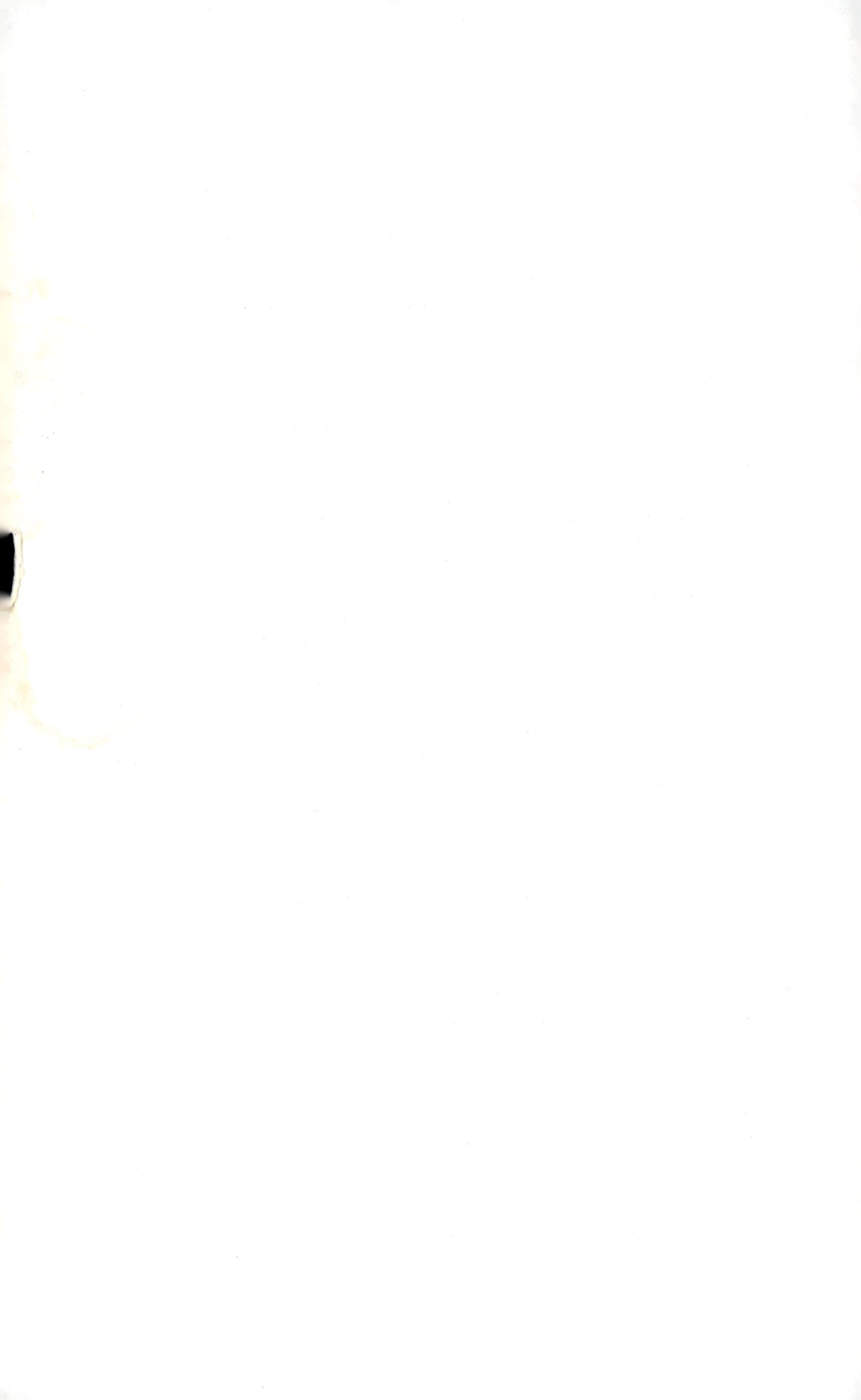

Index

About the Editor

Larry E. Millikan is Professor and Chairman, Department of Dermatology, Tulane University Medical Center, New Orleans, Louisiana. Previously Associate Professor and Vice Chairman, Department of Dermatology, University of Missouri, Columbia, Dr. Millikan is a Fellow of the American College of Physicians and the College of Physicians of Philadelphia, and a member of the International Academy of Cosmetic Dermatology and the Royal Society of Medicine, among others. He received the A.B. degree (1958) from Monmouth College, Illinois, and the M.D. degree (1962) from the University of Missouri, Columbia.